Self-Organizing Map Formation

Computational Neuroscience

Terrence J. Sejnowski and Tomaso A. Poggio, editors

Neural Nets in Electric Fish, Walter Heiligenberg, 1991

The Computational Brain, Patricia S. Churchland and Terrence J. Sejnowski, 1992

Dynamic Biological Networks: The Stomatogastric Nervous System, edited by Ronald M. Harris-Warrick, Eve Marder, Allen I. Selverston, and Maurice Moulins, 1992

The Neurobiology of Neural Networks, edited by Daniel Gardner, 1993

Large-Scale Neuronal Theories of the Brain, edited by Christof Koch and Joel L. Davis, 1994

The Theoretical Foundation of Dendritic Function: Selected Papers of Wilfrid Rall with Commentaries, edited by Idan Segev, John Rinzel, and Gordon M. Shepherd, 1995

Models of Information Processing in the Basal Ganglia, edited by James C. Houk, Joel L. Davis, and David G. Beiser, 1995

Spikes: Exploring the Neural Code, Fred Rieke, David Warland, Rob de Ruyter van Steveninck, and William Bialek, 1997

Neurons, Networks, and Motor Behavior, edited by Paul S. G. Stein, Sten Grillner, Allen I. Selverston, and Douglas G. Stuart, 1997

Methods in Neuronal Modeling: From Ions to Networks, second edition, edited by Christof Koch and Idan Segev, 1998

Fundamentals of Neural Network Modeling: Neuropsychology and Cognitive Neuroscience, edited by Randolph W. Parks, Daniel S. Levine, and Debra L. Long, 1998

Neural Codes and Distributed Representations: Foundations of Neural Computation, edited by Laurence Abbott and Terrence J. Sejnowski, 1999

Unsupervised Learning: Foundations of Neural Computation, edited by Geoffrey Hinton and Terrence J. Sejnowski, 1999

Fast Oscillations in Cortical Circuits, Roger D. Traub, John G. R. Jefferys, and Miles A. Whittington, 1999

Computational Vision: Information Processing in Perception and Visual Behavior, Hanspeter A. Mallot, 2000

Graphical Models: Foundations of Neural Computation, edited by Michael I. Jordan and Terrence J. Sejnowski, 2001

Self-Organizing Map Formation: Foundations of Neural Computation, edited by Klaus Obermayer and Terrence J. Sejnowski, 2001

Self-Organizing Map Formation: Foundations of Neural Computation

Edited by Klaus Obermayer and Terrence J. Sejnowski

A Bradford Book

The MIT Press
Cambridge, Massachusetts
London, England

© 2001 Massachusetts Institute of Technology

All rights reserved. No part of this book may be reproduced in any form by any electronic or mechanical means (including photocopying, recording, or information storage and retrieval) without permission in writing from the publisher.

This book was set in Palatino and printed and bound in the United States of America.

Library of Congress Cataloging-in-Publication Data

Self-organizing map formation : foundations of neural computation / edited by Klaus Obermayer and Terrence J. Sejnowski.
  p. cm. — (Computational neuroscience)
"A Bradford Book."
 ISBN 0-262-65060-6 (pbk. : alk. paper)
 1. Neural computers. 2. Neural networks (Computer science) 3. Self-organizing maps. I. Obermayer, Klaus. II. Sejnowski, Terrence J. (Terrence Joseph) III. Series.
QA76.87 .S46 2001
006.3'2—dc21

2001030329

Contents

Series Foreword	vii
Sources	ix
Introduction	xi

I Receptive Fields — 1

1 Analysis of Linsker's Simulations of Hebbian Rules — 3
  David J. C. MacKay and Kenneth D. Miller

2 Toward a Theory of the Striate Cortex — 19
  Zhaoping Li and Joseph J. Atick

3 Bayesian Self-Organization Driven by Prior Probability Distributions — 39
  Alan L. Yuille, Stelios M. Smirnakis, and Lei Xu

II Models of Topographic Maps in the Brain — 53

4 Dynamics and Formation of Self-Organizing Maps — 55
  Jun Zhang

5 A Unifying Objective Function for Topographic Mappings — 69
  Geoffrey J. Goodhill and Terrence J. Sejnowski

6 Constrained Optimization for Neural Map Formation: A Unifying Framework for Weight Growth and Normalization — 83
  Laurenz Wiskott and Terrence J. Sejnowski

7 How to Generate Ordered Maps by Maximizing the Mutual Information between Input and Output Signals — 129
  Ralph Linsker

III Models of Cortical Feature Maps — 139

8 Models of Orientation and Ocular Dominance Columns in the Visual Cortex: A Critical Comparison — 141
  E. Erwin, K. Obermayer, and K. Schulten

9 Development of Oriented Ocular Dominance Bands as a Consequence of Areal Geometry — 185
  H.-U. Bauer

10 The Joint Development of Orientation and Ocular Dominance: Role of Constraints — 201
  Christian Piepenbrock, Helge Ritter, and Klaus Obermayer

11 A Self-Organizing Model of "Color Blob" Formation — 213
  H. G. Barrow, H. J. Bray, and J. M. L. Budd

12 A Type of Duality between Self-Organizing Maps and Minimal Wiring — 235
  Graeme Mitchison

IV Self-Organizing Maps for Unsupervised Data Analysis — 247

13 A Bayesian Analysis of Self-Organizing Maps — 249
Stephen P. Luttrell

14 Hyperparameter Selection for Self-Organizing Maps — 277
Akio Utsugi

15 GTM: The Generative Topographic Mapping — 291
Christopher M. Bishop, Markus Svensen, and Christopher K. I. Williams

16 Self-Organization as an Iterative Kernel Smoothing Process — 311
Filip Mulier and Vladimir Cherkassky

V Extensions of Self-Organizing Maps — 325

17 A Stochastic Self-Organizing Map for Proximity Data — 327
Thore Graepel and Klaus Obermayer

18 Self-Organized Formation of Various Invariant-Feature Filters in the Adaptive-Subspace SOM — 345
Teuvo Kohonen, Samuel Kaski, and Harri Lappalainen

19 Faithful Representation of Separable Distributions — 369
Juan Lin, David G. Grier, and Jack D. Cowan

20 Dynamic Cell Structure Learns Perfectly Topology Preserving Map — 385
Jörg Bruske and Gerald Sommer

21 An Analysis of the Elastic Net Approach to the Traveling Salesman Problem — 407
Richard Durbin, Richard Szeliski, and Alan Yuille

22 Sorting with Self-Organizing Maps — 419
Marco Budinich

Index — 423

Series Foreword

Computational neuroscience is an approach to understanding the information content of neural signals by modeling the nervous system at many different structural scales, including the biophysical, the circuit, and the systems levels. Computer simulations of neurons and neural networks are complementary to traditional techniques in neuroscience. This book series welcomes contributions that link theoretical studies with experimental approaches to understanding information processing in the nervous system. Areas and topics of particular interest include biophysical mechanisms for computation in neurons, computer simulations of neural circuits, models of learning, representation of sensory information in neural networks, systems models of sensory-motor integration, and computational analysis of problems in biological sensing, motor control, and perception.

Terrence J. Sejnowski
Tomaso A. Poggio

Sources

MacKay, D. J. C., and Miller, K. D. 1990. Analysis of Linsker's simulations of Hebbian rules. *Neural Computation* 2(2), 173–187.

Li, Z., and Atick, J. J. 1994. Toward a theory of the striate cortex. *Neural Computation* 6(1), 127–146.

Yuille, A., Smirnakis, S., and Xu, L. 1995. Bayesian self-organization driven by prior probability distributions. *Neural Computation* 7(3), 580–593.

Zhang, J. 1991. Dynamics and formulation of self-organizing maps. *Neural Computation* 3(1), 54–66.

Goodhill, G. J., and Sejnowski, T. J. 1997. A unifying objective function for topographic mappings. *Neural Computation* 9(6), 1291–1303.

Wiskott, L., and Sejnowski, T. J. 1998. Constrained optimization for neural map formation: A unifying framework for weight growth and normalization. *Neural Computation* 10(3), 671–716.

Linsker, R. 1989. How to generate ordered maps by maximizing the mutual information between input and output signals. *Neural Computation* 1(3), 402–411.

Erwin, E., Obermayer, K., and Schulten, K. 1995. Models of orientation and ocular dominance columns in the visual cortex: A critical comparison. *Neural Computation* 7(1), 425–468.

Bauer, H.-U. 1995. Development of oriented ocular dominance bands as a consequence of areal geometry. *Neural Computation* 7(1), 36–50.

Piepenbrock, C., Ritter, H., and Obermayer, K. 1997. The joint development of orientation and ocular dominance role of constraints. *Neural Computation* 9(5), 959–970.

Barrow, H. G., Bray, A. J., and Budd, J. M. L. 1996. A self-organizing model of "color blob" formation. *Neural Computation* 8(7), 1427–1448.

Mitchison, G. 1995. A type of duality between self-organizing maps and minimal wiring. *Neural Computation* 7(1), 25–35.

Luttrell, S. P. 1994. A Bayesian analysis of self-organizing maps. *Neural Computation* 6(5), 767–794.

Utsugi, A. 1997. Hyperparameter selection for self-organizing maps. *Neural Computation* 9(3), 623–635.

Bishop, C., M. Svensén, M., and Williams, C. K. I. 1998. GTM: The generative topographic mapping. *Neural Computation* 10(1), 215–234.

Mulier, F., and Cherkassky, V. 1995. Self-organization as an iterative kernel smoothing process. *Neural Computation* 6(6), 1165–1177.

Graepel, T., and Obermayer, K. 1999. A stochastic self-organizing map for proximity data. *Neural Computation* 11(1), 139–155.

Kohonen, T., Kaski, S., and Lappalainen, H. 1997. Self-organized formation of various invariant-feature filters in the adaptive-subspace SOM. *Neural Computation* 9(6), 1321–1344.

Lin, J. K., Grier, D. G., and Cowan, J. D. 1997. Faithful representation of separable distributions. *Neural Computation* 9(6), 1305–1320.

Bruske, J., and Sommer, G. 1995. Dynamic cell structure learns perfect topology preserving map. *Neural Computation* 7(4), 845–865.

Durbin, R., Szeliski, R., and Yuille, A. 1989. An analysis of the elastic net approach to the traveling salesman problem. *Neural Computation* **1**(3), 348–358.

Budinich, M. 1995. Sorting with self-organizing maps. *Neural Computation* **7**(6), 1188–1190.

Introduction

The papers on self-organizing map formation collected here have appeared in *Neural Computation* over the past ten years. The papers provide an overview of the field as well as recent developments and can be used by students, researchers, and practitioners. The field of self-organizing maps is a branch of unsupervised learning, whose goal is to determine the statistical properties of input data without explicit feedback from a teacher. A previous volume in this series (Hinton and Sejnowski 1999) collected additional papers from *Neural Computation* on unsupervised learning that are not concerned with self-organizing map formation.

Since much of the original inspiration for the self-organizing maps arose from biological studies, this volume begins with a series of papers that attempts to model the organization of cortical maps and ends with a series of papers on the theory and the applications of the related artificial neural network algorithms. These papers illustrate the fruitfulness of interactions between the modeling of biological systems and the exploration of practical algorithms for solving difficult computational problems. Models of biological systems provide inspiration and a source of new ideas for unsupervised data analysis; the theoretical analyses of the derived algorithms in turn give rise to new hypotheses for the development and function of cortical maps.

Topographic Maps in the Cerebral Cortex

A central organizing principle in the mammalian cerebral cortex is the orderly topographical arrangement of sensory and motor neurons with similar response properties across the cortical surface. Anatomical evidence for cortical maps, based on lesion studies and electrical stimulation, has been available since the early nineteenth century. When methods for recording from single cortical neurons were developed in the 1960s, it became possible to determine how neurons were organized in the cortex. Vernon Mountcastle was the first to report that in a vertical column all neurons tend to have the same properties, based on recording from neurons in the somatosensory cortex. In the visual cortex, David Hubel and Torsten Wiesel reported smooth changes in the response properties of cortical neurons, such as the ocular dominance and orientation of an edge (Hubel and Wiesel 1962). Since then cortical maps have been found and characterized in nearly all of the sensory and motor areas of the brain (Churchland and Sejnowski 1992).

Cortical maps, particularly in the visual cortex, have been the focus of studies into activity-driven mechanisms for synaptic plasticity and their interplay with non-activity-dependent processes based on cell adhesion molecules and diffusible substances (Goodman and Shatz 1993; Quartz and Sejnowski 1997). Recently, new imaging methods (Blasdel and Salama 1986; Grinvald et al. 1986) have made it possible to monitor the distribution of neuronal selectivities across the cortex and over time. These methods have allowed the large-scale development of neuronal response properties to be studied with much greater coverage than previously possible with single-unit recording techniques. Driven by these experimental results, a series of computational studies have attempted to explain the structure of the cortical maps by simulating and analyzing cortical models. One set of studies was concerned with the mechanisms underlying development and plasticity (see chapter 8 and Swindale 1996 for reviews). These approaches were typically based on constrained Hebbian learning and intracortical competition; despite their simplicity, they were able to explain many features of the experimentally observed spatial patterns.

Another set of studies was concerned with the computational advantages of these maps. For example, "minimal wiring" (Durbin and Mitchison 1990), which seeks to reduce the volume of axons needed, has been used to explain the orderly architecture of the cerebral cortex and the patterns of discontinuities (primarily the visual cortex); analogies with parallel computers (Nelson and Bower 1990) have suggested an interpretation of cortical maps in terms local processing, load balancing, and communication requirements. Other approaches based on the goal of efficient coding (Barlow 1961; Field 1994) have attempted to explain the properties of receptive fields (Atick 1992) and their spatial arrangement (Ritter et al. 1991) in terms of the statistics of the signals and the noise. In contrast to the developmental studies, however, most of these modeling studies were less successful in explaining the spatial layout of the maps, and there is still no adequate explanation for why the cortex has such a regular structure.

Self-Organizing Maps

Inspired by the ubiquity of cortical maps in the central nervous system, several mapping algorithms were introduced in the 1970s and early 1980s (Takeuchi and Amari 1979; Whitelaw and Cowan 1981; Grossberg 1976; Malsburg 1973; Kohonen 1982b; Kohonen 1982a; Willshaw and von der Malsburg 1976). It soon became apparent that self-organizing maps are valuable tools for unsupervised data analysis (Kohonen 1987; Ritter, Martinetz, and Schulten 1992). Subsequently, self-organizing maps were applied to real-world problems such as preprocessing for solving classification and regression problems or as a technique for extracting and visualizing salient features in the data (Kohonen 1995; Kohonen 1997).

Although mapping algorithms became widely adopted in the neural network community because of their conceptual simplicity and their computational efficiency, theoretical analysis lagged. Important advances have recently been made by formulating mapping algorithms in terms of cost-functions (Cottrell and Fort 1987; chapter 13; chapter 5), which allow a deeper theoretical understanding and suggest improved optimization procedures. The introduction of cost functions also made it possible to link mapping techniques to methods in classical statistics, which opened new approaches through generative models as well as through statistical techniques such as maximum likelihood and Bayesian analysis (chapter 15).

Receptive Fields

Three papers included here illustrate three aspects of receptive field development that are important for the formation of cortical maps: Hebbian learning, efficient encoding, and statistical relationships. The analysis of constrained Hebbian learning for the activity-driven formation of receptive fields in the primary visual cortex in MacKay and Miller (chapter 1) had a considerable impact on subsequent analyses of map formation. Li and Atick (chapter 2) examine the computational advantages of these emerging receptive fields and show that the filters found in the early visual system, by reducing second-order correlations in the visual input, form an efficient representation of the natural visual environment, which is to some extent invariant under translation and scale. Yuille, Smirnakis and Xu (chapter 3) focus on the emergence of feature detectors based on higher-order correlations in the input data. They examine the receptive fields that emerge by minimizing the Kullback-Leibler divergence between the true probability distribution of a signal amid distracting noise and the output probability distribution of the neurons in the network, thus forming a link with Bayesian theories of visual perception.

Models of Topographic Maps in the Brain

Another group of papers is devoted to an analysis of topographic maps and their formation via objective functions. Zhang (chapter 4) analyzes and extends a continuum model (Amari 1983) and derives point-spread resolution, magnification factors, and bandwidth resolution for topographic maps. Map formation can be characterized by a Lyapunov function that is minimized during map formation. Goodhill and Sejnowski (chapter 5) relate objective functions used by several authors in models of topographic map formation and show that they can be seen as particular cases of a more general cost function that they call the C-measure. Wiskott and Sejnowski (chapter 6) compare objective functions for map formation that use Hebbian learning and relate different models through coordinate transformations. This chapter also discusses additional constraints imposed on the connection strengths and shows how they should be chosen to be consistent with the objective function. Linsker (chapter 7) derives topographic maps from an information-theoretic argument based on "efficiency": maximizing the mutual information between the network input and output. This infomax approach has influenced other unsupervised learning algorithms for extracting higher-order information from the input data (Bell and Sejnowski 1995; Lee, Girolami, and Sejnowski 1999).

Cortical Maps of Stimulus Features

Among the most prominent architectural elements of primary visual cortex are orientation selectivity, ocular dominance, and (in primates) color blobs. The mapping of orientation selectivity and ocular dominance have received most of the attention, although other features such as disparity have also been examined (Berns, Dayan, and Sejnowski 1993). Erwin, Obermayer, and Schulten (chapter 8) provide a systematic review of developmental models for orientation selectivity and ocular dominance and compare model predictions with experimental data from macaque striate cortex. Bauer (chapter 9) considers the influence of areal boundaries on the global map structure for the example of ocular dominance bands, and Piepenbrock, Ritter and Obermayer (chapter 10) revisit constraints in models of Hebbian learning to show that these nonlinearities are essential for the joint development of orientation selectivity and ocular dominance maps. Barrow, Bray, and Bud (chapter 11) apply Hebbian learning to a three-layer recurrent network trained with patches from color photographs of natural scenes and compare the results to a principal component analysis of the image data. Not only did their network develop spatial filters similar to the principal components of the data, but it also grouped the corresponding feature-detecting cells within the cortical layer into color "blobs" embedded in a sea of contrast-sensitive, orientation-selective cells. The resulting pattern is similar to what is seen in the superficial layers of visual cortex area V1 in primates. Mitchison (chapter 12) makes the assumption that local cortical processing occurs within feature spaces and explores the arrangement of computational elements across cortex such that the "wiring length" for connections between them is minimal. The results mathematically relate the elastic net to the self-organizing map approaches.

Self-Organizing Maps for Unsupervised Data Analysis

In a seminal paper, Luttrell (chapter 13) used Bayesian methods to relate self-organizing map formation to the training of probabilistic autoencoders. This insight led to the formulation of a cost function from which Kohonen's original self-organizing map approach could be derived as an approximation of the expectation-maximization (EM) optimization of this cost function; it also paved the way for several extensions of the self-organizing map. Utsugi (chapter 14) formulated a generalized deformable model via a Gaussian mixture model and derived a "mapping" algorithm by a maximum a posteriori estimate of the weight parameters. This is the first paper to apply Bayesian model selection techniques to

Introduction

estimate the hyperparameters for the noise and the prior on the weights. Bishop, Svensen, and Williams (chapter 15) follow up on the idea of generative models. They consider a small number of unobservable, "explanatory" variables that generate the observed distribution of the data, and use statistical techniques to infer their values for each data point, thus performing dimension reduction. Mulier and Cherkassky (chapter 16) relate self-organizing maps to classical nonparametric regression.

Extensions of Self-Organizing Maps

Graepel and Obermayer (chapter 17), following up on Luttrell (chapter 13) and Hofmann and Buhmann (1997), consider dissimilarity values between data items and apply a self-organizing map to combine clustering with metric multidimensional scaling. Kohonen, Kaski, and Lappalainen (chapter 18) combine the mapping property of the self-organizing map with a local projection method, which is similar to principal component analysis, and apply this method to temporal sequences of data. Lin, Grier, and Cowan (chapter 19) successfully use coupled one-dimensional self-organizing maps for the blind separation of sources, while Bruske and Sommer (chapter 20) apply growing and pruning algorithms to self-organizing maps. This section concludes with two surprising applications of mapping algorithms to standard computer science problems: combinatorial optimization and sorting. Durbin, Szeliski, and Yuille (chapter 21) use an elastic net method to find solutions for the traveling salesman problem, and Budinich (chapter 22) shows how self-organizing maps can beat quicksort.

Conclusions

Self-organizing maps occur in both biological and engineering domains. The papers in the collection highlight some of the most important issues that arise in studying the properties of these maps. In particular, maps can be constructed from relatively simple rules governing the local interactions between neighboring elements. This may allow a wide range of properties to be encoded in sensory maps. Most of modeling studies have focused on maps in the earliest stages of sensory processing, where topography is the dominant organizing principle. At higher stages of processing, the sizes of receptive fields become larger, the topography becomes less distinct, and the mapping of higher-order features rather than topography become a dominant organizing principle (Tanaka 1996). Feedback connections between these areas allows the highest levels to influence the earliest levels of processing. Modeling these extrastriate areas and the interactions between them provides a challenge for future studies that build on the papers collected in this volume. A self-organizing multilevel system would have many practical applications.

References

Amari, S. 1983. Field theory of self-organizing neural nets. *IEEE Trans. SMC* **13**, 741–748.

Atick J. J. 1992. Could information theory provide an ecological theory of sensory processing? *Network* **3**, 213–251.

Barlow, H. 1961. The coding of sensory messages. In *Current Problems in Animal Behavior*. Cambridge: Cambridge University Press.

Bell, A. J., and Sejnowski, T. J. 1995. An information-maximization approach to blind separation and blind deconvolution. *Neural. Comp.* **7**, 1129–1159.

Berns, G. S., Dayan, P., and Sejnowski, T. J. 1993. A correlational model for the development of disparity selectivity in visual cortex that depends on prenatal and postnatal phases. *Proceedings of the National Academy of Sciences U.S.A.* **90**, 8277–8281.

Blasdel, G. G., and Salama, G. 1986. Voltage sensitive dyes reveal a modular organization in monkey striate cortex. *Nature* **321**, 579–585.

Churchland, P. S., and Sejnowski, T. J. 1992. *The Computational Brain*. Cambridge, MA: MIT Press.

Cottrell, M., and Fort, J. C. 1987. Etude d'un processus d'auto-organisation. *Ann. Inst. Henri Poincaré* **23**, 1–20.

Durbin, R. and Mitchison, G. 1990. A dimension reduction framework for understanding cortical maps. *Nature* **343**, 644–647.

Field, D. 1994. What is the goal of sensory coding? *Neural Computation* **6**, 559–601.

Goodman, C., and Shatz, C. 1993. Developmental mechanisms that generate precise patterns of neuronal connectivity. *Cell* **72**, 77–89.

Grinvald, A., Lieke, E., Frostig, R. D., Gilbert, C. D., and Wiesel, T. N. 1986. Functional architecture of cortex revealed by optical imaging technique. *Nature* **324**, 361–364.

Grossberg, S. 1976. Adaptive pattern classification and universal recoding, I: Parallel development and coding of neural feature detectors. *Biol. Cybern.* **23**, 121–134.

Hinton, G. E., and Sejnowski, T. J., eds. 1999. *Unsupervised learning: Foundations of neural computation*. Cambridge, MA: MIT Press.

Hofmann, T., and Buhmann, J. 1997. Pairwise data clustering by deterministic annealing. *IEEE PAMI* **19**, 1–14.

Hubel, D., and Wiesel, T. N. 1962. Receptive fields, binocular interaction and functional architecture in the cat's visual cortex. *J. Physiol. (Lond.)* **160**, 106–154.

Kohonen, T. 1982a. Analysis of a simple self-organizing process. *Biol. Cybern.* **44**, 135–140.

Kohonen, T. 1982b. Self-organized formation of topologically correct feature maps. *Biol. Cybern.* **43**, 59–69.

Kohonen, T. 1987. *Self-organization and associative memory*. New York: Springer-Verlag.

Kohonen, T. 1995. *Self-organizing maps*. Berlin, Heidelberg: Springer-Verlag.

Kohonen, T. 1997. Bibliography on the SOM and the LVQ. Available on the Internet at ⟨http://www.cis.hut.fi/nnrc/refs/⟩.

Lee, T.-W., Girolami, M., and Sejnowski, T. J. 1999. Independent component analysis using an extended infomax algorithm for mixed sub-Gaussian and super-Gaussian Sources. *Neural Computation* **11**(2), 417–441.

Malsburg, C. 1973. Self-organization of orientation sensitive cells in the striate cortex. *Kybernetik* **14**, 85–100.

Nelson, M. E., and Bower, J. M. 1990. Brain maps and parallel computers. *Trends in the Neurosciences* **13**, 403–408.

Quartz, S., and Sejnowski, T. J. 1997. The neural basis of cognitive development: A constructivist manifesto. *Behavioral and Brain Sciences* **20**(4), 537–596.

Ritter, H., Martinetz, T., and Schulten, K. 1992. *Neural computation and self-organizing maps: An introduction.* New York: Addison-Wesley.

Ritter, H., Obermayer, K., Schulten, K., and Rubner, J. 1991. Self-organizing maps and adaptive filters. In E. Domani, J. L. van Hemmen, and K. Schulten, eds., *Physics of Neural Networks*, pp. 281–306. New York: Springer-Verlag.

Swindale, N. 1996. The development of topography in the visual cortex: A review of models. *Network* **7**, 161–247.

Takeuchi, A., and Amari, S. 1979. Formation of topographic maps and columnar microstructures. *Biol. Cybern.* **35**, 63–72.

Whitelaw, V., and Cowan, J. 1981. Specificity and plasticity of retinotectal connections: A computational model. *J. Neurosci.* **1**, 1369–1387.

Willshaw, D. J., and von der Malsburg, C. 1976. How patterned neural connections can be set up by self-organization. *Proc. R. Soc. Lond. B* **194**, 431–445.

I

Receptive Fields

1

Analysis of Linsker's Simulations of Hebbian Rules

David J. C. MacKay
*Computation and Neural Systems, Caltech 164-30 CNS,
Pasadena, CA 91125 USA*

Kenneth D. Miller
*Department of Physiology, University of California,
San Francisco, CA 94143-0444 USA*

Linsker has reported the development of center-surround receptive fields and oriented receptive fields in simulations of a Hebb-type equation in a linear network. The dynamics of the learning rule are analyzed in terms of the eigenvectors of the covariance matrix of cell activities. Analytic and computational results for Linsker's covariance matrices, and some general theorems, lead to an explanation of the emergence of center-surround and certain oriented structures. We estimate criteria for the parameter regime in which center-surround structures emerge.

Linsker (1986, 1988) has studied by simulation the evolution of weight vectors under a Hebb-type teacherless learning rule in a feedforward linear network. The equation for the evolution of the weight vector **w** of a single neuron, derived by ensemble averaging the Hebbian rule over the statistics of the input patterns, is[1]

$$\frac{\partial}{\partial t} w_i = k_1 + \sum_j (Q_{ij} + k_2) w_j \quad \text{subject to } -w_{\max} \leq w_i \leq w_{\max} \quad (1.1)$$

---

[1] Our definition of equation 1.1 differs from Linsker's by the omission of a factor of $1/N$ before the sum term, where N is the number of synapses. Also, Linsker allowed more general hard limits, $n_E - 1 \leq w_i \leq n_E$, $0 < n_E < 1$, which he implemented either directly or by allowing a fraction n_E of synapses to be excitatory ($0 \leq w_i^+ \leq 1$) and the remaining fraction $1 - n_E$ to be inhibitory ($-1 \leq w_i^- \leq 0$). These two formulations are essentially mathematically equivalent; this equivalence depends on the fact that the spatial distributions of inputs and correlations in activity among inputs were taken to be independent of whether the inputs were excitatory or inhibitory. Linsker summarized results for $0.35 \leq n_E \leq 0.65$ for his layer $B \to C$, but did not report any dependence of results on n_E within this range and focused discussion on $n_E = 0.5$. At higher layers only $n_E = 0.5$ was discussed. Equation 1.1 is equivalent to $n_E = 0.5$. Our analysis does not depend critically on this choice; what is critical is that the origin be well within the interior of the hypercube of allowed synaptic weights, so that initial development is linear.

where **Q** is the covariance matrix of activities of the inputs to the neuron. The covariance matrix depends on the covariance function, which describes the dependence of the covariance of two input cells' activities on their separation in the input field, and on the location of the synapses, which is determined by a synaptic density function. Linsker used a gaussian synaptic density function. Similar equations have been developed and studied by others (Miller et al. 1986, 1989).

Depending on the covariance function and the two parameters k_1 and k_2, different weight structures emerge. Using a gaussian covariance function (his layer $B \to C$), Linsker reported the emergence of nontrivial weight structures, ranging from saturated structures through center-surround structures to bilobed-oriented structures.

The analysis in this paper examines the properties of equation 1.1. We concentrate on the gaussian covariances in Linsker's layer $B \to C$. We give an explanation of the structures reported by Linsker and discuss criteria for the emergence of center-surround weight structures. Several of the results are more general, applying to any covariance matrix **Q**. Space constrains us to postpone general discussion, technical details, and discussion of other model networks, to a future publication (MacKay and Miller 1990).

2 Analysis in Terms of Eigenvectors

We write equation 1.1 as a first-order differential equation for the weight vector **w**:

$$\dot{\mathbf{w}} = (\mathbf{Q} + k_2 \mathbf{J})\mathbf{w} + k_1 \mathbf{n} \quad \text{subject to} \quad -w_{\max} \leq w_i \leq w_{\max} \qquad (2.1)$$

where **J** is the matrix $J_{ij} = 1 \, \forall i, j$, and **n** is the DC vector $n_i = 1 \, \forall i$. This equation is linear, up to the hard limits on w_i. These hard limits define a hypercube in weight space within which the dynamics are confined. We make the following assumption:

Assumption 1. The principal features of the dynamics are established before the hard limits are reached. When the hypercube is reached, it captures and preserves the existing weight structure with little subsequent change.

The matrix $\mathbf{Q} + k_2 \mathbf{J}$ is symmetric, so it has a complete orthonormal set of eigenvectors[2] $\mathbf{e}^{(a)}$ with real eigenvalues λ_a. The linear dynamics within the hypercube can be characterized in terms of these eigenvectors, each of

---

[2]The indices a and b will be used to denote the eigenvector basis for **w**, while the indices i and j will be used for the synaptic basis.

Linsker's Simulations of Hebbian Rules

which represents an independently evolving weight configuration. First, equation 2.1 has a fixed point at

$$\mathbf{w}^{FP} = -k_1(\mathbf{Q} + k_2\mathbf{J})^{-1}\mathbf{n} = -k_1 \sum_a \frac{\mathbf{e}^{(a)} \cdot \mathbf{n}}{\lambda_a} \mathbf{e}^{(a)} \qquad (2.2)$$

Second, relative to the fixed point, the component of **w** in the direction of an eigenvector grows or decays exponentially at a rate proportional to the corresponding eigenvalue. Writing $\mathbf{w}(t) = \sum_a w_a(t)\mathbf{e}^{(a)}$, equation 2.1 yields

$$w_a(t) - w_a^{FP} = [w_a(0) - w_a^{FP}]e^{\lambda_a t} \qquad (2.3)$$

Thus, the principal emergent features of the dynamics are determined by the following three factors:

1. The principal eigenvectors of $\mathbf{Q} + k_2\mathbf{J}$, that is, the eigenvectors with largest positive eigenvalues. These are the fastest growing weight configurations.

2. Eigenvectors of $\mathbf{Q} + k_2\mathbf{J}$ with negative eigenvalue. Each is associated with an attracting constraint surface, the hyperplane defined by $w_a = w_a^{FP}$.

3. The location of the fixed point of equation 1.1. This is important for two reasons: (a) it determines the location of the constraint surfaces and (b) the fixed point gives a "head start" to the growth rate of eigenvectors $\mathbf{e}^{(a)}$ for which $|w_a^{FP}|$ is large compared to $|w_a(0)|$ (see Fig. 3).

3 Eigenvectors of Q

We first examine the eigenvectors and eigenvalues of $\mathbf{Q}$. The principal eigenvector of $\mathbf{Q}$ dominates the dynamics of equation 2.1 for $k_1 = 0$, $k_2 = 0$. The subsequent eigenvectors of $\mathbf{Q}$ become important as k_1 and k_2 are varied. Some numerical results on the spectrum of $\mathbf{Q}$ have appeared in Linsker (1987, 1990) and Miller (1990). Analyses of the spectrum when output cells are laterally interconnected appear in Miller et al. (1986, 1989).

3.1 Properties of Circularly Symmetric Systems.
If an operator commutes with the rotation operator, its eigenfunctions can be written as eigenfunctions of the rotation operator. For Linsker's system, in the continuum limit, the operator $\mathbf{Q} + k_2\mathbf{J}$ is unchanged under rotation of the system. So the eigenfunctions of $\mathbf{Q} + k_2\mathbf{J}$ can be written as the product of a radial function and one of the angular functions $\cos l\theta$, $\sin l\theta$, $l = 0, 1, 2, \ldots$. To describe these eigenfunctions we borrow from quantum mechanics the notation $n = 1, 2, 3\ldots$ and $l = s, p, d\ldots$ to denote the function's total number of nodes $= 0, 1, 2\ldots$ and number of angular

Name	Eigenfunction	λ/N
1s	$e^{-r^2/2R}$	lC/A
2p	$r\cos\theta e^{-r^2/2R}$	$l^2 C/A$
2s	$(1 - r^2/r_0^2)e^{-r^2/2R}$	$l^3 C/A$

$$R = \frac{C}{2}\left(1 + \sqrt{1 + 4A/C}\right)$$
$$l = \frac{R-C}{R} \quad (0 < l < 1)$$
$$r_0^2 = \frac{2A}{\sqrt{1 + 4A/C}}$$

Table 1: The First Three Eigenfunctions of the Operator $\mathbf{Q}(\mathbf{r}, \mathbf{r}')$. $\mathbf{Q}(\mathbf{r}, \mathbf{r}') = e^{-|\mathbf{r}-\mathbf{r}'|^2/2C} e^{-r'^2/2A}$, where C and A denote the characteristic sizes of the covariance function and synaptic density function. $\mathbf{r}$ denotes two-dimensional spatial position relative to the center of the synaptic arbor, and $r = |\mathbf{r}|$. The eigenvalues λ are normalized by the effective number of synapses $N = 2\pi A$.

nodes $= 0, 1, 2\ldots$, respectively. For example, "2s" and "2p" both denote eigenfunctions with one node, which is radial in 2s and angular in 2p (see Fig. 1).

For monotonic and nonnegative covariance functions, we conjecture that the leading eigenfunctions of $\mathbf{Q}$ are ordered in eigenvalue by their numbers of nodes such that the eigenfunction $[nl]$ has larger eigenvalue than both $[(n+1)l]$ and $[n(l+1)]$. This conjecture is obeyed in analytical and numerical results we have obtained for Linsker's and similar systems. The general validity of this conjecture is under investigation.

3.2 Analytic Calculations for $k_2 = 0$. We have solved analytically for the first three eigenfunctions and eigenvalues of the covariance matrix for layer $\mathcal{B} \to \mathcal{C}$ of Linsker's network, in the continuum limit (Table 1). 1s, the function with no changes of sign, is the principal eigenfunction of $\mathbf{Q}$; 2p, the bilobed-oriented function, is the second eigenfunction; and 2s, the center-surround eigenfunction, is third.[3]

Figure 1a shows the first six eigenfunctions for layer $\mathcal{B} \to \mathcal{C}$ of Linsker (1986).

---

[3] 2s is degenerate with 3d at $k_2 = 0$.

Linsker's Simulations of Hebbian Rules

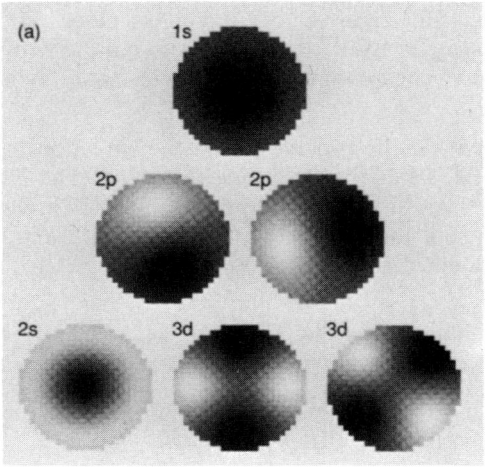

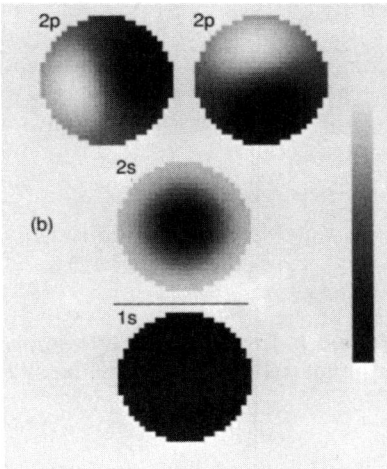

Figure 1: Eigenfunctions of the operator $\mathbf{Q}+k_2\mathbf{J}$. In each row the eigenfunctions have the same eigenvalue, with largest eigenvalue at the top. Eigenvalues (in arbitrary units): (a) $k_2 = 0$: 1s, 2.26; 2p, 1.0; 2s and 3d, 0.41. (b) $k_2 = -3$: 2p, 1.0; 2s, 0.66; 1s, -17.8. The gray scale indicates the range from maximum negative to maximum positive synaptic weight within each eigenfunction. Eigenfunctions of the operator $(e^{-|\mathbf{r}-\mathbf{r'}|^2/2C} + k_2)e^{-r'^2/2A}$ were computed for $C/A = 2/3$ (as used by Linsker for most layer $B \to C$ simulations) on a circle of radius 12.5 grid intervals, with $\sqrt{A} = 6.15$ grid intervals.

4 The Effects of the Parameters k_1 and k_2

Varying k_2 changes the eigenvectors and eigenvalues of the matrix $\mathbf{Q}+k_2\mathbf{J}$. Varying k_1 moves the fixed point of the dynamics with respect to the origin. We now analyze these two changes, and their effects on the dynamics.

Definition. Let $\hat{\mathbf{n}}$ be the unit vector in the direction of the DC vector $\mathbf{n}$. We refer to $(\mathbf{w} \cdot \hat{\mathbf{n}})$ as the *DC component* of $\mathbf{w}$. The DC component is proportional to the sum of the synaptic strengths in a weight vector. For example, 2p and all the other eigenfunctions with angular nodes have zero DC component. Only the s-modes have a nonzero DC component.

4.1 General Theorem: The Effect of k_2.
We now characterize the effect of adding $k_2\mathbf{J}$ to *any* covariance matrix $\mathbf{Q}$.

Theorem 1. *For any covariance matrix $\mathbf{Q}$, the spectrum of eigenvectors and eigenvalues of $\mathbf{Q} + k_2\mathbf{J}$ obeys the following:*

1. *Eigenvectors of $\mathbf{Q}$ with no DC component, and their eigenvalues, are unaffected by k_2.*

2. *The other eigenvectors, with nonzero DC component, vary with k_2. Their eigenvalues increase continuously and monotonically with k_2 between asymptotic limits such that the upper limit of one eigenvalue is the lower limit of the eigenvalue above.*

3. *There is at most one negative eigenvalue.*

4. *All but one of the eigenvalues remain finite. In the limits $k_2 \to \pm\infty$ there is a DC eigenvector $\hat{\mathbf{n}}$ with eigenvalue $\to k_2 N$, where N is the dimensionality of $\mathbf{Q}$, that is, the number of synapses.*

The properties stated in this theorem, whose proof is in MacKay and Miller (1990), are summarized pictorially by the spectral structure shown in Figure 2.

4.2 Implications for Linsker's System.
For Linsker's circularly symmetric systems, all the eigenfunctions with angular nodes have zero DC component and are thus independent of k_2. The eigenvalues that vary with k_2 are those of the s-modes. The leading s-modes at $k_2 = 0$ are 1s, 2s; as k_2 is decreased to $-\infty$, these modes transform continuously into 2s, 3s respectively (Fig. 2).[4] 1s becomes an eigenvector with negative eigenvalue, and it approaches the DC vector $\hat{\mathbf{n}}$. This eigenvector enforces a constraint $\mathbf{w} \cdot \hat{\mathbf{n}} = \mathbf{w}^{FP} \cdot \hat{\mathbf{n}}$, and thus determines that the final average synaptic strength is equal to $\mathbf{w}^{FP} \cdot \mathbf{n}/N$.

---

[4]The 2s eigenfunctions at $k_2 = 0$ and $k_2 = -\infty$ both have one radial node, but are not identical functions.

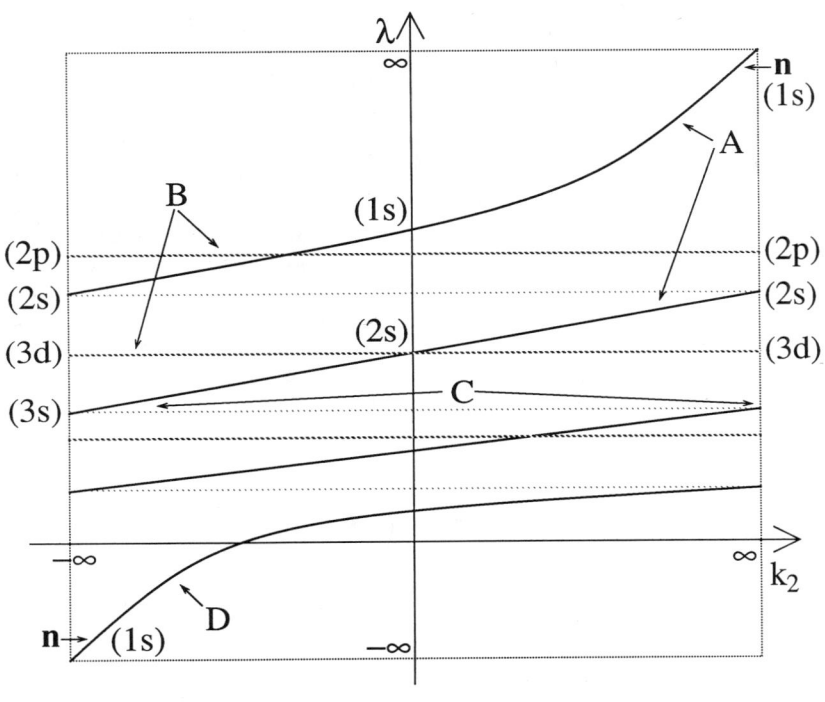

Figure 2: General spectrum of eigenvalues of $Q + k_2 J$ as a function of k_2. A: Eigenvectors with DC component. B: Eigenvectors with zero DC component. C: Adjacent DC eigenvalues share a common asymptote. D: There is only one negative eigenvalue. The annotations in parentheses refer to the eigenvectors of Linsker's system.

Linsker (1986) used $k_2 = -3$. This value of k_2 is sufficiently large that the properties of the $k_2 \to -\infty$ limit hold (MacKay and Miller 1990), and in the following we concentrate interchangeably on $k_2 = -3$ and $k_2 \to -\infty$. The computed eigenfunctions for Linsker's system at layer $B \to C$ are shown in Figure 1b for $k_2 = -3$. The principal eigenfunction is 2p. The center-surround eigenfunction 2s is the principal *symmetric* eigenfunction, but it still has smaller eigenvalue than 2p.

4.3 Effect of k_1. Varying k_1 changes the location of the fixed point of equation 2.1. From equation 2.2, the fixed point is displaced from the origin only in the direction of eigenvectors that have nonzero DC component, that is, only in the direction of the s-modes. This has two important effects, as discussed in Section 2: (1) The s-modes are given a head start in growth rate that increases as k_1 is increased. In particular, the principal s-mode, the center-surround eigenvector 2s, may outgrow the principal eigenvector 2p. (2) The constraint surface is moved when k_1 is changed. For large negative k_2, the constraint surface fixes the average synaptic strength in the final weight vector. To leading order in $1/k_2$, Linsker showed that the constraint is $\sum w_j = k_1/|k_2|$.[5]

4.4 Summary of the Effects of k_1 and k_2. We can now anticipate the explanation for the emergence of center-surround cells: For $k_1 = 0$, $k_2 = 0$, the dynamics are dominated by 1s. The center-surround eigenfunction 2s is third in line behind 2p, the bilobed function. Making k_2 large and negative removes 1s from the lead. 2p becomes the principal eigenfunction and dominates the dynamics for $k_1 \simeq 0$, so that the circular symmetry is broken. Finally, increasing $k_1/|k_2|$ gives a head start to the center-surround function 2s. Increasing $k_1/|k_2|$ also increases the final average synaptic strength, so large $k_1/|k_2|$ also produces a large DC bias. The center-surround regime therefore lies sandwiched between a 2p-dominated regime and an all-excitatory regime. $k_1/|k_2|$ has to be large enough that 2s dominates over 2p, and small enough that the DC bias does not obscure the center-surround structure. We now estimate this parameter regime.

5 Criteria for the Center-Surround Regime

We use two approaches to determine the DC bias at which 2s and 2p are equally favored. This DC bias gives an estimate for the boundary between the regimes dominated by 2s and 2p.

1. **Energy Criterion:** We first estimate the level of DC bias at which the weight vector composed of (2s plus DC bias) and the weight vector composed of (2p plus DC bias) are energetically equally favored. This gives an estimate of the level of DC bias above which 2s will dominate under simulated annealing, which explores the entire space of possible weight configurations.

2. **Time Development Criterion:** Second, we estimate the level of DC bias above which 2s will dominate under simulations of time development of equation 1.1. We estimate the relationship between the parameters such that, starting from a typical random distribution of initial weights, the 2s mode reaches the saturating hypercube at the same time as the 2p mode.

---

[5]To next order, this expression becomes $\sum w_j = k_1/|k_2 + \bar{q}|$, where $\bar{q} = \langle Q_{ij} \rangle$, the average covariance (averaged over i and j). The additional term largely resolves the discrepancy between Linsker's g and $k_1/|k_2|$ in Linsker (1986).

Both criteria will depend on an estimate of the complex effect of the weight limits $-w_{max} \leq w_i \leq w_{max}$. (Without this hypercube of saturation constraints, 2p will always dominate the dynamics of equation 1.1 after a sufficiently long time.) We introduce $g = k_1/(|k_2|Nw_{max})$ as a measure of the average synaptic strength induced by the DC constraint, such that $g = 1$ means all synapses equal w_{max}.[6] Noting that a vector of amplitude $\sqrt{N}w_{max}$ has rms synaptic strength w_{max}, we make the following estimate of the constraint imposed by the hypercube (discussed further in MacKay and Miller 1990):

Assumption 2. When the DC level is constrained to be g, the component $h(g)$ in the direction of a typical unit AC vector at which the hypercube constraint is "reached" is $h(g) = \sqrt{N}w_{max}(1-g)$.

Assumptions 1 and 2 may not adequately characterize the effects of the hypercube on the dynamics, so the numerical estimates of the precise locations of the boundaries between the regions may be in error. However, the qualitative picture presented by these boundaries is informative.

5.1 Energy Criterion. Linsker suggested analysis of equation 1.1 in terms of the energy function on which the dynamics perform constrained gradient descent. The energy of a configuration $\mathbf{w} = \sum w_a \mathbf{e}^{(a)}$ is

$$E = -\frac{1}{2}\sum_a \lambda_a w_a^2 - \sqrt{N} k_1 \sum_a w_a n_a \tag{5.1}$$

where n_a is the DC component of eigenvector $\mathbf{e}^{(a)}$. We consider two configurations, one with w_{2p} equal to its maximum value $h(g)$ and $w_{2s} = 0$, and one with $w_{2p} = 0$ and $w_{2s} = \text{sign}(n_{2s})h(g)$. The component w_{1s} is the same in both cases. All the other components are assumed to be small and to contribute no bias in energy between the two configurations. The energies of these configurations will be our estimates of the energies of saturated configurations obtained by saturating 2p and 2s, respectively, subject to the constraints. We compare these two energies and find the DC level $g = g^E$ at which they are equal:[7]

$$g^E = \frac{1}{1 + 2\frac{|n_{2s}k_2|}{(\lambda_{2p}-\lambda_{2s})/N}}$$

For Linsker's layer $\mathcal{B} \to \mathcal{C}$ connections, our estimate of g^E is 0.16.

5.2 Time Development Criterion. The energy criterion does not take into account the initial conditions from which equation 1.1 starts. We now derive a second criterion that attempts to do this.

---
[6]This is equal to twice Linsker's g.
[7]λ/N is written as a single entity because $\lambda \propto N$. Also $n_{2s} \sim 1/k_2$, so $n_{2s}k_2$ tends to a constant as $k_2 \to \infty$.

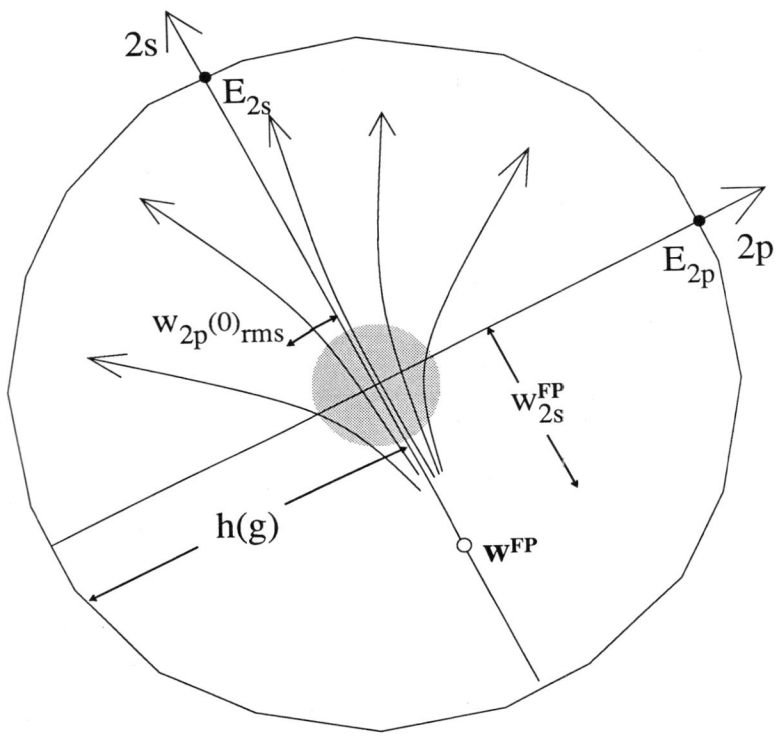

Figure 3: Schematic diagram illustrating the criteria for 2s to dominate. The polygon of size $h(g)$ represents the hypercube. *Energy criterion*: The points marked E_{2p} and E_{2s} show the locations at which the energy estimates were made. *Time development criterion*: The gray cloud surrounding the origin represents the distribution of initial weight vectors. If $w_{2p}(0)$ is sufficiently small compared to w_{2s}^{FP}, and if the hypercube is sufficiently close, then the weight vector reaches the hypercube in the direction of 2s before w_{2p} has grown appreciably.

If the initial random component in the direction of 2p, $w_{2p}(0)$, is sufficiently smallcompared to w_{2s}^{FP}, which provides 2s with a head start, then w_{2p} may never start growing appreciably before the growth of w_{2s} saturates (Fig. 3). The initial component $w_{2p}(0)$ is a random quantity whose typical magnitude can be estimated statistically from the weight initialization parameters. $w_{2p}(0)_{rms}$ scales as $1/\sqrt{N}$ relative to the nonrandom quantity w_{2s}^{FP}. Hence the initial relative magnitude of w_{2p} can be made arbitrarily small by increasing N, and the emergence of center-surround structures may be achieved at any g by using an N sufficiently large to suppress the initial symmetry breaking fluctuations.

We estimate the boundary between the regimes dominated by 2s and 2p by finding the choice of parameters such that $w_{2p}(t)$ and $w_{2s}(t)$ reach the hypercube at the same time. We evaluate the time t_{2s} at which w_{2s} reaches the hypercube.[8] Our estimate of the typical starting component for 2p is $w_{2p}(0)_{rms} = \sqrt{2}\sigma(g)w_{max}$ where $\sigma(g)$ is a dimensionless standard deviation derived in MacKay and Miller (1990). We set $w_{2p}(t_{2s}) = h(g)$, and solve for N^*, the number of synapses above which w_{2s} reaches the hypercube before w_{2p}, in terms of g:

$$\sqrt{N^*} = \frac{\sqrt{2}\sigma(g)}{(1-g)}\left(1 + \frac{1-g}{g}\frac{\lambda_{2s}/N}{|n_{2s}k_2|}\right)^{\lambda_{2p}/\lambda_{2s}} \quad (5.2)$$

5.3 Discussion of the Two Criteria. Figure 4 shows g^E and $N^*(g)$. The two criteria give different boundaries. In regime A, 2p is estimated to both emerge under equation 1.1, and to be energetically favored. Similarly, in regime C, 2s is estimated to dominate equation 1.1, and to be energetically favored. In regime D, the initial fluctuations are so big that although 2s is energetically favored, symmetry breaking structures can dominate equation 1.1.[9] Lastly, in regime B, although 2p is energetically favored, 2s will reach saturation first because N is sufficiently large that the symmetry breaking fluctuations are suppressed. Whether this saturated 2s structure will be stable, or whether it might gradually destabilize into a 2p-like structure, is not predicted by our analysis.[10] The possible difference between simulated annealing and equation 1.1 makes it clear that if initial conditions are important (regimes B and D), the use of simulated annealing on the energy function as a quick way of finding the outcome of equation 1.1 may give erroneous results.

Figure 4 also shows the areas in the parameter space in which Linsker made the simulations he reported. The agreement between experiment and our estimated boundaries is reasonable.

---

[8]We set $w_{2s}(0) = 0$, neglecting its fluctuations, which for large N are negligible compared with w_{2s}^{FP}.

[9]If the initial component of 2s is *toward* the fixed point, the 2s component must first shrink to zero before it can then grow in the opposite direction. Thus, large fluctuations may either hinder or help 2s, while they always help 2p.

[10]In a one-dimensional model system we have found that both cases may be obtained, depending sensitively on the parameters.

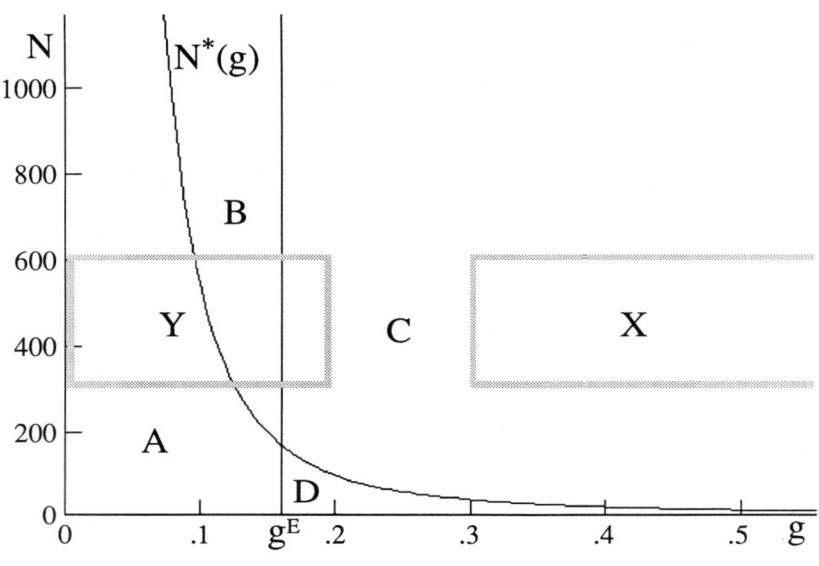

Figure 4: Boundaries estimated by the two criteria for $C/A = 2/3$. To the left of the line labeled g^E, the energy criterion predicts that 2p is favored; to the right, 2s is favored. Above and below the line $N^*(g)$, the time development criterion estimates that 2s and 2p, respectively, will dominate equation 1.1. The regions X, Y, mark the regimes studied by Linsker: (X) $N = 300 - 600$, $g = 0.3$–0.6: the region in which Linsker reported robust center-surround; (Y) $N = 300$–600, $g <\sim 0.2$: asymmetric center-surround structures and (near $g = 0$) bilobed cells.

6 Conclusions and Discussion

For Linsker's $B \to C$ connections, we predict four main parameter regimes for varying k_1 and k_2.[11] These regimes, shown in Figure 5, are dominated by the following weight structures:

$k_2 = 0$, $k_1 = 0$	The principal eigenvector of Q, 1s.
k_2 = large positive and/or k_1 = large	The flat DC weight vector, which leads to the same saturated structures as 1s.

---

[11] not counting the symmetric regimes $(k_1, k_2) \leftrightarrow (-k_1, k_2)$ in which all the weight structures are inverted in sign.

Linsker's Simulations of Hebbian Rules

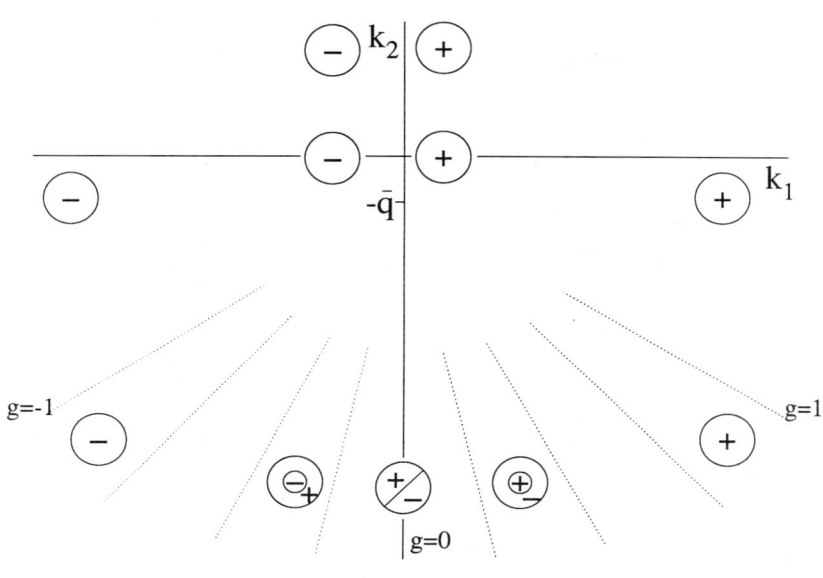

Figure 5: Parameter regimes for Linsker's system. The DC bias is approximately constant along the radial lines, so each of the regimes with large negative k_2 is wedge shaped.

k_2 =large negative, $k_1 \simeq 0$	The principal eigenvector of $\mathbf{Q} + k_2 \mathbf{J}$ for $k_2 \to -\infty$, 2p.
k_2 =large negative, k_1 = intermediate	The principal eigenvector of $\mathbf{Q} + k_2 \mathbf{J}$ for $k_2 \to -\infty$ with nonzero DC component, 2s. The size of this regime can depend on the size of the symmetry-breaking fluctuations, and hence on the number of synapses.

Higher layers of Linsker's network can be analyzed in terms of the same four regimes; the principal eigenvectors are altered, so that different structures can emerge (MacKay and Miller 1990).

Linsker suggested that the emergence of center-surround structures may depend on the peaked synaptic density function that he used (Linsker 1986, p. 7512). However, with a flat ("pillbox") density function, the eigenfunctions are qualitatively unchanged, so we expect that center-surround structures may emerge by the same mechanism.

The development of the interesting cells in Linsker's layer $B \to C$ depends on the use of negative synapses and on the use of the terms k_1 and k_2 to enforce a constraint on the final percentages of positive and negative synapses. Both of these may be biologically problematic (Miller 1990; MacKay and Miller 1990). A linear Hebb rule like Linsker's can be derived without the use of negative synapses by examining the *difference* between the innervation strengths of two equivalent excitatory projections, for example, left-eye and right-eye inputs (Miller et al. 1989) or ON-center and OFF-center inputs (Miller 1989). However, in this case the constants k_1 and k_2 disappear from the equation for the development of the difference of synaptic strengths because these constants take on equal values for each of the two equivalent populations. Therefore, there will only be one regime, in which the principal eigenvector of Q dominates. Such a model can nonetheless develop interesting receptive field structures if oscillations exist in the covariance functions of the input layer, and particularly if lateral interactions are introduced in the output layer (Linsker 1987; Miller et al. 1989; Miller 1989, 1990).

Acknowledgments

D.J.C.M. is supported by a Caltech Fellowship and a Studentship from SERC, UK. K.D.M. thanks M. P. Stryker for encouragement and financial support while this work was undertaken. K.D.M. was supported by an N.E.I. Fellowship and the International Joint Research Project Bioscience Grant to M. P. Stryker (T. Tsumoto, Coordinator) from the N.E.D.O., Japan. This collaboration would have been impossible without the internet/NSFnet.

References

Linsker, R. 1986. From basic network principles to neural architecture (series). *Proc. Natl. Acad. Sci. U.S.A.* **83**, 7508–7512, 8390–8394, 8779–8783.

Linsker, R. 1987. Towards an organizing principle for perception: Hebbian synapses and the principle of optimal neural encoding. *IBM Research Report RC 12830*.

Linsker, R. 1988. Self-organization in a perceptual network. *Computer* **21**(3), 105–117.

Linsker, R. 1990. Designing a sensory processing system: What can be learned from principal components analysis? *Proc. Int. Joint Conf. on Neural Networks, Jan. 1990*, M. Caudill, ed., pp. II:291–97. Lawrence Erlbaum, Hillsdale, NJ.

MacKay, D. J. C., and Miller, K. D. 1990. Analysis of Linsker's application of Hebbian rules to linear networks. *Network*, to appear.

Miller, K. D. 1989. Orientation-selective cells can emerge from a Hebbian mechanism through interactions between ON- and OFF-center inputs. *Soc. Neurosci. Abstr.* **15**, 794.

Miller, K. D. 1990. Correlation-based mechanisms of neural development. In *Neuroscience and Connectionist Theory*, M.A. Gluck and D.E. Rumelhart, eds., pp. 267–353. Lawrence Erlbaum, Hillsdale, NJ.

Miller, K. D., Keller, J. B., and Stryker, M. P. 1986. Models for the formation of ocular dominance columns solved by linear stability analysis. *Soc. Neurosci. Abstr.* **12**, 1373.

Miller, K. D., Keller, J. B., and Stryker, M. P. 1989. Ocular dominance column development: Analysis and simulation. *Science* **245**, 605–615.

2

Toward a Theory of the Striate Cortex

Zhaoping Li
Joseph J. Atick
The Rockefeller University, 1230 York Avenue, New York, NY 10021, USA

We explore the hypothesis that linear cortical neurons are concerned with building a particular type of representation of the visual world—one that not only preserves the information and the efficiency achieved by the retina, but in addition preserves spatial relationships in the input—both in the plane of vision and in the depth dimension. Focusing on the *linear* cortical cells, we classify all transforms having these properties. They are given by representations of the scaling and translation group and turn out to be labeled by rational numbers '$(p+q)/p$' (p, q integers). Any given (p, q) predicts a set of receptive fields that comes at different spatial locations and scales (sizes) with a bandwidth of $\log_2[(p+q)/p]$ octaves and, most interestingly, with a diversity of 'q' cell varieties. The bandwidth affects the trade-off between preservation of planar and depth relations and, we think, should be selected to match structures in natural scenes. For bandwidths between 1 and 2 octaves, which are the ones we feel provide the best matching, we find for each scale a minimum of two distinct cell types that reside next to each other and in phase quadrature, that is, differ by $90°$ in the phases of their receptive fields, as are found in the cortex, they resemble the "even-symmetric" and "odd-symmetric" simple cells in special cases. An interesting consequence of the representations presented here is that the pattern of activation in the cells in response to a translation or scaling of an object remains the same but merely shifts its locus from one group of cells to another. This work also provides a new understanding of color coding changes from the retina to the cortex.

1 Introduction

What is the purpose of the signal processing performed by neurons in the visual pathway? Are there first principles that predict the computations of these neurons? Recently there has been some progress in answering these questions for neurons in the early stages of the visual pathway. In Atick and Redlich (1990, 1992) a quantitative theory, based on the principle of redundancy reduction, was proposed. It hypothesizes that the main goal of retinal transformations is to eliminate redundancy in input signals, particularly that due to pairwise correlations among pixels—second-order statistics.[1] The predictions of the theory agree well with experimental data on processing of retinal ganglion cells (Atick and Redlich 1992; Atick et al. 1992).

Given the successes of this theory, it is natural to ask whether redundancy reduction is a computational strategy continued into the striate cortex. One possibility is that cortical neurons are concerned with eliminating higher-order redundancy, which is due to higher-order statistics. We think this is unlikely. To see why, we recall the facts that make redundancy reduction compelling when applied to the retina and see that these facts are not as relevant for the cortex.

First, the retina has a clear bottleneck problem: the amount of visual data falling on the retina per second is enormous, of the order of tens of megabytes, while the retinal output has to fit into an optic nerve of a dynamic range significantly smaller than that of the input. Thus, the retina must compress the signal, and it can do so without significant loss of information by reducing redundancy. In contrast, after the signal is past the optic nerve, there is no identifiable bottleneck that requires continued redundancy reduction beyond the retina.

Second, even if there were pressure to reduce data,[2] eliminating higher-order statistics does not help. The reason is that higher-order statistics do not contribute significantly to the entropy of images, and hence no significant compression can be achieved by eliminating them (for reviews of information theory see Shannon and Weaver 1949; Atick 1992). The dominant redundancy comes from pairwise correlations.[3]

There is another intrinsic difference between higher- and second-order statistics that suggests their different treatment by the visual pathway. Figure 1 shows image A and another image B that was obtained by randomizing the phases of the Fourier coefficients of A. B thus has the same second-order statistics as A but no higher-order ones. Contrary to A, B has no clear forms or structures (cf. Field 1989). This suggests that for defining forms and for discriminating between images, second-order statistics are useless, while higher-order ones are essential. Actually, eliminating the former highlights the higher-order statistics that should be used to extract form signals from "noise."[4]

---

[1]Since retinal neurons receive noisy signals it is necessary to formulate the redundancy reduction hypothesis carefully taking noise into account. In Atick and Redlich (1990, 1992) a generalized notion of redundancy was defined, whose minimization leads to elimination of pairwise correlations and to noise smoothing.

[2]For example, there could be a computational bottleneck such as an attentional bottleneck occuring deep into the cortex—perhaps in the link between $V4$ and IT (Van Essen et al. 1991).

[3]This fact is well known in the television industry (see, e.g., Schreiber 1956). This is why practical compression schemes for television signals never take into account more than pairwise correlations, and even then, typically nearest neighbor correlations. This fact was also verified for several scanned natural images in our laboratory by N. Redlich and by Z. Li.

[4]Extracting signal from noise can achieve by far more significant data reduction than trying to eliminate higher-order correlations.

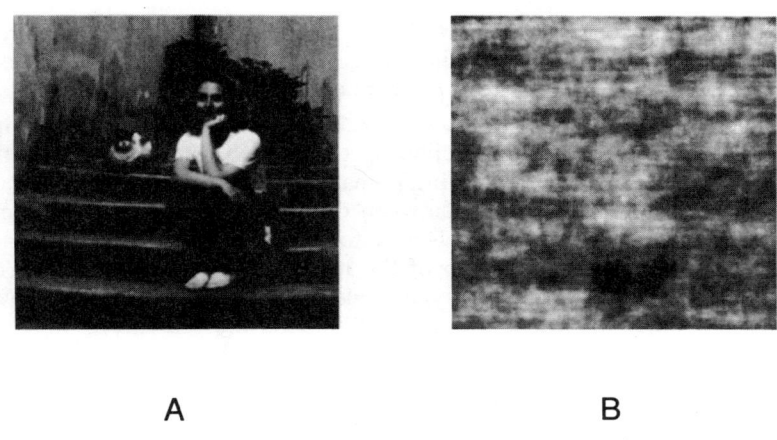

A   B

Figure 1: (A, B) Demonstration of the uselessness of second-order statistics for form definition and discrimination. Following Field (1989), image B is constructed by first Fourier transforming A, randomizing the phases of the coefficients and then taking the inverse Fourier transform. The two images thus have the same second-order statistics but B has no higher-order ones. All relevant object features disappeared from B.

So what is the cortex then trying to do? Ultimately, of course, the cortex is concerned with object and pattern recognition. One promising direction could be to use statistical regularities of images to discover matched filters that lead to better representations for pattern recognition. Research in this direction is currently under way. However, there is another important problem that a perceptual system has to face before the recognition task. This is the problem of *segmentation*, or equivalently, the problem of grouping features according to a hypothesis of which objects they belong to. It is a complex problem, which may turn out not to be solvable independently from the recognition problem. However, since objects are usually localized in space, we think an essential ingredient for its successful solution is a representation of the visual world where *spatial relationships*, both in the plane of vision and in the depth dimension, are preserved as much as possible.

In this paper we hypothesize that the purpose of early cortical processing is to produce a representation that (1) preserves information, (2) is free of second-order statistics, and (3) preserves spatial relationships. The first two objectives are fully achieved by the retina so we merely require that they be maintained by cortical neurons. We think the third objective is attempted in the retina (e.g., retinotopic and scale invariant sampling);

however, it is completed only in the cortex where more computational and organizational resources are available.

Here, we focus on the cortical transforms performed by the relatively linear cells; the first two requirements immediately limit the class of transforms that linear cells can perform on the retinal signals to the class of unitary matrices,[5] $\mathbf{U}$ with $\mathbf{U} \cdot \mathbf{U}^\dagger = \mathbf{1}$. So the principle for deriving cortical cell kernels reduces to finding the $\mathbf{U}$ that best preserves spatial relationships. Actually, preserving planar and depth relationships simultaneously requires a trade-off between the two (see Section 2). This implies that there is a family of $\mathbf{U}$s, one for every possible trade-off. Each $\mathbf{U}$ is labeled by the bandwidth of the resulting cell filters and forms a representation of the scaling and translation group (see Section 3). We show that the requirement of unitarity limits the allowed choices of bandwidths, and for each choice predicts the needed cell diversity. The bandwidth that should ultimately be selected is the one that best matches structures in natural scenes. For bandwidths around 1.6 octaves, which are the ones we feel are most relevant for natural scenes, the predicted cell kernels and cell diversity resemble those observed in the cortex.

The resulting cell kernels also possess an interesting *object constancy* property: when an object in the visual field is translated in the plane or perpendicular to the plane of vision, the pattern of activation it evokes in the cells remains intrinsically the same but shifts its locus from one group of cells to another, leaving the same total number of cells activated. The importance of such representations for pattern recognition has been stressed repeatedly by many people before and recently by Olshausen *et al.* (1992). Furthermore, this work provides a new understanding of color coding change from the single opponency in the retina to the double opponency in the cortex.

2 Manifesting Spatial Relationships

In this section we examine the family of decorrelating maps and see how they differ in the degree with which they preserve spatial relationships. We start with the input, represented by the activities of photoreceptors in the retina, $\{S(\underline{x}_n)\}$ where $\underline{x}_n$ labels the spatial location of the nth photoreceptor in a two-dimensional (2D) grid. For simplicity, we take the grid to be uniform. To focus on the relevant issues without the notational complexity of 2D, we first examine the one-dimensional (1D) problem and then generalize the analysis to 2D in Section 4. The autocorrelator of the signals $\{S(x_n)\}$ is

$$R_{nm} \equiv \langle S(x_n) S(x_m) \rangle \qquad (2.1)$$

---

[5]In this paper we use the term "unitary" instead of "orthogonal" since we find it more convenient to use complex basis [e.g., e^{ifx} instead of $\cos(fx)$]. $\mathbf{U}^\dagger \equiv \mathbf{U}^{*T}$, where the asterisk denotes complex conjugate. For real matrices, unitary means orthogonal.

where brackets denote ensemble average. To eliminate this particular redundancy, one has to decorrelate the output and then apply the appropriate gain control to fit the signals into a limited dynamic range. This can be achieved by a linear transformation

$$O_j = \sum_{n=1}^{N} K_{jn} S(x_n) \qquad (2.2)$$

where $j = 1, \ldots, N$ and the kernel K_{jn} is the product of two matrices. Using boldface to denote matrices:

$$\mathbf{K} = \mathbf{V} \cdot \mathbf{M} \qquad (2.3)$$

M_{jn} is the rotation to the principal components of $\mathbf{R}$: $(\mathbf{M} \cdot \mathbf{R} \cdot \mathbf{M}^T)_{ij} = \lambda_i \delta_{ij}$, where $\{\lambda_i\}$ are the eigenvalues of $\mathbf{R}$. While $\mathbf{V}$ is the gain control which is a diagonal matrix with elements $V_{ii} = 1/\sqrt{\lambda_i}$. Thus the output has the property

$$\langle O_i O_j \rangle = (\mathbf{K} \cdot \mathbf{R} \cdot \mathbf{K}^T)_{ij} = \delta_{ij} \qquad (2.4)$$

An important fact to note is that redefining $\mathbf{K}$ by $\mathbf{K}' = \mathbf{U} \cdot \mathbf{K}$ where $\mathbf{U}$ is a unitary matrix ($\mathbf{U} \cdot \mathbf{U}^\dagger = 1$) does not alter the decorrelation property (equation 2.4). (Actually $\mathbf{U}$ should be an orthogonal matrix for real O_i, but since we will for convenience use complex variables, unitary $\mathbf{U}$ is appropriate.) Therefore, there is a whole family of equally efficient representations parameterized by $\{\mathbf{U}\}$. Any member is denoted by $\mathbf{K}_\mathbf{U}$

$$\mathbf{K}_\mathbf{U} = \mathbf{U} \cdot (\mathbf{V} \cdot \mathbf{M}) \equiv \mathbf{U} \cdot \mathbf{K}^{(p)} \qquad (2.5)$$

where $\mathbf{K}^{(p)} \equiv \mathbf{V} \cdot \mathbf{M}$ is the transformation to the principal components. Without compromising efficiency, this nonuniqueness allows one to look for a specific $\mathbf{U}$ that leads to $\mathbf{K}_\mathbf{U}$ with other desirable properties such as manifest spatial relationships.[6]

To see this, let us exhibit the transformation $\mathbf{K}^{(p)}$ more explicitly. For natural signals, the autocorrelator is translationally invariant, in the sense that $R_{nm} = R(n-m)$. One can then define the autocorrelator by its Fourier transform or its power spectrum, which in 2D is $R(f) \sim 1/|f|^2$, where f is the 2D spatial frequency (Field 1987; Ruderman and Bialek 1993). For illustration purposes, we take in this section the analogous 1D "scale

---

[6]It should be noted that this nonuniqueness in receptive field properties is due to the fact that the principle used is decorrelation. If one insists on minimization of pixel entropy (which for gaussian signals is equivalent to decorrelation) this symmetry formally does not exist for ensembles of nongaussian signals. In other words some choice of $\mathbf{U}$ may be selected over others. However, for the ensemble of 40 images that we have considered, we found that the pixel entropy varied only by few percent for different $\mathbf{U}$s. This is consistent with the idea that natural scenes are dominated by second-order statistics that do not select any particular $\mathbf{U}$. In other systems it is possible that higher order statistics do select a special $\mathbf{U}$, see, for example, Hopfield (1991). For another point of view see Linsker (1992).

invariant" spectrum, namely, $R(f) \sim 1/f$. In the 2D analysis of Section 4 we use the measured spectrum $\sim 1/|f|^2$.

For a translationally invariant autocorrelator, the transformation to principal components is a Fourier transform. This means, the principal components of natural scenes or the row vectors of the matrix **M** are sine waves of different frequencies

$$M_{jn} = \frac{1}{\sqrt{N}} e^{-if_j x_n} \tag{2.6}$$

where

$$j = (0, 1, 2, \ldots, N-1)$$

$$f_j = \begin{cases} \frac{2\pi}{N} \frac{j+1}{2}, & \text{if } j \text{ is odd} \\ -\frac{2\pi}{N} \frac{j}{2}, & \text{if } j \text{ is even} \end{cases}$$

While the gain control matrix **V** is $V_{jj} = 1/\sqrt{R(f_j)} = 1/\sqrt{|f_j|}$. The total transform then becomes

$$K_{jn}^{(p)} = \frac{1}{\sqrt{N}} \cdot \frac{1}{\sqrt{|f_j|}} e^{-if_j x_n} \tag{2.7}$$

This performs a Fourier transform and at the same time normalizes the output such that the power is equalized among frequency components $\langle O_i^2 \rangle = \text{const.}$ (i.e., output is whitened). One undesirable feature of the transformation $\mathbf{K}^{(p)}$ is that it does not preserve spatial relationships in the plane. As an object is translated in the field of view, the locus of response $\{O_i\}$ will not simply translate. Also two objects separated in the input do not activate two separate groups of cells in the output. Typically all cells respond to a mixture of features of all objects in the visual field. Segmentation is thus not easily achievable in this representation.

Mathematically, we say that the output $\{O_i\}$ preserves planar spatial relationships in the input if

$$O_i[S] = O_{i-m}[S'] \quad \text{when} \quad S'(x_n) = S(x_{n+m}) \tag{2.8}$$

where $O_i[S] \equiv \sum_{n=1}^{N} K_{in} S(x_n)$. In other words, a translation in the input merely shifts the output from one group of cells to another. Implicitly, preserving planar spatial relationship also requires, and we will therefore enforce, that the cell receptive fields be local, so a spatially localized object evokes activities only in a local cell group, which shifts its location when the object moves and is separated from another cell group evoked by another spatially disjoint object in the image plane. Technically speaking, an $\{O_i\}$ that satisfies equation 2.8 is said to form a representation of the discrete "translation group."

Theory of the Striate Cortex

Insisting on equation 2.8 picks up a unique choice of **U**. In fact in this case **U** is given by

$$U_{nj} = M^*_{nj} = \frac{1}{\sqrt{N}} e^{if_j x_n} \tag{2.9}$$

which is just the inverse Fourier transform. The resulting transformation $\mathbf{K}^{(t)} = \mathbf{U} \cdot \mathbf{V} \cdot \mathbf{U}^\dagger$ gives translationally invariant center-surround cell kernels

$$K^{(t)}_{nm} = K^{(t)}(n - m) = \sum_j U_{nj} V_{jj} U^*_{mj} \propto \sum_f \cos[f(x_n - x_m)] / \sqrt{R(f)}$$

In two dimensions, taking into account optical properties of the eye medium and the noise, these kernels were shown to account well for properties of retinal ganglion cells (Atick and Redlich 1992).

Although the representation defined by $\mathbf{K}^{(t)}$ is ideal for preserving spatial relationships in the plane, it completely destroys spatial relations **in scale or** depth dimension. The change in the patterns of activation in $\{O_i\}$ in response to a change in the object distance is very complicated. To preserve depth relations the output should form a representation of another group the so-called "scaling group." This is because when an object recedes or approaches, the image it projects goes from $S(x)$ to $S(\lambda x)$ for some scale factor λ. The requirement of object invariance under scaling dictates that

$$O_i[S(\lambda x)] = O_{i+l}[S(x)] \tag{2.10}$$

for some shift l depending on λ. It is not difficult to see that $\mathbf{K}^{(t)}$, which satisfies equation 2.8 all the way down to the smallest possible translation, violates this condition. Actually, satisfying equations 2.8 and 2.10 for the smallest possible translation and scale changes simultaneously is not possible. A compromise between them has to be found.

The problem of finding the kernels that lead to $\{O_i\}$ with the best compromise between equations 2.8 and 2.10 is equivalent to the mathematical problem of constructing simultaneous representations of the translation and scaling group, which is what we do next.

3 Representations of Translation and Scaling Group

To satisfy equations 2.8 and 2.10 the cells must carry two different labels. One is a spatial position label "n" and the other is a scale label "a." The idea is that under translations of the input the output translates over the "n" index, while under scaling by some scale factor λ the output shifts over the "a" index. Such cell groups can be obtained from $\mathbf{O} = \mathbf{U} \cdot \mathbf{K}^{(p)}$ using a $\mathbf{U}$ that is block diagonal:

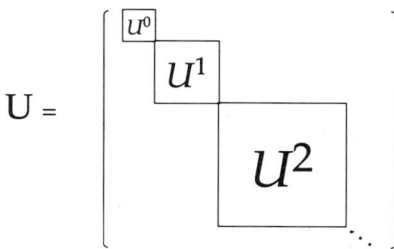

Each submatrix $\mathbf{U}^a$ has dimension N^a and gives rise to N^a cells with outputs O_n^a located at lattice points $x_n^a = (N/N^a)n$ for $n = 1, 2, \ldots, N^a$. Since the block matrices $\mathbf{U}^a$ act on $\mathbf{K}^{(p)}$, which are the Fourier modes of the inputs, the resulting cells in any given block a filter the inputs through a limited and exclusive frequency band with frequencies f_j for $\sum_{a'<a} N^{a'} \leq j < \sum_{a'\leq a} N^{a'}$. Since $N^a < N$ these cells sample more sparsely on the original visual field. Notice the cells from different blocks a are spatially mingled with each other, and their total number add up to $N = \sum_a N^a$. The hope is to have translation invariance within each block and scale invariance between blocks, that is,

$$O_n^a[S] = O_{n+\delta n}^a[S'] \text{ for } S'(x) = S(x + \delta x) \text{ and } \delta x = (N/N^a)\delta n \quad (3.1)$$
$$O_n^a[S] = O_n^{a+1}[S'] \text{ for } S'(x) = S(\lambda x) \quad (3.2)$$

Each block 'a' thus represents a particular scale, the translation invariance within that scale can be achieved with a resolution $\delta x \propto N/N^a$, inversely proportional to N^a. Larger blocks or larger N^a thus give better translation invariance, and the single block matrix $\mathbf{U} = \mathbf{U}^0 = \mathbf{M}^\dagger$ achieves this symmetry to the highest possible resolution. On the other hand, a higher resolution in scaling invariance calls for a smaller $\lambda > 1$. As we will see below, $(\lambda - 1) \propto N^a/f^a$, where f^a is the smallest frequency sampled by the ath block. Hence a better scaling invariance requires smaller block sizes N^a. A trade-off between better translation and scaling invariance reduces to choosing the scaling factor λ, or the bandwidth depending on it. This will become clearer as we now follow the detailed construction of U. The unitarity condition now requires having $\mathbf{U}^a(\mathbf{U}^a)^\dagger = 1$ for each a, resulting in output cells uncorrelated within each scale and between scales.

To construct $\mathbf{U}^a$, one notices that the requirement of translation invariance is equivalent to having identical receptive fields, except for a spatial shift of the centers, within each scale a. It forces $\mathbf{U}_{nj}^a \propto e^{if_j x_n^a}$. For a general λ, it turns out that the constraint $\mathbf{U}^a(\mathbf{U}^a)^\dagger = 1$ for $a > 0$ cannot be satisfied if one insists on only one cell or receptive field type within the scale. However, if one allows the existence of several say, 'q', cell types within the scale, $\mathbf{U}^a(\mathbf{U}^a)^\dagger = 1$ is again possible. In this case, each cell is identical to (or is the off-cell type of) the one that is q lattice spaces away in the same scale lattice (i.e., $x_n^a \to x_{n+q}^a$). The most general choice for real receptive fields is then

$$U_{nj}^a = \begin{cases} \frac{1}{\sqrt{N^a}} e^{i(f_j x_n^a - \phi^a n + \theta)} & \text{if } f_j > 0 \\ \frac{1}{\sqrt{N^a}} e^{-i(|f_j| x_n^a - \phi^a n + \theta)} & \text{if } f_j < 0 \end{cases} \quad (3.3)$$

where θ is an arbitrary phase that can be thought of as zero for simplicity at the moment, and

$$\phi^a = \frac{p}{q}\pi \quad (3.4)$$

for two relatively prime integers p and q. This means the number of cell types in any given scaling block will be q. The frequencies sampled by this cell group are $f_j = \pm(2\pi/N)j$ for $j^a < j \leq j^{a+1}$. Including both the positive and the negative frequencies, the total number of frequencies sampled, and, since U^a is a square matrix, the total number of cells in this scale, is $N^a = 2(j^{a+1} - j^a)$.

The constraint of unitarity for $a > 0$ leads to the equation

$$\sum_{j=2j^a+1}^{2j^{a+1}} U_{nj}^a (U_{n'j}^a)^* = \sum_{j=j^a+1}^{j^{a+1}} \frac{1}{N^a} e^{i\Delta n[(2\pi/N^a)j - \phi^a]} + c.c. = \delta_{nn'} \quad (3.5)$$

whose solution is

$$\phi^a = \frac{2j^a + 1}{j^{a+1} - j^a} \cdot \frac{\pi}{2} \quad (3.6)$$

The condition $\phi^a = (p/q)\pi$ then leads to the nontrivial consequence

$$j^{a+1} = \frac{(q+p)}{p} j^a + \frac{q}{2p} \quad (3.7)$$

In a discrete system, the only acceptable solutions are those where $q/2p$ is an integer. For example, the choice of $q = 2$ and $p = 1$ leads to the scaling $j^{a+1} = 3j^a + 1$. This is the most interesting solution as discussed below. Mathematically speaking, in the continuum limit a large class of solutions exists, since in that limit one takes $j^a \to \infty$ and $N \to \infty$ such that $f^a = (2\pi/N)j^a$ remains finite, then we are simply lead to $f^{a+1} = f^a(q+p)/p$ for any q and p. Thus representations of the scaling and translation group are possible for all rational scaling factors $\lambda = (q+p)/p$. The bandwidth, B_{oct}, of the corresponding cells is $\log_2[(q+p)/p]$.

Interesting consequences follow from the relationship between cell bandwidth and diversity:

$$B_{oct} = \log_2\left[\frac{q+p}{p}\right]$$

$$\text{Cell types} = q$$

For example, a bandwidth of one octave or a scaling factor $(q+p)/p = 2$ needs only one cell type in each scale, when $q = p = 1$. If it turns out to be necessary to have B_{oct} greater than 1 octave, then at least two classes of cells are needed to faithfully represent information in each scale, with $q = 2$ and $p = 1$ giving scaling factor of 3 or B_{oct} close to 1.6 octaves.

It is interesting to compare our solutions to the so called "wavelets" that, constructed in the mathematical literature, also form representations of the translation and scaling group. In the standard construction of Grossman and Morlet (1984) and Meyer (1985), the representations could be made orthonormal (i.e., unitary in the case of real matrices) only for limited choice of scaling factors given by $1 + 1/m$ where $m \geq 1$ is an integer. Such constructions need only one filter type in each scale and give scale factors no larger than 2 [equivalently the largest bandwidth is 1 octave—e.g., the well-known Haar basis wavelets (Daubechies 1988)]. This agrees with what we derived above for the special case of $q = 1$ where $B_{\text{oct}} = \log_2(1 + 1/p)$. However, allowing $q > 1$ gives more bandwidth choices in our construction. For example, $q = 2$ gives $B_{\text{oct}} = \log_2(1 + 2/p)$, however, no larger than 1.6 octaves, and $q = 3$ gives $\log_2(1 + 3/p)$, no larger than 2 octaves, etc. These results also agree with the recent theorem of Auscher (1992) who proved that multiscale representations can exist for scalings by any rational number k/l, provided $k - l$ filter types are allowed in each scale. Our conclusion above yields exactly the same result by redefining $k = p + q$ and $l = q$. We arrived at our conclusion independently through the explicit construction presented above.[7]

The connection between the number of cell types and the bandwidth that is possible to achieve is significant. We believe the bandwidth needed by cortical cells is determined by properties of natural images. Its value should be the best compromise between planar and depth resolution preservation for the distribution of structures in natural scenes. Actually, Field (1987, 1989) examined the issue of best bandwidth for filters that modeled cortical cells and found that bandwidths between 1 and 2 octaves best matched natural scene structures. Our results here show that cortical cells cannot achieve bandwidths more than one octave without having more than one cell type.

Next we show what the predicted cell kernels look like. For generality, we give the expression for the kernels in the continuum limit for any scale factor $\lambda = (q+p)/p$ or equivalently with any allowed bandwidth— although the ones we think are most relevant to the cortex are the discrete $p = 1, q = 2$ kernels. The cell kernels are given by $\{K^a(x_n^a - x), a > 0\}$ and $\{K^0(x_n^0 - x)\}$. For any given $a > 0$, the kernels sample the frequency in the range $f \in (f^a, \lambda f^a) = (f^a, f^{a+1})$. For $a = 0$, K^0 samples only frequencies $f \in (0, f^1)$, and $\mathbf{U}^0$ is given by $\mathbf{U}^0 = \mathbf{M}^\dagger$ in equation 2.9 with N replaced by

---

[7]We thank Ingrid Daubechies for pointing out the result of P. Auscher to us.

Theory of the Striate Cortex

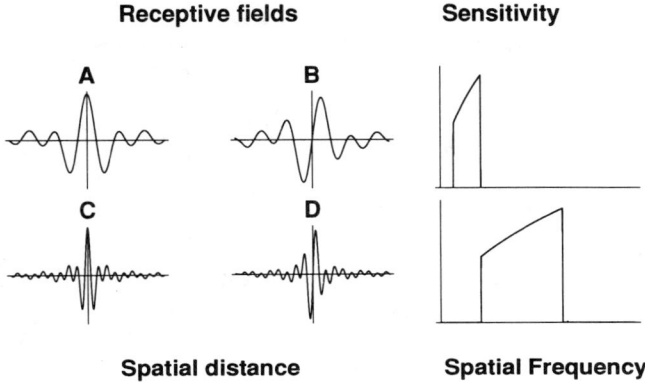

Figure 2: "Even-symmetric" (A, C) and "odd-symmetric" (B, D) kernels predicted for the scale factor 3 (equivalently for $B_{oct} = 1.6$ octaves) for two neighboring scales (top and bottom rows, respectively), together with their spectra (frequency sensitivities or selectivities).

N^0. Including both the positive and negative frequencies the predicted kernels are

$$K^a(x_n^a - x) = \frac{1}{\sqrt{N^a}} \int_{f^a}^{f^{a+1}} df \sqrt{f} \, e^{i(f(x_n^a - x) - (p/q)\pi n + \theta)} + c.c.$$

$$= \frac{2}{\sqrt{N^a}} \int_{f^a}^{f^{a+1}} df \sqrt{f} \, \cos\left[f(x_n^a - x) - \frac{p}{q}\pi n + \theta\right] \quad (3.8)$$

$$K^0(x_n^a - x) = \frac{2}{\sqrt{N^0}} \int_0^{f^1} df \sqrt{f} \, \cos\left[f(x_n^a - x)\right] \quad (3.9)$$

For any given p and q the kernels for $a > 0$ come in q varieties. Even and odd varieties are immediately apparent when one sets $q = 2$, $p = 1$, and $\theta = 0$ [$K^a(x_n^a - x)$ are even or odd functions of $x_n^a - x$ for even or odd n]. In Figure 2 we exhibit the even and odd kernels in two adjacent scales and their spectra. The $a = 0$ kernels, where $\theta = 0$ is chosen, are similar to the center-surround retinal ganglion cells (however, they are larger in size), and hence we need not exhibit them here. In general, though, θ can take any value, and the neighboring cells will simply differ by a 90° phase shift, or in quadrature, without necessarily having even or odd symmetry in their receptive field shapes.

From equation 3.8, it is easy to show that the kernels for $a > 0$ satisfy the following recursive relations:

$$K^a(x_n^a - \lambda x) = \frac{1}{\lambda} K^{a+1}(x_n^{a+1} - x) \tag{3.10}$$

$$K^a[x_n^a - (x + x_q^a)] = K^a(x_{n-q}^a - x) \tag{3.11}$$

To prove these one needs to use the following facts, $f^{a+1} = \lambda f^a$, $N^{a+1} = \lambda N^a$, and $\lambda x_n^{a+1} = x_{\lambda n}^{a+1} = x_n^a$. (Equation 3.11 also applies for K^0.) The above relations imply that, except shifted in space, each cell has the same receptive field as its qth neighbor within the same scale block, for example, when $q = 2$ in the example above, all the even (or odd) cells are identical. Furthermore, except for the lowest scale $a = 0$, the nth cell in all scales has the same receptive field except for a factor of λ expansion in size and a λ reduction in amplitude. Actually, since $x_n^a \neq x_n^{a+1}$, these cells are located at different spatial locations.

Now it is straightforward to see that the translation invariance (equation 3.1) for $\delta n = q$ and scale invariance (equation 3.2) are the direct consequence of the translation and scaling relationships, 3.11 and 3.10, respectively, between the receptive fields. This is exactly our goal of object constancy. Notice that the scaling constancy would not have been possible if the whitening factor $\sqrt{f}$ was not there in equation 3.8. These results can be extended to 2D where the whitening factor is $1/\sqrt{R(f)} = |\underline{f}|$ as we will see next.

4 Extension to 2D and Color Vision: Oriented Filters and Color Opponent Cells

The extension to two dimensions of the above construction is not difficult but involves a new subtlety. In this case, the constraint of unitarity on the matrices $\mathbf{U}^a, a > 0$ is hard to satisfy even if we allow for the phase factor ϕ that leads ultimately to different classes of cells. This constraint is considered in more detail in the Appendix; here we only state the conclusions of that analysis.

What one finds is that to ensure unitarity of $\mathbf{U}^a$, one needs to allow for cell diversity of a different kind—cells in the ath scale need to be further broken down into different types or orientations, each sampling from a limited region of the frequency space in that scale. Three examples of acceptable unitary breakings are shown in Figure 3A, B, C. In A (B) filters are broken into two classes in any scale $a > 0$—in addition to the q-cell diversity discussed in 1D. One filter type is a lowpass-bandpass in the x–y direction, and the other is a bandpass-lowpass in the x–y direction, which are denoted by "lb" and "bl." In C there are three classes of filters, "lb," "bl," and finally a class of filters which are bandpass in both x and y, "bb." The "lb" and "bl" filters are oriented while the "bb" ones

Theory of the Striate Cortex

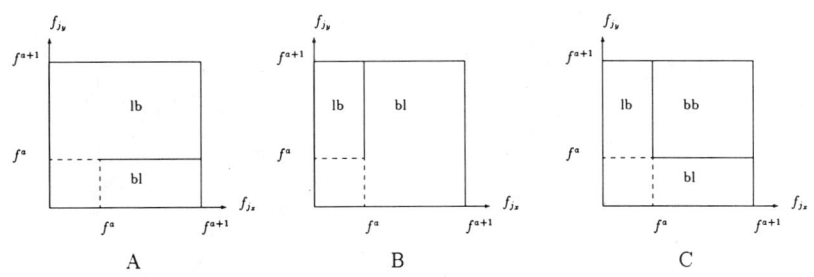

Figure 3: (A–C) Proliferation of more cell types by the break-down of the frequency sampling region in 2D within a given scale a. Ignoring the negative frequencies, the frequencies f within the scale are inside the large solid box but outside the small dashed box. The solid lines within the large solid box further partition the sampling into subregions denoted by "bl," "lb," and "bb," which indicate bandpass–lowpass, lowpass–bandpass, and bandpass–bandpass, respectively, in x–y directions. (A, B) Asymmetric breakdown between x and y directions, the "lb" cells are not equivalent to a 90° rotation of the "bl" cells. (C) Symmetric breakdown between x and y directions. The "bb" cells are significantly different from the others (see Fig. 4).

are not.[8] Figure 4A and B shows the five cell types one encounters for the breaking in Figure 3B and the nine cell types for the breaking in Figure 3C, respectively, for a choice of scaling factor 3.

Finally, the object constancy equations 3.1 and 3.2 still hold since equations 3.10 and 3.11 extend to 2D as

$$K^a(\underline{x}_n^a - \lambda \underline{x}) = \frac{1}{\lambda^2} K^{a+1}(\underline{x}_n^{a+1} - \underline{x})$$
$$K^a[\underline{x}_n^a - (\underline{x} + \underline{x}_q^a)] = K^a(\underline{x}_{n-q}^a - \underline{x})$$

where $\underline{x}$ and $\underline{x}_n^a$ are 2D vectors, and $\underline{n}$ and q are 2D indices.

These relationships are understood to hold between cells belonging to the same frequency sampling category ("lb," "bl," or "bb"). The factor of $1/\lambda^2$ comes because the whitening factor in 2D is $1/\sqrt{R(|f|)} = |\underline{f}|$.

---

[8]One notices that this extension to 2D requires a choice of orientations such as the x–y axes, breaking the rotational symmetry. Furthermore, it is natural to ask if the object constancy by translations and scalings should be extended to the object rotations in the image plane—requiring the cells be representations of the rotation group. At this point, it is not clear whether the rotational invariance is necessary (noting that we usually tilt our heads to read a tilted book or fail to recognize a face upside down), and whether the rotational invariance can be incorporated simultanously with the translation and scaling ones without increasing the number of cells. We will leave this outside the paper.

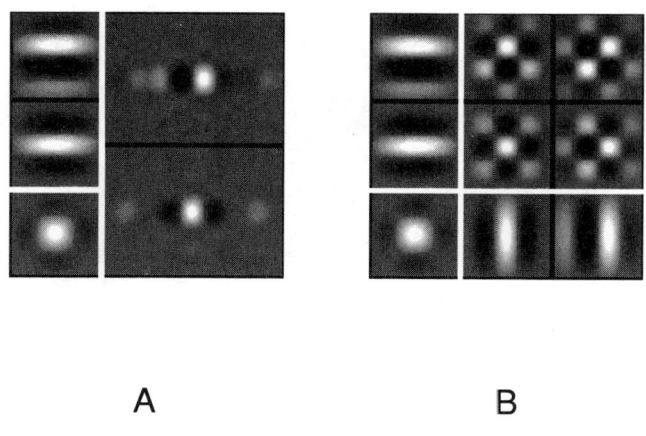

A   **B**

Figure 4: (A, B) The predicted variety of cell receptive fields in 2D. The five cell types in (A) and the nine cell types in (B) arise from the frequency partitioning schemes in Figure 3B and C, respectively. The kernels in the lower-left corner of both images demonstrate the lowpass–lowpass filter K^0 in 2D and they are nonoriented. All others are bandpass in at least one direction. Those are actually significantly smaller but are expanded in size in this figure for demonstration. The "bb" cells in the upper-right part of (B) come in four varieties (even–even, odd–odd, even–odd, and odd–even when $\theta = 0$ is taken for both x and y directions) and should exist in the cortex if the scheme in Figure 3C is favored. All kernels are constructed taking into account the optical MTF of the eye.

From equations 3.8 and 3.9, it is clear that the cortical kernels $K^a(x) \propto \int_{f_a}^{f_{a+1}} df [1/\sqrt{R(f)}] \cos(fx + \phi_a)$ differ from the retinal kernel

$$K(x) \propto \int_0^{f_{max}} df [1/\sqrt{R(f)}] \cos(fx + \phi)$$

only by the range of the frequency integration or selectivity. The cortical receptive fields are lowpass or bandpass versions of the retinal ones. One immediate consequence of this is that most cortical cells, especially the lowpass ones like those in the cytochrome oxidase blob cells, have larger receptive fields than the retinal ones. Second, when considering color vision, the power spectrums $R_l(f)$ and $R_c(f)$ for the luminance and chrominance channels, respectively, differ in their magnitudes. In reality when noises are considered, the receptive field filters are not simply $1/\sqrt{R(f)}$, which would have simply resulted in identical receptive field forms for luminance and chrominance except for their different strengths, but instead, the filter for luminance is more of a bandpass and the filter for chrominance a relatively lowpass. Since the retinal cells carry luminance and chrominance information simultanously by multiplexing the signals from both channels, the resulting retinal cells are of red-center-green-surround (or green-center-red-surround) types (Atick et al. 1992). This is because at low spatial frequencies, the chrominance filter dominates, while at higher spatial frequencies, the luminance one dominates. As we argued above, the cortical cells simply lowpass or bandpass the signals from the retinal cells; thus the lowpass version will carry mostly the chrominance signals while the bandpass or highpass ones the luminance signals. This is indeed observed in the cortex (Livingstone and Hubel 1984; Ts'o and Gilbert 1988) where the large (lowpass) blob cells are more color selective, while the smaller (higher-pass) nonblob cells, which are also more orientation selective by our results above, are less color sensitive. Furthermore, since the luminance signals are negligible at low frequencies, when one only considers the linear cell properties, the color sensitive blob cells are double-opponent (e.g. red-excitatory-green-inhibitory center and the red-inhibitory-green-excitatory surround) or color-opponent-center-only (type II), depending on the noise levels. This is apparent when one tries to spatially lowpass the signals from a group of single-opponent retinal cells (Fig. 5).

5 Discussion: Comparison with Other Work

The types of cells that we arrive at in constructing unitary representations of the translation and scaling group (see Figs. 2 and 4) are similar to simple cells in cat and monkey striate cortex. The analysis also predicts an interesting relationship between bandwidths of cells and their diversity as was discussed in Sections 3 and 4. One consequence of that relationship is that for cells to achieve a representation of the world with sampling bandwidth between 1 and 2 octaves there must be at least two cell types adjacent to each other and differ by $90°$ in their receptive field phases (Fig. 2). This bandwidth range is the range of measured bandwidths of simple cells (e.g., Kulikowski and Bishop 1981; Andrews and Pollen 1979) and also, we think, is best suited for matching structures in natural scenes (cf. Field 1987, 1989). This analysis thus explains the presence of phase quadrature (e.g., paired even-odd simple cells) observed in the cortex (Pollen and Ronner 1981): such cell diversity is needed to build a faithful multiscale representation of the visual world.

The analysis also requires breaking orientation symmetry. Here we do not wish to advocate scaling symmetry as an explanation for the existence of oriented cells in the cortex. It may be that orientation symmetry is broken for a more fundamental reason and that scaling symmetry takes advantage of that. Either way, orientation symmetry breaking is an important ingredient in building these multiscale representations.

In the past, there has been a sizeable body of work on trying to model simple cells in terms of "Gabor" and "log Gabor" filters (Kulikowski *et al.* 1982; Daugman 1985, Field 1987, 1989). Such filters are qualitatively close to those derived here, and they describe some of the properties of simple cells well. Our work differs from previous work in many ways. The two most important differences are the following. First, the filters here are derived by unitary transforms on retinal filters that reduce

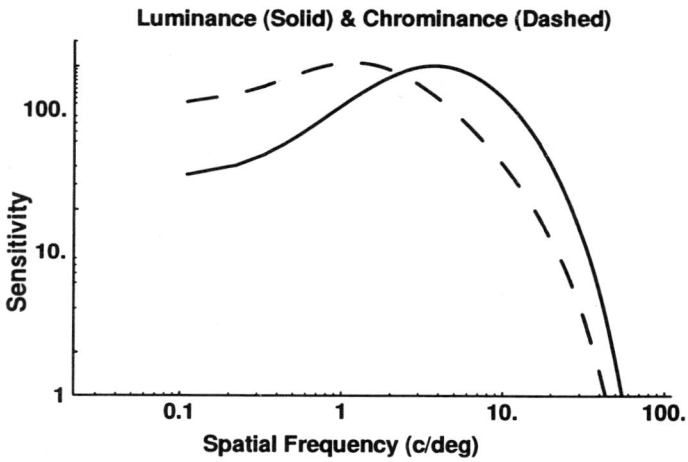

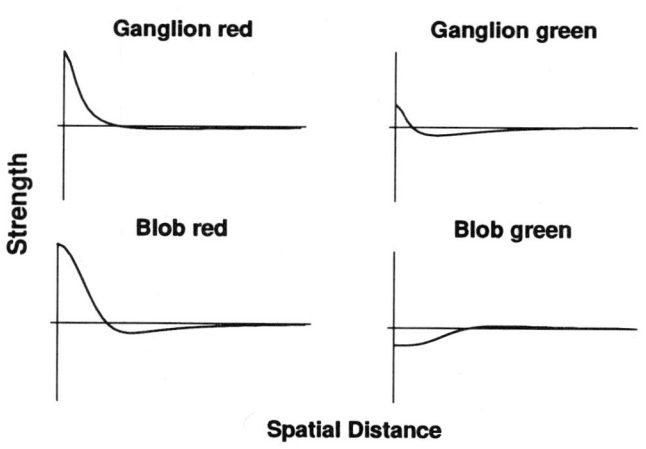

redundancy in inputs by whitening. By selecting the unitary transformation that manifests spatial-scale relationships in signals, one arrives at a representation that exhibits object constancy—the output response to an input $S(x)$ and its planar and depth translated version [i.e., $S(x) \to S[\lambda(x + \delta x)]$] are related by

$$O_n^a[S(x)] = O_{n+\delta n}^{a+1}[S[\lambda(x + \delta x)]] \tag{5.1}$$

Hence, a visual object moved in space simply shifts the outputs from one group of cells to another. Second, we find a direct linkage between cell bandwidth and diversity. Such linkage does not appear in previous works where orthonormality or unitarity was not required.

More recently there has also been a lot of work on orthonormal multiscale representations of the scaling and the translation group, alternatively known as wavelets (Meyer 1985; Daubechies 1988; Mallat 1989). The relationship of our work to wavelets was discussed in Section 3. Here we should add that in this paper we provide explicit construction of these representations for any rational scaling factor. Furthermore, our filters satisfy $K^a(\lambda x) = (1/\lambda^d)K^{a+1}(x)$ where d is the dimension of the space (e.g., $d = 1$ or 2), while those in the wavelet construction satisfy $K^a(\lambda x) = (1/\lambda^{d/2})K^{a+1}(x)$. This difference stems from the fact that our filters are the convolution of the whitening filter <u>and</u> the standard-type wavelet. The whitening filter—given by $\sim 1/\sqrt{R(f)}$ where $R(f)$ is the scale-invariant power spectrum of natural scenes—is what ultimately leads to the object constancy property that is absent from the standard-type wavelets.

The question at this stage is whether we could identify the pieces in our mathematical construction with classes of cells in the cortex. First, there is the class of lowpass cells $a = 0$, which have large receptive fields, and no orientation tuning (actually since their kernels have a whitening factor, they are not completely lowpass but an incomplete bandpass–weak surround). We think a good candidate for these cells are the cells in the cytochrome oxidase blob areas in the cortex. When we add color

---

Figure 5: *Facing page.* Change of color coding from retina to cortex. The top plot shows the visual contrast sensitivities to the luminance and chrominance signals. The bottom plot demonstrates the receptive field profiles (sensitivity to red or green cone inputs) of the color selective cells in the retina (or ganglion) and the cortex. The parameters used for the ganglion cells are the same as those in Atick et al. (1992). The blob cells are constructed by lowpass filtering the ganglion cell outputs with a filter frequency sensitivity of $e^{-f^2/(2f_{\text{low}}^2)}$ where $f_{\text{low}} = 1.5$ c/deg. The strengths of the cell profiles are individually normalized for both the ganglion and the blob cells. The range of the spatial distance axes, or the size, of the blob cells is 3.7 times larger than that of ganglion cells. This means that each blob cell sums the outputs from (on the order of) at least about $(3.7)^2 \sim 16$ local ganglion cells.

to our analysis, this class will come out to be color opponent.[9] These cells, a lowpass version of the single opponent retinal cells, turn out to be double opponent or color-opponent-center-only (see Fig. 5) from this mathematical construction, in agreement with observations. Second, the representation requires several orientation classes in every choice of higher scale; they are not as likely to be color selective and, within each orientation and scale, there are two types of cells—in phase quadrature (e.g., even and odd symmetric)—if the bandwidth of the cells is greater than one octave. These have kernels similar to simple cells. Also, in some choices of division of the two-dimensional frequency space into bands (see Fig. 4), one encounters cells that are very different from simple cells. These cells come from the bandpass region in both the x and y directions (the "bb" region in Fig. 3C) and as such possess relatively small receptive fields in space. It is amusing to note their resemblance to the type of cells that Van Essen discovered in $V4$ (private communication).

It is important at this stage to look in detail for evidence that cortical neurons are building a multiscale, translationally invariant representation of the input along the lines described in this paper. However, in looking for those we must allow for the possibility that these representations are formed in an active process starting as early as the striate cortex, as was proposed recently by Olshausen et al. (1992). We also must keep in mind that to perform detailed comparison with real cortical filters, our filters have to be modified to take noise into account.

Appendix

In this appendix we examine the condition of unitarity on the matrix $\mathbf{U}^a$. The matrix elements of $\mathbf{U}^a$ in the scale $a > 0$ are generalized from the 1D case simply as (taking $\theta = 0$)

$$U^a_{\underline{n}\underline{j}} = e^{i(\underline{\phi}\underline{n} + \underline{f}_{\underline{j}} \underline{x}^a_{\underline{n}})} \tag{A.1}$$

where $\underline{n} = (n_x, n_y)$, $\underline{x}^a_{\underline{n}} = (x^a_{n_x}, x^a_{n_y})$, $\underline{j} = (j_x, j_y)$, $\underline{f}_{\underline{j}} = (f_{j_x}, f_{j_y})$, and $\underline{\phi} = [(f_{j_x}/|f_{j_x}|)\phi_x, (f_{j_y}/|f_{j_y}|)\phi_y]$. A priori the cells in $\mathbf{U}^a$ sample from the frequency region inside the big solid box but outside the dashed box in Figure 3. The critical fact that makes the 2D case different from 1D is that there are $(N^a)^2 = 4(j^{a+1})^2 - 4(j^a)^2$ cells in the ath class, while the total number of cells is $(N)^2$, then

$$(x^a_{n_x}, x^a_{n_y}) = \left(\frac{N}{N^a}n_x, \frac{N}{N^a}n_y\right)$$

---

[9] It is easy to see why: since they are roughly lowpass—large receptive fields—they have higher signal-to-noise in space, and hence they can afford to have a low signal-to-noise in color. While opponent cells in space have low signal-to-noise, they need to integrate in color to improve their signal-to-noise (see Atick et al. 1992).

Theory of the Striate Cortex

The unitarity requirement $\mathbf{U}^a(\mathbf{U}^a)^\dagger = 1$ ($a > 0$) can be shown to be equivalent to

$$\cos\left[\left(\frac{j^{a+1} + j^a + 1}{N^a}\pi + \phi_x\right)\Delta n_x\right] \sin\left[\frac{j^{a+1} - j^a}{N^a}\pi\Delta n_x\right] = 0 \quad \text{(A.2)}$$

where Δn_x is any integer $\neq 0$. A similar condition in the y direction should also hold. To satisfy equation A.2 one can only hope that the cosine factor is zero for odd Δn_x and the sine factor is zero for the rest. This is impossible in 2D although possible in 1D. To see this difference, note that in 1D, $N^a = 2(j^{a+1} - j^a)$ and the argument of the sine is $\Delta n\pi/2$, which leads to vanishing sine for even Δn. One then makes cosine term zero for odd Δn by choosing ϕ such that $[(j^{a+1} + j^a + 1)/N^a]\pi + \phi_x = \pm\pi/2$. This is exactly how equation 3.6 is reached. In 2D, $N^a = 2\sqrt{(j^{a+1})^2 - (j^a)^2}$, and hence the sine term is

$$\sin[\Delta n_x(\sqrt{(j^{a+1} - j^a)/(j^{a+1} + j^a)}\pi/2] \neq 0$$

for even Δn_x. Although we cannot prove that the negative result in 2D is not caused by the fact that we have a Euclidean grid, we think it not possible to construct the representation even when using a radially symmetric lattice.

To ensure unitarity of $\mathbf{U}^a$, we need to allow for cell diversity of a different kind—cells in ath scale need to be further broken down into different types or orientations, each type sampling from a limited region of the frequency space as shown, for example, in Figure 3.

Acknowledgments

We would like to thank D. Field, C. Gilbert, and N. Redlich for useful discussions, and the Seaver Institute for its support.

References

Andrews, B. W., and Pollen, D. A. 1979. Relationship between spatial frequency selectivity and receptive field profile of simple cells. *J. Physiol. (London)* **287**, 163–176.

Atick, J. J. 1992. Could information theory provide an ecological theory of sensory processing? *Network* **3**, 213–251.

Atick, J. J., and Redlich, A. N. 1990. Towards a theory of early visual processing. *Neural Comp.* **2**, 308–320.

Atick, J. J., and Redlich, A. N. 1992. What does the retina know about natural scenes? *Neural Comp.* **4**, 196–210.

Atick, J. J., Li, Z., and Redlich, A. N. 1992. Understanding retinal color coding from first principles. *Neural Comp.* **4**, 559–572.

Auscher, P. 1992. Wavelet bases for $L^2(R)$ with rational dilation factor. In *Wavelets and their applications*, M. B. Ruskai, ed., pp. 439–451. Jones and Bartlett, Boston.

Daubechies, I. 1988. Orthonormal bases of compactly supported waves. *Commun. Pure Appl. Math.* **41**, 909–996.

Daugman, J. G. 1985. Uncertainty relations for resolution in space, spatial frequency and orientation optimized by two-dimensional visual cortical filters. *J. Opt. Soc. Am.* **A 2**, 1160–1169.

Field, D. J. 1987. Relations between the statistics of natural images and the response properties of cortical cells. *J. Opt. Soc. Am.* **A 4**, 2379–2394.

Field, D. J. 1989. What the statistics of natural images tell us about visual coding. SPIE Vol. **1077**, Human Vision, Visual Processing, and Digital Display, 269–276.

Grossmann, A., and Morlet, J. 1984. Decomposition of hardy functions into square integrable wavelets of constant shape. *SIAM J. Math.* **15**, 17–34.

Hopfield, J. J. 1991. Olfactory computation and object perception. *Proc. Natl. Acad. Sci. U.S.A.* **88**, 6462–6466.

Kulikowski, J. J., and Bishop, P. 1981. Linear analysis of the responses of simple cells in the cat visual cortex. *Exp. Brain Res.* **44**, 386–400.

Kulikowski, J. J., Marcelja, S., and Bishop, P. 1982. Theory of spatial position and spatial frequency relations in the receptive fields of simple cells in the visual cortex. *Biol. Cybern.* **43**, 187–198.

Linsker, R. 1992. Private communication. See also, talk at NIPS 92.

Livingstone M. S., and Hubel, D. H. 1984. Anatomy and physiology of a color system in the primate visual cortex. *J. Neurosci.* **4**(1), 309–356.

Mallat, S. 1989. A theory of multiresolution signal decomposition: The wavelet representation. *IEEE Transact. Pattern Anal. Machine Intelligence* **11**, 674–693.

Meyer, Y. 1985. Principe d'incertitude, bases hilbertiennes et algebres d'operateurs *Sem. Bourbaki* **662**, 209–223.

Olshausen, B., Anderson, C. H., and Van Essen, D. C. 1992. A neural model of visual attention and invariant pattern recognition. Caltech Report no. CNS MEMO 18, August.

Pollen, D. A., and Ronner, S. F. 1981. Phase relationships between adjacent simple cells in the cat. *Science* **212**, 1409–1411.

Ruderman, D. L., and Bialek, W. 1993. Statistics of natural images: scaling in the woods. Private communication and to appear.

Schreiber, W. F. 1956. The measurement of third order probability distributions of television signals. *IRE Trans. Inform. Theory* **IT-2**, 94–105.

Shannon, C. E., and Weaver, W. 1949. *The Mathematical Theory of Communication.* University of Illinois Press, Urbana, IL.

Ts'o, D. Y., and Gilbert, C. D. 1988. The organization of chromatic and spatial interactions in the primate striate cortex. *J. Neurosci.* **8**(5), 1712–1727.

Van Essen, D. C., Olshausen B., Anderson, C. H., and Gallant, J. L. 1991. Pattern recognition, attention, and information bottlenecks in the primate visual system. *Conf. on Visual Information Processing: From Neurons to Chips (SPIE Proc. 1473).*

3

Bayesian Self-Organization Driven by Prior Probability Distributions

Alan L. Yuille
Stelios M. Smirnakis
Lei Xu
Division of Applied Sciences, Harvard University, Cambridge, MA 02138, USA

Recent work by Becker and Hinton (1992) shows a promising mechanism, based on maximizing mutual information assuming spatial coherence, by which a system can self-organize to learn visual abilities such as binocular stereo. We introduce a more general criterion, based on Bayesian probability theory, and thereby demonstrate a connection to Bayesian theories of visual perception and to other organization principles for early vision (Atick and Redlich 1990). Methods for implementation using variants of stochastic learning are described.

1 Introduction

The input intensity patterns received by the human visual system are typically complicated functions of the object surfaces and light sources in the world. It seems probable, however, that humans perceive the world in terms of surfaces and objects (Nakayama and Shimojo 1987). Thus the visual system must be able to extract information from the input intensities that is relatively independent of the actual intensity values. Such abilities may not be present at birth and hence must be learned. It seems, for example, that binocular stereo develops at about the age of 2 to 3 months (Held 1987).

Becker and Hinton (1992) describe an interesting mechanism for self-organizing a system to achieve this. The basic idea is to assume spatial coherence of the structure to be extracted and to train a neural network by maximizing the mutual information between neurons with spatially disjoint receptive fields (see Fig. 1). For binocular stereo, for example, the surface being viewed is assumed flat (see Becker and Hinton 1992, for generalizations of this assumption) and hence has spatially constant disparity. The intensity patterns, however, do not have any simple spatial behavior. Adjusting the synaptic strengths of the network to maximize the mutual information between neurons with nonoverlapping receptive fields, for an ensemble of images, causes the neurons to extract features that are spatially coherent, thereby obtaining the disparity.

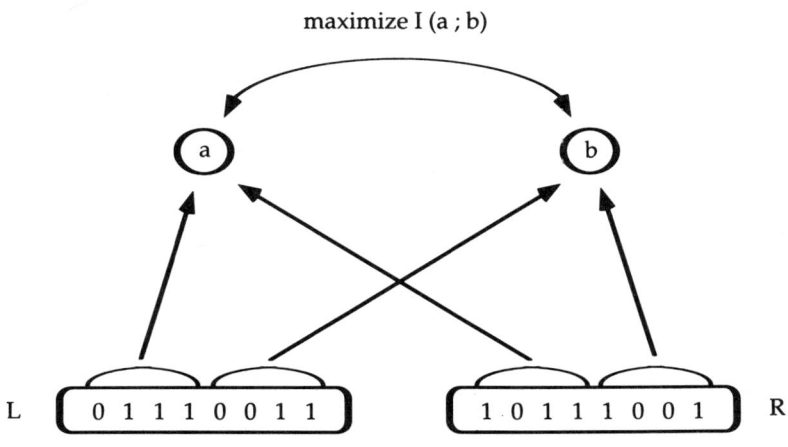

Figure 1: In Hinton and Becker's initial scheme, maximization of mutual information between neurons with spatially disjoint receptive fields leads to disparity tuning, provided they train on spatially coherent patterns (i.e., those for which disparity changes slowly with spatial position).

We argue that this approach has three key ingredients:

1. It uses strong prior knowledge about the output variables, i.e., it assumes that the disparities are spatially constant. If this assumption is not valid then the performance of the system will degrade.

2. It represents the desired outputs as functions of the inputs by a multilayer perceptron with adjustable weights.

3. It proposes a criterion, mutual information maximization, motivated by the prior knowledge (see point 1) to determine the weights.

The approach relies heavily on prior assumptions about the form of the outputs. This is similar to Bayesian theories of visual perception that also rely (Clark and Yuille 1990) on prior assumptions about properties of the world, such as binocular disparities. Such priors are needed because of the ill-posed nature of vision (Poggio et al. 1985) and can be thought of as *natural constraints* (Marr 1982).

This similarity motivates the following questions. Can we reformulate Becker and Hinton's theory so that it can be applied directly to learning Bayesian theories of vision? More precisely, assuming a prior of the type commonly used in vision, can we find an optimization criterion and learning algorithm such that we can learn the corresponding Bayesian theory?

This note shows that it is indeed possible to reformulate Becker and Hinton to make it compatible with Bayesian theories. In particular, their algorithm for stereo corresponds to one of the standard priors used for Bayesian stereo theories (see Section 3). The key idea is to force the activity distribution of the outputs, **S**, to be close to a prespecified prior distribution $P_p(\mathbf{S})$. Our approach is general and is related to the work performed by Atick and Redlich (1990) for modeling the early visual system. In previous work (Yuille *et al.* 1993) we proved that applying our approach to linear filtering problems leads to a solution that is the square root of the Wiener filter in Fourier space. A similar result has been derived (Redlich, private communication) from the principles described in Atick and Redlich (1990).

We should clarify what we mean by "learning a Bayesian theory." A Bayesian theory for estimating a scene property **S** from input **D** consists of three elements: (1) a prior for the property $P_p(\mathbf{S})$, (2) a likelihood function $P_l(\mathbf{D} \mid \mathbf{S})$, and (3) an algorithm for estimating $\mathbf{S}^*(\mathbf{D}) = \arg\max_\mathbf{S} P_l(\mathbf{D} \mid \mathbf{S}) P_p(\mathbf{S})$.[1] Because we assume that the prior is known we are essentially learning the likelihood function and the algorithm. Our approach, after training, will yield a neural net, or some other function approximation scheme, that computes $\mathbf{S}^*(\mathbf{D})$. In related work (Smirnakis and Yuille 1994) we assume that both prior and likelihood are known and train a network to learn the algorithm.

This can be contrasted to alternative ways for learning Bayesian theories. Hidden Markov models (Paul 1990) (see Section 5) learn both the priors and the likelihood functions. A general purpose optimization algorithm, dynamic programming, is then used to compute the MAP, or some alternative, estimator. This approach can be highly effective, though dynamic programming is efficient only for one-dimensional problems and functional forms for the prior and likelihood are required. Kersten *et al.* (1987) describe Bayesian learning with a teacher that yields the algorithm $\mathbf{S}^*(\mathbf{D}) = \arg\max_\mathbf{S} P_l(\mathbf{D} \mid \mathbf{S}) P_p(\mathbf{S})$. But as Becker and Hinton have shown, a teacher is not always necessary.

We will take the viewpoint that the prior $P_p(\mathbf{S})$ is assumed known in advance by the visual system (perhaps by being specified genetically) and will act as a self-organizing principle. Later we will discuss ways that this might be relaxed.

2 Theory

We assume that the input **D** is a function $F(\mathbf{n}, \boldsymbol{\alpha})$ of a *signal* $\boldsymbol{\alpha}$ that the system wants to determine and a *distractor* **n**. These quantities are vectors indexed by spatial location (see Fig. 2). For example, $\boldsymbol{\alpha}$ might correspond to the disparities of a pair of binocular stereo images and **n** to the intensity

---

[1]This corresponds to the commonly used maximum a posteriori (MAP) estimator. Other estimators may be preferable, but we will consider only MAP in this paper.

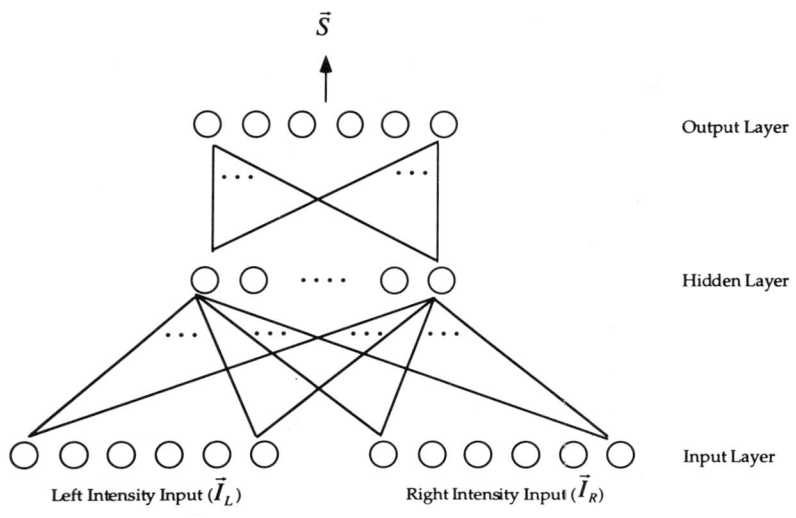

Figure 2: Note that the vectors I_L and I_R represent the intensities falling on the left and right retinas respectively, and are indexed by spatial location. S represents the vector of the disparities to be extracted. That is, the output S_i of output unit i represents the disparity at spatial location i. By setting some of the synapses to zero we obtain the disjoint receptive fields of the Becker and Hinton paradigm (Fig. 1).

patterns. The variables have distributions $P_n(\mathbf{n})$ and $P_p(\alpha)$, respectively. Note that **D** and $P_p(\alpha)$ are assumed to be known but $P_n(\mathbf{n})$ and the functional form of $F(\mathbf{n}, \alpha)$ are unknown.

The input distribution is given by

$$P_D(\mathbf{D}) = \int\int \delta[\mathbf{D} - F(\mathbf{n},\alpha)]P_n(\mathbf{n})P_p(\alpha)[d\alpha][d\mathbf{n}]$$

and can be observed by the system.

Let the output of the system be $\mathbf{S} = G(\mathbf{D}, \gamma)$ where **G** is a function of a set of parameters γ to be determined. For example, the function $G(\mathbf{D}, \gamma)$ could be represented by a multilayer perceptron with γ being the synaptic weights. By approximation theory, it can be shown that a large variety of neural networks can approximate any input–output function arbitrarily well given enough hidden nodes (Hornik *et al.* 1991). We can combine these formulas to give

$$\mathbf{S} = G[F(\mathbf{n}, \alpha), \gamma] \tag{2.1}$$

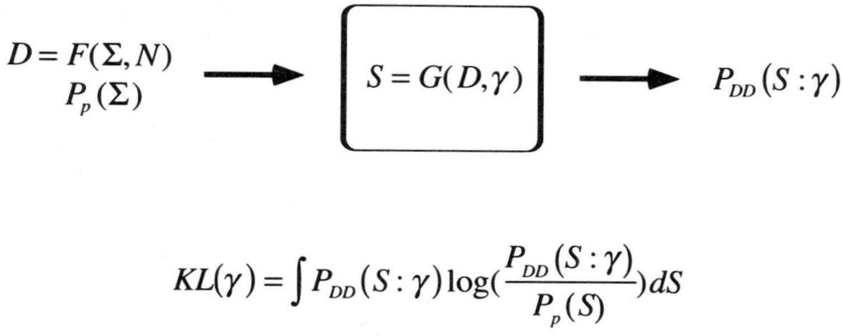

Bayesian Self-Organization

$$D = F(\Sigma, N)$$
$$P_p(\Sigma)$$
$$\longrightarrow \boxed{S = G(D, \gamma)} \longrightarrow P_{DD}(S : \gamma)$$

$$KL(\gamma) = \int P_{DD}(S : \gamma) \log(\frac{P_{DD}(S : \gamma)}{P_p(S)}) dS$$

Figure 3: The parameters γ are adjusted to minimize the Kullback–Leibler distance between the prior (P_p) distribution of the true signal (Σ) and the derived distribution (P_{DD}) of the network output (S).

The aim of self-organizing the network is to ensure that the parameters γ are chosen so that the outputs $\mathbf{S}$ are as close to the α (or some simple transformation of the αs) as possible. We claim that this can be achieved by adjusting the parameters γ so as to make the derived distribution of the outputs $P_{DD}(\mathbf{S} : \gamma) = \int \delta[\mathbf{S} - \mathbf{G}(\mathbf{D}, \gamma)] P_D(\mathbf{D})[d\mathbf{D}]$ as close as possible to $P_p(\mathbf{S})$.

This can be seen to be a consistency condition for a Bayesian theory. From Bayes's formula we obtain the condition:

$$\int P(\mathbf{S} \mid \mathbf{D}) P_D(\mathbf{D})[d\mathbf{D}] = \int P(\mathbf{D} \mid \mathbf{S}) P_p(\mathbf{S})[d\mathbf{D}] = P_p(\mathbf{S}) \qquad (2.2)$$

This is equivalent to our condition provided we identify $P(\mathbf{S} \mid \mathbf{D})$ with $\delta[\mathbf{S} - \mathbf{G}(\mathbf{D}, \gamma)]$.

To make this more precise we must define a measure of similarity between the two distributions $P_p(\mathbf{S})$ and $P_{DD}(\mathbf{S} : \gamma)$. An attractive measure is the Kullback–Leibler distance (the entropy of P_{DD} relative to P_p):

$$KL(\gamma) = \int P_{DD}(\mathbf{S} : \gamma) \log \frac{P_{DD}(\mathbf{S} : \gamma)}{P_p(\mathbf{S})} [d\mathbf{S}] \qquad (2.3)$$

Thus our theory (see Fig. 3) corresponds to adjusting the parameters γ to minimize the Kullback–Leibler distance between $P_p(\mathbf{S})$ and $P_{DD}(\mathbf{S} : \gamma)$. This measure can be divided into two parts: (1) $-\int P_{DD}(\mathbf{S} : \gamma) \log P_p(\mathbf{S})[d\mathbf{S}]$ and (2) $\int P_{DD}(\mathbf{S} : \gamma) \log P_{DD}(\mathbf{S} : \gamma)[d\mathbf{S}]$. As we now show both terms have very intuitive interpretations.

Suppose that $P_p(\mathbf{S})$ can be expressed as a Markov random field [i.e., the spatial distribution of $P_p(\mathbf{S})$ has a local neighborhood structure, as is commonly assumed in Bayesian models of vision]. Then, by the

Hammersely–Clifford theorem, we can write $P_p(S) = e^{-\beta E_p(S)}/Z$ where $E_p(S)$ is an energy function with local connections [for example, $E_p(S) = \sum_i (S_i - S_{i+1})^2$], β is an inverse temperature, and Z is a normalization constant.

Then the first term can be written as

$$-\int P_{DD}(S:\gamma) \log P_p(S)[dS]$$
$$= \int\int \delta[S - G(D,\gamma)] P_D(D) \beta E_p(S)[dD][dS] + \log Z$$
$$= \int \beta E_p[G(D,\gamma)] P_D(D)[dD] + \log Z$$
$$= \beta \langle E_p[G(D,\gamma)] \rangle_D + \log Z \qquad (2.4)$$

We can ignore the $\log Z$ term since it is a constant (independent of γ). Minimizing the first term with respect to γ will therefore try to minimize the energy of the outputs averaged over the inputs—$\langle E_p[G(D,\gamma)]\rangle_D$—which is highly desirable [since it has a close connection to the minimal energy principles in Poggio et al. (1985), and Clark and Yuille (1990)]. It is important, however, to avoid the trivial solution $G(D,\gamma) = $ *constant* or solutions where $G(D,\gamma)$ is very small for most inputs. Fortunately these solutions will be discouraged by the second term.

The second term $\int P_{DD}(D,\gamma) \log P_{DD}(D,\gamma)[dD]$ can be interpreted as the negative of the entropy of the derived distribution of the output. Minimizing it with respect to γ is a maximum entropy principle that will encourage variability in the outputs $G(D,\gamma)$ and hence prevent the trivial solutions.

The two terms combine to determine the γ so that the energy of the output variables is minimized while maximizing their variability. This is closely related to Becker and Hinton's method of maximizing the mutual information between pairs of output variables—essentially assuming a spatially constant prior distribution for S. At the same time it is reminiscent of other organizational principles for early vision based on information theory (Atick and Redlich 1990).

How can one guarantee that the optimal solution to our criteria will indeed extract the signal? This will depend on a number of factors: (1) the forms of the functions F and G, (2) the forms of the probability distributions $P_n(n)$ and $P_p(\alpha)$, and (3) whether the prior P_p is indeed correct or not.

It is straightforward to write down the conditions for the derived distribution to be equal to the prior distribution (assuming that the prior is correct). This is a stronger condition than requiring the Kullback–Leibler distance to be minimal (though, if equality is possible, minimizing Kullback–Leibler would lead to it). It is

$$P_p(S) = \int\int \delta\{S - G[F(n,\alpha),\gamma]\} P_n(n) P_p(\alpha)[d\alpha][dn] \qquad (2.5)$$

If one could find γ^* so that $G[F(n,\alpha),\gamma^*] = \alpha$, $\forall n, \alpha$ then the equation could be solved exactly. The condition $G[F(n,\alpha),\gamma^*] = \alpha$, however, is

Bayesian Self-Organization

too strong. It requires that the function **G**, which can be thought of as a nonlinear filter, is able to completely eliminate the dependence on **n**.

We have assumed that the correct prior is known by the system, perhaps by being specified genetically. An alternative possibility is that the prior itself is learned by a method reminiscent of Occam's razor: the goodness of the prior is evaluated based on the Kullback–Leibler distance after self-organization, and a more complex prior is chosen if this distance is large (see also Mumford 1992).

3 Connection to Becker and Hinton

In this section, we show that the case of disparity extraction implemented by Becker and Hinton based on their principle of mutual information maximization arises as a special case of our formalism, by choosing a particular prior. The Becker and Hinton method (Becker and Hinton 1992) for extracting the disparity involves maximizing the mutual information between two network output units S_1, S_2 with spatially disjoint receptive fields, under the assumption that disparity is spatially coherent. S_1 and S_2 denote the scalar values of two units in the output layer of a neural network, indexed by spatial location. The mutual information between S_1, S_2 is given by

$$\begin{aligned} I(S_1, S_2; \gamma) &= -\langle \log P_{\text{DD}}(S_1; \gamma) \rangle - \langle \log P_{\text{DD}}(S_2; \gamma) \rangle \\ &\quad + \langle \log P_{\text{DD}}(S_1, S_2; \gamma) \rangle \\ &= H(S_1; \gamma) - H(S_1 \mid S_2; \gamma) \end{aligned} \quad (3.1)$$

From this equation we see that we want to maximize the entropy, $H(S_1; \gamma)$, of S_1 while minimizing the conditional entropy, $H(S_1 \mid S_2; \gamma)$, of S_1 given S_2, which forces S_1 to be a deterministic function of S_2 (alternatively, by symmetry, we can interchange the roles of S_1 and S_2). For the discussion below we will use our criterion to reproduce the case in which this last term forces $S_1 \approx S_2$.

By contrast, in our version (see Fig. 4) we propose to minimize the expression $\langle \log P_{\text{DD}}(S_1, S_2; \gamma) \rangle - \int \log P_{\text{p}}(S_1, S_2) P_{\text{DD}}(S_1, S_2; \gamma)[d\mathbf{S}]$. If we ensure that the prior $P_{\text{p}}(S_1, S_2) \propto e^{-\tau(S_1-S_2)^2}$, then, for large τ, our second term will force $S_1 \approx S_2$ and our first term will maximize the entropy of the joint distribution of S_1, S_2. We argue that this is effectively the same as Becker and Hinton (1992), since maximizing the joint entropy of S_1, S_2 with S_1 constrained to equal S_2 is equivalent to maximizing the individual entropies of S_1 and S_2 with the same constraint.

To be more concrete, we consider Becker and Hinton's implementation of the mutual information maximization principle in the case of units with continuous outputs. They assume that the outputs of units 1, 2 are gaussian[2] and perform steepest descent to maximize the symmetrized

---
[2]We assume for simplicity that these gaussians have zero mean.

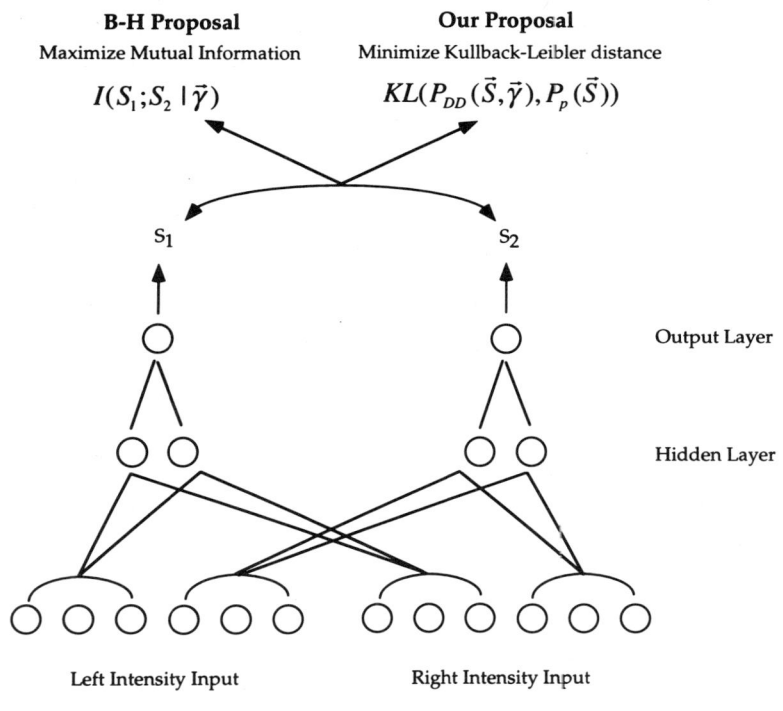

Figure 4: Comparing our theory with Becker and Hinton's. Observe that setting $P_p(S_1, S_2) \propto e^{-\tau(S_1-S_2)^2}$ forces $S_1 \approx S_2$ for large τ, implementing their assumption that the disparity is spatially coherent.

form of the mutual information between S_1 and S_2:

$$I(S_1, S_2) = \log \frac{V(S_1)}{V(S_1 - S_2)} + \log \frac{V(S_2)}{V(S_1 - S_2)}$$
$$= \log V(S_1) + \log V(S_2) - 2 \log V(S_1 - S_2) \quad (3.2)$$

where $V(\cdot)$ stands for variance over the set of inputs. They assume that the difference between the two outputs can be expressed as uncorrelated additive noise, $S_1 = S_2 + N$. Therefore, their criterion amounts to maximizing

$$E_{BH}[V(S_2), V(N)] = \log\{V(S_2) + V(N)\} + \log V(S_2) - 2 \log V(N) \quad (3.3)$$

For our scheme we make similar assumptions about the distributions of S_1 and S_2. We then see that, up to additive constants independent of γ,

Bayesian Self-Organization

$\langle \log P_{DD}(S_1, S_2) \rangle = -1/2 \log\{\langle S_1^2\rangle\langle S_2^2\rangle - \langle S_1 S_2\rangle^2\} = -1/2 \log\{V(S_2)V(N)\}$ [since $\langle S_1 S_2\rangle = \langle(S_2+N)S_2\rangle = V(S_2)$ and $\langle S_1^2\rangle = V(S_2) + V(N)$]. We now observe that if we choose the prior distribution $P_p(S_1, S_2) \propto e^{-\tau(S_1-S_2)^2}$ our criterion corresponds to minimizing $E_{YSX}[V(S_2), V(N)]$ where

$$E_{YSX}[V(S_2), V(N)] = -\log V(S_2) - \log V(N) + \tau V(N) \qquad (3.4)$$

It is easy to see that maximizing $E_{BH}[V(S_2), V(N)]$ will try to make $V(S_2)$ as large as possible and force $V(N)$ to zero [recall that, by definition, $V(N) \geq 0$]. On the other hand, minimizing our energy will try to make $V(S_2)$ as large as possible and will force $V(N)$ to $1/\tau$. Since τ appears as the inverse of the variance of the gaussian prior for $\mathbf{S} = (S_1, S_2)$, making τ large will force the prior distribution to approach $\delta(S_1 - S_2)$. Thus, in the case of large τ, our method has the same effect as the Becker and Hinton algorithm.

For this to be true, it is important to choose a network architecture satisfying the requirement that the output units representing disparity have spatially disjoint receptive fields (see Fig. 4). If this were not the case, the output units would run the risk of getting entrained on the receptive field overlap, provided it has the right probability structure. Even though we did not pursue this issue in the above analysis, it is, in principle, possible to implement such architectural constraints by defining a prior distribution on the weights of the network.

Note that, in principle, maximizing the mutual information between S_1, S_2 can only determine the network output up to transformations that leave the mutual information invariant. Which solution the network will settle at depends on the specifics of the implementation and on initial conditions. For instance, in the Becker and Hinton example the network sometimes settles so that $S_1 \approx S_2$, and sometimes so that $S_1 \approx -S_2$. This may not be always desirable. In this context, the ability to choose a prior affords a natural way to restrict the possible space of solutions.

4 Reformulating for Implementation in a General Setting

Our proposal requires us to minimize the Kullback–Leibler distance (equation 2.3) with respect to γ. In the previous section, we showed that Becker and Hinton's implementation of the mutual information maximization principle for disparity extraction arose as a special case of our formalism, for a particular prior. Therefore, their simulation already represents a concrete example of how our scheme can be implemented. In the present section, we endeavor to expand further by outlining two general implementation strategies based on variants of stochastic learning:

First observe that by substituting the form of the derived distribution, $P_{DD}(\mathbf{S} : \boldsymbol{\gamma}) = \int \delta[\mathbf{S} - \mathbf{G}(\mathbf{D}, \boldsymbol{\gamma})] P_D(\mathbf{D})[d\mathbf{D}]$, into equation 2.3 and integrating out the $\mathbf{S}$ variable we obtain

$$KL(\boldsymbol{\gamma}) = \int P_D(\mathbf{D}) \log \frac{P_{DD}[\mathbf{G}(\mathbf{D}, \boldsymbol{\gamma}) : \boldsymbol{\gamma}]}{P_p[\mathbf{G}(\mathbf{D}, \boldsymbol{\gamma})]}[d\mathbf{D}] \qquad (4.1)$$

This is the form of the Kullback–Liebler distance that we assume in the implementation strategies we describe below:

1. Assuming a representative sample $\{\mathbf{D}^\mu : \mu \in \Lambda\}$ of inputs we can approximate $KL(\gamma)$ by $\sum_{\mu \in \Lambda} \log\{P_{DD}[\mathbf{G}(\mathbf{D}^\mu, \gamma) : \gamma]/P_P[\mathbf{G}(\mathbf{D}^\mu, \gamma)]\}$. We can now, in principle, perform stochastic learning using backpropagation: pick inputs $\mathbf{D}^\mu$ at random and update the weights γ using $\log\{P_{DD}[\mathbf{G}(\mathbf{D}^\mu, \gamma) : \gamma]/P_P[\mathbf{G}(\mathbf{D}^\mu, \gamma)]\}$ as the error function.

To do this, however, we need expressions for $P_{DD}[\mathbf{G}(\mathbf{D}^\mu, \gamma) : \gamma]$ and its derivative with respect to γ. If the function $\mathbf{G}(\mathbf{D}, \gamma)$ can be restricted to being 1-1 (artificially increasing the dimensionality of the output space if necessary) then we can obtain analytic expressions $P_{DD}[\mathbf{G}(\mathbf{D}, \gamma) : \gamma] = P_D(\mathbf{D})/|\det(\partial \mathbf{G}/\partial \mathbf{D})|$ and $\{\partial \log P_{DD}[\mathbf{G}(\mathbf{D}, \gamma) : \gamma]/\partial \gamma\} = -(\partial \mathbf{G}/\partial \mathbf{D})^{-1}(\partial^2 \mathbf{G}/\partial \mathbf{D} \partial \gamma)$, where -1 denotes the matrix inverse.

To see this we observe that

$$P_{DD}(\mathbf{S} : \gamma) = \int \delta[\mathbf{S} - \mathbf{G}(\mathbf{D}, \gamma)] P_D(\mathbf{D})[d\mathbf{D}]$$
$$= \frac{P_D(\mathbf{D}^*)}{|\det(\partial \mathbf{G}/\partial \mathbf{D})(\mathbf{D}^*, \gamma)|} \quad (4.2)$$

where $\mathbf{D}^* = G^{-1}(\mathbf{S}, \gamma)$ and we assume that the function G is 1-1. It follows directly that

$$P_{DD}[\mathbf{G}(\mathbf{D}, \gamma) : \gamma] = \frac{P_D(\mathbf{D})}{|\det(\partial \mathbf{G}/\partial \mathbf{D})(\mathbf{D}, \gamma)|} \quad (4.3)$$

Substituting back into the K–L measure (equation 4.1) means that we must minimize with respect to γ the cost function $E[\gamma, \mathbf{D}]$ averaged over a sample of $\mathbf{D}$ (where we have dropped terms that are independent of γ):

$$E[\gamma, \mathbf{D}] = -\log \left|\det \frac{\partial \mathbf{G}}{\partial \mathbf{D}}(\mathbf{D}, \gamma)\right| + \beta E_P[\mathbf{G}(\mathbf{D}, \gamma)] \quad (4.4)$$

We implement this by stochastic learning. Pick an input $\mathbf{D}$ at random, set $\gamma_{\text{new}} = \gamma_{\text{old}} - \zeta(\partial E/\partial \gamma)$ (where ζ is the learning rate), and repeat.

This involves calculating $\partial E/\partial \gamma$. After some algebra we find that

$$\frac{\partial}{\partial \gamma_a} \log \left|\det\left\{\frac{\partial \mathbf{G}}{\partial \mathbf{D}}(\mathbf{D}, \gamma)\right\}\right| = \sum_{j,k} \left(\frac{\partial G_j}{\partial D_k}\right)^{-1} \frac{\partial^2 G_k}{\partial D_j \partial \gamma_a} \quad (4.5)$$

where -1 denotes the matrix inverse.

The contribution from the second term will simply be $\beta(\partial E/\partial \mathbf{G})(\partial \mathbf{G}/\partial \gamma_a)$.

This analysis has assumed that $\mathbf{G}$ is a 1-1 function and requires, as a necessary condition, that the input and output spaces have the same dimension. This could often be ensured by adding additional output units or input units with fixed synaptic strengths.

2. Alternatively we can perform additional sampling to estimate $P_{DD}[\mathbf{G}(\mathbf{D}, \boldsymbol{\gamma}) : \boldsymbol{\gamma}]$ and $\{\partial \log P_{DD}[\mathbf{G}(\mathbf{D}, \boldsymbol{\gamma}) : \boldsymbol{\gamma}]/\partial \boldsymbol{\gamma}\}$ directly from their integral representations. [This second approach is similar to Becker and Hinton (1992), though they are concerned with estimating only the first and second moments of these distributions.] The Kullback–Leibler measure corresponds to minimizing $KL(\boldsymbol{\gamma}) = \sum_\mu E(\boldsymbol{\gamma}, \mathbf{D}^\mu)$, where $E(\boldsymbol{\gamma}, \mathbf{D}^\mu) = \log P_{DD}[\mathbf{G}(\mathbf{D}^\mu, \boldsymbol{\gamma}) : \boldsymbol{\gamma}] + \beta E_p[\mathbf{G}(\mathbf{D}^\mu, \boldsymbol{\gamma})]$.

Thus calculating the gradient of $E(\boldsymbol{\gamma}, \mathbf{D}^\mu)$ requires evaluating the expression $\{\partial P_{DD}[\mathbf{G}(\mathbf{D}^\mu, \boldsymbol{\gamma}) : \boldsymbol{\gamma}]/\partial \boldsymbol{\gamma}\}/P_{DD}[\mathbf{G}(\mathbf{D}^\mu, \boldsymbol{\gamma}) : \boldsymbol{\gamma}]$. To estimate these quantities we make the approximation:

$$P_{DD}[\mathbf{G}(\mathbf{D}^\mu, \boldsymbol{\gamma}) : \boldsymbol{\gamma}] \approx \sum_\nu \frac{1}{\left[\sqrt{(2\pi)}\sigma\right]^N} e^{-(1/2\sigma^2)|\mathbf{G}(\mathbf{D}^\mu, \boldsymbol{\gamma}) - \mathbf{G}(\mathbf{D}^\nu, \boldsymbol{\gamma})|^2} \qquad (4.6)$$

where $\{\mathbf{D}^\nu\}$ are a representative set of samples from $P_D(\mathbf{D})$ and σ is a constant. This reduces to the previous expression, the first part of equation 4.2, in the limit as $\sigma \mapsto 0$ and as the size of the sample set tends to infinity.

A formula for $\{\partial P_{DD}[\mathbf{G}(\mathbf{D}^\mu, \boldsymbol{\gamma}) : \boldsymbol{\gamma}]/\partial \boldsymbol{\gamma}\}$ can be obtained by differentiating (4.6) with respect to $\boldsymbol{\gamma}$. This gives

$$\frac{\partial P_{DD}[\mathbf{G}(\mathbf{D}^\mu, \boldsymbol{\gamma}) : \boldsymbol{\gamma}]}{\partial \gamma_a}$$

$$\approx \sum_\nu \frac{1}{\left[\sqrt{(2\pi)}\sigma\right]^N} \times \left\{-\frac{1}{\sigma^2}\right\}$$

$$\times \sum_i \left\{\frac{\partial G_i(\mathbf{D}^\mu, \boldsymbol{\gamma})}{\partial \gamma_a} - \frac{\partial G_i(\mathbf{D}^\nu, \boldsymbol{\gamma})}{\partial \gamma_a}\right\} \{G_i(\mathbf{D}^\mu, \boldsymbol{\gamma}) - G_i(\mathbf{D}^\nu, \boldsymbol{\gamma})\}$$

$$\times e^{-(1/2\sigma^2)|\mathbf{G}(\mathbf{D}^\mu, \boldsymbol{\gamma}) - \mathbf{G}(\mathbf{D}^\nu, \boldsymbol{\gamma})|^2} \qquad (4.7)$$

The learning proceeds by picking a sample $\mathbf{D}^\mu$ from $P_D(\mathbf{D})$ and then an additional set of samples $\{\mathbf{D}^\nu\}$ to approximate the integrals 4.6 and 4.7 and hence enable us to calculate the gradient of $E(\boldsymbol{\gamma}, \mathbf{D}^\mu)$ and update the weights. Then the process repeats.

Note that this approach has the advantage of circumventing the demand that the dimensions of the input and output spaces be equal, i.e., that $\mathbf{G}$ be 1-1, and is more generally applicable.

5 Relationship to Hidden Markov Models and Maximum Likelihood Estimation

It is instructive to contrast our work to alternative learning approaches and, in particular, to hidden Markov models (HMMs)[3] (Paul 1990).

---

[3] Approaches closely related to HMMs are being used for learning stereo (Geiger, personal communication).

HMMs have been very successful in speech processing where models are trained for each recognizable speech segment. Here, however, we are considering training only a single HMM.

In an HMM there are hidden states and observables that, in our notation, correspond to **S** and **D**, respectively. An HMM assumes (1) a prior model $P(\mathbf{S} \mid \beta)$, where the β are parameters to be learned, and (2) an imaging model $P(\mathbf{D} \mid \mathbf{S}, \alpha)$, where the α are parameters to be learned. Together these generate probabilities $P(\mathbf{D} \mid \alpha, \beta) = \sum_S P(\mathbf{D} \mid \mathbf{S}, \alpha) P(\mathbf{S} \mid \beta)$ for the observables as functions of the parameters.[4] Similar expressions arise in MLE parameter estimation (Ripley 1992).

To learn the priors and likelihood functions we must estimate the parameters α and β. This requires a set of data $\{\mathbf{D}^\mu\}$, indexed by μ, that we assume is a representative sample from the distribution $P(\mathbf{D})$ of the observables. We then train the system by maximum likelihood estimation (MLE). More precisely, we select the parameters α and β that maximize $\prod_\mu P(\mathbf{D}^\mu \mid \alpha, \beta)$ or, equivalently, that maximize $\sum_\mu \log P(\mathbf{D}^\mu \mid \alpha, \beta)$. As the sample size tends to infinity this becomes equivalent to maximizing $\sum_\mathbf{D} P(\mathbf{D}) \log[P(\mathbf{D} \mid \alpha, \beta)$ or, equivalently, to maximizing $\sum_\mathbf{D} P(\mathbf{D}) \log P(\mathbf{D} \mid \alpha, \beta)/P(\mathbf{D})]$ [since $P(\mathbf{D})$ is independent of α and β]. Thus, in the infinite sample size limit, we are simply *minimizing* the Kullback–Leibler measure $(\sum_\mathbf{D} P(\mathbf{D}) \log[P(\mathbf{D})/P(\mathbf{D} \mid \alpha, \beta)])$ between the observed distribution $P(\mathbf{D})$ and the distribution $P(\mathbf{D} \mid \alpha, \beta)$ derived by the model.

By contrast, we propose a Kullback–Leibler measure of similarity on the outputs, or hidden states, **S**, rather than on the input states. The MLE justification for this leads to minimizing the Kullback–Leibler distance $\sum_S P(\mathbf{S}) \log[P(\mathbf{S})/P(\mathbf{S} \mid \gamma)]$, where γ represents the parameters of the network.

HMMs assume a class of prior probabilities, parameterized by β, rather than the single model that we have assumed. However, we can readily generalize our model to deal with this case by replacing $P_p(\mathbf{S})$ by a parameterized family of distributions $P_p(\mathbf{S} \mid \tau)$. We must now minimize the Kullback–Leibler distance between $P_p(\mathbf{S} \mid \tau)$ and the derived distribution $P_{DD}(\mathbf{S} : \gamma)$ with respect to γ and τ simultaneously.

6 Conclusion

The goal of this note was to introduce a Bayesian approach to self-organization using prior assumptions about the signal as an organizing principle. We argued that it was a natural generalization of the criterion of maximizing mutual information assuming spatial coherence (Becker and Hinton 1992). Using our principle it should be possible to

---

[4]HMMs have other important properties that are not directly relevant here. For example, the functional forms of $P(\mathbf{S} \mid \beta)$ and $P(\mathbf{D} \mid \mathbf{S}, \alpha)$ are chosen to ensure that highly efficient algorithms are available to perform these computations (Paul 1990).

self-organize Bayesian theories of vision, assuming that the priors are known, the network is capable of representing the appropriate functions, and the learning algorithm converges. There will also be problems if the probability distributions of the true signal and the distractor are too similar.

If the prior is not correct then it may be possible to detect this by evaluating the goodness of the Kullback–Leibler fit after learning.[5] This suggests a strategy whereby the system increases the complexity of the priors until the Kullback–Leibler fit is sufficiently good [this is somewhat similar to an idea proposed by Mumford (1992)]. This is related to the idea of competitive priors in vision (Clark and Yuille 1990). One way to implement this would be for the prior probability itself to have a set of adjustable parameters that would enable it to adapt to different classes of scenes.

Our approach differs from standard MLE by acting on the distributions of the output variables rather than the inputs. Unlike MLE our approach will directly yield an algorithm for computing the outputs. It is still unclear, however, for what class of problems our approach is applicable. For example, it seems unlikely to work if the dimensions of the outputs is a lot lower than that of the inputs.

We proposed two variants of stochastic learning that are suitable for implementing our theory. They relate, in particular, to Becker and Hinton's approach. As a further illustration of our approach we derived elsewhere (Yuille *et al.* 1993) the filter that our criterion would give for filtering out additive gaussian noise (possibly the only analytically tractable case). This turned out to be the square root of the Wiener filter in Fourier space.

Acknowledgments

We would like to thank ARPA for an Air Force contract F49620-92-J-0466. Conversations with Dan Kersten and David Mumford were highly appreciated. We would also like to thank the reviewers for their insightful comments.

References

Atick, J. J., and Redlich, A. N. 1990. Towards a theory of early visual processing. *Neural Comp.* **2**, 308–320.

Barlow, H. B. 1993. What is the computational goal of the neocortex? In *Large Scale Neuronal Theories of the Brain*, C. Koch, ed. MIT Press, Cambridge, MA.

---

[5]This is reminiscent of Barlow's suspicious coincidence detectors (Barlow 1993), where we might hope to determine if two variables x and y are independent or not by calculating the Kullback–Leibler distance between the joint distribution $P(x,y)$ and the product of the individual distributions $P(x)P(y)$.

Becker, S., and Hinton, G. E. 1992. Self-organizing neural network that discovers surfaces in random-dot stereograms. *Nature (London)* **355**, 161–163.

Clark, J. J., and Yuille, A. L. 1990. *Data Fusion for Sensory Information Processing Systems*. Kluwer, Boston.

Held, R. 1987. Visual development in infants. In *The Encyclopedia of Neuroscience*, Vol. 2. Birkhauser, Boston.

Hornik, K., Stinchcombe, S., and White, H. 1991. Multilayer feed-forward networks are universal approximators. *Neural Networks* **4**, 251–257.

Kersten, D., O'Toole, A. J., Sereno, M. E., Knill, D. C., and Anderson, J. A. 1987. Associative learning of scene parameters from images. *Opt. Soc. Am.* **26**, 4999–5006.

Marr, D. 1982. *Vision*. W. H. Freeman, San Francisco.

Mumford, D. 1992. *Pattern Theory: A Unifying Perspective*. Mathematics Preprint. Harvard University.

Nakayama, K., and Shimojo, S. 1987. Experiencing and perceiving visual surfaces. *Science* **257**, 1357–1363.

Paul, D. B. 1990. Speech recognition using hidden Markov models. *Lincoln Lab. J.* **3**, 41–62.

Poggio, T., Torre, V., and Koch, C. 1985. Computational vision and regularization theory. *Nature (London)* **317**, 314–319.

Ripley, B. D. 1992. Classification and clustering in spatial and image data. In *Analyzing and Modeling Data and Knowledge*, M. Schader, ed. Springer-Verlag, Berlin.

Smirnakis, S. M., and Yuille, A. L. 1994. Neural implementation of Bayesian vision theories by unsupervised learning. *CNS Conf. Proc.*, in press.

Yuille, A. L., Smirnakis, S. M., and Xu, L. 1993. Bayesian self-organization. *NIPS Conf. Proc.*

II

Models of Topographic Maps in the Brain

4

Dynamics and Formation of Self-Organizing Maps

Jun Zhang
Neurobiology Group, 3210 Tolman Hall, University of California, Berkeley, CA 94720 USA

Amari (1983, 1989) proposed a mathematical formulation on the self-organization of synaptic efficacies and neural response fields under the influence of external stimuli. The dynamics as well as the equilibrium properties of the cortical map were obtained analytically for neurons with binary input–output transfer functions. Here we extend this approach to neurons with arbitrary sigmoidal transfer function. Under the assumption that both the intracortical connection and the stimulus-driven thalamic activity are well localized, we are able to derive expressions for the cortical magnification factor, the point-spread resolution, and the bandwidth resolution of the map. As a highlight, we show analytically that the receptive field size of a cortical neuron in the map is inversely proportional to the cortical magnification factor at that map location, the experimentally well-established rule of inverse magnification in retinotopic and somatotopic maps.

1 Introduction

The self-organization of the nervous system and the consequential formation of cortical maps have been studied quite extensively (von der Malsburg 1973; Swindale 1980; Kohonen 1982; Linsker 1986; Miller *et al.* 1989). A cortical map, or more generally, a computational map refers to the neural structure of representing a continuous stimulus parameter by a place-coded populational response, whose peak location reflects the mapped parameter (Knudsen *et al.* 1987). The cortical neurons in the map, each with a slightly different range of stimulus selectivity established during developmental course, operate as preset parallel filters on the afferent stimulus almost simultaneously. The stimulus parameter, now coded as the location of the most active neuron(s), can be accessed by higher processing centers via relatively simple neural connections.

The network models for such cortical maps are usually composed of several layers of neurons from sensory receptors to cortical units, with feedforward excitations between the layers and lateral (or recurrent) connection within the layer. Standard techniques include (1) Hebbian rule and its variations for modifying synaptic efficacies, (2) lateral inhibition (in the general sense) for establishing topographical organization of the cortex as well as sharpening the cells' tuning properties, and (3) adiabatic approximation in decoupling the dynamics of relaxation (which is on the fast time scale) and the dynamics of learning (which is on the slow time scale) of the network. However, in most cases, only computer simulation results were obtained and therefore provided limited mathematical understanding of the self-organizing neural response fields.

In Takeuchi and Amari (1979) and Amari (1983, 1989), a general mathematical formulation was presented to study analytically the existence conditions, the resolution and magnification properties, as well as the dynamic stability of cortical maps. This rather rigorous approach yielded very illuminating results. In particular, they suggested by perturbation analysis that, in the presence of periodic boundary conditions of the mapping, the relative values of the afferent spread size and the receptive field size will determine the emergence of a block-like, columnar structure as opposed to a continuous, topographic organization. Since their analysis was restricted to binary-valued neurons only, that is, neurons with step-function as their input–output transfer function, it is certainly desirable to extend this approach to the more general case of neurons with arbitrary sigmoidal transfer functions.

2 Dynamics of Self-Organization Revisited

The network that Amari and colleagues investigated consists of three layers, a sensory receptor layer, a thalamic layer, and a cortical layer, with feedforward connections between the layers and lateral inhibition within the cortical layer only (Fig. 1). Following Takeuchi and Amari (1979), the activity of the cortical neuron at location $\mathbf{x}$ (a 2D vector in general) and time t may be described by its net input $u(\mathbf{x},t)$ (postsynaptic membrane potential with respect to the resting state) and output $v(\mathbf{x},t)$ (average firing rate of the spike train) interrelated via some monotone increasing (sigmoidal) input–output function: $v = f(u)$, $u \in (-\infty,\infty)$, $v \in (0,1)$. To further indicate that these variables are functions of stimulus parameter $\mathbf{y}$ (a vector) and time parameter of the learning dynamics τ, we shall write in this article $u(\mathbf{x},\mathbf{y},t,\tau)$ and $v(\mathbf{x},\mathbf{y},t,\tau)$ instead. The receptors have delta-function tuning to the stimulus parameter, and they feed into the thalamic layer with localized afferent spread. Notice that $\mathbf{y}$ is used to denote the stimulus variable *as well as* to index cells in the thalamic layer according to their optimal stimulus parameter (i.e., according to their connections from the receptor layer). The cortical neurons in the model receive both thalamocortical afferent projections as well as intracortical

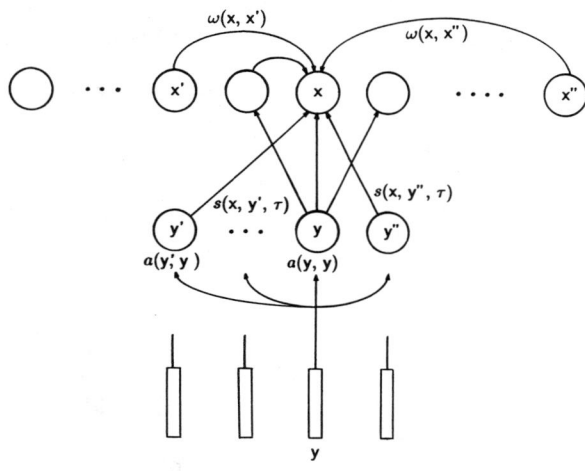

Figure 1: The three layered network model for the self-organizing cortical maps. The receptors, having delta-function tuning for the stimulus **y**, feed into thalamic neurons, with the stimulus-driven thalamic activity denoted by $a(\mathbf{y'}, \mathbf{y})$. The cortical neurons receive both the intracortical interaction characterized by the weighting function $w(\mathbf{x}, \mathbf{x'})$ and the thalamocortical input with synaptic connection $s(\mathbf{x}, \mathbf{y}, \tau)$ modifiable (based on Hebbian learning rule) during development. Note that each thalamic neuron is indexed by its optimal driving stimulus (according to the connections from the receptor layer).

lateral connections. The relaxation of the system is dictated, on the fast time scale t, by the equation

$$\frac{\partial}{\partial t} u(\mathbf{x}, \mathbf{y}, t, \tau) = -u(\mathbf{x}, \mathbf{y}, t, \tau) + \int w(\mathbf{x}, \mathbf{x'}) f[u(\mathbf{x'}, \mathbf{y}, t, \tau)] \, d\mathbf{x'} + \int s(\mathbf{x}, \mathbf{y'}, \tau) a(\mathbf{y'}, \mathbf{y}) \, d\mathbf{y'} \quad (2.1)$$

where $w(\mathbf{x}, \mathbf{x'})$ characterizes the weighting of lateral connections within the cortex from location $\mathbf{x'}$ to location $\mathbf{x}$, assumed to be unchanged with time; $a(\mathbf{y'}, \mathbf{y})$ represents the thalamocortical afferent activity at $\mathbf{y'}$ [the first argument in the function $a(\cdot, \cdot)$] on the presentation of the stimulus $\mathbf{y}$ [the second argument in $a(\cdot, \cdot)$]; and $s(\mathbf{x}, \mathbf{y}, \tau)$ is the synaptic efficacy from the thalamocortical afferent $\mathbf{y}$ to the cortical neuron $\mathbf{x}$, which varies on a slow time scale τ and is thus treated as constant on the fast time scale t. This "adiabatic approximation" allows Amari (1989) to construct a global Lyapunov function $L[u]$ that is a function of $\mathbf{y}, t, \tau$ (**x** having been integrated) and thus represents the overall pattern of cortical activity. It was proved that, on the stimulus presentation $\mathbf{y}$ at time τ, the value of $L[u]$ monotonously decreases, on the fast time scale t, as $u(\mathbf{x}, \mathbf{y}, t, \tau)$ evolves according to equation 2.1 until $L[u] = L(\mathbf{y}, t, \tau)$ reaches a minimum value $L_{\min}(\mathbf{y}, \tau)$ while $u(\mathbf{x}, \mathbf{y}, t, \tau)$ reaches its "equilibrium" solution $\bar{u}[\mathbf{x}, \mathbf{y}, \tau, s(\cdot), a(\cdot)]$ [$\bar{u}$ is a functional of $s(\mathbf{x}, \mathbf{y}, \tau)$ and $a(\mathbf{y}', \mathbf{y})$, and the bar denotes the equilibrium of the relaxation phase]. This establishes a cortical response field $\bar{u} = \bar{u}(\mathbf{x}, \mathbf{y}, \tau)$ relating the external stimulus $\mathbf{y}$ to the cortical activity at $\mathbf{x}$ at time τ. To study the self-organization of this mapping, the synaptic efficacy $s(\mathbf{x}, \mathbf{y}, \tau)$ is assumed to be modifiable, on the slow time scale τ, according to the following equation of learning (Hebbian rule):

$$\frac{\partial}{\partial \tau} s(\mathbf{x}, \mathbf{y}, \tau) = -s(\mathbf{x}, \mathbf{y}, \tau) + \eta \int a(\mathbf{y}, \mathbf{y}') f[\bar{u}(\mathbf{x}, \mathbf{y}', \tau)] p(\mathbf{y}') \, d\mathbf{y}' \quad (2.2)$$

Note that, for the dynamics of learning, stimuli presentations are considered to be stochastically independent at each time τ with some prescribed probability distribution $p(\mathbf{y}')$. Here we set $p(\mathbf{y}') = constant$ (and thus let absorbed into the constant η) to indicate the normal developmental course. Note that the integration is with respect to the second slot of $a(\cdot, \cdot)$, the argument representing stimulus parameter. At the end of the network learning, synapses get "matured" so that $s(\mathbf{x}, \mathbf{y}, \tau)$ becomes the time-independent $S(\mathbf{x}, \mathbf{y})$:

$$S(\mathbf{x}, \mathbf{y}) = \eta \int a(\mathbf{y}, \mathbf{y}') f[U(\mathbf{x}, \mathbf{y}')] \, d\mathbf{y}' \quad (2.3)$$

whereas $\bar{u}(\mathbf{x}, \mathbf{y}, \tau)$ becomes the time-independent $U(\mathbf{x}, \mathbf{y})$:

$$\begin{aligned} U(\mathbf{x}, \mathbf{y}) &= \int \omega(\mathbf{x}, \mathbf{x}') f[U(\mathbf{x}', \mathbf{y})] \, d\mathbf{x}' + \int S(\mathbf{x}, \mathbf{y}') a(\mathbf{y}', \mathbf{y}) \, d\mathbf{y}' \\ &= \int \omega(\mathbf{x}, \mathbf{x}') f[U(\mathbf{x}', \mathbf{y})] d\mathbf{x}' + \int \kappa(\mathbf{y}, \mathbf{y}') f[U(\mathbf{x}, \mathbf{y}')] d\mathbf{y}' \quad (2.4) \end{aligned}$$

Here $\kappa(\mathbf{y}, \mathbf{y}')$ is the autocorrelation between the thalamocortical afferents defined as

$$\kappa(\mathbf{y}, \mathbf{y}') = \eta \int a(\mathbf{y}'', \mathbf{y}) a(\mathbf{y}'', \mathbf{y}') \, d\mathbf{y}'' \quad (2.5)$$

Equivalently, we may write

$$f^{-1}[V(\mathbf{x}, \mathbf{y})] = \int \omega(\mathbf{x}, \mathbf{x}') V(\mathbf{x}', \mathbf{y}) \, d\mathbf{x}' + \int \kappa(\mathbf{y}, \mathbf{y}') V(\mathbf{x}, \mathbf{y}') \, d\mathbf{y}' \quad (2.6)$$

3 Reduced Equation of Cortical Map Formation

The master equation (equation 2.4 or 2.6) developed by Amari and colleagues describes the formation of cortical maps as equilibrium solutions to the dynamic self-organization of layered neural systems. In Amari

Self-Organizing Maps

(1989), the resolution and magnification properties were studied for neurons with binary input–output transfer function, where $f(\cdot)$ assumes the value of either 1 or 0 and thus the integral in equation 2.4 can be explicitly evaluated. In Chernjavsky and Moody (1990), the case of linear transfer function $f(u) = au + b$ was studied. Here we relax these restrictions and consider arbitrary transfer function $f(u)$. We will derive approximations of equation 2.6 for well-localized, translation-invariant functions of the intracortical connection $w(\mathbf{x}, \mathbf{x}')$ and the stimulus-driven thalamic activity $a(\mathbf{y}, \mathbf{y}')$:

$$w(\mathbf{x}, \mathbf{x}') = w(\mathbf{x} - \mathbf{x}') \tag{3.1}$$
$$a(\mathbf{y}, \mathbf{y}') = a(\mathbf{y} - \mathbf{y}') \tag{3.2}$$

It follows from equations 2.5 and 3.2 that the afferent autocorrelation $\kappa(\mathbf{y}, \mathbf{y}')$ must also be translation invariant:

$$\kappa(\mathbf{y}, \mathbf{y}') = \kappa(\mathbf{y} - \mathbf{y}') \tag{3.3}$$

Now we consider the first integral term in equation 2.6. For simplicity, $\mathbf{x}, \mathbf{y}$ are taken as real numbers x, y here (i.e., the mapping is one-dimensional). Expanding $V(x', y)$ into the Taylor series around point (x, y)

$$\begin{aligned} V(x', y) &= V(x, y) + \frac{\partial V(x, y)}{\partial x}(x' - x) + \cdots \\ &+ \frac{1}{n!} \frac{\partial^n V(x, y)}{\partial x^n}(x' - x)^n + \cdots \end{aligned} \tag{3.4}$$

we have

$$\int w(x - x') V(x', y)\, dx' = a_0 V(x, y) + a_1 \frac{\partial V}{\partial x} + \cdots + a_n \frac{\partial^n V}{\partial x^n} + \cdots \tag{3.5}$$

where

$$\begin{aligned} a_k &= \frac{1}{k!} \int w(x - x')(x' - x)^k\, dx' \\ &= \frac{(-1)^k}{k!} \int w(t)\, t^k\, dt \end{aligned} \tag{3.6}$$

Similarly,

$$\int \kappa(y - y') V(x, y')\, dy' = b_0 V(x, y) + b_1 \frac{\partial V}{\partial y} + \cdots + b_n \frac{\partial^n V}{\partial y^n} + \cdots \tag{3.7}$$

with

$$b_k = \frac{(-1)^k}{k!} \int \kappa(t)\, t^k\, dt \tag{3.8}$$

Therefore, the master equation 2.6 is transformed into[1]

$$f^{-1}(x,y) = (a_0 + b_0)V + \left(a_1\frac{\partial V}{\partial x} + b_1\frac{\partial V}{\partial y}\right) + \cdots$$
$$+ \left(a_n\frac{\partial^n V}{\partial x^n} + b_n\frac{\partial^n V}{\partial y^n}\right) + \cdots \quad (3.9)$$

By assuming that $\omega(t)$ and $a(t)$ are well localized, we imply a_k, b_k converge rapidly to 0 as $k \to \infty$. Taking only a few leading terms in the expansion, and further assuming that $\omega(x,x') = \omega(|x - x'|)$ and $a(y,y') = a(|y - y'|)$ are both even functions of their arguments, therefore making $a_1 = 0$ and $b_1 = 0$, we obtain

$$f^{-1}[V(x,y)] = (a_0 + b_0)V + \left(a_2\frac{\partial^2 V}{\partial x^2} + b_2\frac{\partial^2 V}{\partial y^2}\right) \quad (3.10)$$

or

$$G(V) = a_2\frac{\partial^2 V}{\partial x^2} + b_2\frac{\partial^2 V}{\partial y^2} \quad (3.11)$$

with

$$G(V) = f^{-1}(V) - (a_0 + b_0)V \quad (3.12)$$

If the cortical lateral connection is balanced in its total excitation and total inhibition, $a_0 = 0$. If the afferent autocorrelation is normalized, $b_0 = \eta > 0$. Equation 3.11 is a semilinear second-order partial differential equation. When $a_2 b_2 > 0$, it is of elliptic type; when $a_2 b_2 < 0$, it is of hyperbolic type. The standard techniques of solving equation 3.11 can be found in mathematical textbooks, such as Chester (1971). In particular, 3.11 may be linearized and transformed into the canonical forms of (when $a_2 b_2 < 0$) $\partial_{XY} V + cV = 0$, known as the telegraph equation, or (when $a_2 b_2 > 0$) $\nabla^2 V + cV = 0$, known as the Helmholtz equation. These linear second-order partial differential equations have closed-form solutions when given appropriate boundary conditions.

4 Resolution and Magnification of the Map

The solution of equation 3.11 $V = V(x,y)$ represents the response of the neuron at location x due to stimulus parameter y after the cortical map matures. When x is fixed, that is, at a particular cortical location x_0, the neuron's response is a function of stimulus parameter y. Maximal

---

[1] This simplified derivation of equation 3.9 is suggested to the author by Dr. S. Amari. This equation was earlier obtained by expanding $\omega(x - x')$ into the sum of $\delta(x - x')$ and its derivatives $\delta^{(n)}(x - x')$, where the delta-function is envisioned as the limiting case (i.e., with zero width) of a normalized gaussian function and its successive derivatives represent derivatives of gaussian that become less and less localized (Zhang 1990).

Self-Organizing Maps

response is achieved for some optimal stimulus y_0, which is determined by

$$\left.\frac{\partial V(x,y)}{\partial y}\right|_{x=x_0} = 0 \tag{4.1}$$

Obviously the optimal stimulus thus obtained is different for each location x_0. The optimal stimulus parameter y as a function of cortical locations x may be written as

$$y = \mu(x) \tag{4.2}$$

so that equation 4.1 holds identically for all x

$$V_2[x, \mu(x)] = 0 \tag{4.3}$$

Here and in the sequel, we use the subscript(s) 1, 2 of V to denote partial derivative(s) with respect to the first and/or second argument(s) in $V(\cdot, \cdot)$. Upon the presentation of an optimal stimulus, the maximal response of the neuron at x is

$$V_{\max}(x) = V[x, \mu(x)] \tag{4.4}$$

Suppose that this maximal response is everywhere the same (i.e., cortical neurons are indistinguishable)

$$V_{\max}(x) = \text{constant} \tag{4.5}$$

or

$$\frac{d}{dx}V[x, \mu(x)] = V_1[x, \mu(x)] + V_2[x, \mu(x)]\mu'(x) = 0 \tag{4.6}$$

It follows from equations 4.6 and 4.3 that

$$V_1[x, \mu(x)] = 0 \tag{4.7}$$

or equivalently

$$\left.\frac{\partial V(x,y)}{\partial x}\right|_{y=\mu(x)} = 0 \tag{4.8}$$

Hence $x = \mu^{-1}(y)$ defines the location of maximal response (i.e., center of the cortical map) as a function of the stimulus variable. Differentiating equations 4.7 and 4.3 yields, respectively,

$$\frac{d}{dx}V_1[x, \mu(x)] = V_{11}[x, \mu(x)] + V_{12}[x, \mu(x)]\mu'(x) = 0 \tag{4.9}$$

$$\frac{d}{dx}V_2[x, \mu(x)] = V_{21}[x, \mu(x)] + V_{22}[x, \mu(x)]\mu'(x) = 0 \tag{4.10}$$

Remembering that the order of partial differentiations is interchangeable $V_{12} = V_{21}$, we immediately have

$$V_{11}[x, \mu(x)] - V_{22}[x, \mu(x)] \, [\mu'(x)]^2 = 0 \, . \tag{4.11}$$

On the other hand, equation 3.11 should always be satisfied:

$$G(V_{\max}) = a_2 V_{11}[x, \mu(x)] + b_2 V_{22}[x, \mu(x)] \tag{4.12}$$

From 4.11 and 4.12, we finally obtain

$$V_{11}[x, \mu(x)] = \frac{G(V_{\max}) \, [\mu'(x)]^2}{a_2 \, [\mu'(x)]^2 + b_2} \tag{4.13}$$

$$V_{22}[x, \mu(x)] = \frac{G(V_{\max})}{a_2 \, [\mu'(x)]^2 + b_2} \tag{4.14}$$

The above results can be understood intuitively. Recall that the cortical magnification factor (CMF) is defined as the ratio of a resulting shift of the mapped location in the cortex over a change in the stimulus parameter. In the present context, it is simply equal to $[\mu'(x)]^{-1} = [d\mu(x)/dx]^{-1}$, the reciprocal of the derivative of the function $y = \mu(x)$, which is solvable from equation 4.3 or 4.7. The cortical magnification factor is apparently a function of cortical location x.

The resolution of the map can be described by two related measures. For a fixed stimulus parameter, the extent of cortical regions being excited is a measure of the stimulus localization in a populational response ("point-spread resolution"). At a particular cortical location, the range of effective stimuli is a measure of the stimulus selectivity of a single cell ("bandwidth resolution"). To get the intuitive picture, we draw a family of "isoclines" of $V(x, y)$ in the (x, y)-coordinates whereby $V(x, y) = $ constant along each curve (Fig. 2a). The variation of $V(x, y)$ in the vertical direction indicates to look at cells' response at a fixed cortical location ($x = x_0$) while changing the stimulus parameter — the vertical bar measures, in reciprocal, the bandwidth resolution. The variation of $V(x, y)$ in the horizontal direction indicates to fix the stimulus parameter while looking at responses of cells at different cortical locations — the horizontal bar measures, in reciprocal, the point-spread resolution. In both cases, of course, one needs to specify a criterion (in terms of percentage of maximal response, for instance) to discuss the magnitude of each resolution measure. From the graph, it is obvious that these two measures are interrelated.

If we take a slice (cross-section) along the vertical direction, the value of $V(x_0, y)$ may be schematically plotted (Fig. 2b). Note that this is a plot of response amplitude V versus the stimulus parameter y, with the cortical location x_0 fixed. The peak location of this curve corresponds to $V_{\max} = V(x_0, y_0)$, with $y_0 = \mu(x_0)$ representing the optimal stimulus for the cell located at x_0. The "width" of this tuning curve represents the extent

Self-Organizing Maps

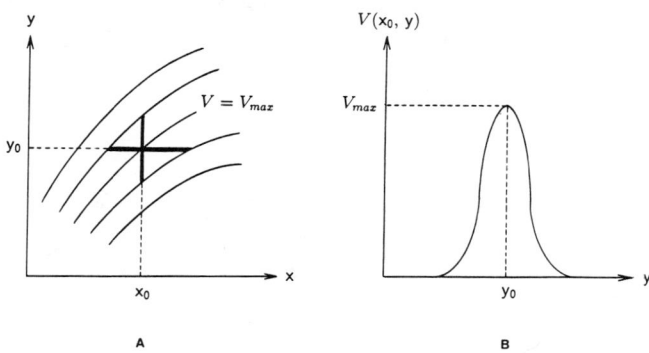

Figure 2: (a) The "isoclines" of V are plotted on the (x, y)-coordinates, whereby along each curve $V(x, y) = $ constant. In particular, the curve $y = \mu(x)$ corresponding to $V(x, y) = V_{\max}$ was labeled. The vertical bar is a measure of the bandwidth resolution of the cortical map, while the horizontal bar is a measure of the point-spread resolution of the map (see text for details). (b) Taking a slice (cross-section) along the vertical direction in (a), the value of $V(x_0, y)$ is plotted as a function of the stimulus parameter y, representing the tuning curve of the cell at a particular cortical location x_0.

of stimulus selectivity, or the reciprocal of the bandwidth resolution of the map. If the cell's tuning curve is symmetric about its peak, it may be approximated by a quadratic function (at least near the peak location $y_0 = \mu(x_0)$, where $\partial V(x_0, y_0)/\partial y$ according to equation 4.3)

$$V(x_0, y) \simeq V(x_0, y_0) + \frac{1}{2} \frac{\partial^2 V(x_0, y_0)}{\partial y^2} (y - y_0)^2 + \cdots \qquad (4.15)$$

The "width" of this parabola is inversely related to the quadratic coefficient $\partial^2 V(x_0, y_0)/\partial y^2$, or simply $V_{22}[x_0, \mu(x_0)]$. We may replace x_0 with x to indicate that this analysis applies to all cortical locations. Therefore $V_{22}[x, \mu(x)]$ as calculated in 4.14 is nothing but the bandwidth resolution of the map. Similarly, $V_{11}[x, \mu(x)]$ can be viewed as the point-spread resolution of the cortical map. These two resolutions are linked to the cortical magnification factor via equation 4.11.

It is interesting to note that equations 4.9 and 4.10 yield

$$V_{11}[x, \mu(x)] V_{22}[x, \mu(x)] - V_{12}[x, \mu(x)] V_{21}[x, \mu(x)] = 0 \qquad (4.16)$$

or that the graph $z = V(x, y)$ is parabolic at its peak points $[x, \mu(x)]$. This, along with the restrictions that $V_{11}[x, \mu(x)]$ and $V_{22}[x, \mu(x)]$ are both negative, constitutes the conditions of a continuous, homogeneous map.

Similarly, the occurrence of a discontinuous, columnar-like structure of the map corresponds to having isolated peak points at which the elliptic graph $z = V(x, y)$ attains the maximal value:

$$V_{11}(x_0, y_0) V_{22}(x_0, y_0) - V_{12}^2(x_0, y_0) < 0 \tag{4.17}$$

5 Rule of Inverse Magnification

The continuous and homogeneous cortical map as discussed in the previous section is a topographic map that uniformly associates a cortical location with each stimulus. The retinotopic map is an example where the stimulus parameter being mapped is the position in the frontal-parallel visual field. The somatotopic map is another example where the stimulus parameter is the location in the skin surface. In both cases, the receptive field size (RF) is a synonym of our previously defined "bandwidth" of a cortical neuron, be it an effective area of the visual space or an effective patch of the skin surfaces. In terms of the square-root of areal measurement, RF is simply $(-V_{22})^{-1/2}$, or

$$\text{RF}(x) = \sqrt{\frac{a_2 \left[\mu'(x)\right]^2 + b_2}{-G(V_{\max})}} \tag{5.1}$$

If $b_2 = 0$ or b_2 is very small (for a discussion, see Appendix), then 5.1 becomes

$$\text{RF}(x) \propto \mu'(x) = \text{CMF}^{-1}(x) \tag{5.2}$$

or finally

$$\text{RF}(x) \cdot \text{CMF}(x) = constant \tag{5.3}$$

The product of the receptive field size and the cortical magnification factor is nothing but the size (in terms of cortical distance) that a cell receives its total input and would be activated. From equation 4.11, this product also equals $(-V_{11})^{-1/2}$, the "point-image" of a stimulus (McIlwain 1986). That the total cortical distance to influence (drive) a cell and the overall size of cortical point-image are constant imply that the cortex is uniform in neuronal connections to implement its computations.

The physiological uniformity of the cortex has long been observed experimentally. In monkey striate visual cortex, Hubel and Weisel (1974) reported that, despite the large scattering of cells' receptive field sizes of cells at each eccentricity (now believed to correspond to functionally different cell groups), the average size (in square-root of areal measurement) is roughly proportional to the inverse of the cortical magnification factor. This inverse magnification rule was also revealed in monkey somatosensory cortex (Sur et al. 1980), and was demonstrated most convincingly in the studies of reorganization of the hand-digit representation under various surgical and behavioral manipulations (Jenkins *et al.* 1990). This remarkable relationship $\text{RF}(x) \cdot \text{CMF}(x) = constant$ is compatible with the anatomical uniformity of the cortex, in particular the uniform dendritic field sizes (which is the anatomical substrate of receptive field) of each cell type across the cortex.

In Grajski and Merzenich (1990), the self-organization of somatotopic map was simulated using a three-layered network essentially the same as the one being discussed here. These authors demonstrated that the general principles of Hebbian rule, lateral inhibition, and adiabatic approximation are sufficient to account for the inverse relationship between the receptive field size and the cortical magnification factor. A similar result was also obtained by a probabilistic analysis of the Kohonen-type network (Obermayer *et al.* 1990). These empirical and computer studies are all consistent with our analytical result, and therefore nicely complement each other in helping us understand the principles as well as properties such as the inverse magnification rule of self-organizing cortical maps.

6 Conclusions

The analytic power of this approach toward a unified description of self-organization of cortical maps, as developed by Amari and colleagues and extended here, greatly facilitates mathematical appreciations of the dynamics as well as the equilibrium behavior of the neural system. The present formulation embodies the general scheme of layered neural networks with feedforward (thalamocortical) excitations and lateral (intracortical) connections, and takes into account features such as the autocorrelation in the stimulus-driven activities of the thalamic afferents and the Hebbian rule of synaptic modification. The magnification and the resolution of the map are derived analytically to allow comparisons with experimental data. In particular, the linear relationship between the receptive field size and the inverse cortical magnification factor (namely the inverse magnification rule) as derived under this formulation is consistent with both experimental observations and results from computer simulations.

Appendix A

We discuss the condition $b_2 = 0$ in this appendix. From equation 3.8,

$$b_2 = \frac{1}{2} \int_{-\infty}^{\infty} \kappa(t)\, t^2\, dt \qquad (A.1)$$

According to equations 2.5 and 3.2,

$$\kappa(y - y') = \int a(y'' - y) a(y'' - y') \, dy''$$
$$= \int a(y'') a[y'' + (y - y')] \, dy'' \quad (A.2)$$

which is simply the autocorrelation operation

$$\kappa(t) = \int_{-\infty}^{\infty} a(t') a(t' + t) \, dt' \quad (A.3)$$

So,[2]

$$b_2 = \frac{1}{2} \int_{-\infty}^{\infty} \int_{-\infty}^{\infty} t^2 a(t') a(t + t') \, dt' \, dt$$
$$= \frac{1}{2} \int_{-\infty}^{\infty} a(t') \, dt' \int_{-\infty}^{\infty} (y - t')^2 a(y) \, dy \quad (A.4)$$

where we put $y = t + t'$. Denoting

$$A_k = \int_{-\infty}^{\infty} a(y) y^k \, dy, \quad k = 0, 1, 2 \quad (A.5)$$

we have

$$b_2 = \frac{1}{2} \int_{-\infty}^{\infty} a(t') \, dt' \int_{-\infty}^{\infty} (y^2 - 2yt' + t'^2) a(y) \, dy$$
$$= \frac{1}{2} \left(A_0 A_2 - 2 A_1^2 + A_2 A_0 \right)$$
$$= A_0 A_2 - A_1^2 \quad (A.6)$$

For an even-symmetric $a(t)$, $A_1 = 0$. We finally obtain

$$b_2 = \left[\int_{-\infty}^{\infty} a(t) \, dt \right] \left[\int_{-\infty}^{\infty} t^2 a(t) \, dt \right] \quad (A.7)$$

Therefore, the condition $b_2 = 0$ implies that the integral of $a(t)$, either weighted by t^2 or not, should be zero. Physiologically, the ON/OFF regions in the response fields of the thalamic (geniculate) neurons must be balanced in its total excitation and total inhibition.

Acknowledgments

This work was supported by PHS Grant EY–00014. The author especially thanks Dr. S. Amari for his helpful comments and for simplifying proofs that have enhanced this manuscript. Thanks are also extended to Drs. K. K. De Valois and R. L. De Valois for their generous support and constant encouragement.

---

[2] The following simplified proof is provided by Dr. S. Amari, and replaces a previous proof using Fourier transform techniques.

References

Amari, S. 1983. Field theory of self-organizing neural nets. *IEEE Trans. SMC* **SMC-13**, 741–748.

Amari, S. 1989. Dynamical study of formation of cortical maps. In *Dynamic Interactions in Neural Networks: Models and Data*, M. A. Arbib and S. Amari, eds., pp. 15–34. Springer-Verlag, New York.

Chernjavsky, A., and Moody, J. 1990. Spontaneous development of modularity in simple cortical models. *Neural Comp.* **2**, 334–350.

Chester, C. R. 1971. *Techniques in Partial Differential Equations*. McGraw-Hill, New York.

Grajski, K. A., and Merzenich, M. M. 1990. Hebb-type dynamics is sufficient to account for the inverse magnification rule in cortical somatotopy. *Neural Comp.* **2**, 71–84.

Hubel, D. H., and Wiesel, T. N. 1974. Uniformity of monkey striate cortex: A parallel relationship between field size, scatter, and magnification factor. *J. Comp. Neurol.* **158**, 295–306.

Jenkins, W. M., Merzenich, M. M., Ochs, M. T., Allard, T., and Guíc-Robles, E. 1990. Functional reorganization of primary somatosensory cortex in adult owl monkeys after behaviorally controlled tactile stimulation. *J. Neurophys.* **63**, 82–104.

Kohonen, T. 1982. Self-organized formation of topologically correct feature maps. *Biol. Cybern.* **43**, 59–69.

Knudsen, E. I., du Lac, S., and Esterly, S. D. 1987. Computational maps in the brain. *Annu. Rev. Neurosci.* **10**, 41–65.

Linsker, R. 1986. From basic network principles to neural architecture. *Proc. Natl. Acad. Sci. U.S.A.* **83**, 7508–7512, 8390–8394, 8779–8783.

Malsburg, Ch. von der 1973. Self-organization of orientation sensitive cells in the striate cortex. *Kybernetik* **14**, 85–100.

McIlwain, J. T. 1986. Point images in the visual system: New interest in an old idea. *Trends Neurosci.* **9**, 354–358.

Miller, K. D., Keller, J. B., and Stryker, M. P. 1989. Ocular dominance column development: Analysis and simulation. *Science* **245**, 605–615.

Obermayer, K., Ritter, H., and Schulten, K. 1990. A neural network model for the formation of topographic maps in the CNS: Development of receptive fields. In *Proc. Int. Joint Conf. Neural Networks (IJCNN'90), San Diego*, **II**, 423–429.

Sur, M., Merzenich, M. M., and Kaas, J. H. 1980. Magnification, receptive-field area, and "hypercolumn" size in area 3b and 1 of somatosensory cortex in owl monkeys. *J. Neurophys.* **44**, 295–311.

Swindale, N. V. 1980. A model for the formation of ocular dominance stripes. *Proc. R. Soc. London Ser. B.* **208** 243–264.

Takeuchi, A., and Amari, S. 1979. Formation of topographic maps and columnar microstructures in nerve fields. *Biol. Cybern.* **35**, 63–72.

Zhang, J. 1990. Dynamical self-organization and formation of cortical maps. In *Proc. Int. Joint Conf. Neural Networks (IJCNN'90), San Diego*, **III**, 487–492.

5

A Unifying Objective Function for Topographic Mappings

Geoffrey J. Goodhill
Sloan Center for Theoretical Neurobiology, Salk Institute for Biological Studies, La Jolla, CA 92037, U.S.A. and Georgetown Institute for Cognitive and Computational Sciences, Georgetown University Medical Center, Washington, DC 20007, U.S.A.

Terrence J. Sejnowski
The Howard Hughes Medical Institute, Salk Institute for Biological Studies, La Jolla, CA 92037, U.S.A. and Department of Biology, University of California San Diego, La Jolla, CA 92037, U.S.A.

Many different algorithms and objective functions for topographic mappings have been proposed. We show that several of these approaches can be seen as particular cases of a more general objective function. Consideration of a very simple mapping problem reveals large differences in the form of the map that each particular case favors. These differences have important consequences for the practical application of topographic mapping methods.

1 Introduction

The notion of a topographic mapping that takes nearby points in one space to nearby points in another appears in many domains, both biological and practical. A number of algorithms have been proposed that claim to construct such mappings (reviewed in Goodhill & Sejnowski, 1996). However, a fundamental problem with these claims, or the claim that a particular given mapping is topographic, is that the computational-level meaning of topography has not been formally defined. Given the wide variety of contexts in which topography or degrees of topography are discussed, it is unlikely that an application-independent definition would be generally useful. A more productive goal is to attempt to lay bare the assumptions behind different approaches to topographic mappings, and thus clarify the relationships among them. In this way, the hope is to make it easier to choose the appropriate approach for a particular problem.

In this article, we introduce an objective function we call the C measure and show that it has the capacity to unify several different approaches to topographic mapping. These approaches constitute particular instantiations of the functions from which the C measure is constructed. We then consider a simple mapping problem and explicitly optimize different versions of the C measure. It becomes apparent that the "optimally topographic" map can radically change depending on the particular measure employed.

2 The C measure

For the purposes of this article, we consider only bijective (1-1) mappings and a finite number of points in each space. Some mapping problems intrinsically have this form, and many others can be reduced to this by separating out a clustering or vector quantization step from the mapping step.

Consider an input space V_{in} and an output space V_{out}, each of which contains N points (see Figure 1). Let M be the mapping from points in V_{in} to points in V_{out}. We use the word *space* in a general sense: either or both of V_{in} and V_{out} may not have a geometric interpretation. Assume that for each space there is a symmetric similarity function that, for any given pair of points in the space, specifies by a nonnegative scalar value how similar (or dissimilar) they are. Call these functions F for V_{in} and G for V_{out}. Then we define a cost function C as follows,

$$C = \sum_{i=1}^{N} \sum_{j<i} F(i,j) G(M(i), M(j)), \qquad (2.1)$$

where i and j label points in V_{in}, and $M(i)$ and $M(j)$ are their respective images in V_{out}. The sum is over all possible pairs of points in V_{in}. Since we have assumed that M is a bijection, it is therefore invertible, and C can equivalently be written as

$$C = \sum_{i=1}^{N} \sum_{j<i} F(M^{-1}(i), M^{-1}(j)) G(i,j), \qquad (2.2)$$

where i and j label points in V_{out}, and M^{-1} is the inverse map. A good mapping is one with a high value of C. However, if one of F or G is given

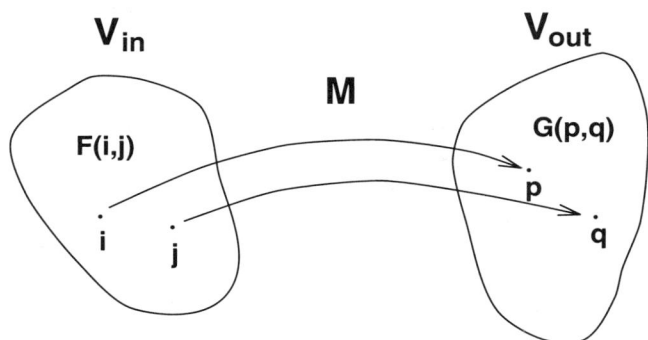

Figure 1: The mapping framework.

Unifying Objective Function

as a dissimilarity function (i.e., increasing with decreasing similarity), then a good mapping has a low value of C. How F and G are defined is problem specific. They could be Euclidean distances in a geometric space, some (possibly nonmonotonic) function of those distances, or they could just be given, in which case it may not be possible to interpret the points as lying in some geometric space. C measures the correlation between the F's and the G's. It is straightforward to show that if a mapping that preserves orderings exists, then maximizing C will find it. This is equivalent to saying that for two vectors of real numbers, their inner product is maximized over all permutations within the two vectors if the elements of the vectors are identically ordered, a proof of which can be found in Hardy, Littlewood, and Pólya (1934, p. 261).

3 Measures Related to C

Several objective functions for topographic mapping can be seen as versions of the C measure, given particular instantiations of the F and G functions.

3.1 Metric Multidimensional Scaling. Metric multidimensional scaling (metric MDS) is a technique originally developed in the context of psychology for representing a set of N entities (e.g., subjects in an experiment) by N points in a low- (usually two-) dimensional space. For these entities one has a matrix that gives the numerical dissimilarity between each pair of entities. The aim of metric MDS is to position points representing entities in the low-dimensional space so that the set of distances between each pair of points matches as closely as possible the given set of dissimilarities. The particular objective function optimized is the summed squared deviations of distances from dissimilarities. The original method was presented in Torgerson (1952); for reviews, see Shepard (1980) and Young (1987).

In terms of the framework presented earlier, the MDS dissimilarity matrix is F. Note that there may not be a geometric space of any dimensionality for which these dissimilarities can be represented by distances (for instance, if the dissimilarities do not satisfy the triangle inequality), in which case V_{in} does not have a geometric interpretation. V_{out} is the low-dimensional, continuous space in which the points representing entities are positioned, and G is Euclidean distance in V_{out}. Metric MDS selects the mapping M by adjusting the positions of points in V_{out}, which minimizes

$$\sum_{i=1}^{N} \sum_{j<i} (F(i,j) - G(M(i), M(j)))^2. \tag{3.1}$$

Under our assumptions, this objective function is identical to the C measure. Expanding out the square in equation 3.1 gives

$$\sum_{i=1}^{N}\sum_{j<i}(F(i,j)^2 + G(M(i),M(j))^2 - 2F(i,j)G(M(i),M(j))). \quad (3.2)$$

The last term is twice the C measure. The entries in F are fixed, so the first term is independent of the mapping. In metric MDS, the sum over the G's varies as the entities are moved in the output space. If one instead considers the case where the positions of the points in V_{out} are fixed, and the problem is to find the assignment of entities to positions that minimize equation 3.1, then the sum over the G's is also independent of the map. In this case the metric MDS measure becomes exactly equivalent to C.

3.2 Minimal Wiring. In minimal wiring (Mitchison & Durbin, 1986; Durbin & Mitchison, 1990), a good mapping is defined as one that maps points that are nearest neighbors in V_{in} as close as possible in V_{out}, where closeness in V_{out} is measured by, for instance, Euclidean distance raised to some power. The motivation here is the idea that it is often useful in sensory processing to perform computations that are local in some space of input features V_{in}. To do this in V_{out} (e.g., the cortex) the images of neighboring points in V_{in} need to be connected; the dissimilarity function in V_{out} is intended to capture the cost of the wire (e.g., axons) required to do this. Minimal wiring is equivalent to the C measure for

$$F(i,j) = \begin{cases} 1 & : \ i,j \text{ neighboring} \\ 0 & : \ \text{otherwise} \end{cases}$$

$$G(M(i),M(j)) = ||M(i) - M(j)||^p.$$

For the cases of one- or two-dimensional square arrays investigated in Mitchison and Durbin (1986) and Durbin and Mitchison (1990), neighbors are taken to be just the two or four adjacent points in the array, respectively.

3.3 Minimal Path Length. In this scheme, a good map is one such that, in moving between nearest neighbors in V_{out}, one moves the least possible distance in V_{in}. This is, for instance, the mapping required to solve the traveling salesman problem (TSP), where V_{in} is the distribution of cities and V_{out} is the one-dimensional tour. This goal is implemented by the elastic net algorithm (Durbin & Willshaw, 1987; Durbin & Mitchison, 1990; Goodhill & Willshaw, 1990), which measures dissimilarity in V_{in} by squared distances:

$$F(i,j) = ||\mathbf{v}_i - \mathbf{v}_j||^2$$

$$G(p,q) = \begin{cases} 1 & : \ p,q \text{ neighboring} \\ 0 & : \ \text{otherwise} \end{cases}$$

where $\mathbf{v}_k$ is the position of point k in V_{in} (we have only considered here the regularization term in the elastic net energy function, which also includes a term matching input points to output points). Thus, minimal wiring and minimal path length are symmetrical cases under equation 2.1, with respect to exchange of V_{in} and V_{out}. Their relationship is discussed further in Durbin & Mitchison (1990), where the abilities of minimal wiring and minimal path length are compared with regard to reproducing the structure of the map of orientation selectivity in the primary visual cortex (see also Mitchison, 1995).

3.4 The Approach of Jones, Van Sluyters, and Murphy (1991). Jones, Van Sluyters, and Murphy (1991) investigated the effect of the shape of the cortex (V_{out}) relative to the lateral geniculate nuclei (V_{in}) on the overall pattern of ocular dominance columns in the cat and monkey, using an optimization approach. They desired to keep both neighboring cells in each LGN (as defined by a hexagonal array), and anatomically corresponding cells between the two LGNs, nearby in the cortex (also a hexagonal array). Their formulation of this problem can be expressed as a maximization of C when

$$F(i, j) = \begin{cases} 1 & : \quad i, j \text{ neighboring, corresponding} \\ 0 & : \quad \text{otherwise} \end{cases}$$

and

$$G(p, q) = \begin{cases} 1 & : \quad p, q \text{ first or second nearest neighbors} \\ 0 & : \quad \text{otherwise.} \end{cases}$$

For two-dimensional V_{in} and V_{out} they found a solution such that if $F(i, j) = 1$, then $G(M(i), M(j)) = 1$, $\forall i, j$. Alternatively this problem could be expressed as a minimization of C when $G(p, q)$ is the stepping distance (see below) between positions in the V_{out} array. They found this gave appropriate behavior for the problem addressed.

3.5 Minimal Distortion. Luttrell and Mitchison have introduced mapping functionals for the continuous case. Under appropriate assumptions to reduce them to the discrete case, these are equivalent to C. Luttrell (1990, 1994) defined a minimal distortion principle that can be interpreted as a measure of mapping quality. He defined "distortion" D as

$$D = \int d\mathbf{x}\, P(\mathbf{x})\, d\{\mathbf{x}, \mathbf{x}'[\mathbf{y}(\mathbf{x})]\}.$$

$\mathbf{x}$ and $\mathbf{y}$ are vectors in the input and output spaces, respectively. $\mathbf{y}$ is the map in the input to output direction, $\mathbf{x}'$ is the (in general different) map back again, and $P(\mathbf{x})$ is the probability of occurrence of $\mathbf{x}$. $\mathbf{x}'$ and $\mathbf{y}$ are suitably adjusted to minimize D. An augmented version of D includes additive noise in the output space,

$$D = \int d\mathbf{x}\, P(\mathbf{x}) \int d\mathbf{n}\, \pi(\mathbf{n})\, d\{\mathbf{x}, \mathbf{x}'[\mathbf{y}(\mathbf{x}) + \mathbf{n}]\},$$

where $\pi(\mathbf{n})$ is the probability density of the noise vector $\mathbf{n}$. Intuitively, the aim is now to find the forward and backward maps so that the reconstructed value of the input vector is as close as possible to its original value after being corrupted by noise in the output space. In Luttrell (1990), the d function was taken to be $\{\mathbf{x} - \mathbf{x}'[\mathbf{y}(\mathbf{x}) + \mathbf{n}]\}^2$. In this case, Luttrell showed that the minimal distortion measure can be differentiated to produce a learning rule that is almost the self-organizing map rule of Kohonen (1982).

For the discrete version of this, it is necessary to assume that appropriate quantization has occurred so that $\mathbf{y}(\mathbf{x})$ defines a 1-1 map, and $\mathbf{x}'(\mathbf{y})$ defines the same map in the opposite direction. In this case the minimal distortion measure becomes equivalent to the C measure, with $F(i, j)$ the squared Euclidean distance between the positions of vectors i and j (assuming these to lie in a geometric space) and $G(p, q)$ the noise process in the output space (generally assumed gaussian).

The minimal distortion principle was generalized in Mitchison (1995) by allowing the noise process and reconstruction error to take arbitrary forms. For instance, they can be reversed, so that F is a gaussian and G is Euclidean distance. In this case, the measure can be interpreted as a version of the minimal wiring principle, establishing a connection between minimal distortion (and hence the SOM algorithm) and minimal wiring. This identification also yields a self-organizing algorithm similar to the SOM for solving minimal wiring problems, the properties of which are briefly explored in Mitchison (1995).

Luttrell (1994) generalized minimal distortion to allow a probabilistic match between points in the two spaces, which in the discrete case can be expressed as

$$D = \sum_i \sum_j F(i, j) \sum_k P(k|i) P(j|k),$$

where D is the distortion to be minimized, F is Euclidean distance in the input space, $P(k|i)$ is the probability that output state k occurs given that input state i occurs, and $P(j|k)$ is the corresponding Bayes inverse probability that input state j occurs given that output state k occurs. This reduces to C in the special case that $P(k|i) = P(i|k)$, which is true for bijections.

3.6 Dynamic Link Matching. Bienenstock and von der Malsburg (1987a, 1987b) considered position-invariant pattern recognition as a problem of graph matching. Their formalism consists of two sets of nodes, one with links expressing neighborhood relationships given by $F(i, j)$ and one with analogous links given by $G(p, q)$. The aim is to find the bijective mapping between the two sets of nodes that optimally preserves the link structure. By

Unifying Objective Function

approximating the Hamiltonian for a particular type of spin neural network, they derived an objective function H that in our notation (taking $p = M(i)$, $q = M(j)$) can be written as

$$H = \sum_{i,j=1}^{N} \sum_{p,q=1}^{N} F(i,j) G(p,q) w_{ip} w_{jq}$$

$$+ \gamma \left(\sum_{i=1}^{N} \left(\sum_{p=1}^{N} w_{ip} - a \right)^2 + \sum_{p=1}^{N} \left(\sum_{i=1}^{N} w_{ip} - a \right)^2 \right). \qquad (3.3)$$

Here γ and a are constants, and w_{ip} is the strength of connection between node i and node p. The first term is a generalized version of the C measure, which allows a weighted match between all pairs of nodes i and p. The second term enforces the regularization constraint that the sum of the weights from or to each node is equal to a. When $a = 1$ and γ is large, the minima of H are clearly the same as the maxima of C. More recent work has investigated its potential as a general objective function for topographic mappings (Wiskott & Sejnowski, 1997).

4 Application to a Simple Mapping Problem

To show the range of optimal maps that the C measure implies for different F and G, we consider the very simple case of mapping between a regular 10×10 square array of points (V_{in}) and a regular 1×100 linear array of points (V_{out}). This is a paradigmatic example of dimension reduction (also used in Durbin & Mitchison, 1990 and Mitchison, 1995). It has the virtue that solutions are easily represented (see Figures 2 and 3) and easily compared with intuition. Calculation of the global optimum for this problem by exhaustive search is clearly impractical, since there are of the order of 100! possible mappings. Instead we employ simulated annealing (Kirkpatrick, Gelatt, & Vecchi, 1983) to find a solution close to optimal. The parameters used are given in the legend to Figure 2.

Figure 2 shows the best maps obtained by this method for the minimal path, minimal wiring, and metric MDS versions of the C measure. Also shown for comparison is a solution to this problem produced by the elastic net algorithm, taken from Durbin & Mitchison (1990). An optimal map for the minimal path version (A) is one with no diagonal segments. Our simulated annealing algorithm found one with three diagonal segments and a cost of 100.243, 1.3 percent larger than the optimal of 99.0. The optimal map for the minimal wiring measure has been explicitly calculated (Mitchison & Durbin, 1986), and has a cost of 914.0. Our algorithm found the map shown in (B), which is similar in shape and has a cost of 917.0 (0.3 percent larger than the optimal value). These results confirm that the simulated annealing algorithm employed can find close to optimal solutions. The cost for the

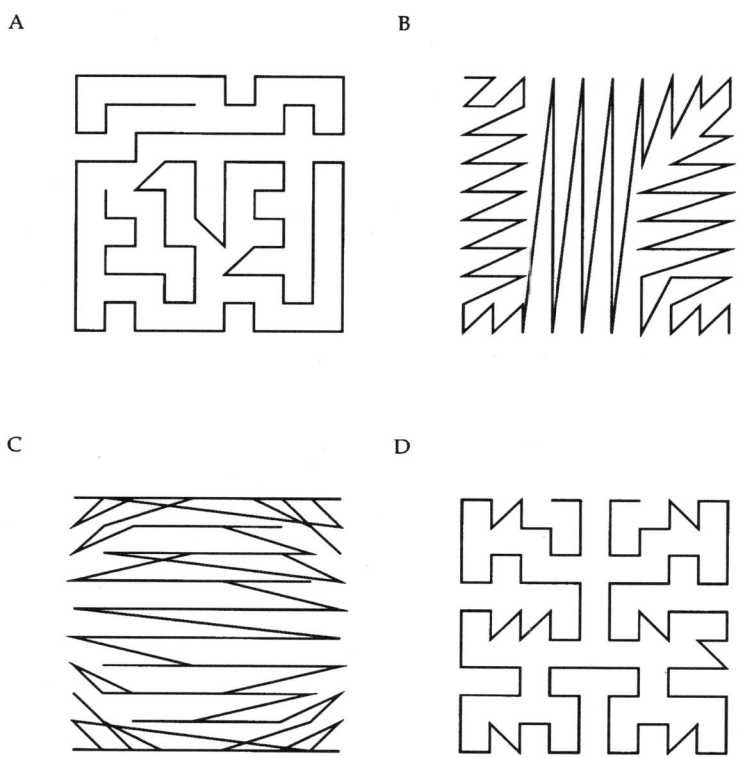

Figure 2: Maps found by optimizing using simulated annealing. (A) Minimal path length solution. (B) Minimal wiring solution. (C) Metric MDS solution. (D) Map found by the elastic net algorithm (see Durbin & Mitchison, 1990). Parameters used for simulated annealing were as follows (for further explanation, see van Larhoven & Aarts, 1987). Initial map: random. Move set: pairwise interchanges. Initial temperature: 3 × the mean energy difference over 10,000 moves. Cooling schedule: exponential. Cooling rate: 0.998. Acceptance criterion: 1000 moves at each temperature. Upper bound: 10,000 moves at each temperature. Stopping criterion: zero acceptances at upper bound.

metric MDS map (C) is 6,352,324. The illusion of multiple ends to the line is due to the map frequently doubling back on itself. For instance, in the fourth row up the square, the horizontal component for neighboring points in the line progresses in the order 5, 6, 4, 7, 3, 8, 2, 9, 10. Local discontinuity arises because this measure takes into account neighborhood preservation at all scales: local continuity is not privileged over global continuity. The costs of the map produced by the elastic net (D) are 102.3 for the minimal

Unifying Objective Function

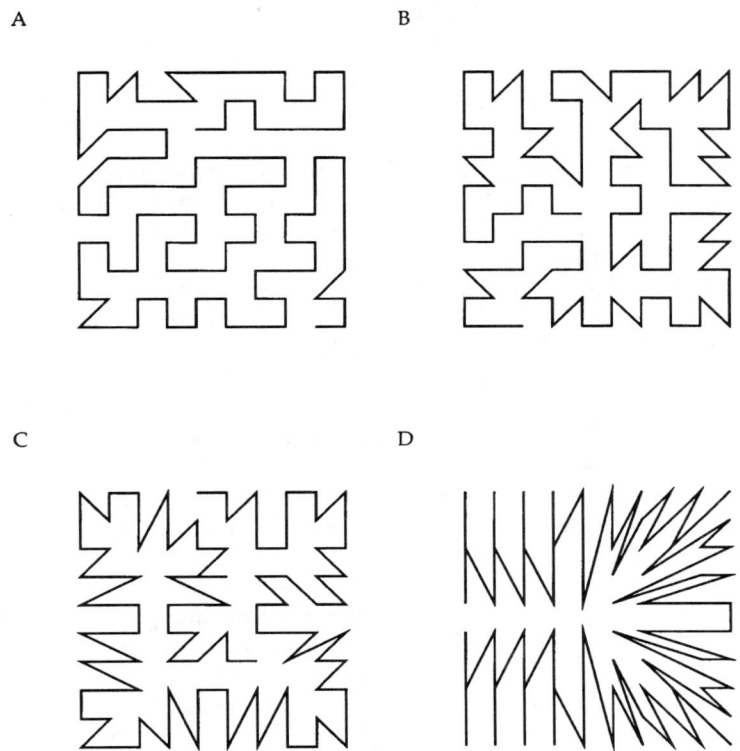

Figure 3: Minimal distortion solutions. (A) $\sigma = 1.0$, cost = 43.3. (B) $\sigma = 2.0$, cost = 214.7. (C) $\sigma = 4.0$, cost = 833.2. (D) $\sigma = 20.0$, cost = 18467.1. Simulated annealing parameters as in Figure 2.

path function, 1140 for the minimal wiring function, and 6,455,352 for the metric MDS function. In each case this is a higher cost than for the maps shown in (A), (B), and (C), respectively.

Figure 3 shows close-to-optimal maps for the minimal distortion version of the C measure (F is squared Euclidean distance in the square, G is given by e^{-d^2/σ^2} where d is Euclidean distance along the line), for varying σ. For small σ, the solution resembles the minimal path optimum of Figure 2A, since the contribution from more distant neighbors on the line compared to nearest neighbors is negligible. However, as σ increases, the map changes form. Local continuity becomes less important compared to continuity at the scale of σ, the map becomes spikier, and the number of large-scale folds in the map gradually decreases until at $\sigma = 20$ there is just one. This last map also shows some of the frequent doubling back behavior seen in Figure 2C.[1]

5 Discussion

5.1 Types of Mappings. Several qualitatively different types of map are apparent in Figures 2 and 3. For the metric MDS measure, Figure 2C, the line progresses through the square by a series of locally discontinuous jumps along one axis of the square and a comparatively smooth progression in the orthogonal direction. One consequence is that nearby points in the square never map too far apart on the line. For the minimal distortion measure with $\sigma = 20$ (see Figure 3D), the strategy is similar except that there is now one fold to the map. This decreases the size of local jumps in following the line through the square, at the cost of introducing a seam across which nearby points in the square map a very long way apart on the line. For the minimal distortion measure with small σ (see Figures 3A–C), the strategy is to introduce several folds. This gives strong local continuity, at the cost that now many points that are nearby in the square map to points that are far apart on the line.

What do these maps suggest about which measures are most appropriate for different problems? If it is desired that generally nearby points should always map to generally nearby points as much as possible in both directions, and one is not concerned about very local continuity, then something like the MDS measure is useful. This may be appropriate for some data visualization applications where the overall structure of the map is more important than the fine detail. If, on the other hand, one desires a smooth progression through the output space to imply a smooth progression through the input space, one should choose something like minimal path or minimal distortion for small σ. This may be important for data visualization where it is believed the data actually lie on a lower-dimensional manifold in the high-dimensional space. However, an important weakness of this representation is that some neighborhood relationships between points in the input space may be completely lost in the resulting representation. For understanding the structure of cortical mappings, self-organizing algorithms that optimize objectives of this type have proved useful (Durbin & Mitchison, 1990; Obermayer, Blasdel, & Schulten, 1992). However, very few other objectives have been applied to this problem, so it is still an open question which are most appropriate. The type of map seen in Figure 3D has not been much investigated. There may be some applications for which such maps are worthwhile, perhaps in a neurobiological context for understand-

---

[1] We have also explicitly optimized the objective functions proposed by Sammon (1969) and Bezdek and Pal (1995). The former produces a map similar to that of Figure 2C, while the latter resembles Figure 3D (for more details, see Goodhill & Sejnowski, 1996).

ing why different input variables are sometimes mapped into different areas rather than interdigitated in the same area.

5.2 Relation of C to Quadratic Assignment Problems. Formulating neighborhood preservation in terms of the C measure sets it within the well-studied class of quadratic assignment problems (QAPs). These occur in many different practical contexts and take the form of finding the minimal or maximal value of an equation similar to C (see Burkard, 1984, for a general review and Lawler, 1963, and Finke, Burkard, & Rendl, 1987, for more technical discussions). An illustrative example is the optimal design of typewriter keyboards (Burkard, 1984). If $F(i, j)$ is the average time it takes a typist to sequentially press locations i and j on the keyboard, while $G(p, q)$ is the average frequency with which letters p and q appear sequentially in the text of a given language (note that in this example F and G are not necessarily symmetrical), then the keyboard that minimizes average typing time will be the one that minimizes the product

$$\sum_{i=1}^{N}\sum_{j=1}^{N} F(i, j) G(M(i), M(j))$$

(see equation 2.1), where $M(i)$ is the letter that maps to location i. The substantial amount of theory developed for QAPs is directly applicable to the C measure. As a concrete example, QAP theory provides several different ways of calculating bounds on the minimum and maximum values of C for each problem. This could be very useful for the problem of assessing the quality of a map relative to the unknown best possible. One particular case is the eigenvalue bound (Finke et al., 1987). If the eigenvalues of symmetric matrices F and G are λ_i and μ_i, respectively, such that $\lambda_1 \leq \lambda_2 \leq \cdots \leq \lambda_n$ and $\mu_1 \geq \mu_2 \geq \cdots \geq \mu_n$, then it can be shown that $\sum_i \lambda_i \mu_i$ gives a lower bound on the value of C.

QAPs are in general known to be of complexity NP-hard. A large number of algorithms for both exact and heuristic solution have been studied (see, e.g., Burkard, 1984; the references in Finke et al., 1987; and Simić, 1991). However, particular instantiations of F and G may allow efficient algorithms for finding good local optima, or alternatively may beset C with many bad local optima. Such considerations provide an additional practical constraint on what choices of F and G are most appropriate.

5.3 Many-to-One Mappings. In many practical contexts, there are many more points in V_{in} than V_{out}, and it is necessary also to specify a many-to-one mapping from points in V_{in} to N exemplar points in V_{in}, where N = number of points in V_{out}. It may be desirable to do this adaptively while simultaneously optimizing the form of the map from V_{in} to V_{out}. For instance, shifting a point from one cluster to another may increase the clustering cost, but by moving the positions of the cluster centers decrease the sum of this and the continuity cost. The elastic net, for instance, trades off these two contributions explicitly with a ratio that changes during the minimization, so that finally each cluster contains only one point and the continuity cost dominates (Durbin & Willshaw, 1987; for discussions, see Simíc, 1990, and Yuille, 1990). The self-organizing map of Kohonen (1982) trades off these two contributions implicitly. Luttrell (1994) discusses allowing each point in the input space to map to many in the output space in a probabilistic manner, and vice-versa. The H function (Bienenstock & von der Malsburg, 1987a, 1987b) offers an alternative way of introducing a weighted match between input and output points.

Acknowledgments

We thank Steve Finch for very useful discussions at an earlier stage of this work. We are grateful to Graeme Mitchison, Steve Luttrell, Hans-Ulrich Bauer, and Laurenz Wiskott for helpful discussions and comments on the manuscript. Research was supported by the Sloan Center for Theoretical Neurobiology at the Salk Institute and the Howard Hughes Medical Institute.

References

Bezdek, J. C., & Pal, N. R. (1995). An index of topological preservation for feature extraction. *Pattern Recognition* 28:381–391.

Bienenstock, E., & von der Malsburg, C. (1987a). A neural network for the retrieval of superimposed connection patterns. *Europhys. Lett.* 3:1243–1249.

Bienenstock, E., & von der Malsburg, C. (1987b). A neural network for invariant pattern recognition. *Europhys. Lett.* 4:121–126.

Burkard, R. E. (1984). Quadratic assignment problems. *Europ. J. Oper. Res.* 15:283–289.

Durbin, R., & Mitchison, G. (1990). A dimension reduction framework for understanding cortical maps. *Nature* 343:644–647.

Durbin, R., & Willshaw, D. J. (1987). An analogue approach to the traveling salesman problem using an elastic net method. *Nature* 326:689–691.

Finke, G., Burkard, R. E., & Rendl, F. (1987). Quadratic assignment problems. *Annals of Discrete Mathematics* 31:61–82.

Goodhill, G. J., & Sejnowski, T. J. (1996). Quantifying neighbourhood preservation in topographic mappings. In *Proceedings of the 3rd Joint Symposium on Neural Computation* (pp. 61–82). Pasadena: California Institute of Technology. Available from http://www.cnl.salk.edu/~geoff/.

Goodhill, G. J., & Willshaw, D. J. (1990). Application of the elastic net algorithm to the formation of ocular dominance stripes. *Network* 1:41–59.

Hardy, G. H., Littlewood, J. E., & Pólya, G. (1934). *Inequalities*. Cambridge: Cambridge University Press.

Jones, D. G., Van Sluyters, R. C., & Murphy, K. M. (1991). A computational model for the overall pattern of ocular dominance. *J. Neurosci.* 11:3794–3808.

Kirkpatrick, S., Gelatt, C. D., & Vecchi, M. P. (1983). Optimization by simulated annealing. *Science* 220:671-680.
Kohonen, T. (1982). Self-organized formation of topologically correct feature maps. *Biol. Cybern.* 43:59-69.
Lawler, E. L. (1963). The quadratic assignment problem. *Management Science* 9:586-599.
Luttrell, S. P. (1990). Derivation of a class of training algorithms. *IEEE Trans. Neural Networks* 1:229-232.
Luttrell, S. P. (1994). A Bayesian analysis of self-organizing maps. *Neural Computation* 6:767-794.
Mitchison, G. (1995). A type of duality between self-organizing maps and minimal wiring. *Neural Computation* 7:25-35.
Mitchison, G., & Durbin, R. (1986). Optimal numberings of an $N \times N$ array. *SIAM J. Alg. Disc. Meth.* 7:571-581.
Obermayer, K., Blasdel, G. G., & Schulten, K. (1992). Statistical-mechanical analysis of self-organization and pattern formation during the development of visual maps. *Phys. Rev. A* 45:7568-7589.
Sammon, J. W. (1969). A nonlinear mapping for data structure analysis. *IEEE Trans. Comput.* 18:401-409.
Shepard, R. N. (1980). Multidimensional scaling, tree-fitting and clustering. *Science* 210:390-398.
Simić, P. D. (1990). Statistical mechanics as the underlying theory of "elastic" and "neural" optimizations. *Network* 1:89-103.
Simić, P. D. (1991). Constrained nets for graph matching and other quadratic assignment problems. *Neural Computation* 3:268-281.
Torgerson, W. S. (1952). Multidimensional scaling, I: Theory and method. *Psychometrika* 17:401-419.
van Laarhoven, P. J. M., & Aarts, E. H. L. (1987). *Simulated annealing: Theory and applications*. Dordrecht: Reidel.
Wiskott, L., & Sejnowski, T. J. (1997). Objective functions for neural map formation (Tech. Rep. INC-9701). Institute for Neural Computation.
Young, F. W. (1987). *Multidimensional scaling: History, theory, and applications*. Hillsdale, NJ: Erlbaum.
Yuille, A. L. (1990). Generalized deformable models, statistical physics, and matching problems. *Neural Computation* 2:1-24.

6

Constrained Optimization for Neural Map Formation: A Unifying Framework for Weight Growth and Normalization

Laurenz Wiskott
Computational Neurobiology Laboratory, Salk Institute for Biological Studies, San Diego, CA 92186-5800, U.S.A. http://www.cnl.salk.edu/CNL/

Terrence Sejnowski
Computational Neurobiology Laboratory, Howard Hughes Medical Institute, Salk Institute for Biological Studies, San Diego, CA 92186-5800, U.S.A.
Department of Biology, University of California, San Diego, La Jolla, CA 92093, U.S.A.

Computational models of neural map formation can be considered on at least three different levels of abstraction: detailed models including neural activity dynamics, weight dynamics that abstract from the neural activity dynamics by an adiabatic approximation, and constrained optimization from which equations governing weight dynamics can be derived. Constrained optimization uses an objective function, from which a weight growth rule can be derived as a gradient flow, and some constraints, from which normalization rules are derived. In this article, we present an example of how an optimization problem can be derived from detailed nonlinear neural dynamics. A systematic investigation reveals how different weight dynamics introduced previously can be derived from two types of objective function terms and two types of constraints. This includes dynamic link matching as a special case of neural map formation. We focus in particular on the role of coordinate transformations to derive different weight dynamics from the same optimization problem. Several examples illustrate how the constrained optimization framework can help in understanding, generating, and comparing different models of neural map formation. The techniques used in this analysis may also be useful in investigating other types of neural dynamics.

1 Introduction

Neural maps are an important motif in the structural organization of the brain. The best-studied maps are those in the early visual system. For example, the retinotectal map connects a two-dimensional array of ganglion cells in the retina to a corresponding map of the visual field in the optic tectum of vertebrates in a neighborhood-preserving fashion. These are called topographic maps. The map from the lateral geniculate nucleus (LGN) to the primary visual cortex (V1) is more complex because the inputs coming from

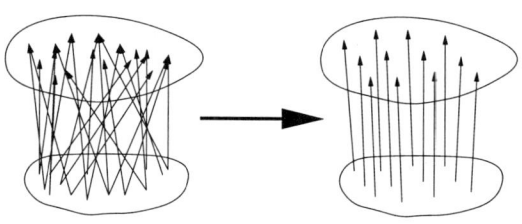

Figure 1: Goal of neural map formation: The initially random all-to-all connectivity self-organizes into an orderly connectivity that appropriately reflects the correlations within the input stimuli and the induced correlations within the output layer. The output correlations also depend on the connectivity within the output layer.

LGN include signals from both eyes and are unoriented, but most cells in V1 are tuned for orientation, an emergent property. Neurons with preferred orientation and ocular dominance in area V1 form a columnar structure, where neurons responding to the same eye or the same orientation tend to be neighbors. Other neural maps are formed in the somatosensory, the auditory, and the motor systems. All neural maps connect an input layer, possibly divided into different parts (e.g., left and right eye), to an output layer. Each neuron in the output layer can potentially receive input from all neurons in the input layer (here we ignore the limits imposed by restricted axonal arborization and dendritic extension). However, particular receptive fields develop due to a combination of genetically determined and activity-driven mechanisms for self-organization. Although cortical maps have many feedback projections (for example, from area V1 back to the LGN), these are disregarded in most models of map formation and will not be considered here.

The goal of neural map formation is to self-organize from an initial random all-to-all connectivity a regular pattern of connectivity, as in Figure 1, for the purpose of producing a representation of the input on the output layer that is of further use to the system. The development of the structure depends on the architecture, the lateral connectivity, the initial conditions, and the weight dynamics, including growth rule and normalization rules.

The first model of map formation, introduced by von der Malsburg (1973), was for a small patch of retina stimulated with bars of different orientation. The model self-organized orientation columns, with neighboring neurons having receptive fields tuned to similar orientation. This model already included all the crucial ingredients important for map formation: (1) characteristic correlations within the stimulus patterns, (2) lateral interactions within the output layer, inducing characteristic correlations there

Neural Map Formation

as well, (3) Hebbian weight modification, and (4) competition between synapses by weight normalization. Many similar models have been proposed since then for different types of map formation (see Erwin, Obermayer, & Schulten, 1995; Swindale, 1996; and Table 2 for examples). We do not consider models that are based on chemical markers (e.g., von der Malsburg & Willshaw, 1977). Although they may be conceptionally similar to those based on neural activities, they can differ significantly in the detailed mathematical formulation. Nor do we consider in detail models that treat the input layer as a low-dimensional space, say two-dimensional for the retina, from which input vectors are drawn (e.g., Kohonen, 1982, but see section 6.8). The output neurons then receive only two synapses per neuron, one for each input dimension.

The dynamic link matching model (e.g., Bienenstock & von der Malsburg, 1987; Konen, Maurer, & von der Malsburg, 1994) is a form of neural map formation that has been developed for pattern recognition. It is mathematically similar to the self-organization of retinotectal projections; in addition, each neuron has a visual feature attached, so that a neural layer can be considered as a labeled graph representing a visual pattern. Each synapse has associated with it an individual value, which affects the dynamics and expresses the similarity between the features of connected neurons. The self-organization process then not only tends to generate a neighborhood preserving map, it also tends to connect neurons having similar features. If the two layers represent similar patterns, the map formation dynamics finds the correct feature correspondences and connects the corresponding neurons.

Models of map formation have been investigated by analysis (e.g., Amari, 1980; Häussler & von der Malsburg, 1983) and computer simulations. An important tool for both methods is the objective function (or energy function) from which the dynamics can be generated as a gradient flow. The objective value (or energy) can be used to estimate which weight configurations would be more likely to arise from the dynamics (e.g., MacKay & Miller, 1990). In computer simulations, the objective function is maximized (or the energy function is minimized) numerically in order to find stable solutions of the dynamics (e.g., Linsker, 1986; Bienenstock & von der Malsburg, 1987).

Objective functions, which can also serve as a Lyapunov function, have many advantages. First, the existence of an objective function guarantees that the dynamics does not have limit cycles or chaotic attractors as solutions. Second, an objective function often provides more direct and intuitive insight into the behavior of a dynamics, and the effects of each term can be understood more easily. Third, an objective function allows additional mathematical tools to be used to analyze the system, such as methods from statistical physics. Finally, an objective function provides connections to more abstract models, such as spin systems, which have been studied in depth.

Although objective functions have been used before in the context of neural map formation, they have not yet been investigated systematically. The goal of this article is to derive objective functions for a wide variety of models. Although growth rules can be derived from objective functions as gradient flows, normalization rules are derived from constraints by various methods. Thus, objective functions and constraints have to be considered in conjunction and form a constrained optimization problem. We show that although two models may differ in the formulation of their dynamics, they may be derived from the same constrained optimization problem, thus providing a unifying framework for the two models. The equivalence between different dynamics is revealed by coordinate transformations. A major focus of this article is therefore on the effects of coordinate transformations on weight growth rules and normalization rules.

1.1 Model Architecture. The general architecture considered here consists of two layers of neurons, an input and an output layer, as in Figure 2. (We use the term *layer* for a population of neurons without assuming a particular geometry.) Input neurons are indicated by ρ (retina) and output neurons by τ (tectum); the index ν can indicate a neuron in either layer. Neural activities are indicated by a. Input neurons are connected all-to-all to output neurons, but there are no connections back to the input layer. Thus, the dynamics in the input layer is completely independent of the output layer and can be described by mean activities $\langle a_\rho \rangle$ and correlations $\langle a_\rho, a_{\rho'} \rangle$. Effective lateral connections within a layer are denoted by $D_{\rho\rho'}$ and $D_{\tau\tau'}$; connections projecting from the input to the output layer are denoted by $w_{\tau\rho}$. The second index always indicates the presynaptic neuron and the first index the postsynaptic neuron. The lateral connections defined here are called *effective*, because they need not correspond to physical connections. For example, in the input layer, the effective lateral connections represent the correlations between input neurons regardless of what induced the correlations, $D_{\rho\rho'} = \langle a_\rho, a_{\rho'} \rangle$. In the example below, the output layer has short-term excitatory and long-term inhibitory connections; the effective lateral connections, however, are only excitatory. The effective lateral connections thus represent functional properties of the lateral interactions and not the anatomical connectivity itself.

To make the notation simpler, we use the definitions $i = \{\rho, \tau\}$, $j = \{\rho', \tau'\}$, $A_{ij} = D_{\tau\tau'} A_{\rho'} = D_{\tau\tau'} \langle a_{\rho'} \rangle$, and $D_{ij} = D_{\tau\tau'} D_{\rho\rho'} = D_{\tau\tau'} \langle a_\rho, a_{\rho'} \rangle$ in section 3 and later. We assume symmetric matrices $A_{ij} = A_{ji}$ and $D_{ij} = D_{ji}$, which requires some homogeneity of the architecture, that is, $\langle a_\rho \rangle = \langle a_{\rho'} \rangle$, $\langle a_\rho, a_{\rho'} \rangle = \langle a_{\rho'}, a_\rho \rangle$, and $D_{\tau\tau'} = D_{\tau'\tau}$.

In the next section, a simple model is used to demonstrate the basic procedure for deriving a constrained optimization problem from detailed neural dynamics. This procedure has three steps. First, the neural dynamics is transformed into a weight dynamics, where the induced correlations are expressed directly in terms of the synaptic weights, thus eliminating neu-

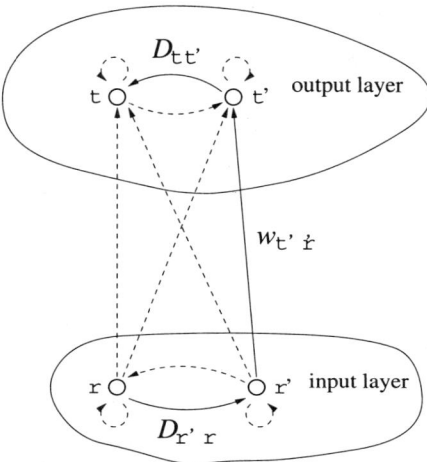

Figure 2: General architecture: Neurons in the input layer are connected all-to-all to neurons in the output layer. Each layer has effective lateral connections D representing functional aspects of the lateral connectivity (e.g., characteristic correlations). As an example, a path through which activity can propagate from neuron ρ to neuron τ is shown by solid arrows. Other connections are shown as dashed arrows.

ral activities from the dynamics by an adiabatic approximation. Second, an objective function is constructed, which can generate the dynamics of the growth rule as a gradient flow. Third, the normalization rules need to be considered and, if possible, derived from constraint functions. The last two steps depend on each other insofar as growth rule, as well as normalization rules, must be inferred under the same coordinate transformation. The three important aspects of this example—deriving correlations, constructing objective functions, and considering the constraints—are then discussed in greater detail in the following three sections, respectively. Readers may skip section 2 and continue directly with these more abstract considerations beginning in section 3. In section 6, several examples are given for how the constrained optimization framework can be used to understand, generate, and compare models of neural map formation.

2 Prototypical System

As a concrete example, consider a slightly modified version of the dynamics proposed by Willshaw and von der Malsburg (1976) for the self-organization of a retinotectal map, where the input and output layer correspond to retina and tectum, respectively. The dynamics is qualitatively described by the following set of differential equations:

Neural activity dynamics

$$\dot{m}_\rho = -m_\rho + (k * a_{\rho'})_\rho \tag{2.1}$$

$$\dot{m}_\tau = -m_\tau + (k * a_{\tau'})_\tau + \sum_{\rho'} w_{\tau\rho'} a_{\rho'} \tag{2.2}$$

Weight growth rule

$$\dot{w}_{\tau\rho} = a_\tau a_\rho \tag{2.3}$$

Weight normalization rules

$$\text{if } w_{\tau\rho} < 0 : w_{\tau\rho} = 0 \tag{2.4}$$

$$\text{if } \sum_{\rho'} w_{\tau\rho'} > 1 : w_{\tau\rho} = \tilde{w}_{\tau\rho} + \frac{1}{M_\tau}\left(1 - \sum_{\rho'} \tilde{w}_{\tau\rho'}\right) \quad \text{for all } \rho \tag{2.5}$$

$$\text{if } \sum_{\tau'} w_{\tau'\rho} > 1 : w_{\tau\rho} = \tilde{w}_{\tau\rho} + \frac{1}{M_\rho}\left(1 - \sum_{\tau'} \tilde{w}_{\tau'\rho}\right) \quad \text{for all } \tau \tag{2.6}$$

where m denotes the membrane potential, $a_\nu = \sigma(m_\nu)$ is the mean firing rate determined by a nonlinear input-output function σ, $(k * a_{\nu'})$ indicates a convolution of the neural activities with the kernel k representing lateral connections with local excitation and global inhibition, $\tilde{w}_{\tau\rho}$ indicates weights as obtained by integrating the differential equations for one time step, that is, $\tilde{w}_{\tau\rho}(t+\Delta t) = w_{\tau\rho}(t) + \Delta t\, \dot{w}_{\tau\rho}(t)$, M_τ is the number of links terminating on output neuron τ, and M_ρ is the number of links originating from input neuron ρ. Equations 2.1 and 2.2 govern the neural activity dynamics on the two layers, equation 2.3 is the growth rule for the synaptic weights, and equations 2.4–2.6 are the normalization rules that keep the sums over synaptic weights originating from an input neuron or terminating on an output neuron equal to 1 and prevent the weights from becoming negative. Notice that since the discussion is qualitative, we included only the basic terms and discarded some parameters required to make the system work properly. One difference from the original model is that subtractive instead of multiplicative normalization rules are used.

2.1 Correlations. The dynamics within the neural layers is well understood (Amari, 1977; Konen et al., 1994). Local excitation and global inhibition lead to the development of a local patch of activity, called a *blob*. The shape and size of the blob depend on the kernel k and other parameters of the

Neural Map Formation

system and can be described by $B_{\rho'\rho_0}$ if centered on input neuron ρ_0 and $B_{\tau'\tau_0}$ if centered on output neuron τ_0. The location of the blob depends on the input, which is assumed to be weak enough that it does not change the shape of the blob. Assume the input layer receives noise such that the blob arises with equal probability $p(\rho_0) = 1/R$ centered on any of the input neurons, where R is the number of input neurons. For simplicity we assume cyclic boundary conditions to avoid boundary effects. The location of the blob in the output layer, on the other hand, is affected by the input,

$$i_{\tau'}(\rho_0) = \sum_{\rho'} w_{\tau'\rho'} B_{\rho'\rho_0}, \tag{2.7}$$

received from the input layer and therefore depends on the position ρ_0 of the blob in the input layer. Only one blob can occur in each layer, and the two layers need to be reset before new blobs can arise. A sequence of blobs is required to induce the appropriate correlations.

Konen et al. (1994) have shown that without noise, blobs in the output layer will arise at location τ_0 with the largest overlap between input $i_{\tau'}(\rho_0)$ and the final blob profile $B_{\tau'\tau_0}$, that is, the location for which $\sum_{\tau'} B_{\tau'\tau_0} i_{\tau'}(\rho_0)$ is maximal. This winner-take-all behavior makes it difficult to analyze the system. We therefore make the assumption that in contrast to this deterministic dynamics, the blob arises at location τ_0 with a probability equal to the overlap between the input and blob activity,

$$p(\tau_0|\rho_0) = \sum_{\tau'} B_{\tau'\tau_0} i_{\tau'}(\rho_0) = \sum_{\tau'\rho'} B_{\tau'\tau_0} w_{\tau'\rho'} B_{\rho'\rho_0}. \tag{2.8}$$

Assume the blobs are normalized such that $\sum_{\rho'} B_{\rho'\rho_0} = 1$ and $\sum_{\tau_0} B_{\tau'\tau_0} = 1$ and that the connectivity is normalized such that $\sum_{\tau'} w_{\tau'\rho'} = 1$, which is the case for the system above if the input layer does not have more neurons than the output layer. This implies $\sum_{\tau'} i_{\tau'}(\rho_0) = 1$ and $\sum_{\tau_0} p(\tau_0|\rho_0) = 1$ and justifies the interpretation of $p(\tau_0|\rho_0)$ as a probability.

Although it is plausible that such a probabilistic blob location could be approximated by noise in the output layer, it is difficult to develop a concrete model. For a similar but more algorithmic activity model (Obermayer, Ritter, & Schulten, 1990), an exact noise model for the probabilistic blob location can be formulated (see the appendix). With equation 3.8 the probability for a particular combination of blob locations is

$$p(\tau_0, \rho_0) = p(\tau_0|\rho_0) p(\rho_0) = \sum_{\tau'\rho'} B_{\tau'\tau_0} w_{\tau'\rho'} B_{\rho'\rho_0} \frac{1}{R}, \tag{2.9}$$

and the correlation between two neurons defined as the average product of their activities is

$$\langle a_\tau a_\rho \rangle = \sum_{\tau_0 \rho_0} p(\tau_0, \rho_0) B_{\tau\tau_0} B_{\rho\rho_0} \tag{2.10}$$

$$= \sum_{\tau_0 \rho_0} \sum_{\tau' \rho'} B_{\tau' \tau_0} w_{\tau' \rho'} B_{\rho' \rho_0} \frac{1}{R} B_{\tau \tau_0} B_{\rho \rho_0} \qquad (2.11)$$

$$= \frac{1}{R} \sum_{\tau' \rho'} \left(\sum_{\tau_0} B_{\tau' \tau_0} B_{\tau \tau_0} \right) w_{\tau' \rho'} \left(\sum_{\rho_0} B_{\rho' \rho_0} B_{\rho \rho_0} \right) \qquad (2.12)$$

$$= \frac{1}{R} \sum_{\tau' \rho'} \bar{B}_{\tau \tau'} w_{\tau' \rho'} \bar{B}_{\rho' \rho}, \qquad \text{with } \bar{B}_{\nu' \nu} = \sum_{\nu_0} B_{\nu' \nu_0} B_{\nu \nu_0}, \qquad (2.13)$$

where the brackets $\langle \cdot \rangle$ indicate the ensemble average over a large number of blob presentations. $\frac{1}{R} \bar{B}_{\rho' \rho}$ and $\bar{B}_{\tau \tau'}$ are the effective lateral connectivities of the input and the output layer, respectively, and are symmetrical even if the individual blobs $B_{\rho \rho_0}$ and $B_{\tau \tau_0}$ are not, that is, $D_{\rho' \rho} = \frac{1}{R} \bar{B}_{\rho' \rho}, D_{\tau \tau'} = \bar{B}_{\tau \tau'}$, and $D_{ij} = D_{ji} = D_{\tau \tau'} D_{\rho' \rho} = \frac{1}{R} \bar{B}_{\tau \tau'} \bar{B}_{\rho' \rho}$. Notice the linear relation between the weights $w_{\tau' \rho'}$ and the correlations $\langle a_\tau a_\rho \rangle$ in the probabilistic blob model (see equation 2.13).

Substituting the correlation into equation 2.3 for the weight dynamics leads to:

$$\langle \dot{w}_{\tau \rho} \rangle = \langle a_\tau a_\rho \rangle = \frac{1}{R} \sum_{\tau' \rho'} \bar{B}_{\tau \tau'} w_{\tau' \rho'} \bar{B}_{\rho' \rho}. \qquad (2.14)$$

The same normalization rules given above (equations 2.4–2.6) apply to this dynamics. Since there is little danger of confusion, we neglect the averaging brackets for $\langle \dot{w}_{\tau \rho} \rangle$ in subsequent equations and simply write $\dot{w}_{\tau \rho} = \langle a_\tau, a_\rho \rangle$.

Although we did not give a mathematical model of the mechanism by which the probabilistic blob location as given in equation 2.8 could be implemented, it may be interesting to note that the probabilistic approach can be generalized to other activity patterns, such as stripe patterns or hexagons, which can be generated by Mexican hat interaction functions (local excitation, finite-range inhibition) (von der Malsburg, 1973; Ermentrout & Cowan, 1979). If the probability for a stripe pattern's arising in the output layer is linear in its overlap with the input, the same derivation follows, though the indices ρ_0 and τ_0 will then refer to phase and orientation of the patterns rather than location of the blobs.

Using the probabilistic blob location in the output layer instead of the deterministic one is analogous to the soft competitive learning proposed by Nowlan (1990) as an alternative to hard (or winner-take-all) competitive learning. Nowlan demonstrated superior performance of soft competition over hard competition for a radial basis function network tested on recognition of handwritten characters and spoken vowels, and suggested there might be a similar advantage for neural map formation. The probabilistic blob location induced by noise might help improve neural map formation by avoiding local optima.

2.2 Objective Function.

The next step is to find an objective function that generates the dynamics as a gradient flow. For the above example, a suitable objective function is

$$H(\mathbf{w}) = \frac{1}{2R} \sum_{\tau\rho\tau'\rho'} w_{\tau\rho} \bar{B}_{\rho\rho'} \bar{B}_{\tau\tau'} w_{\tau'\rho'}, \qquad (2.15)$$

since it yields equation 2.14 from $\dot{w}_{\tau\rho} = \frac{\partial H(\mathbf{w})}{\partial w_{\tau\rho}}$, taking into account that $\bar{B}_{vv'} = \bar{B}_{v'v}$.

2.3 Constraints.

The normalization rules given above ensure that synaptic weights do not become negative and that the sums over synaptic weights originating from an input neuron or terminating on an output neuron do not become larger than 1. This can be written in the form of inequalities for constraint functions g:

$$g_{\tau\rho}(\mathbf{w}) = w_{\tau\rho} \geq 0, \qquad (2.16)$$

$$g_\tau(\mathbf{w}) = 1 - \sum_{\rho'} w_{\tau\rho'} \geq 0, \qquad (2.17)$$

$$g_\rho(\mathbf{w}) = 1 - \sum_{\tau'} w_{\tau'\rho} \geq 0. \qquad (2.18)$$

These constraints define a region within which the objective function is to be maximized by steepest ascent. While the constraints follow uniquely from the normalization rules, the converse is not true. In general, there are various normalization rules that would enforce or at least approximate the constraints, but only some of them are compatible with the constrained optimization framework. As shown in section 5.2.1, compatible normalization rules can be obtained by the method of Lagrangian multipliers. If a constraint g_x, $x \in \{\tau\rho, \tau, \rho\}$ is violated, a normalization rule of the form

$$\text{if } g_x(\tilde{\mathbf{w}}) < 0: \quad w_{\tau\rho} = \tilde{w}_{\tau\rho} + \lambda_x \frac{\partial g_x}{\partial \tilde{w}_{\tau\rho}} \quad \text{for all } \tau\rho, \qquad (2.19)$$

has to be applied, where λ_x is a Lagrangian multiplier and determined such that $g_x(\mathbf{w}) = 0$. This method actually leads to equations 2.4–2.6, which are therefore a compatible set of normalization rules for the constraints above. This is necessary to make the formulation as a constrained optimization problem (see equations 2.15–2.18) an appropriate description of the original dynamics (see equations 2.3–2.6).

This example illustrates the general scheme by which a detailed model dynamics for neural map formation can be transformed into a constrained optimization problem. The correlations, objective functions, and constraints are discussed in greater detail and for a wide variety of models below.

3 Correlations

In the above example, correlations in a highly nonlinear dynamics led to a linear relationship between synaptic weights and the induced correlations. We derived effective lateral connections in the input as well as the output layer mediating these correlations. Corresponding equations for the correlations have been derived for other, mostly linear activity models (e.g., Linsker, 1986; Miller, 1990; von der Malsburg, 1995), as summarized here.

Assume the dynamics in the input layer is described by neural activities $a_\rho(t) \in \mathbb{R}$, which yield mean activities $\langle a_\rho \rangle$ and correlations $\langle a_\rho, a_{\rho'} \rangle$. The input received by the output layer is assumed to be a linear superposition of the activities of the input neurons:

$$i_{\tau'} = \sum_{\rho'} w_{\tau'\rho'} a_{\rho'}. \tag{3.1}$$

This input then produces activity in the output layer through effective lateral connections in a linear fashion:

$$a_\tau = \sum_{\tau'} D_{\tau\tau'} i_{\tau'} = \sum_{\tau'\rho'} D_{\tau\tau'} w_{\tau'\rho'} a_{\rho'}. \tag{3.2}$$

As seen in the above example, this linear behavior could be generated by a nonlinear model. Thus, the neurons need not be linear, only the effective behavior of the correlations (cf. Sejnowski, 1976; Ginzburg & Sompolinsky, 1994). The mean activity of output neurons is

$$\langle a_\tau \rangle = \sum_{\tau'\rho'} D_{\tau\tau'} w_{\tau'\rho'} \langle a_{\rho'} \rangle = \sum_j A_{ij} w_j. \tag{3.3}$$

Assuming a linear correlation function ($\langle a_\rho, \alpha(a_{\rho'} + a_{\rho''}) \rangle = \alpha \langle a_\rho, a_{\rho'} \rangle + \alpha \langle a_\rho, a_{\rho''} \rangle$ with a real constant α) such as the average product or the covariance (Sejnowski, 1977), the correlation between input and output neurons is

$$\langle a_\tau, a_\rho \rangle = \sum_{\tau'\rho'} D_{\tau\tau'} w_{\tau'\rho'} \langle a_{\rho'}, a_\rho \rangle = \sum_j D_{ij} w_j. \tag{3.4}$$

Note that $i = \{\rho, \tau\}$, $j = \{\rho', \tau'\}$, $A_{ij} = A_{ji} = D_{\tau\tau'} A_{\rho'} = D_{\tau\tau'} \langle a_{\rho'} \rangle$, and $D_{ij} = D_{ji} = D_{\tau\tau'} D_{\rho'\rho} = D_{\tau\tau'} \langle a_{\rho'}, a_\rho \rangle$. Since the right-hand sides of equations 3.3 and 3.4 are formally equivalent, we will consider only the latter one in the further analysis, bearing in mind that equation 3.3 is included as a special case.

In this linear correlation model, all variables may assume negative values. This may not be plausible for the neural activities a_ρ and a_τ. However,

Neural Map Formation

equation 3.4 can be derived also for nonnegative activities, and a similar equation as equation 3.3 can be derived if the mean activities $\langle a_\rho \rangle$ are positive. The difference for the latter would be an additional constant, which can always be compensated for in the growth rule.

The correlation model in Linsker (1986) differs from the linear one introduced here in two respects. The input (see equation 3.1) has an additional constant term, and correlations are defined by subtracting positive constants from the activities. However, it can be shown that correlations in the model in Linsker (1986) are a linear combination of a constant and the terms of equations 3.3 and 3.4.

4 Objective Functions

In general, there is no systematic way of finding an objective function for a particular dynamical system, but it is possible to determine whether there exists an objective function. The necessary and sufficient condition is that the flow field of the dynamics be curl free. If there exists an objective function $H(\mathbf{w})$ with continuous partial derivatives of order two that generates the dynamics $\dot{w}_i = \partial H(\mathbf{w})/\partial w_i$, then

$$\frac{\partial \dot{w}_i}{\partial w_j} = \frac{\partial^2 H(\mathbf{w})}{\partial w_j \partial w_i} = \frac{\partial^2 H(\mathbf{w})}{\partial w_i \partial w_j} = \frac{\partial \dot{w}_j}{\partial w_i}. \tag{4.1}$$

The existence of an objective function is thus equivalent to $\partial \dot{w}_i/\partial w_j = \partial \dot{w}_j/\partial w_i$, which can be checked easily. For the dynamics given by

$$\dot{w}_i = \sum_j D_{ij} w_j \tag{4.2}$$

(cf. equation 2.14), for example, $\partial \dot{w}_i/\partial w_j = D_{ij} = \partial \dot{w}_j/\partial w_i$, which shows that it can be generated as a gradient flow. A suitable objective function is

$$H(\mathbf{w}) = \frac{1}{2} \sum_{ij} w_i D_{ij} w_j \tag{4.3}$$

(cf. equation 2.15), since it yields $\dot{w}_i = \partial H(\mathbf{w})/\partial w_i$.

A dynamics that cannot be generated by an objective function directly is

$$\dot{w}_i = w_i \sum_j D_{ij} w_j, \tag{4.4}$$

as used in Häussler and von der Malsburg (1983), since for $i \neq j$ we obtain $\partial \dot{w}_i/\partial w_j = w_i D_{ij} \neq w_j D_{ji} = \partial \dot{w}_j/\partial w_i$, and $\dot{w}_i$ is not curl free. However, it is sometimes possible to convert a dynamics with curl into a curl-free dynamics by a coordinate transformation. Applying the transformation $w_i = \frac{1}{4}v_i^2$ ($\mathcal{C}^w$) to equation 4.4 yields

$$\dot{v}_i = \frac{dv_i}{dw_i}\dot{w}_i = \sqrt{w_i}\sum_j D_{ij}w_j = \frac{1}{2}v_i\sum_j D_{ij}\frac{1}{4}v_j^2, \qquad (4.5)$$

which is curl free, since $\partial \dot{v}_i/\partial v_j = \frac{1}{2}v_i D_{ij}\frac{1}{2}v_j = \partial \dot{v}_j/\partial v_i$. Thus, the dynamics of $\dot{v}_i$ in the new coordinate system $\mathcal{V}^w$ can be generated as a gradient flow. A suitable objective function is

$$H(\mathbf{v}) = \frac{1}{2}\sum_{ij}\frac{1}{4}v_i^2 D_{ij}\frac{1}{4}v_j^2, \qquad (4.6)$$

since it yields $\dot{v}_i = \partial H(\mathbf{v})/\partial v_i$. Transforming the dynamics of $\mathbf{v}$ back into the original coordinate system $\mathcal{W}$, of course, yields the original dynamics in equation 4.4:

$$\dot{w}_i = \frac{dw_i}{dv_i}\dot{v}_i = \frac{1}{4}v_i^2\sum_j D_{ij}\frac{1}{4}v_j^2 = w_i\sum_j D_{ij}w_j. \qquad (4.7)$$

Coordinate transformations thus can provide objective functions for dynamics that are not curl free. Notice that $H(\mathbf{v})$ is the same objective function as $H(\mathbf{w})$ (see equation 4.3) evaluated in $\mathcal{V}^w$ instead of $\mathcal{W}$. Thus $H(\mathbf{v}) = H(\mathbf{w}(\mathbf{v}))$ and H is a Lyapunov function for both dynamics.

More generally, for an objective function H and a coordinate transformation $w_i = w_i(v_i)$,

$$\dot{w}_i = \frac{d}{dt}[w_i(v_i)] = \frac{dw_i}{dv_i}\dot{v}_i = \frac{dw_i}{dv_i}\frac{\partial H}{\partial v_i} = \left(\frac{dw_i}{dv_i}\right)^2 \frac{\partial H}{\partial w_i}, \qquad (4.8)$$

which implies that the coordinate transformation simply adds a factor $(dw_i/dv_i)^2$ to the original growth term obtained in the original coordinate system $\mathcal{W}$. For the dynamics in equation 4.4 derived under the coordinate transformation $w_i = \frac{1}{4}v_i^2$ ($\mathcal{C}^w$) relative to the dynamics of equation 4.2, we verify that $(dw_i/dv_i)^2 = w_i$. Equation 4.8 also shows that fixed points are preserved under the coordinate transformation in the region where dw_i/dv_i is defined and finite but that additional fixed points may be introduced if $dw_i/dv_i = 0$.

This effect of coordinate transformations is known from the general theory of relativity and tensor analysis (e.g., Dirac, 1996). The gradient of a potential (or objective function) is a covariant vector, which adds the factor

Neural Map Formation

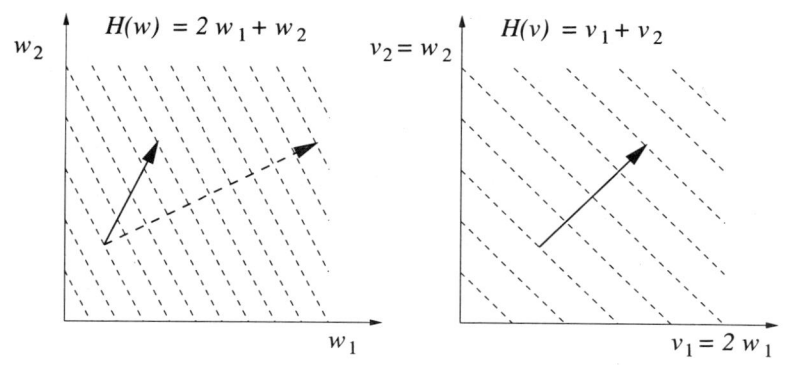

Figure 3: The effect of coordinate transformations on the induced dynamics. The figure shows a simple objective function H in the original coordinate system $\mathcal{W}$ (left) and the new coordinate system $\mathcal{V}$ (right) with $w_1 = v_1/2$ and $w_2 = v_2$. The gradient induced in $\mathcal{W}$ (dashed arrow) and the gradient induced in $\mathcal{V}$ and then backtransformed into $\mathcal{W}$ (solid arrows) have the same component in the w_2 direction but differ by a factor of four in the w_1 direction (cf. equation 4.8). Notice that the two dynamics differ in amplitude and direction, but that H is a Lyapunov function for both.

dw_i/dv_i through the transformation from $\mathcal{W}$ to $\mathcal{V}$. Since $\dot{v}$ as a kinematic description of the trajectory is a contravariant vector, this adds another factor dw_i/dv_i through the transformation back from $\mathcal{V}$ to $\mathcal{W}$. If both vectors were either covariant or contravariant, the back-and-forth transformation between the different coordinate systems would have no effect. The same argument holds for the constraints in section 5.2. In some cases, it may also be useful to consider more general coordinate transformations $w_i = w_i(\mathbf{v})$ where each weight w_i may depend on all variables v_j, as is common in the general theory of relativity and tensor analysis. Equation 4.8 would have to be modified correspondingly. In Figure 3, the effect of coordinate transformations is illustrated by a simple example.

Table 1 shows two objective functions and the corresponding dynamics terms they induce under different coordinate transformations. The first objective function, L, is linear in the weights and induces constant weight growth (or decay) under coordinate transformation $\mathcal{C}^1$. The growth of one weight does not depend on other weights. This term can be useful for dynamic link matching to introduce a bias for each weight depending on the similarity of the connected neurons. The second objective function, Q, is a quadratic form. The induced growth rule for one weight includes other weights and is usually based on correlations between input and output neurons, $\langle a_\tau a_\rho \rangle = \sum_j D_{ij} w_j$, and possibly also the mean activities of output neurons, $\langle a_\tau \rangle = \sum_j A_{ij} w_j$. This term is, for instance, important to form topographic maps. Functional aspects of term Q are discussed in section 6.3.

5 Constraints

A constraint is either an inequality describing a surface (of dimensionality $RT - 1$ if RT is the number of weights) between valid and invalid region or an equality describing the valid region as a surface. A normalization rule is a particular prescription for how the constraint has to be enforced. Thus, constraints can be uniquely derived from normalization rules but not vice versa.

5.1 Orthogonal Versus Nonorthogonal Normalization Rules.
Normalization rules can be divided into two classes: those that enforce the constraints orthogonal to the constraint surface, that is, along the gradient of the constraint function, and those that also have a component tangential to the constraint surface (see Figure 4). We refer to the former ones as *orthogonal* and to the latter ones as *nonorthogonal*.

Only the orthogonal normalization rules are compatible with an objective function, as is illustrated in Figure 5. For a dynamics induced as an ascending gradient flow of an objective function, the value of the objective function constantly increases as long as the weights change. If the weights cross a constraint surface, a normalization rule has to be applied iteratively to the growth rule. Starting from the constraint surface at point $\mathbf{w}'$, the gradient ascent causes a step to point $\tilde{\mathbf{w}}$ in the invalid region, where $\tilde{\mathbf{w}} - \mathbf{w}'$ is in general nonorthogonal to the constraint surface. A normalization rule causes a step back to $\mathbf{w}$ on the constraint surface. If the normalization rule is orthogonal, that is, $\mathbf{w} - \tilde{\mathbf{w}}$ is orthogonal to the constraint surface, $\mathbf{w} - \tilde{\mathbf{w}}$ is shorter than or equal to $\tilde{\mathbf{w}} - \mathbf{w}'$ and the cosine of the angle between the combined step $\mathbf{w} - \mathbf{w}'$ and the gradient $\tilde{\mathbf{w}} - \mathbf{w}'$ is nonnegative, that is, the value of the objective function does not decrease. This cannot be guaranteed for nonorthogonal normalization rules, in which case the objective function of the unconstrained dynamics may not even be a Lyapunov function for the combined system, including weight dynamics and normalization rules. Thus, only orthogonal normalization rules can be used in the constrained optimization framework.

The term *orthogonal* is not well defined away from the constraint surface. However, the constraints used in this article are rather simple, and a natural orthogonal direction is usually available for all weight vectors. Thus, the term *orthogonal* will also be used for normalization rules that do not project back exactly onto the constraint surface but keep the weights close to the surface and affect the weights orthogonal to it. For more complicated constraint surfaces, more careful considerations may be required.

Neural Map Formation

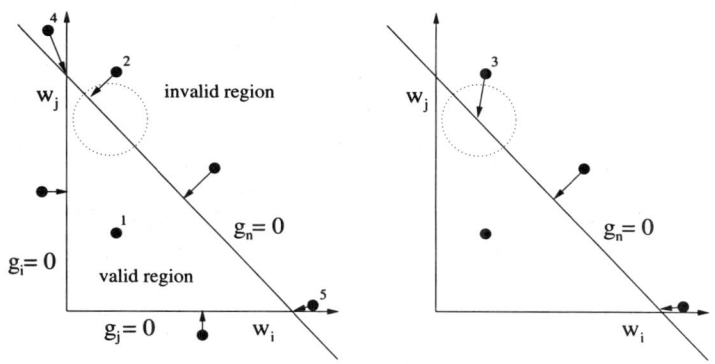

Figure 4: Different constraints and different ways in which constraints can be violated and enforced. The constraints along the axes are given by $g_i = w_i \geq 0$ and $g_j = w_j \geq 0$, which keep the weights w_i and w_j nonnegative. The constraint $g_n = 1 - (w_i + w_j) \geq 0$ keeps the sum of the two weights smaller or equal to 1. Black dots indicate points in state-space that may have been reached by the growth rule. Dot 1: None of the constraints is violated, and no normalization rule is applied. Dot 2: $g_n \geq 0$ is violated, and an orthogonal subtractive normalization rule is applied. Dot 3: $g_n \geq 0$ is violated, and a nonorthogonal multiplicative normalization rule is applied. Notice that the normalization does not follow the gradient of g_n; it is not perpendicular to the line $g_n = 0$. Dot 4: Two constraints are violated, and the respective normalization rules must be applied simultaneously. Dot 5: $g_n \geq 0$ is violated, but the respective normalization rule violates $g_j \geq 0$. Again both rules must be applied simultaneously. The dotted circles indicate regions considered in greater detail in Figure 5.

Whether a normalization rule is orthogonal depends on the coordinate system in which it is applied. This is illustrated in Figure 6 and discussed in greater detail below. The same rule can be nonorthogonal in one coordinate system but orthogonal in another. It is important to find the coordinate system in which an objective function can be derived and the normalization rules are orthogonal. This then is the coordinate system in which the model can be most conveniently analyzed. Not all nonorthogonal normalization rules can be transformed into orthogonal ones. In Wiskott and von der Malsburg (1996), for example, a normalization rule is used that affects a group of weights if single weights grow beyond their limits. Since the constraint surface depends on only one weight, only that weight can be affected by an orthogonal normalization rule. Thus, this normalization rule cannot be made orthogonal.

5.2 Constraints Can Be Enforced in Different Ways. For a given constraint, orthogonal normalization rules can be derived using various meth-

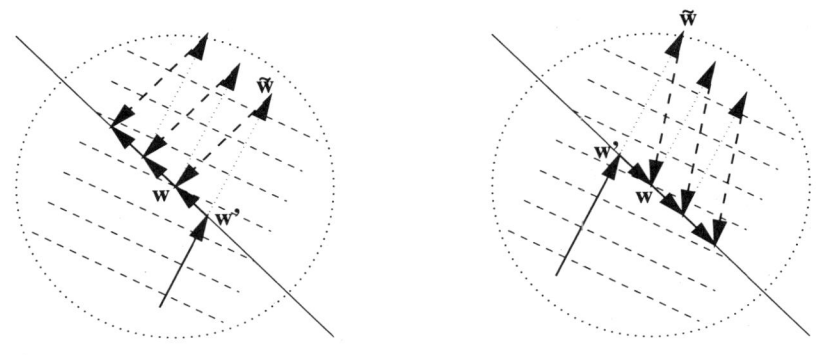

Figure 5: The effect of orthogonal versus nonorthogonal normalization rules. The two circled regions are taken from Figure 4. The effect of the orthogonal subtractive rule is shown on the left, and the nonorthogonal multiplicative rule is shown on the right. The growth dynamics is assumed to be induced by an objective function, the equipotential curves of which are shown as dashed lines. The objective function increases to the upper right. The growth rule (dotted arrows) and normalization rule (dashed arrows) are applied iteratively. The net effect is different in the two cases. For the orthogonal normalization rule, the dynamics increases the value of the objective function, while for the nonorthogonal normalization, the value decreases and the objective function that generates the growth rule is not even a Lyapunov function for the combined system.

ods. These include the method of Lagrangian multipliers, the inclusion of penalty terms, and normalization rules that are integrated into the weight dynamics without necessarily having any objective function. The former two methods are common in optimization theory. The latter is more specific to a model of neural map formation. It is also possible to substitute a constraint by a coordinate transformation.

5.2.1 Method of Lagrangian Multipliers. Lagrangian multipliers can be used to derive explicit normalization rules, such as equations 2.4–2.6. If the constraint $g_n(\mathbf{w}) \geq 0$ is violated for $\tilde{\mathbf{w}}$ as obtained after one integration step of the learning rule, $\tilde{w}_i(t + \Delta t) = w_i(t) + \Delta t \dot{w}_i(t)$, the weight vector has to be corrected along the gradient of the constraint function g_n, which is orthogonal to the constraint surface $g_n(\mathbf{w}) = 0$,

$$\text{if } g_n(\tilde{\mathbf{w}}) < 0: \quad w_i = \tilde{w}_i + \lambda_n \frac{\partial g_n}{\partial \tilde{w}_i} \quad \text{for all } i, \tag{5.1}$$

where $(\partial g_n/\partial \tilde{w}_i) = (\partial g_n/\partial w_i)$ at $\mathbf{w} = \tilde{\mathbf{w}}$ and $\lambda_n = \lambda_n(\tilde{\mathbf{w}})$ is a Lagrangian multiplier and determined such that $g_n(\mathbf{w}) = 0$ is obtained. If no constraint

Neural Map Formation

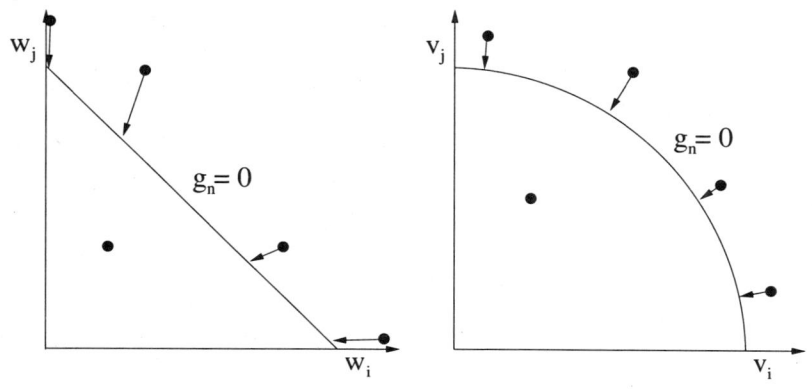

Figure 6: The effect of a coordinate transformation on a normalization rule. The constraint function is $g_n = 1 - (w_i + w_j) \geq 0$, and the coordinate transformation is $w_i = \frac{1}{4} v_i^2$, $w_j = \frac{1}{4} v_j^2$. In the new coordinate system $\mathcal{V}^w$ (right), the constraint becomes $g_n = 1 - \frac{1}{4}(v_i^2 + v_j^2) \geq 0$ and leads there to an orthogonal multiplicative normalization rule. Transforming back into $\mathcal{W}$ (left) then yields a nonorthogonal multiplicative normalization rule.

is violated, the weights are simply taken to be $w_i = \tilde{w}_i$. The constraints that must be taken into account, either because they are violated or because they become violated if a violated one is enforced, are called *operative*. All others are called *inoperative* and do not need to be considered for that integration step. If there is more than one operative constraint, the normalization rule becomes

$$\text{if } g_n(\tilde{\mathbf{w}}) < 0: \qquad w_i = \tilde{w}_i + \sum_{n \in N_O} \lambda_n \frac{\partial g_n}{\partial \tilde{w}_i} \qquad \text{for all } i, \qquad (5.2)$$

where N_O denotes the set of operative constraints. The Lagrangian multipliers λ_n are determined such that $g_{n'}(\mathbf{w}) = 0$ for all $n' \in N_O$ (cf. Figure 4). Computational models of neural map formation usually take another strategy and simply iterate the normalization rules (see equation 5.1) for the operative constraints individually, which is in general not accurate but may be sufficient for most practical purposes. It should also be mentioned that in the standard method of Lagrangian multipliers as usually applied in physics or optimization theory, the two steps, weight growth and normalization, are combined in one dynamical equation such that $\mathbf{w}$ remains on the constraint surface. The steps were split here to obtain explicit normalization rules independent of growth rules.

Consider now the effect of coordinate transformations on the normalization rules derived by the method of Lagrangian multipliers. The constraint in equation 2.17 can be written as $g_n(\mathbf{w}) = \theta_n - \sum_{i \in I_n} w_i \geq 0$ and leads to a subtractive normalization rule as in the example above (see equation 2.5). Under the coordinate transformation C^w ($w_i = \frac{1}{4} v_i^2$), the constraint becomes $g_n(\mathbf{v}) = \theta_n - \sum_{i \in I_n} \frac{1}{4} v_i^2 \geq 0$, and in the coordinate system $\mathcal{V}^w$, the normalization rule is:

$$\text{if } g_n(\tilde{\mathbf{v}}) < 0: \quad v_i = \tilde{v}_i - 2 \left(\frac{\sqrt{\theta_n}}{\sqrt{\sum_{j \in I_n} \frac{1}{4} \tilde{v}_j^2}} - 1 \right) \left(-\frac{1}{2} \tilde{v}_i \right) \quad (5.3)$$

$$= \frac{\sqrt{\theta_n}\, \tilde{v}_i}{\sqrt{\sum_{j \in I_n} \frac{1}{4} \tilde{v}_j^2}} \quad \text{for all } i \in I_n. \quad (5.4)$$

Taking the square on both sides and applying the backtransformation from $\mathcal{V}^w$ to $\mathcal{W}$ leads to

$$\text{if } g_n(\tilde{\mathbf{w}}) < 0: \quad w_i = \frac{\theta_n \tilde{w}_i}{\sum_{j \in I_n} \tilde{w}_j} \quad \text{for all } i \in I_n. \quad (5.5)$$

This is a multiplicative normalization rule in contrast to the subtractive one obtained in the coordinate system $\mathcal{W}$ (see also Figure 6). It is listed as normalization rule $N^w_\geq$ in Table 1 (or $N^w_=$ for constraint $g(\mathbf{w}) = 0$). This multiplicative rule is commonly found in the literature (cf. Table 2), but it is not orthogonal in $\mathcal{W}$, though it is in $\mathcal{V}^w$.

For a more general coordinate transformation $w_i = w_i(v_i)$ and a constraint function $g(\mathbf{w})$, an orthogonal normalization rule can be derived in $\mathcal{V}$ with the method of Lagrangian multipliers and transformed back into $\mathcal{W}$, which results in general in a nonorthogonal normalization rule:

$$\text{if constraint is violated:} \quad w_i = \tilde{w}_i + \lambda \left(\frac{dw_i}{d\tilde{v}_i} \right)^2 \frac{\partial g}{\partial \tilde{w}_i} + O(\lambda^2). \quad (5.6)$$

The λ actually would have to be calculated in $\mathcal{V}$, but since $\lambda \propto \Delta t$, second- and higher-order terms can be neglected for small Δt and λ calculated such that $g(\mathbf{w}) = 0$. Notice the similar effect of the coordinate transformation on the growth rules (see equation 4.8), as well as on the normalization rules (see equation 5.6). In both cases, a factor $(dw_i/dv_i)^2$ is added to the modification rate. As for gradient flows derived from objective functions, for a more general coordinate transformation $w_i = w_i(\mathbf{v})$, equation 5.6 would have to be modified accordingly.

We indicate these normalization rules by a subscript $=$ (for an equality) and $\geq$ (for an inequality), because the constraints are enforced immediately and exactly.

Neural Map Formation

5.2.2 Integrated Normalization Without Objective Function. Growth rule and explicit normalization rule as derived by the method of Lagrangian multipliers can be combined in one dynamical equation. As an example, consider the growth rule $\dot{w}_i = f_i$, that is, $\tilde{w}_i(t + \Delta t) = w_i(t) + \Delta t f_i(t)$, where f_i is an arbitrary function in $\mathbf{w}$ and can be interpreted as a fitness of a synapse. Together with the normalization rule $N_{\simeq}^w$ (see equation 5.5) and assuming $\sum_{j \in I} w_j(t) = \theta$, it follows that (von der Malsburg & Willshaw, 1981):

$$w_i(t + \Delta t) = \frac{\theta \left[w_i(t) + \Delta t f_i(t) \right]}{\sum_{j \in I} \left[w_j(t) + \Delta t f_j(t) \right]} \tag{5.7}$$

$$= w_i(t) + \Delta t f_i(t) - \Delta t \frac{w_i(t)}{\theta} \sum_{j \in I} f_j(t) + O(\Delta t^2) \tag{5.8}$$

$$\implies \dot{w}_i(t) = f_i(t) - \frac{w_i(t)}{\theta} \sum_{j \in I} f_j(t), \tag{5.9}$$

and with $W(t) = \sum_{i \in I} w_i(t)$

$$\dot{W}(t) = \left(1 - \frac{W(t)}{\theta} \right) \sum_{j \in I} f_j(t), \tag{5.10}$$

which shows that $W = \theta$ is indeed a stable fixed point under the dynamics of equation 5.9. However, this is not always the case. The same growth rule combined with the subtractive normalization rule $N_{\simeq}^1$ (see equation 2.5) would yield a dynamics that provides only a neutrally stable fixed point for $W = \theta$. An additional term $(\theta - \sum_{j \in I} w_j(t))$ would have to be added to make the fixed point stable. This is the reason that this type of normalization rule is listed in Table 1 only for C^w. We indicate these kinds of normalization rules by the subscript $\simeq$ because the dynamics smoothly approaches the constraint surface and will stay there exactly.

Notice that this method differs from the standard method of Lagrangian multipliers, which also yields a dynamics such that $\mathbf{w}$ remains on the constraint surface. The latter applies only to the dynamics at $g(\mathbf{w}) = 0$ and always produces neutrally stable fixed points because $\sum_i \dot{w}_i(t) \frac{\partial g}{\partial w_i} = 0$ is required by definition. If applied to a weight vector outside the constraint surface, the standard method of Lagrangian multipliers yields $g(\mathbf{w}) = \text{const} \neq 0$.

An advantage of this method is that it provides one dynamics for the growth rule as well as the normalization rule and that the constraint is enforced exactly. However, difficulties arise when interfering constraints are combined; that is, different constraints affect the same weights. This type of formulation is required for certain types of analyses (e.g., Häussler & von der Malsburg, 1983). A disadvantage is that in general there no longer exists an objective function for the dynamics, though the growth term itself without the normalization term still has an objective function that is a Lyapunov function for the combined dynamics.

5.2.3 Penalty Terms. Another method of enforcing the constraints is to add penalty terms to the objective function (e.g., Bienenstock & von der Malsburg). For instance, if the constraint is formulated as an equality $g(\mathbf{w}) = 0$, then add $-\frac{1}{2}g^2(\mathbf{w})$; if the constraint is formulated as an inequality $g(\mathbf{w}) \leq 0$ or $g(\mathbf{w}) \geq 0$, then add $\ln|g(\mathbf{w})|$. Other penalty functions, such as g^4 and $1/g$, are possible as well, but those used here induce the required terms as used in the literature.

The effect of coordinate transformations is the same as in the case of objective functions. Consider, for example, the simple constraint $g_i(\mathbf{w}) = w_i \geq 0$ ($I_\geq$ in Table 1), which keeps weights w_i nonnegative. The respective penalty term is $\ln|w_i|$ ($I_>$) and the induced dynamics under the four different transformations considered in Table 1 are $\frac{1}{w_i}, \frac{\alpha_i}{w_i}, 1$, and α_i.

An advantage of this approach is that a coherent objective function, as well as a weight dynamics, is available, including growth rules and normalization rules. A disadvantage may be that the constraints are only approximate and not enforced strictly, so that $g(\mathbf{w}) \approx 0$ and $g(\mathbf{w}) < 0$ or $g(\mathbf{w}) > 0$. We therefore indicate these kinds of normalization rules by subscripts $\approx$ and $>$. However, the approximation can be made arbitrarily precise by weighting the penalty terms accordingly.

5.2.4 Constraints Introduced by Coordinate Transformations. An entirely different way by which constraints can be enforced is by means of a coordinate transformation. Consider, for example, the coordinate transformation $\mathcal{C}^w$ ($w_i = \frac{1}{4}v_i^2$). Negative weights are not reachable under this coordinate transformation because the factor $(dw_i/dv_i)^2 = w_i$ added to the growth rules (see equation 4.8) as well as to the normalization rules (see equation 5.6) allows the weight dynamics of weight w_i to slow down as it approaches zero, so that positive weights always stay positive (This can be generalized to positive and negative weights by the coordinate transformation $w_i = \frac{1}{4}v_i|v_i|$.) Thus the coordinate transformation $\mathcal{C}^w$ (and also $\mathcal{C}^{\alpha w}$) implicitly introduces limitation constraint $I_>$. This is interesting because it shows that a coordinate transformation can substitute for a constraint, which is well known in optimization theory.

The choice of whether to enforce the constraints by explicit normalization, an integrated dynamics without an objective function, penalty terms, or even implicitly a coordinate transformation depends on the system as well as the methods applied to analyze it. Table 1 shows several constraint functions and their corresponding normalization rules as derived in different coordinate systems and by the three different methods discussed above. Not shown is normalization implicit in a coordinate transformation. It is

Neural Map Formation

interesting that there are only two types of constraints. All variations arise from using different coordinate systems and different methods by which the normalization rules are implemented. The first type is a limitation constraint I, which limits the range of individual weights. The second type is a normalization constraint N, which affects a group of weights, usually the sum, very rarely the sum of squares as indicated by Z. In the next section we show how to use Table 1 for analyzing models of neural map formation and give some examples from the literature.

6 Examples and Applications

6.1 How to Use Table 1. The aim of Table 1 is to provide an overview of the different objective functions and derived growth terms as well as the constraint functions and derived normalization rules and terms discussed in this article. The terms and rules are ordered in columns belonging to a particular coordinate transformation $\mathcal{C}$. Only entries in the same column may be combined to obtain a consistent, constrained optimization formulation for a system. However, some terms can be derived under different coordinate transformations. For instance, the normalization rule $I_=$ is the same for all coordinate transformations, and term $L^{\alpha w}$ with $\beta_i = 1/\alpha_i$ is the same as term L^w with $\beta_i = 1$.

To analyze a model of neural map formation, first identify possible candidates in Table 1 representing the different terms of the desired dynamics. Notice that the average activity of output neurons is represented by $\langle a_\tau \rangle = \sum_j A_{ij} w_j$ and that the correlation between input and output neurons is represented by $\langle a_\tau, a_\rho \rangle = \sum_j D_{ij} w_j$. Usually both terms will be only an approximation of the actual mean activities and correlations of the system under consideration (cf. section 2.1). Notice also that normalization rules $N^w_=$, $N^{\alpha w}_=$, $Z^1_=$, and $Z^\alpha_=$ are actually multiplicative normalization rules and not subtractive ones, as might be suggested by the special form in which they are written in Table 1.

Next identify the column in which all terms of the weight dynamics can be represented. This gives the coordinate transformation under which the model can be analyzed through the objective functions and constraint or penalty functions listed on the left side of the table. Equivalent models (cf. section 6.4) can be derived by moving from one column to another and by using normalization rules derived by a different method. Thus, Table 1 provides a convenient tool for checking whether a system can be analyzed within the constrained optimization framework presented here and for identifying the equivalent models. The function of each term can be coherently interpreted with respect to the objective, constraint, and penalty functions on the left side. The table can be extended with respect to additional objective, constraint, and penalty functions, as well as additional coordinate transformations. Although the table is compact, it suffices to

Table 1: Objective Functions, Constraint Functions, and the Dynamics Terms Induced in Different Coordinate Systems.

	Coordinate Transformations			
	$\mathcal{C}^1$	$\mathcal{C}^\alpha$	$\mathcal{C}^w$	$\mathcal{C}^{\alpha w}$
	$w_i = v_i$	$w_i = \sqrt{\alpha_i} v_i$	$w_i = \frac{1}{2} v_i^2$	$w_i = \frac{1}{4}\alpha_i v_i^2$
	$\left(\frac{dw_i}{dv_i}\right)^2 = 1$	$\left(\frac{dw_i}{dv_i}\right)^2 = \alpha_i$	$\left(\frac{dw_i}{dv_i}\right)^2 = w_i$	$\left(\frac{dw_i}{dv_i}\right)^2 = \alpha_i w_i$
Objective Functions $H(\mathbf{w})$	Growth Terms: $\dot{w}_i = \cdots + \cdots$ or $\tilde{w}_i = w_i + \Delta t(\cdots + \cdots)$			
L	$\sum_i \beta_i w_i$	β_i	$\beta_i w_i$	$\alpha_i \beta_i w_i$
Q	$\frac{1}{2}\sum_{ij} w_i D_{ij} w_j$	$\sum_j D_{ij} w_j$	$\alpha_i \sum_j D_{ij} w_j$	$w_i \sum_j D_{ij} w_j$	$\alpha_i w_i \sum_j D_{ij} w_j$
Constraint Functions $g(\mathbf{w})$	Normalization Rules (if constraint is violated): $w_i = \cdots$ $\forall i \in I_n$			
$I_=, I_\geq$	$\theta_i - w_i$	θ_i	θ_i	θ_i
$N_=, N^1_\geq$	$\theta_n - \sum_{j \in I_n} \beta_j w_j$	$\tilde{w}_i + \lambda_n \beta_i$	$\tilde{w}_i + \lambda_n \alpha_i \beta_i$	$\tilde{w}_i + \lambda_n \beta_i \tilde{w}_i$	$\tilde{w}_i + \lambda_n \alpha_i \beta_i \tilde{w}_i$
$Z_=, Z_\geq$	$\theta_n - \sum_{j \in I_n} \beta_j w_j^2$	$\tilde{w}_i + \lambda_n \beta_i \tilde{w}_i$	$\tilde{w}_i + \lambda_n \alpha_i \beta_i \tilde{w}_i$	$\tilde{w}_i + \lambda_n \beta_i \tilde{w}_i^2$	$\tilde{w}_i + \lambda_n \alpha_i \beta_i \tilde{w}_i^2$
Constraint Functions $g(\mathbf{w})$	Normalization Terms: $\dot{w}_i = \cdots$ or $\tilde{w}_i = w_i + \Delta t(\cdots)$			
$N_\simeq$	$\theta_n - \sum_{j \in I_n} w_j$			$f_i - \frac{w_i}{\theta_n}\sum_j f_j$	
Penalty Functions $H(\mathbf{w})$	Normalization Terms: $\dot{w}_i = \cdots + \cdots$ or $\tilde{w}_i = w_i + \Delta t(\cdots + \cdots)$			
$I_\approx$	$-\frac{1}{2}\gamma_i(\theta_i - w_i)^2$	$\gamma_i(\theta_i - w_i)$	$\alpha_i \gamma_i(\theta_i - w_i)$	$\gamma_i w_i(\theta_i - w_i)$	$\alpha_i \gamma_i w_i(\theta_i - w_i)$
$I_>$	$\gamma_i \ln|\theta_i - w_i|$	$-\frac{\gamma_i}{\theta_i - w_i}$	$-\frac{\alpha_i \gamma_i}{\theta_i - w_i}$	$-\frac{\gamma_i w_i}{\theta_i - w_i}$	$-\frac{\alpha_i \gamma_i w_i}{\theta_i - w_i}$
$N_\approx$	$-\frac{1}{2}\gamma_i(\theta_n - \sum_{j \in I_n}\beta_j w_j)^2$	$\beta_i \gamma_n \times$	$\alpha_i \beta_i \gamma_n \times$	$\beta_i \gamma_n w_i \times$	$\alpha_i \beta_i \gamma_n w_i \times$
		$(\theta_n - \sum_j \beta_j w_j)$	$(\theta_n - \sum_j \beta_j w_j)$	$(\theta_n - \sum_j \beta_j w_j)$	$(\theta_n - \sum_j \beta_j w_j)$

Note: C indicates a coordinate transformation that is specified by a superscript. L indicates a linear term. Q indicates a quadratic term that is usually induced by correlations $(a_\tau, a_\rho) := \sum_\tau D_{ij} w_j$. But it can also account for mean activities $(a_\tau) := \sum_\tau A_{ij} w_j$. I indicates a limitation constraint that limits the range for individual weights (I may stand for "interval"). N indicates a normalization constraint that limits the sum over a set of weights. Z is a rarely used variation of N (the symbol Z can be thought of as a rotated N). Subscript signs distinguish between the different ways in which constraints can be enforced. $\approx$, for instance, indicates the normalization term $\gamma_i w_i(\theta_i - w_i)$ induced by the penalty function $-\frac{1}{2}\gamma_i(\theta_i - w_i)^2$ under the coordinate transformation C^w. Subscripts n and i for θ, λ, and γ denote different constraints of the same type, for example, the same constraint applied to different output neurons. Normalization terms are integrated into the dynamics directly, while normalization rules are applied iteratively to the dynamics of the growth rule. f_i denotes a fitness by which a weight would grow without any normalization (cf. section 5.2.2).

Neural Map Formation

explain a wide range of representative examples from the literature, as discussed in the next section.

6.2 Examples from the Literature. Table 2 shows representative models from the literature. The original equations are listed, as well as the classification in terms of growth rules and normalization rules listed in Table 1. Detailed comments for these models and the model in Amari (1980) follow below. The latter is not listed in Table 2 because it cannot be interpreted within our constrained optimization framework. The dynamics of the introductory example of section 2 can be classified as Q^1 (see equation 2.3), $I^1_{\geq}$ (see equation 2.4), and $N^1_{\geq}$ (see equations 2.5 and 2.6).

The models are discussed here mainly with respect to whether they can be consistently described within the constrained optimization framework, that is, whether growth rules and normalization rules can be derived from objective functions and constraint functions under one coordinate transformation (that does not imply anything about the quality of a model). Another important issue is whether the linear correlation model introduced in section 3 is an appropriate description for the activity dynamics of these models. It is an accurate description for some of them, but others are based on nonlinear models, and the approximations discussed in section 2.1 and appendix A have to be made.

Models typically contain three components: the quadratic term Q to induce neighborhood-preserving maps, a limitation constraint I to keep synaptic weights positive, and a normalization constraint N (or Z) to induce competition between weights and to keep weights limited. The limitation constraint can be waived for systems with positive weights and multiplicative normalization rules (Konen & von der Malsburg, 1993; Obermayer et al., 1990; von der Malsburg, 1973) (cf. section 5.2.4). A presynaptic normalization rule can be introduced implicitly by the activity dynamics (cf. section A.2 in the appendix). In that case, it may be necessary to use an explicit presynaptic normalization constraint in the constrained optimization formulation. Otherwise the system may have a tendency to collapse on the input layer (see section 6.3), a tendency it does not have in the original formulation as a dynamical system. Only few systems contain the linear term L, which can be used for dynamic link matching. In Häussler and von der Malsburg (1983) the linear term was introduced for analytical convenience and does not differentiate between different links. The two models of dynamic link matching (Bienenstock & von der Malsburg, 1987; Konen & von der Malsburg, 1993) introduce similarity values implicitly and not through the linear term. The models are now discussed individually in chronological order.

von der Malsburg (1973): The activity dynamics of this model is nonlinear and based on hexagon patterns in the output layer. Thus, the applicability of the linear correlation model is not certain (cf. section 2.1). The weight

Table 2: Examples of Weight Dynamics from Previous Studies.

Reference	Weight Dynamics	Equation	Classification
von der Malsburg (1973)	$\tilde{w}_{\tau\rho} = w_{\tau\rho} + ha_\rho a_\tau$ $\quad \tilde{w}_\tau = \sum_{\rho=1}^{19} \tilde{w}_{\tau\rho}$ $w_{\tau\rho} = \tilde{w}_{\tau\rho} \cdot 19 \cdot \frac{w}{2} / \tilde{w}_\tau$		Q^1 $N_=^w$
Whitelaw and Cowan (1981)	$\dot{w}_{\tau\rho} = \alpha_{\tau\rho} a_\rho a_\tau - \alpha a_\tau + \Omega \quad$ (Ω: small noise term) $\sum_\rho w_{\tau\rho'} = 1, \sum_\tau w_{\tau'\rho} = 1$	(2) (5)	$Q^a - Q^1 + ?$ $N_=^?$
Häussler and von der Malsburg (1983)	$\dot{w}_{\tau\rho} = f_{\tau\rho} - \frac{1}{2N} w_{\tau\rho} \left(\sum_{\tau'} f_{\tau'\rho} + \sum_{\rho'} f_{\tau\rho'} \right)$ $f_{\tau\rho} = \alpha + \beta w_{\tau\rho} C_{\tau\rho}$ $C_{\tau\rho} = \sum_{\tau'\rho'} D_{\tau\tau'} D_{\rho\rho'} w_{\tau'\rho'}$	(2.1) (2.2) (2.3)	$(I_>^w + Q^w) - (L^w + N_{\cong}^w)$
Linsker (1986)	$\dot{w}_{\tau\rho} = k_1 + \frac{1}{N_G} \sum_{\rho'} \left(Q_{\rho\rho'}^F + k_2 \right) w_{\tau\rho'}$ $\quad + R_b \sum_{\tau'} f_{\tau\tau'} \left[k_{1a} + \frac{1}{N_G} \sum_{\rho'} \left(Q_{\rho\rho'}^F + k_2 \right) w_{\tau\rho'} \right]$ $= k_1' - \frac{A_\rho - k_2}{N_G} \sum_{\tau'\rho'} D_{\tau\tau'} A_{\rho'} w_{\tau\tau'} + \frac{1}{N_G} \sum_{\tau'\rho'} D_{\tau\tau'} D_{\rho\rho'} w_{\tau'\rho'}$ $(k_1' = k_1 + R_b k_{1a} \sum_{\tau'} f_{\tau\tau'}, \; D_{\tau\tau'} = R_b f_{\tau\tau'} + \delta_{\tau\tau'}$ (δ: Kronecker), $D_{\rho\rho'} = (a_\rho a_{\rho'}), \; A_\rho = (a_\rho), \; k_2 < 0)$ some $w_{\tau\rho} \in [0,1]$ and some $w_{\tau\rho} \in [-1,0]$ or all $w_{\tau\rho} \in [-0.5, 0.5]$	(5)	$L^1 + Q^1$ $I_{\geq}^1$
Bienenstock and von der Malsburg (1987)	$H = -\sum_{\tau\tau'\rho\rho'} D_{\tau\tau'} w_{\tau\rho} w_{\tau\rho} D_{\rho\rho'}$ $\quad + \gamma' \sum_\tau \left(\sum_\rho w_{\tau\rho} - p' \right)^2 + \gamma' \sum_\rho \left(\sum_\tau w_{\tau\rho} - p' \right)^2$ $w_{\tau\rho} \in [0, T_{\tau\rho}]$	(2)	Q^1 $+ N_{\approx}^1$ $I_{\geq}^1$

Table 2: Continued.

Reference	Weight Dynamics	Equation	Classification
Miller, Keller, and Stryker, 1989	$\dot{w}_{\tau\rho}^L = \lambda\alpha_{\tau\rho}\sum_{\tau'\rho'}D_{\tau\tau'}\left[D_{\rho\rho'}^{LL}w_{\tau'\rho'}^L + D_{\rho\rho'}^{LR}w_{\tau'\rho'}^R\right] - \left[\gamma w_{\tau\rho}^L + \epsilon\alpha_{\tau\rho}\right]$ a) $\sum_\rho(w_{\tau\rho'}^L + w_{\tau\rho'}^R) = 2\sum_{\rho'}\alpha_{\tau\rho'}, \quad w_{\tau\rho}^L = \tilde{w}_{\tau\rho}^L + \lambda_\tau\alpha_{\tau\rho}$ b) $\sum_\tau w_{\tau'\rho}^L = \text{const}, \quad w_{\tau\rho}^L = \tilde{w}_{\tau\rho}^L + \lambda_\tau\alpha_{\tau\rho}$ $w_{\tau\rho}^L \in [0, 8\alpha_{\tau\rho}]$ (If weights were cut due to $I_{\geqq}^\alpha: w_{\tau\rho}^L = \tilde{w}_{\tau\rho}^L + \lambda_\tau\tilde{w}_{\tau\rho}^L$) Interchanging L (left eye) and R (right eye) yields equations for $w_{\tau\rho}^R$.	(1) (Note 23)	Q^α - $I_{\approx}^\alpha$ $N_=$ $N_=$ $I_\geqq^\alpha$ ($N_=^w$)
Obermayer et al. (1990)	$w_{\tau\rho}(t+1) = \dfrac{w_{\tau\rho}(t) + \epsilon(t)a_\tau(t)a_\rho}{\sqrt{\sum_{\rho'}\left(w_{\tau\rho'}(t) + \epsilon(t)a_\tau(t)a_{\rho'}\right)^2}}$	(4)	$Q^1_=$ $Z^1_=$
Tanaka (1990)	$\dot{w}_{\tau\rho} = w_{\tau\rho}\left[\kappa_0 - \kappa_1\sum_{\rho'}\beta_{\rho'}w_{\tau\rho'}\right] + gm_\tau w_{\tau\rho}a_\rho + \gamma_{\tau\rho}$ (later in the article $\beta_{\rho'} = 1$)	(2.1)	$N_{\approx}^{\alpha w} + Q^w + I_>^w$ ($N_{\approx}^{\alpha w} = N_{\approx}^w$)
Goodhill (1993)	$w_{\tau\rho} = w_{\tau\rho} + \alpha a_\rho a_\tau$ a) $w_{\tau\rho} = \begin{cases} w_{\tau\rho} - t & \text{if } w_{\tau\rho} - t > 0 \\ 0 & \text{otherwise} \end{cases}, \quad t = \dfrac{\sum_{\rho'}w_{\tau\rho'} - N_\tau}{n_\tau}, \quad n_\tau = \sum_{\{\rho'\|0<w_{\tau\rho'}\}}1$ (if some weights have become zero due to $I_{\geqq}^1$: $w_{\tau\rho} = \dfrac{N_\tau w_{\tau\rho}}{\sum_{\rho'}w_{\tau\rho'}}$) b) $w_{\tau\rho} = \dfrac{N_\rho w_{\tau\rho}}{\sum_{\tau'}w_{\tau'\rho}}$		$Q^1_=$ $\begin{cases} N^1_= \\ I^1_\geqq \\ (N^w_=) \end{cases}$ $N^w_=$
Konen and von der Malsburg (1993)	$w_{\tau\rho} \to w_{\tau\rho} + \epsilon w_{\tau\rho}\alpha_{\tau\rho}a_\tau a_\rho$ $\to w_{\tau\rho} / \sum_{\rho'}\dfrac{w_{\tau\rho'}}{\alpha_{\tau\rho'}}$ $\to w_{\tau\rho} / \sum_{\tau'}\dfrac{w_{\tau'\rho}}{\alpha_{\tau'\rho}}$ ($w_{\tau\rho}$ are the "effective couplings" $J_{\tau\rho}T_{\tau\rho}$)	(3.5)	$Q^{\alpha w}$ $N^{\alpha w}_=$ $N^{\alpha w}_=$

Note: The original equations are written in a form that uses the notation of this article. The classification of the original equations by means of the terms and coordinate transformations listed in Table 1 are shown in the right column (the coordinate transformations are indicated by superscripts). See section 6.2 for further comments on these models.

dynamics is inconsistent in its original formulation. However, Miller and MacKay (1994) have shown that constraints $N_=^w$ and $Z_=^1$ have a very similar effect on the dynamics, so that the weight dynamics could be made consistent by using $Z_=^1$ instead of $N_=^w$. No limitation constraint is necessary because neither the growth rule nor the multiplicative normalization rule can lead to negative weights, and the normalization rule limits the growth of positive weights.

Amari (1980): This is a particularly interesting model not listed in Table 2. It is based on a blob dynamics, but no explicit normalization rules are applied, so that the derivation of correlations and mean activities as discussed in section 3 cannot be used. Weights are prevented from growing infinitely by a simple decay term, which is possible because correlations induced by the blob model are finite and do not grow with the total strength of the synapses. Additional inhibitory inputs received by the output neurons from a constantly active neuron ensure that the average activity is evenly distributed in the output layer, which also leads to expanding maps. In this respect, the architecture deviates from Figure 2. Thus, this model cannot be formulated within our framework.

Whitelaw and Cowan (1981): The activity dynamics is nonlinear and based on blobs. Thus, the linear correlation model is only an approximation (cf. section 2.1). The weight dynamics is difficult to interpret in the constrained optimization framework. The normalization rule is not specified precisely, but it is probably multiplicative because a subtractive one would lead to negative weights and possibly infinite weight growth. The quadratic term $-Q^1$ is based on mean activities and would lead by itself to zero weights. The Ω term was introduced only to test the stability of the system.

Häussler and von der Malsburg (1983): This model is directly formulated in terms of weight dynamics; thus, the linear correlation model is accurate. The weight dynamics is consistent; however, as argued in section 5.2.2, there is usually no objective function for the normalization rule $N_=^w$, but by replacing $N_=^w$ by $N_\simeq^w$ or $N_\approx^w$, the system can be expressed as a constrained optimization problem without qualitatively changing the model behavior. The limitation term $I_>^w$ and the linear term L^w are induced by the constant α and were introduced for analytical reasons. The former is meant to allow weights to grow from zero strength, and the latter limits this growth. α needs to be small for neural map formation, and for a stable one-to-one mapping, α strictly should be zero. Thus, these two terms could be discarded if all weights would be initially larger than zero. Notice that the linear term does not differentiate between different links and thus does not have a function as suggested for dynamic link matching (cf. sections 4 and 6.5).

Linsker (1986): This model is also directly formulated in terms of weight dynamics; thus, the linear correlation model is accurate. The weight dynamics is consistent. Since the model uses negative and positive weights

Neural Map Formation

and weights have a lower and an upper bound, no normalization rule is necessary. The weights converge to their upper or lower limit.

Bienenstock and von der Malsburg (1987): This is a model of dynamic link matching and was originally formulated in terms of an energy function. Thus the classification is accurate. The energy function does not include the linear term. The features are binary, black versus white, and the similarity values are therefore 0 and 1 and do not enter the dynamics as continuous similarity values. The $T_{\tau\rho}$ in the constraint $I_\geq^1$ represent the stored patterns in the associative memory, not similarity values.

Miller et al. (1989): This model is directly formulated in terms of weight dynamics; thus, the linear correlation model is accurate. One inconsistent part in the weight dynamics is the multiplicative normalization rule $N_=^w$, which is applied when subtractive normalization leads to negative weights. But it is only an algorithmic shortcut to solve the problem of interfering constraints (limitation and subtractive normalization). A more systematic treatment of the normalization rules could replace this inconsistent rule (cf. section 5.2.1). Another inconsistency is that weights that reach their upper or lower limit become frozen, or fixed at the limit value. With some exception, this seems to have little effect on the resulting maps (Miller et al., 1989, n. 23). Thus, this model has only two minor inconsistencies, which could be modified to make the system consistent. Limitation constraints enter the weight dynamics in two forms, $I_\approx^\alpha$ and $I_\geq^\alpha$. The former tends to keep $w_{\tau\rho}^L = -\frac{\epsilon}{\gamma}\alpha_{\tau\rho}$ while the latter keeps $w_{\tau\rho}^L \in [0, 8\alpha_{\tau\rho}]$, which can unnecessarily introduce conflicts. However, $\gamma = \epsilon = 0$, so that only the latter constraint applies and the $I_\approx^\alpha$ term is discarded in later publications. In principle, the system can be simplified by using coordinate transformation $\mathcal{C}^1$ instead of $\mathcal{C}^\alpha$, thereby eliminating $\alpha_{\tau\rho}$ in the growth rule Q^α as well as in the normalization rule $N_=^\alpha$, but not in the normalization rule $I_\geq^\alpha$. This is different from setting $\alpha_{\tau\rho}$ to a constant in a certain region. Using coordinate transformation $\mathcal{C}^1$ would result in the same set of stable solutions, though the trajectories would differ. Changing $\alpha_{\tau\rho}$ generates a different set of solutions. However, the original formulation using $\mathcal{C}^\alpha$ is more intuitive and generates the "correct" trajectories—those that correspond to the intuitive interpretation of the model.

Obermayer et al. (1990): This model is based on an algorithmic blob model and the linear correlation model is only an approximation (cf. the appendix). The weight dynamics is consistent. It employs the rarely used normalization constraint Z, which induces a multiplicative normalization rule under the coordinate transformation $\mathcal{C}^1$. No limitation constraint is necessary because neither the growth rule nor the multiplicative normalization rule can lead to negative weights, and positive weights are limited by the normalization rule.

Tanaka (1990): This model uses a nonlinear input-output function for the neurons, which makes a clear distinction between membrane potential and firing rate. However, this nonlinearity does not seem to play a specific functional role and is partially eliminated by linear approximations. Thus, the linear correlation model seems to be justified. The weight dynamics includes parameters $\beta_{\rho'}$ (f_{SP} in the original notation), which make it inconsistent. The penalty term $N_{\approx}^{\alpha w}$, which induces the first terms of the weight dynamics, is $-\frac{1}{2\kappa_1} \sum_{\tau'} (\kappa_0 - \kappa_1 \sum_{\rho'} \beta_{\rho'} w_{\tau'\rho'})^2$, which has to be evaluated under the coordinate transformation $\mathcal{C}^{\alpha w}$ with $\alpha_{\tau\rho} = 1/\beta_\rho$. Later in the article, the parameters $\beta_{\rho'}$ are set to 1, so that the system becomes consistent. Tanaka gives an objective function for the dynamics, employing a coordinate transformation for this purpose. The objective function is not listed here because it is derived under a different set of assumptions, including the nonlinear input-output function of the output neurons and a mean field approximation.

Goodhill (1993): This model is based on an algorithmic blob model and the linear correlation model is only an approximation (cf. the appendix). Like the model in Miller et al. (1989), this model uses an inconsistent normalization rule as a backup, and it freezes weights that reach their upper or lower limit. In addition, it uses an inconsistent normalization rule for the input neurons. But since this inconsistent multiplicative normalization for the input neurons is applied after a consistent subtractive normalization for the output neurons, its effect is relatively weak, and substituting it by a subtractive one would make little difference (G. J. Goodhill, personal communication). To avoid dead units (neurons in the output layer that never become active), Goodhill (1993) divides each output activity by the number of times each output neuron has won the competition for the blob in the output layer. This guarantees a roughly equal average activity of the output neurons. With the probabilistic blob model (cf. the appendix), dead units do not occur as long as output neurons have any input connections. The specific parameter setting of the model even guarantees a roughly equal average activity of the output neurons under the probabilistic blob model because the sum over the weights converging on an output neuron is roughly the same for all neurons in the output layer. Thus, despite some inconsistencies, this model can probably be well approximated within the constrained optimization framework.

Konen and von der Malsburg (1993): The activity dynamics is nonlinear and based on blobs. Thus the linear correlation model is only an approximation (cf. section 2.1). The weight dynamics is consistent. Although this is a model of dynamic link matching, it does not contain the linear term to bias the links. It introduces the similarity values in the constraints and through the coordinate transformation $\mathcal{C}^{\alpha w}$ (see section 6.4). No limitation constraint is necessary because neither the growth rule nor the multiplicative normalization rule can lead to negative weights, and positive weights are limited by the normalization rule.

6.3 Some Functional Aspects of Term Q. So far the focus of the considerations has been only on formal aspects of models of neural map formation.

Neural Map Formation

In this section some remarks on functional aspects of the quadratic term Q are made.

Assume the effective lateral connectivities in the output layer, and in the input layer are sums of positive and/or negative contributions. Each contribution can be either a constant, C, or a centered gaussian-like function, G, which depends on only the distance of the neurons, for example, $D_{\rho\rho'} = D_{|\rho-\rho'|}$ if ρ is a spatial coordinate. The contributions can be indicated by subscripts to the objective function Q. First index indicates the lateral connectivity of the input layer, the second index the one of the output layer. A negative gaussian (constant) would have to be indicated by $-G$ ($-C$). $Q_{(-C)G}$, for instance, would indicate a negative constant $D_{\rho\rho'}$ and a positive gaussian $D_{\tau\tau'}$. $Q_{G(G-G')}$ would indicate a positive gaussian $D_{\rho\rho'}$ and a $D_{\tau\tau'}$ that is a difference of gaussians. Notice that negative signs can cancel each other, for example $Q_{(G-C)G} = -Q_{(C-G)G} = -Q_{(G-C)(-G)}$. We thus discuss the terms only in their simplest form: $-Q_{CG}$ instead of $Q_{(-C)G}$. All feedforward weights are assumed to be positive. Assuming all weights to be negative would lead to equivalent results because Q does not change if all weights change their sign. The situation becomes more complex if some weights were positive and others negative. A term Q is called positive if it can be written in a form where it has a positive sign and only positive contributions; for example, $-Q_{(-C)G} = Q_{CG}$ is positive, while $Q_{(G-C)G}$ is not. Since Q is symmetrical with respect to $D_{\rho\rho'}$ and $D_{\tau\tau'}$, a term such as $Q_{(G-C)G}$ has the same effect as $Q_{G(G-C)}$ with the role of input layer and output layer exchanged. A complicated term can be analyzed most easily by splitting it into its elementary components. For instance, the term $Q_{G(G-C)}$ can be split into $Q_{GG}-Q_{GC}$ and analyzed as a combination of these two simpler terms.

Some elementary terms are now discussed in greater detail. The effect of the terms is considered under two types of constraints. In constraint A, the total sum of weights is constrained, $\sum_{\rho'\tau'} w_{\rho'\tau'} = 1$. In constraint B, the sums of weights originating from an input neuron, $\sum_{\tau'} w_{\rho\tau'} = 1/R$, or terminating on an output neuron, $\sum_{\rho'} w_{\rho'\tau} = 1/T$, are constrained, where R and T denote the number of input and output neurons, respectively. Without further constraints, a positive term always leads to infinite weight growth and a negative term to weight decay.

Terms $\pm Q_{CC}$ simplify to $\pm Q_{CC} = \pm D_{\rho\rho}D_{\tau\tau}(\sum_{\rho'\tau'} w_{\rho'\tau'})^2$ and depend on only the sum of weights. Thus, neither term has any effect under constraints A or B.

Term $+Q_{CG}$ takes its maximum value under constraint A if all links terminate on one output neuron. The map has the tendency to collapse. This is because the lateral connections in the output layer are higher for smaller distances and maximal for zero distance between connected neurons. Under the constraint $\sum_{\tau'} w_{\rho\tau'} \leq 1, \sum_{\rho'} w_{\rho'\tau} \leq 1$, for instance, the resulting map connects the input layer to a region in the output layer that is of the size of the input layer even if the output layer is much larger. No topography is taken into account because $D_{\rho\rho'}$ is constant and does not differentiate between different input neurons. Thus, this term has no effect under constraint B.

Term $-Q_{CG}$ has the opposite effect of $+Q_{CG}$. Consider the induced growth term $\dot{w}_{\rho\tau} = -D_{\rho\rho} \sum_{\tau'} D_{\tau\tau'} \sum_{\rho'} w_{\tau'\rho'}$. This is a convolution of $D_{\tau\tau'}$ with $\sum_{\rho'} w_{\tau'\rho'}$ and induces the largest decay in regions where the weighted sum over terminating links is maximal. A stable solution would require equal decay for all weights because constraint A can compensate only for equal decay. Thus, the convolution of $D_{\tau\tau'}$ with $\sum_{\rho'} w_{\tau'\rho'}$ must be a constant. Since $D_{\tau\tau'}$ is a gaussian, this is possible only if $\sum_{\rho'} w_{\tau'\rho'}$ is a constant, as can be easily seen in Fourier space. Thus, the map expands over the output layer, and each output neuron receives the same sum of weights. Constraint A could be substituted by a constant growth term L, in which case the expansion effect could be obtained without any explicit constraint. As $+Q_{CG}$, this term has no effect under constraint B.

Term $+Q_{GG}$ takes its maximum value under constraint A if all but one weight are zero. The map collapses on the input and the output layer. Under constraint B, the map becomes topographic because links that originate from neighboring neurons (high $D_{\rho\rho'}$ value) favorably terminate on neighboring neurons (high $D_{\tau\tau'}$ value). A more rigorous argument would require a definition of topography, but as argued in section 6.7, the term $+Q_{GG}$ can be directly taken as a generalized measure for topography.

Term $-Q_{GG}$ has the opposite effect of $+Q_{GG}$. Thus, it leads under constraint A to a map that is expanded over input and output layer. In addition, the map becomes antitopographic. Further analytical or numerical investigations are required to show whether the expansion is as even as for the term $-Q_{CG}$ and how an antitopographic map may look. Constraint B also leads to an antitopographic map.

6.4 Equivalent Models. The effect of coordinate transformations has been considered so far only for single growth terms and normalization rules. Coordinate transformations can be used to generate different models that are equivalent in terms of their constrained optimization problem. Consider the system in Konen and von der Malsburg (1993). Its objective function and constraint function are Q and $N_\geq$,

$$H(\mathbf{w}) = \frac{1}{2} \sum_{ij} w_i D_{ij} w_j, \qquad g_n(\mathbf{w}) = 1 - \sum_{j \in I_n} \frac{w_j}{\alpha_j} = 0, \qquad (6.1)$$

which must be evaluated under the coordinate transformation $\mathcal{C}^{\alpha w}$ to induce the original weight dynamics $Q^{\alpha w}$ and $N_\geq^{\alpha w}$,

$$\dot{w}_i = \alpha_i w_i \sum_j D_{ij} w_j, \qquad w_i = \frac{\tilde{w}_i}{\sum_{j \in I_n} \frac{\tilde{w}_j}{\alpha_j}}. \qquad (6.2)$$

Neural Map Formation

If evaluated directly (i.e., under the coordinate transformation C^1), one would obtain

$$\dot{w}_i = \sum_j D_{ij} w_j, \qquad w_i = \tilde{w}_i + \frac{1}{\sum_{j \in I_n} \alpha_j^{-2}} \left(1 - \sum_{j \in I_n} \frac{\tilde{w}_j}{\alpha_j}\right) \frac{1}{\alpha_i}. \qquad (6.3)$$

As argued in section 5.2.4, an additional limitation constraint $I_>^1$ (or $I_>^1$) has to be added to this system to account for the limitation constraint implicitly introduced by the coordinate transformation $C^{\alpha w}$ for the dynamics above (see equation 6.2).

It follows from equation 4.8 that the flow fields of the weight dynamics in equations 6.2 and 6.3 differ, but since $dw_i/dv_i \neq 0$ for positive weights, the fixed points are the same. That means that the resulting maps to which the two systems converge, possibly from different initial states, are the same. In this sense, these two dynamics are equivalent.

This also holds for other coordinate transformations within the defined region as long as dw_i/dv_i is finite ($dw_i/dv_i = 0$ may introduce additional fixed points). Thus, this method of generating equivalent models makes it possible to abstract the objective function from the dynamics. Different equivalent dynamics may have different convergence properties, their attractor basins may differ, and some regions in state space may not be reachable under a particular coordinate transformation. In any case, within the reachable state space, the fixed points are the same. Thus, coordinate transformations make it possible to optimize the dynamics without changing its objective function.

Normalization rules derived by different methods can substitute each other without changing the qualitative behavior of a system. For instance, $I_=$ can be replaced by $I_\approx$, or $N_\geq$ can be replaced by $N_>$ under any coordinate transformation. These replacements will also generate equivalent systems in a practical sense.

6.5 Dynamic Link Matching. In the previous section, the similarity values α_i entered the weight dynamics in two places. In equation 6.2, the differential effect of α_i enters only the growth rule, while in equation 6.3, it enters only the normalization rule. Growth and normalization rules can, to some extent, be interchangeably used to incorporate feature information in dynamic link matching. However, the objective function (see equation 6.1) shows that the similarity values are introduced through the constraints and that they are transferred to the growth rule only by the coordinate transformation $C^{\alpha w}$. Similarity values can enter the growth rule more directly through the linear term L. An alternative objective function for dynamic link matching is

$$H(\mathbf{w}) = \sum_i \beta_i w_i + \frac{1}{2} \sum_{ij} w_i D_{ij} w_j, \quad g_n(\mathbf{w}) = 1 - \sum_{j \in I_n} w_j = 0, \quad (6.4)$$

with $\beta_i = \alpha_i$. The first term now directly favors links with high similarity values. This may be advantageous because it allows better control over the influence of the topography versus the feature similarity term. Furthermore, this objective function is more closely related to the similarity function of elastic graph matching in Lades et al. (1993), which has been developed as an algorithmic abstraction of dynamic link matching (see section 6.7).

6.6 Soft versus Hard Competitive Normalization. Miller and MacKay (1994) have analyzed the role of normalization rules for neural map formation. They consider a linear Hebbian growth rule Q^1 and investigate the dynamics under a subtractive normalization rule $N_=^1$ (S1 in their notation) and two types of multiplicative normalization rules, $N_=^w$ and $Z_=^1$ (M1 and M2 in their notation, respectively). They show that when considering an isolated output neuron with the multiplicative normalization rules, the weight vector tends to the principal eigenvector of the matrix D, which means that many weights can maintain some finite value. Under the subtractive normalization rule, a winner-take-all behavior occurs, and the weight vector tends to saturate with each single weight having either its minimal or maximal value producing a more compact receptive field. If no upper bound is imposed on individual weights, only one weight survives, corresponding to a point receptive field.

von der Malsburg and Willshaw (1981) have performed a similar, though less comprehensive, analysis using a different approach. Instead of modifying the normalization rule, they considered different growth rules with the same multiplicative normalization rule $N_=^w$. They also found two qualitatively different behaviors: a highly competitive case in which only one link survives (or several if single weights are limited in growth by individual bounds) (case $\mu=1$ or $\mu=2$ in their notation) and a less competitive case in which each weight is eventually proportional to the correlation between pre- and postsynaptic neuron (case $\mu=0$).

Hence, one can either change the normalization rule and keep the growth rule or, vice versa, modify the growth rule and keep the normalization rule the same. Either choice generates the two different behaviors. As shown above, by changing both the growth and normalization rules consistently by a coordinate transformation, it is possible to obtain two different weight dynamics with qualitatively the same behavior. More precisely, the system (Q^w, N^w) is equivalent to (Q^1, N^1, I^1) and has the same fixed points; the former one uses a multiplicative normalization rule, and the latter uses a subtractive one. This also explains why changing the growth rule or changing the normalization rule can be equivalent.

Neural Map Formation

It may therefore be misleading to refer to the different cases by the specific normalization rules (subtractive versus multiplicative), because that is valid only for the linear Hebbian growth rule Q^1. We suggest using a more generally applicable nomenclature that refers to the different behaviors rather than the specific mathematical formulation. Following the terminology of Nowlan (1990) in a similar context, the term *hard competitive* normalization could be used to denote the case where only one link survives (or a set of saturated links, which are limited by upper bounds); the term *soft competitive* normalization could be used to denote the case where each link has some strength proportional to its fitness.

6.7 Related Objective Functions. Objective functions also provide means for comparing weight dynamics with other algorithms or dynamics of a different origin for which an objective function exists.

First, maximizing the objective functions L and Q under linear constraints I and N is the quadratic programming problem, and finding an optimal one-to-one mapping between two layers of same size for objective function Q is the quadratic assignment problem. These problems are known to be NP-complete. However, there is a large literature on algorithms that efficiently solve special cases or find good approximate solutions in polynomial time (e.g., Horst, Pandalos, & Thoai, 1995).

Many related objective functions are defined only for maps for which each input neuron terminates on exactly one output neuron with weight 1, which makes the index $\tau = \tau(\rho)$ a function of index ρ. An objective function of this kind may have the form

$$H = \sum_{\rho\rho'} G_{\tau\rho\tau'\rho'}, \tag{6.5}$$

where G encodes how well a pair of links from ρ to $\tau(\rho)$ and from ρ' to $\tau'(\rho')$ preserves topography. A pair of parallel links, for instance, would yield high G values, while others would yield lower values. Now define a particular family of weights **w** that realize one-to-one connectivities:

$$\bar{w}_{\tau\rho} = \begin{cases} 1 & \text{if } \tau = \tau(\rho) \\ 0 & \text{otherwise.} \end{cases} \tag{6.6}$$

$\bar{\mathbf{w}}$ is a subset of **w** with $\bar{w}_{\tau\rho} \in \{0, 1\}$ as opposed to $w_{\tau\rho} \in [0, 1]$. It indicates that an objective function was originally defined for a one-to-one map rather than the more general case of an all-to-all connectivity. Then objective functions of one-to-one maps can be written as

$$H(\bar{\mathbf{w}}) = \sum_{\tau\rho\tau'\rho'} \bar{w}_{\tau\rho} G_{\tau\rho\tau'\rho'} \bar{w}_{\tau'\rho'} = \sum_{ij} \bar{w}_i G_{ij} \bar{w}_j, \tag{6.7}$$

with $i = \{\rho, \tau\}, j = \{\rho', \tau'\}$ as defined above. Simply replacing $\bar{\mathbf{w}}$ by $\mathbf{w}$ then yields a generalization of the original objective function to all-to-all connectivities.

Goodhill, Finch, and Sejnowski (1996) have compared 10 different objective functions for topographic maps and have proposed another, the C measure. They show that for the case of an equal number of neurons in the input and the output layer, most other objective functions can be either reduced to the C measure, or they represent a closely related objective function. This suggests that the C measure is a good unifying measure for topography. The C measure is equivalent to our objective function Q with $\bar{\mathbf{w}}$ instead of $\mathbf{w}$. Adapted to the notation of this article the C measure has the form

$$C(\bar{\mathbf{w}}) = \sum_{ij} \bar{w}_i G_{ij} \bar{w}_j, \tag{6.8}$$

with a separable G_{ij}, that is, $G_{ij} = G_{\rho\tau\rho'\tau'} = G_{\tau\tau'} G_{\rho\rho'}$. Thus, the objective function Q is the typical term for topographic maps in other contexts as well.

Elastic graph matching is an algorithmic counterpart to dynamic link matching and has been used for applications such as object and face recognition (Lades et al., 1993). It is based on a similarity function that in its simplest version is

$$H(\bar{\mathbf{w}}) = \sum_i \beta_i \bar{w}_i + \frac{1}{2} \sum_{ij} \bar{w}_i G_{ij} \bar{w}_j, \tag{6.9}$$

where $G_{ij} = -[(\mathbf{p}_\rho - \mathbf{p}_{\rho'}) - (\mathbf{p}_\tau - \mathbf{p}_{\tau'})]^2$, and $\mathbf{p}_\rho$ and $\mathbf{p}_\tau$ are two-dimensional position vectors in the image plane. This similarity function corresponds formally to the objective function in equation 6.4. The main difference between these two functions is hidden in G and D. The latter ought to be separable into two factors $D_{\rho\tau\rho'\tau'} = D_{\rho\rho'} D_{\tau\tau'}$ while the former is clearly not. G actually favors a metric map, which tends to preserve not only neighborhood relations but also distances, whereas with D, the maps always tend to collapse.

6.8 Self-Organizing Map Algorithm. Models of the self-organizing map (SOM) algorithm can be high-dimensional or low-dimensional, and two different learning rules, which we have called weight dynamics, are commonly used. The validity of the probabilistic blob model for the high-dimensional models is discussed in the appendix. A classification of the high-dimensional model by Obermayer et al. (1990) is given in Table 2. The low-dimensional models do not fall into the class of one-to-one mappings considered in the previous section, because the input layer is represented as a continuous space and not as a discrete set of neurons.

Neural Map Formation

One learning rule for the high-dimensional SOM algorithm is given by

$$\tilde{w}_{\tau\rho}(t) = w_{\tau\rho}(t-1) + \epsilon B_{\tau\tau_0} B_{\rho\rho_0} \tag{6.10}$$

$$w_{\tau\rho}(t) = \frac{\tilde{w}_{\tau\rho}(t)}{\sqrt{\sum_{\rho'} \tilde{w}^2_{\tau\rho'}(t)}}, \tag{6.11}$$

as used, for example, in Obermayer et al. (1990). $B_{\tau\tau_0}$ denotes the neighborhood function (commonly indicated by h) and $B_{\rho\rho_0}$ denotes the stimulus pattern (sometimes indicated by x) with index ρ_0. $B_{\rho\rho_0}$ does not need to have a blob shape, so that ρ_0 may be an arbitrary index. Output neuron τ_0 is the winner neuron in response to stimulus pattern ρ_0. This learning rule is a consistent combination of growth rule Q^1 and normalization rule $Z^1_=$ and an objective function exists, which is a good approximation to the extent that the probabilistic blob model is valid.

The second type of learning rule is given by

$$w_{\tau\rho}(t+1) = w_{\tau\rho}(t) + \epsilon B_{\tau\tau_0}(B_{\rho\rho_0} - w_{\tau\rho}(t)), \tag{6.12}$$

as used, for example, in Bauer, Brockmann, and Geisel (1997). For this learning rule, the weights and the input stimuli are assumed to be sum normalized: $\sum_\rho w_{\tau\rho} = 1$ and $\sum_\rho B_{\rho\rho_0} = 1$. For small ϵ this learning rule is equivalent to

$$\tilde{w}_{\tau\rho}(t) = w_{\tau\rho}(t-1) + \epsilon B_{\tau\tau_0} B_{\rho\rho_0} \tag{6.13}$$

$$w_{\tau\rho}(t) = \frac{\tilde{w}_{\tau\rho}(t)}{\sum_{\rho'} \tilde{w}_{\tau\rho'}(t)}, \tag{6.14}$$

which shows that it is a combination of growth rule Q^1 and normalization rule $N^w_=$. Thus, this system is inconsistent, and to formulate it within our constrained optimization framework $N^w_=$ would have to be approximated by $Z^1_=$, which leads back to the learning rule in equations 6.10 and 6.11.

There are two ways of going from these high-dimensional models to the low-dimensional models. The first is simply to use fewer input neurons (e.g., two). A low-dimensional input vector is then represented by the activities of these few neurons. However, since the low-dimensional input vectors are usually not normalized to homogeneous mean activity of the input neurons and since the receptive and projective fields of the neurons do not codevelop in a homogeneous way, the probabilistic blob model is usually not valid.

A second way of going from a high-dimensional model to a low-dimensional model is by considering the low-dimensional input vectors and weight vectors as abstract representatives of the high-dimensional ones (Ritter, Martinetz, & Schulten, 1991; Behrmann, 1993). Consider, for example, the weight dynamics in equation 6.12 and a two-dimensional input layer. Let $\mathbf{p}_\rho$ be a position vector of input neuron ρ. The center of the receptive field of neuron τ can be defined as

$$\mathbf{m}_\tau(\mathbf{w}) = \sum_\rho \mathbf{p}_\rho w_{\tau\rho}, \tag{6.15}$$

and the center of the input blob can be defined similarly,

$$\mathbf{x}(\mathbf{B}_{\rho_0}) = \sum_\rho \mathbf{p}_\rho B_{\rho\rho_0}. \tag{6.16}$$

Notice that the input blobs as well as the weights are normalized, that is, $\sum_\rho B_{\rho\rho_0} = 1$ and $\sum_\rho w_{\tau\rho} = 1$. Using these definitions and given a pair of blobs at locations ρ_0 and τ_0, the high-dimensional learning rule (see equation 6.12) yields the low-dimensional learning rule

$$\mathbf{m}_\tau(\mathbf{w}(t+1)) = \sum_\rho \mathbf{p}_\rho \left(w_{\tau\rho}(t) + \epsilon B_{\tau\tau_0}(B_{\rho\rho_0} - w_{\tau\rho}(t)) \right) \tag{6.17}$$

$$= \mathbf{m}_\tau(\mathbf{w}(t)) + \epsilon B_{\tau\tau_0} \left(\mathbf{x}(\mathbf{B}_{\rho_0}) - \mathbf{m}_\tau(\mathbf{w}(t)) \right) \tag{6.18}$$

$$\iff \mathbf{m}_\tau(t+1) = \mathbf{m}_\tau(t) + \epsilon B_{\tau\tau_0} \left(\mathbf{x}_{\rho_0} - \mathbf{m}_\tau(t) \right). \tag{6.19}$$

One can first calculate the centers of the receptive fields of the high-dimensional model and then apply the low-dimensional learning rule, or one can first apply the high-dimensional learning rule and then calculate the centers of the receptive fields; the result is the same. Notice that the low-dimensional learning rule is even formally equivalent to the high-dimensional one and that it is the rule commonly used in low-dimensional models (Kohonen, 1990). Even though the high- and the low-dimensional learning rules are equivalent for a given pair of blobs, the overall behavior of the models is not. This is because the positioning of the output blobs is different in the two models (Behrmann, 1993). It is clear that many different high-dimensional weight configurations having different output blob positioning can lead to the same low-dimensional weight configuration. However, for a high-dimensional model that self-organizes a topographic map with point receptive fields, the positioning may be similar for the high- and the low-dimensional models, so that the stable maps may be similar as well.

These considerations show that only the high-dimensional model in equations 6.10 and 6.11 can be consistently described within our constrained optimization framework. The high-dimensional model of equation 6.12 is inconsistent. The probabilistic blob model in general is not applicable to low-dimensional models, because some assumptions required for its derivation are not valid. The simple relation between the high- and the low-dimensional model sketched above holds only for the learning step but not for the blob positioning, though the positioning and thus the resulting maps may be very similar for topographic maps with point receptive fields.

7 Conclusions and Future Perspectives

The results presented here can be summarized:

- A probabilistic nonlinear blob model can behave like a linear correlation model under fairly general conditions (see section 2.1 and the appendix). This clarifies the relationship between deterministic nonlinear blob models and linear correlation models and provides an approximation of the former by the latter.

- Coordinate transformations can transform dynamics with curl into curl-free dynamics, allowing the otherwise impossible formulation of an objective function (see section 4). A similar effect exists for normalization rules. Coordinate transformations can transform nonorthogonal normalization rules into orthogonal ones, allowing the normalization rule to be formulated as a constraint (see section 5.1).

- Growth rules and normalization rules must have a special relationship in order to make a formulation of the system dynamics as a constrained optimization problem possible: the growth rule must be a gradient flow, and the normalization rules must be orthogonal under the same coordinate transformation (see section 5.1).

- Constraints can be enforced by various types of normalization rules (see section 5.2), and they can even be implicitly introduced by coordinate transformations (see section 5.2.4) or the activity dynamics (see section A.2).

- Many all-to-all connected models from the literature can be classified within our constrained optimization framework based on only four terms: L, Q, I, and N (Z) (see section 6.2). The linear term L has rarely been used, but it can have a specific function that may be useful in future models (see section 6.5).

- Models may differ considerably in their weight dynamics and still solve the same optimization problem. This can be revealed by coordinate transformations and by comparing the different but possibly equivalent types of normalization rules (see section 6.4). Coordinate transformations make it in particular possible to optimize the dynamics without changing the stable fixed points.

- The constrained optimization framework provides a convenient formalism to analyze functional aspects of the models (see sections 6.3, 6.5, and 6.6).

- The constrained optimization framework for all-to-all connected models presented here is closely related to approaches for finding optimal one-to-one maps (see section 6.7) but is not easily adapted to the self-organizing map algorithm (see section 6.8).

- Models of neural map formation formulated as constrained optimization problems provide a unifying framework. It abstracts from arbitrary differences in the design of models and leaves only those differences that are likely to be crucial for the different structures that emerge by self-organization.

It is important to note that our constrained optimization framework is unifying in the sense that it provides a canonical formulation independent of most arbitrary design decisions, for example, due to different coordinate transformations or different types of normalization rules. This does not mean that most models are actually equivalent. But with the canonical formulation of the models as constrained optimization problems, it should be possible to focus on the crucial differences and to understand better what the essentials of neural map formation are.

Based on the constrained optimization framework presented here, a next step would be to consider specific architectures with particular effective lateral connectivities and to investigate the structures that emerge. The role of parameters and effective lateral connectivities might be investigated analytically for a variety of models by means of objective functions, similar to the approach sketched in section 6.3 or the one taken in MacKay and Miller (1990).

We have considered here only three levels of abstraction: detailed neural dynamics, abstract weight dynamics, and constrained optimization. There are even higher levels of abstraction, and the relationship between our constrained optimization framework and these more abstract models should be explored. For example, in section 6.7 our objective functions were compared with other objective functions defined only for one-to-one connectivities. Another possible link is with Bienenstock and von der Malsburg (1987) and Tanaka (1990), who have proposed spin models for neural map formation. An interesting approach is that taken by Linsker (1986), who analyzed the receptive fields of the output neurons, which were oriented edge filters of arbitrary orientation. He derived an energy function to evaluate how the different orientations would be arranged in the output layer due to lateral interactions. The only variables of this energy function were the orientations of the receptive fields, an abstraction from the connectivity. Similar models were proposed earlier in Swindale (1980), though not derived from a receptive field model, and more recently in Tanaka (1991). These approaches and their relationships to our constrained optimization framework need to be investigated more systematically.

A neural map formation model of Amari (1980) could not be formulated within the constrained optimization framework presented here (cf. section 6.2). The weight growth in this model is limited by weight decay rather than explicit normalization rules, which is possible because the blob dynamics provides only limited correlation values even if the weights would grow large. This model is particularly elegant with respect to the

Neural Map Formation

way it indirectly introduces constraints and should be investigated further. Our discussion in section 6.3 indicates that the system L+Q might also show map expansion and weight limitation without any explicit constraints, but further analysis is needed to confirm this.

The objective functions listed in Table 1 have a tendency to produce either collapsing or expanding maps. It is unlikely that the terms can be counterbalanced such that they have the tendency to preserve distances directly, independent of normalization rules and the size of the layers, as does the algorithmic objective function in equation 6.9. A solution to this problem might be found by examining propagating activity patterns in the input as well as the output layer, such as traveling waves (Triesch, 1995) or running blobs (Wiskott & von der Malsburg, 1996). Waves and blobs of activity have been observed in the developing retina (Meister, Wong, Baylor, & Shatz, 1991). If the waves or blobs have the same intrinsic velocity in the two layers, they would tend to generate metric maps, regardless of the scaling factor induced by the normalization rules. It would be interesting to investigate this idea further and derive correlations for this class of models.

Another limitation of the framework discussed here is that it is confined to second-order correlations. As von der Malsburg (1995) has pointed out, this is appropriate only for a subset of phenomena of neural map formation, such as retinotopy and ocular dominance. Although orientation tuning can arise by spontaneous symmetry breaking (e.g., Linsker, 1986), a full understanding of the self-organization of orientation selectivity and other phenomena may require taking higher-order correlations into account. It would be interesting as a next step to consider third-order terms in the objective function and the conditions under which they can be derived from detailed neural dynamics. There may also be an interesting relationship to recent advances in algorithms for independent component analysis (Bell & Sejnowski, 1995), which can be derived from a maximum entropy method and is dominated by higher-order correlations.

Finally, it may be interesting to investigate the extent to which the techniques used in the analysis presented here can be applied to other types of neural dynamics, such as learning rules. The existence of objective functions for dynamics with curl may make it possible to formulate more learning rules within the constrained optimization framework, which could lead to new insights. Optimizing the dynamics of a learning rule without changing the set of stable fixed points may be an interesting application for coordinate transformations.

Appendix: Probabilistic Blob Model

A.1 Noise Model. Consider the activity model of Obermayer et al. (1990) as an abstraction of the neural activity dynamics in section 2.1 (see equations 2.1 and 2.2). Obermayer et al. use a high-dimensional version of the self-organizing map algorithm (Kohonen, 1982). A blob $B_{\rho'\rho_0}$ is located at a random position ρ_0 in the input layer, and the input $i_{\tau'}(\rho_0)$ received by the output neurons is calculated as in equation 2.7. A blob $\bar{B}_{\tau'\tau_0}$ in the output layer is located at the position τ_0 of highest input, that is, $i_{\tau_0}(\rho_0) = \max_{\tau'} i_{\tau'}(\rho_0)$. Only the latter step differs in its outcome from the dynamics in section 2, the maximal input instead of the maximal overlap determining the location of the output blob.

The transition to the probabilistic blob location can be done by assuming that the blob $\bar{B}_{\tau'\tau_0}$ in the output layer is located at τ_0 with probability

$$p(\tau_0|\rho_0) = i_{\tau_0}(\rho_0) = \sum_{\rho'} w_{\tau_0\rho'} B_{\rho'\rho_0}. \tag{A.1}$$

For the following considerations, the same normalization assumptions as in section 2.1 are made, which leads to $\sum_{\tau'} i_{\tau'}(\rho_0) = 1$ and $\sum_{\tau_0} p(\tau_0|\rho_0) = 1$ and justifies the interpretation of $p(\tau_0|\rho_0)$ as a probability. The effect of different normalization rules, like those used by Obermayer et al. (1990), is discussed in the next section. The probabilistic blob location can be achieved by multiplicative noise η_τ with the cumulative density function $f(\eta) = \exp(-1/\eta)$, which leads to a modified input $l_\tau = \eta_\tau i_\tau$ with a cumulative density function

$$f_\tau(l_\tau) = \exp\left(-\frac{i_\tau(\rho_0)}{l_\tau}\right), \tag{A.2}$$

and a probability density function

$$p_\tau(l_\tau) = \frac{\partial f_\tau}{\partial l_\tau} = \frac{i_\tau(\rho_0)}{l_\tau^2} \exp\left(-\frac{i_\tau(\rho_0)}{l_\tau}\right). \tag{A.3}$$

Notice that the noise is different for each output neuron but always from the same distribution. The probability of neuron τ_0 having larger input l_{τ_0} than all other neurons τ', that is, the probability of the output blob being located at τ_0, is

$$p(\tau_0|\rho_0) = p(l_{\tau_0} > l_{\tau'} \ \forall \tau' \neq \tau_0) \tag{A.4}$$

$$= \int_0^\infty p_{\tau_0}(l_{\tau_0}) \prod_{\tau' \neq \tau_0} f_{\tau'}(l_{\tau_0}) \, dl_{\tau_0} \tag{A.5}$$

$$= \int_0^\infty \frac{i_{\tau_0}(\rho_0)}{l_{\tau_0}^2} \exp\left(-\frac{1}{l_{\tau_0}} \sum_{\tau'} i_{\tau'}(\rho_0)\right) dl_{\tau_0} \tag{A.6}$$

$$= \frac{i_{\tau_0}(\rho_0)}{\sum_{\tau'} i_{\tau'}(\rho_0)} \tag{A.7}$$

$$= i_{\tau_0}(\rho_0) \quad \left(\text{since } \sum_{\tau'} i_{\tau'}(\rho_0) = 1\right), \tag{A.8}$$

Neural Map Formation

which is the desired result. Thus, the model by Obermayer et al. (1990) can be modified by multiplicative noise to yield the probabilistic blob location behavior. A problem is that the modified input l_τ has an infinite mean value, but this can be corrected by consistently transforming the cumulative density functions by the substitution $l_\tau = k_\tau^2$, yielding

$$f_\tau(k_\tau) = \exp\left(-\frac{i_\tau(\rho_0)}{k_\tau^2}\right) \tag{A.9}$$

for the new modified inputs k_τ, the means of which are finite. Due to the nonlinear transformation $l_\tau = k_\tau^2$, the modified inputs k_τ are no longer a product of the original input i_τ with noise, whose distribution is the same for all neurons, but each input i_τ generates a modified input k_τ with a nonlinearly distorted version of the cumulative density function in equation A.2.

The probability for a particular combination of blob locations is

$$p(\tau_0, \rho_0) = p(\tau_0|\rho_0)p(\rho_0) = \sum_{\rho'} w_{\tau_0\rho'} B_{\rho'\rho_0} \frac{1}{R}, \tag{A.10}$$

and the correlation between two neurons defined as the average product of their activities is

$$\langle a_\tau a_\rho \rangle = \sum_{\tau_0\rho_0} p(\tau_0, \rho_0) \bar{B}_{\tau\tau_0} B_{\rho\rho_0} \tag{A.11}$$

$$= \sum_{\tau_0\rho_0} \sum_{\rho'} w_{\tau_0\rho'} B_{\rho'\rho_0} \frac{1}{R} \bar{B}_{\tau\tau_0} B_{\rho\rho_0} \tag{A.12}$$

$$= \frac{1}{R} \sum_{\tau'\rho'} \bar{B}_{\tau\tau'} w_{\tau'\rho'} \left(\sum_{\rho_0} B_{\rho'\rho_0} B_{\rho\rho_0} \right) \tag{A.13}$$

$$= \frac{1}{R} \sum_{\tau'\rho'} \bar{B}_{\tau\tau'} w_{\tau'\rho'} \bar{B}_{\rho'\rho}, \quad \text{with} \quad \bar{B}_{\rho'\rho} = \sum_{\rho_0} B_{\rho'\rho_0} B_{\rho\rho_0}, \tag{A.14}$$

where the brackets $\langle \cdot \rangle$ indicate the ensemble average over a large number of blob presentations. This is equivalent to equation 2.13 if $\bar{B}_{\tau'\tau} = \sum_{\tau_0} B_{\tau'\tau_0} B_{\tau\tau_0}$. Thus, the two probabilistic dynamics are equivalent, though the blobs in the output layer must be different.

A.2 Different Normalization Rules. The derivation of correlations in the probabilistic blob model given above assumes explicit presynaptic normalization of the form $\sum_{\tau'} w_{\tau'\rho'} = 1$. This assumption is not valid for some models that use only postsynaptic normalization (e.g., von der Malsburg, 1973). The model by Obermayer et al. (1990) postsynaptically normalizes the square sum, $\sum_{\rho'} w_{\tau'\rho'}^2 = 1$, instead of the sum, which may make the applicability of the probabilistic blob model even more questionable.

To investigate the effect of these different normalization rules on the probabilistic blob model, assume that the projective (or receptive) fields of the input (or output) neurons codevelop in such a way that, at any given moment, all neurons in a layer have the same weight histogram. Neuron ρ, for instance, would have the weight histogram $w_{\tau'\rho}$ taken over τ', and it would be the same as those of the other neurons ρ'. Two neurons of same weight histogram have the same number of nonzero weights, and the square sums over their weights differ from the sums by the same factor c, for example, $\sum_{\tau'} w_{\tau'\rho'}^2 = c \sum_{\tau'} w_{\tau'\rho'} = 1$ for all ρ' with $c \leq 1$. The weight histogram, and with it the factor c, may change over time. For instance, if point receptive fields develop from an initial all-to-all connectivity, the histogram has a single peak at $1/T$ in the beginning and has a peak at 0 and one entry at 1 at the end of the self-organization process, and $c(t)$ grows from $1/T$ up to 1, where T is the number of output neurons.

Consider first the effect of the square sum normalization under the assumption of homogeneous codevelopment of receptive and projective fields. The square sum normalization differs from the sum normalization by a factor $c(t)$ common to all neurons in the layer. Since the nonlinear blob model is insensitive to such a factor, the derived correlations and the learning rule are off by this factor c. Since this factor is common to all weights, the trajectories of the weight dynamics are identical, though the time scales differ by c between the two types of normalization.

Consider now the effect of pure postsynaptic normalization under the assumption of homogeneous codevelopment of receptive and projective fields. Assume a pair of blobs is located at ρ_0 and τ_0. With a linear growth rule, the sum over weights originating from an input neuron would change according to

$$\dot{W}_\rho = \sum_\tau \dot{w}_{\tau\rho} = \sum_\tau B_{\tau\tau_0} B_{\rho\rho_0} = B_{\rho\rho_0}, \qquad (A.15)$$

since the blob $B_{\tau\tau_0}$ is normalized to one. Averaging over all input blob positions yields an average change of

$$\langle \dot{W}_\rho \rangle = \frac{1}{R} \sum_{\rho_0} B_{\rho\rho_0} = \frac{1}{R}, \qquad (A.16)$$

since we assume a homogeneous average activity in the input layer, that is, $\sum_{\rho_0} B_{\rho\rho_0} = 1$. A similar expression follows for the postsynaptic sum:

$$\langle \dot{W}_\tau \rangle = \sum_{\rho_0 \tau_0} p(\tau_0, \rho_0) \sum_\rho B_{\tau\tau_0} B_{\rho\rho_0} \qquad (A.17)$$

$$= \sum_{\rho_0 \tau_0} \left(\frac{1}{R} \sum_{\tau'\rho'} B_{\tau'\tau_0} w_{\tau'\rho'} B_{\rho'\rho_0} \right) \sum_\rho B_{\tau\tau_0} B_{\rho\rho_0} \qquad (A.18)$$

Neural Map Formation

$$= \frac{1}{R} \sum_{\tau_0} B_{\tau\tau_0} \sum_{\tau'} B_{\tau'\tau_0} \sum_{\rho'} w_{\tau'\rho'} \sum_{\rho_0} B_{\rho'\rho_0} \sum_{\rho} B_{\rho\rho_0} \qquad (A.19)$$

$$= \frac{1}{T}, \qquad (A.20)$$

where $\sum_{\rho'} w_{\tau'\rho'} = R/T$ is assumed due to the postsynaptic normalization rule and the blobs are normalized with respect to both of their indices. R and T are the number of neurons in the input and output layer, respectively. This equation shows that each output neuron has to normalize its sum of weights by the same amount, and it has to do that by a subtractive normalization rule if the system is consistent. The amount by which each single weight $w_{\tau\rho}$ is changed depends on the number of nonzero weights an output neuron receives. Since we assume the weight histograms are the same, each output neuron has the same number of nonzero weights, and each weight gets corrected by the same amount. Since we also assume same weight histograms for the projective fields, the sum over all weights originating from an input neuron is corrected by the same amount for each input neuron, namely, by $1/R$ per time unit. Thus, the postsynaptic normalization rule preserves presynaptic normalization.

It can even be argued that a postsynaptic normalization rule stabilizes presynaptic normalization. Assume that an input neuron has a larger (or smaller) sum over its weights than the other input neurons. Then this neuron is likely to have more (fewer) nonzero weights than the other input neurons. This results in a larger (smaller) negative compensation by the postsynaptic normalization rule, since each weight is corrected by the same amount. This then reduces the difference between the input neuron under consideration and the others. It is important to notice that this effect of stabilizing the presynaptic normalization is not preserved in the constrained optimization formulation. It may be necessary to use explicit presynaptic normalization in the constrained optimization formulation to account for the implicit presynaptic normalization in the blob model.

If the postsynaptic constraint is based on the square sum, then the normalization rule is multiplicative, and the projective fields of the input neurons need not have the same weight histograms. The system would still preserve the presynaptic normalization. Notice that the derivation given above does not hold for a nonlinear Hebbian rule, for example, $\dot{w}_{\tau\rho} = w_{\tau\rho} a_\tau a_\rho$.

These considerations show that the probabilistic blob model may be a good approximation even if the constraints are based on the square sum instead of the sum and if only the postsynaptic neurons are constrained and not the presynaptic neurons, as was required in the derivation of the probabilistic blob model above. The homogeneous codevelopment of receptive and projective fields is probably a reasonable assumption for high-dimensional models with a homogeneous architecture. For low-dimensional models, such as the low-dimensional self-organizing map algorithm (Kohonen, 1982), the assumption is less likely to be valid. However, numerical simulations or more detailed analytical considerations are needed to verify the assumption for any given concrete model.

Acknowledgments

We are grateful to Geoffrey J. Goodhill, Thomas Maurer, Jozsef Fiser, and two anonymous referees for carefully reading the manuscript and offering useful comments. L. W. has been supported by a Feodor-Lynen fellowship by the Alexander von Humboldt-Foundation, Bonn, Germany.

References

Amari, S. (1977). Dynamics of pattern formation in lateral-inhibition type neural fields. *Biol. Cybern.*, 27, 77–87.

Amari, S. (1980). Topographic organization of nerve fields. *Bulletin of Mathematical Biology*, 42, 339–364.

Bauer, H.-U., Brockmann, D., & Geisel, T. (1997). Analysis of ocular dominance pattern formation in a high-dimensional self-organizing-map model. *Network: Computation in Neural Systems*, 8(1), 17–33.

Behrmann, K. (1993). *Leistungsuntersuchungen des "Dynamischen Link-Matchings" und Vergleich mit dem Kohonen-Algorithmus* (Internal Rep. No. IR-INI 93–05). Bochum: Institut für Neuroinformatik, Ruhr-Universität Bochum.

Bell, A. J., & Sejnowski, T. J. (1995). An information-maximization approach to blind separation and blind deconvolution. *Neural Computation*, 7, 1129–1159.

Bienenstock, E., & von der Malsburg, C. (1987). A neural network for invariant pattern recognition. *Europhysics Letters*, 4(1), 121–126.

Dirac, P. A. M. (1996). *General theory of relativity*. Princeton, NJ: Princeton University Press.

Ermentrout, G. B., & Cowan, J. D. (1979). A mathematical theory of visual hallucination patterns. *Biological Cybernetics*, 34(3), 137–150.

Erwin, E., Obermayer, K., & Schulten, K. (1995). Models of orientation and ocular dominance columns in the visual cortex: A critical comparison. *Neural Computation*, 7, 425–468.

Ginzburg, I., & Sompolinsky, H. (1994). Theory of correlations in stochastic neural networks. *Physical Review E*, 50(4), 3171–3191.

Goodhill, G. J. (1993). Topography and ocular dominance: A model exploring positive correlations. *Biol. Cybern.*, 69, 109–118.

Goodhill, G. J., Finch, S., & Sejnowski, T. J. (1996). Optimizing cortical mappings. In D. Touretzky, M. Mozer, & M. Hasselmo (Eds.), *Advances in neural information processing systems* (Vol. 8, pp. 330–336). Cambridge, MA: MIT Press.

Häussler, A. F., & von der Malsburg, C. (1983). Development of retinotopic projections—An analytical treatment. *J. Theor. Neurobiol.*, 2, 47–73.

Horst, R., Pardalos, P. M., & Thoai, N. V. (1995). *Introduction to global optimization*. Dordrecht: Kluwer.

Kohonen, T. (1982). Self-organized formation of topologically correct feature maps. *Biol. Cybern.*, 43, 59–69.

Kohonen, T. (1990). The self-organizing map. *Proc. of the IEEE, 78*(9), 1464–1480.
Konen, W., Maurer, T., & von der Malsburg, C. (1994). A fast dynamic link matching algorithm for invariant pattern recognition. *Neural Networks, 7*(6/7), 1019–1030.
Konen, W., & von der Malsburg, C. (1993). Learning to generalize from single examples in the dynamic link architecture. *Neural Computation, 5*(5), 719–735.
Lades, M., Vorbrüggen, J. C., Buhmann, J., Lange, J., von der Malsburg, C., Würtz, R. P., & Konen, W. (1993). Distortion invariant object recognition in the dynamic link architecture. *IEEE Transactions on Computers, 42*(3), 300–311.
Linsker, R. (1986). From basic network principles to neural architecture: Emergence of orientation columns. *Ntl. Acad. Sci. USA, 83*, 8779–8783.
MacKay, D. J. C., & Miller, K. D. (1990). Analysis of Linsker's simulations of Hebbian rules. *Neural Computation, 2*, 173–187.
Meister, M., Wong, R. O. L., Baylor, D. A., & Shatz, C. J. (1991). Synchronous bursts of action potentials in ganglion cells of the developing mammalian retina. *Science, 252*, 939–943.
Miller, K. D. (1990). Derivation of linear Hebbian equations from nonlinear Hebbian model of synaptic plasticity. *Neural Computation, 2*, 321–333.
Miller, K. D., Keller, J. B., & Stryker, M. P. (1989). Ocular dominance column development: Analysis and simulation. *Science, 245*, 605–615.
Miller, K. D., & MacKay, D. J. C. (1994). The role of constraints in Hebbian learning. *Neural Computation, 6*, 100–126.
Nowlan, S. J. (1990). Maximum likelihood competitive learning. In D. S. Touretzky (Ed.), *Advances in neural information processing systems* (Vol. 2, pp. 574–582). San Mateo, CA: Morgan Kaufmann.
Obermayer, K., Ritter, H., & Schulten, K. (1990). Large-scale simulations of self-organizing neural networks on parallel computers: Application to biological modelling. *Parallel Computing, 14*, 381–404.
Ritter, H., Martinetz, T., & Schulten, K. (1991). *Neuronale Netze*. Reading, MA: Addison-Wesley.
Sejnowski, T. J. (1976). On the stochastic dynamics of neuronal interaction. *Biol. Cybern., 22*, 203–211.
Sejnowski, T. J. (1977). Storing covariance with nonlinearly interacting neurons. *J. Math. Biology, 4*, 303–321.
Swindale, N. V. (1980). A model for the formation of ocular domance stripes. *Proc. R. Soc. Lond. B, 208*, 243–264.
Swindale, N. V. (1996). The development of topography in the visual cortex: A review of models. *Network: Comput. in Neural Syst., 7*(2), 161–247.
Tanaka, S. (1990). Theory of self-organization of cortical maps: Mathematical framework. *Neural Networks, 3*, 625–640.
Tanaka, S. (1991). Theory of ocular dominance column formation. *Biol. Cybern., 64*, 263–272.
Triesch, J. (1995). *Metrik im visuellen System* (Internal Rep. No. IR-INI 95-05). Bochum: Institut für Neuroinformatik, Ruhr-Universität Bochum.
von der Malsburg, C. (1973). Self-organization of orientation sensitive cells in the striate cortex. *Kybernetik, 14*, 85–100.
von der Malsburg, C. (1995). Network self-organization in the ontogenesis of

the mammalian visual system. In S. F. Zornetzer, J. Davis, and C. Lau (Eds.), *An introduction to neural and electronic networks* (pp. 447–463). San Diego: Academic Press.

von der Malsburg, C., & Willshaw, D. J. (1977). How to label nerve cells so that they can interconnect in an ordered fashion. *Proc. Natl. Acad. Sci. (USA), 74*, 5176–5178.

von der Malsburg, C., & Willshaw, D. J. (1981). Differential equations for the development of topological nerve fibre projections. *SIAM-AMS Proceedings, 13*, 39–47.

Whitelaw, D. J., & Cowan, J. D. (1981). Specificity and plasticity of retinotectal connections: A computational model. *J. Neuroscience, 1*(12), 1369–1387.

Willshaw, D. J., & von der Malsburg, C. (1976). How patterned neural connections can be set up by self-organization. *Proc. R. Soc. London, B194*, 431–445.

Wiskott, L., & von der Malsburg, C. (1996). Face recognition by dynamic link matching. In J. Sirosh, R. Miikkulainen, & Y. Choe (Eds.), *Lateral interactions in the cortex: structure and function* (Chap. 11) [Electronic book]. Austin, TX: UTCS Neural Networks Research Group. Available from http://www.cs.utexas.edu/users/nn/web-pubs/htmlbook96/.

7

How to Generate Ordered Maps by Maximizing the Mutual Information between Input and Output Signals

Ralph Linsker
*IBM Research Division, T.J. Watson Research Center,
P.O. Box 218, Yorktown Heights, NY 10598 USA*

A learning rule that performs gradient ascent in the average mutual information between input and output signals is derived for a system having feedforward and lateral interactions. Several processes emerge as components of this learning rule: Hebb-like modification, and cooperation and competition among processing nodes.

Topographic map formation is demonstrated using the learning rule. An analytic expression relating the average mutual information to the response properties of nodes and their geometric arrangement is derived in certain cases. This yields a relation between the local map magnification factor and the probability distribution in the input space. The results provide new links between unsupervised learning and information-theoretic optimization in a system whose properties are biologically motivated.

1 Introduction

A great deal is known experimentally about the complex organization of certain biological perceptual systems such as the visual system in cat and monkey. One way to study these systems theoretically is to explore whether there are optimization principles that can correctly predict what signal transformations are carried out at various stages of a perceptual pathway. I have proposed a principle of "maximum information preservation" (Linsker 1988a,b) according to which a processing stage has the property that the values of the output signals from that stage optimally discriminate, in an information-theoretic sense, among the possible sets of input signals to that stage. [See (Linsker 1990) for a review of earlier ideas relating information theory and sensory processing.]

The principle in its basic form states: Given a statistically stationary ensemble of input patterns L (to a processing stage) having probability density function (pdf) $P_L(L)$, and a set S of allowed input-output mappings $S = \{f : L \to M\}$, where each f is characterized by a conditional pdf $P(M \mid L)$, choose an $f \in S$ that maximizes the Shannon information rate or average mutual information (Shannon 1949)

$$R \equiv \int dL\, P_L(L) \int dM\, P(M\mid L) \log[P(M\mid L)/P_M(M)] \qquad (1.1)$$

where $P_M(M) \equiv \int dL\, P_L(L) P(M\mid L)$. In this paper we study some consequences of R-maximization for a processing stage in which the choice of set S is relatively simple yet biologically motivated.

2 Information Rate and Gradient Ascent

The type of processing stage we shall consider has the following properties. Each input pattern is denoted by a vector in a space L. There is a set of output "nodes" M, each characterized by a vector $x(M)$ in L space. The response to an input L occurs in three steps: (1) Feedforward activation: Each node M' receives activation $A(L, M') \geq 0$; this quantity depends on L and the position $x(M')$ of node M'. (2) Lateral interaction: The activity of each node M at this step is given by $B(L, M) = \sum_{M'} g(M', M) A(L, M')$ where $g(M', M) \geq 0$ and $\sum_M g(M', M) = 1$ for all M'. (3) Selection of single output node to be fired: Node M is selected with probability $P(M\mid L) = B(L, M)/\sum_{M'} B(L, M')$. (If we view the system as a network, A corresponds to the feedforward connection strengths, and g to lateral excitatory strengths. Lateral inhibitory connections are implicit in the selection of a single firing node at step 3. The requirement that a single node fire makes it easier to compute the information rate, but deprives the system of much of the richness of biological network response.) Thus

$$P(M\mid L) = [\Sigma_{M'} g(M', M) A(L, M')]/\Sigma_{M'} A(L, M') \qquad (2.1)$$

The functions A and g are specified. We wish to maximize R over all choices of the set of vectors $\{x(M)\}$.

We derive a learning rule that, when averaged over the input ensemble, performs gradient ascent on R. The derivative of R with respect to the ith coordinate of $x(M_0)$ is $\partial R/\partial[x_i(M_0)] = \int dL\, P_L(L) Z_i(L, M_0)$ where

$$\begin{aligned} Z_i(L, M_0) &= [\partial A(L, M_0)/\partial x_i(M_0)][\Sigma_{M'} A(L, M')]^{-1} \\ &\quad \times \Sigma_M [\log P(M\mid L) - \log P_M(M)] \\ &\quad \times [g(M_0, M) - P(M\mid L)] \end{aligned} \qquad (2.2)$$

The learning rule is: Select input presentations L according to the pdf $P_L(L)$. For each L in turn, move each node position $x(M_0)$ by a small amount $kZ(L, M_0)$ where $k > 0$. The rule makes use of one item of "historical" information at each node: $P_M(M)$. If the $\{x(M)\}$ change slowly over many presentations, an average of the firing incidence of M over an appropriate number of recent presentations can provide a suitable approximation to $P_M(M)$.

We can interpret equation 2.2 as follows. Consider each node M in turn. Suppose that (1) $P(M\mid L) > P_M(M)$; that is, the occurrence of pattern L conduces to the firing of M. Suppose also that (2) $g(M_0, M) > P(M \mid L)$. In network terms, $g(M_0, M)$ is the strength of the lateral connection from M_0 to M. By equation 2.1, $P(M \mid L)$ equals the average strength of the *active* connections to node M, defined by weighting each $g(M', M)$ by the activity $A(L, M')$ of node M'. If both inequalities hold, then the effect of that M term in the right-hand side of equation 2.2 is to tend to move $x(M_0)$ in the direction of increase of $A(L, M_0)$. Reversing the second inequality tends to move $x(M_0)$ so as to decrease $A(L, M_0)$.

Stated informally, the derived learning rule has the effect that each node M_0 develops to become more (respectively less) responsive to L if it is relatively strongly (respectively weakly) connected to nodes M that are themselves relatively strongly responsive to L. Three elements — Hebb-like modification, and cooperation and competition among output nodes for "territory" in the input signal space — are apparent in this description.

I emphasize that while we specified the *activity dynamics* of the processing stage — that is, the relationship between input and output (equation 2.1) as a function of the parameters $\{x(M)\}$ — we made no assumptions concerning the form of the *learning rule* by which the $\{x(M)\}$ are to be adjusted. It is striking that a learning rule combining Hebb-like modification and cooperative and competitive learning in a specific way emerges as the gradient of an important information-theoretic function — the average mutual information between input and output.

Our model and result can be mapped directly onto a simple ecological problem in which, for example, different organisms M are differently suited to obtain various types of food L, or food at different locations L. Rather than denoting a rate of transfer of signaling information, R in this case provides a measure of the extent to which the statistical structure of M space reflects, or is matched to, the structure of L space. The R function is thus a candidate for a function that may be locally optimized (subject to developmental constraints) by familiar mechanisms such as adaptation and competition, at least in sufficiently simple ecological models.

3 Neighbor-Preserving Map Formation

Figure 1 shows the emergence of a neighbor-preserving or "topographic" map as the result of performing gradient ascent in R, for a case in which the L and M spaces are both two-dimensional. (To reduce boundary effects, periodic boundary conditions are imposed; each space can thus be regarded as the surface of a torus.) For this computation $P_L(L)$ is uniform, $A(L, M') \propto \exp(-\alpha \mid L - x(M') \mid^2)$, $g(M', M) \propto \exp(-\beta \mid M' - M \mid^2)$, and $\mid \cdots \mid$ denotes Euclidean distance going the "short way around" the periodic L or M space. The generation of a neighbor-preserving map by a connection modification rule is of course not new (e.g., von der Malsburg and Willshaw 1977; Kohonen 1982). The point of interest

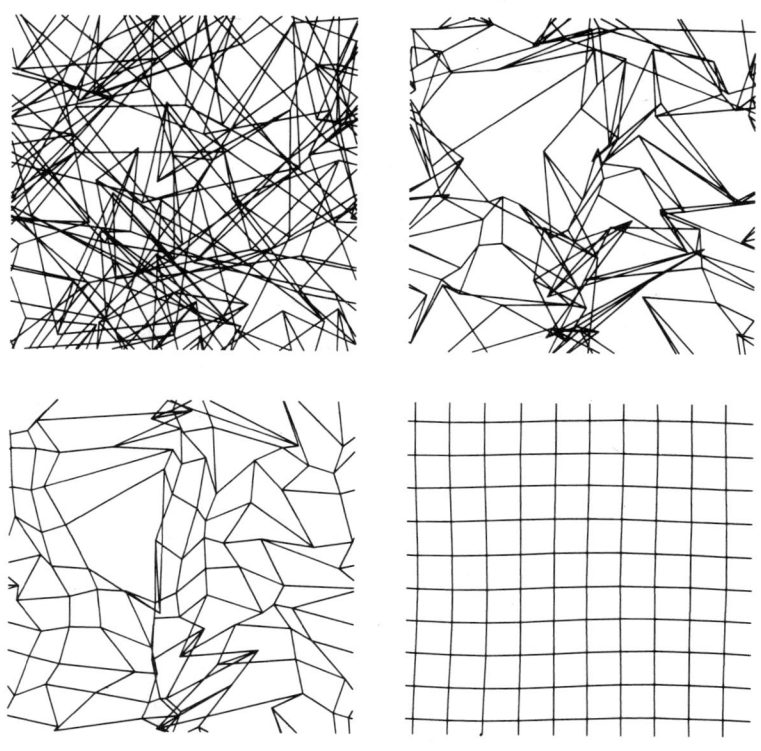

Figure 1: Gradient ascent in the information rate R induces a neighbor-preserving map. The input space L is a unit square. The M space consists of a 10×10 square array of nodes. Periodic boundary conditions are imposed (see text). Each node $(i,j)(i,j = 1,\ldots,10)$ is initially mapped onto a point $x(i,j)$ in L space, which is randomly chosen from a uniform distribution on a square of side $s = 0.7$ centered at $x = (0.1i, 0.1j)$. Thus, a very coarse topographic ordering is initially present. [If the initial $\{x(i,j)\}$ are entirely random ($s = 1$), a map having partially disrupted topographic order and a lower lying local maximum of R is obtained.] At each iteration, $x(i,j)$ is changed by $\Delta x(i,j) \equiv (\gamma/K)\Sigma_{k=1}^{K} Z[L_k, M(i,j)]$ (see equation 2.2) where $\{L_k\}$ is an ensemble of input vectors. Parameter values are $\alpha = 20$, $\beta = 4/9$, $\gamma = 1$, and $K = 900$ ($\{L_k\}$ is a 30×30 array of points). Plots show the links connecting each $x(i,j)$ with $x(i+1,j)$ and $x(i,j+1)$, after 0 (upper left), 10 (upper right), 15 (lower left), and 40 (lower right) iterations.

Maximizing Mutual Information

is rather that an optimization principle and learning rule yielding this result have emerged from information-theoretic considerations.

Figure 1 shows that a square grid in M space is optimally mapped onto a square grid in L space. That is, the "magnification factors" of the mapping $M \to x(M)$ are the same in both coordinate directions, and orthogonality of the coordinate axes is preserved. In the next section we prove that this is a consequence of the principle of maximum information preservation under conditions that are more general than those of Figure 1.

4 Coarse-Grained Information Rate

We can derive a useful "coarse-grained" version of equations 1.1 and 2.1 under certain conditions. Suppose that $A(L, M')$ is negligible for $|L - x(M')| > a_0$ and that $g(M', M)$ is negligible for $|M' - M| > g_0$. Suppose also that the following approximations can be made: (1) The mapping $M \to x(M)$ — which we will call the embedding of the M space in L space — is linear over a local region that is large compared with the length scales a_0 and g_0. (2) For each L, firing is confined to a single such local region in M space. (3) The firing rate is uniform over such a local region. (We will consider a two-dimensional M space, but the generalization to other dimensionalities is straightforward.) Figure 2a shows an orthogonal coordinate grid and unit vectors u, v in M space, and Figure 2b shows a disk cut from the (arbitrary) linear mapping of this grid onto a two-dimensional subspace of L. The mapping is characterized by the lengths f and g of the images of u and v under the mapping, and by the angle θ between them. An area element dM in M space is thus mapped onto an area $dL = c\, dM$ in L space, where $c \equiv fg \sin \theta$.

For definiteness we choose $A(L, M') \propto \exp(-\alpha\, |\, L - x(M')\, |^2)$ and $g(M', M) = (\beta/\pi) \exp(-\beta\, |\, M' - M\, |^2)$. The density of nodes in M space is uniform, and we pass to the continuum limit, so that sums over M become integrals over area elements in M space.

4.1 Derivation — Qualitative Aspects. We can now express R-maximization as a geometric optimization problem. We first describe qualitatively the main geometric effects that arise. (1) By equation 1.1 we have $R = R_1 + R_2$ where $R_1 = -\int dM\, P_M(M) \log P_M(M)$ and $R_2 = \int dL\, P_L(L) \int dM\, P(M \mid L) \log P(M \mid L)$. (2) The quantity R_1 is the entropy of the pdf $P_M(M)$, and is a maximum when $P_M(M)$ is uniform over M. An example of an embedding that achieves this maximum is one in which the density of nodes M mapped to each region of L space is proportional to $P_L(L)$. (3) The quantity R_2 is the average over input vectors L of the negative of the entropy of the pdf $P(M \mid L)$. Its value is greater when the embedding is chosen so that the $P(M \mid L)$ distribution for each L is more sharply localized to a small region of M space. (The intuitive

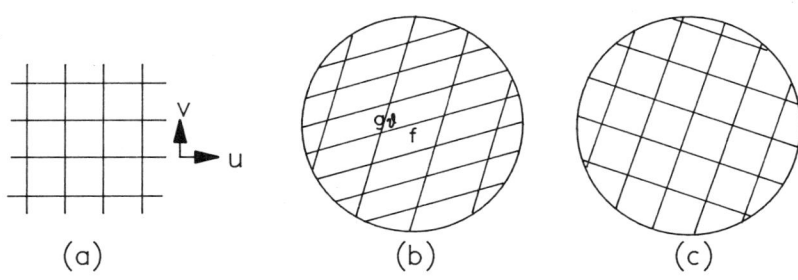

Figure 2: Locally linear mapping of the M-space coordinate system onto a region of L space. (a) Orthonormal vectors u, v and coordinate grid in M space. (b) Arbitrary linear mapping of this grid onto region of L space. (c) A mapping that maximizes information rate under conditions stated in text.

idea is that if each input vector activates fewer nodes, then one's ability to discriminate among the possible input vectors, given knowledge of which node fired, is improved.) This sharpened localization of $P(M \mid L)$ is achieved in two ways: (a) Since the spread of activation due to the feedforward process $A(L, M')$ has fixed extent in L space, lowering the density of nodes M' in the vicinity of L tends to localize $A(L, M')$, and thereby $P(M \mid L)$, to a smaller region of M space. This effect favors spreading out the embedding over a larger region of L space. The balance between this effect and the tendency to cluster the nodes in regions of high $P_L(L)$ (item 2 above) determines the "magnification factor" of the mapping (next section). (b) When viewed in L space (Fig. 2b), the contour lines of $A(L, M')$ are circular, but those of $g(M', M)$ are in general elliptical. When $f = g$ and $\sin \theta = 1$ (Fig. 2c) the contour lines of $g(M', M)$ become circular in L space, and $P(M \mid L)$ — which is proportional to the convolution of $A(L, M')$ and $g(M', M)$ — becomes more sharply localized, as shown at the end of this section.

4.2 Mathematical Details. To derive the coarse-grained information rate R we need to express R_2 in terms of the geometric properties of the embedding, such as the values of (f, g, θ) at each M. The qualitative statements of the previous paragraph apply to a variety of functional forms for $A(L, M')$ and $g(M', M)$, and one can, in general, compute the entropy of the $P(M \mid L)$ distribution numerically. However, when $A(L, M')$ and $g(M', M)$ have the gaussian forms assumed above, we can proceed analytically. The derivation is outlined in the remainder of this paragraph, which may be skipped by the reader interested only in the result and its consequences. (1) Rewriting $P(M \mid L)$ of equation 2.1 as a ratio of integrals in L space (using $dL' = c\,dM'$), we find that $P(M \mid L)$ is a two-dimensional gaussian function of distance: $P(M \mid L) = (c/\pi)(a_+ a_-)^{1/2}\exp(-a_+\xi^2 - a_-\eta^2)$, where $a_\pm^{-1} \equiv \alpha^{-1} + \beta^{-1}[h \pm (h^2 - c^2)^{1/2}]$ and $h \equiv (f^2 + g^2)/2$. We define L_0 as the point in the embedded M sheet that lies closest to the input vector L, and (ξ, η) as the components of the vector $[x(M) - L_0]$ along the major and minor axes of the elliptical contour lines of $g(M', M)$ in L space. The values of (f, g, θ) at L_0 are used, since the activation for given L is confined to a local region of the embedding centered at L_0. (2) The negative of the entropy of the $P(M \mid L)$ distribution for given L is $u(L) \equiv \int dM\, P(M \mid L)\log P(M \mid L) = \log[(a_+ a_-)^{1/2}c/(\pi e)]$. (3) Note that $u(L)$ depends on L only through L_0, and that the integral of $P_L(L)$ over all L sharing the same L_0 is $P_M(M_0)/c(M_0)$, where M_0 is a node in the vicinity of L_0. Therefore $R_2 = \int dL\, P_L(L)u(L) = \int dM_0\, P_M(M_0)u$. Some algebraic manipulation then yields the result stated below.

4.3 Results. The coarse-grained information rate we derive is $R = \int dM\, r(M)$ with

$$r(M) = -P_M(M)\left\{\log P_M(M) + \log\frac{\pi e}{\alpha\beta}\right.$$
$$\left. + \frac{1}{2}\log\left[\alpha^2 + \frac{\beta^2 + \alpha\beta(f^2 + g^2)}{(fg\sin\theta)^2}\right]\right\} \qquad (4.1)$$

where (f, g, θ) are functions of M, and $P_M(M)$ is the firing probability per unit area in M space. The firing probability per unit area of the embedding *in L space* is $q(M) \equiv P_M(M)/c$, which depends on the $P_L(L)$ distribution and the shape of the embedded surface in L space but is independent of (f, g, θ). When the stated approximations are valid, we see that rate maximization has become a geometric problem: that of embedding an M sheet in L space subject to constraints (such as boundary conditions) so as to maximize the integral over M of equation 4.1. (Only a portion of the mapping from M to L might satisfy the stated approximations. In that case only the contribution of that portion to R is being considered here.)

The bracket in equation 4.1 can be written as $X \equiv [(\alpha + \beta\rho)^2 + 2\alpha\beta\epsilon\rho^2]$, where $\rho \equiv 1/c$ and $\epsilon \equiv -c + (f^2 + g^2)/2$. When L and M have the same dimension, ρ is called the "magnification factor." Note that $\epsilon \geq 0$, with $\epsilon = 0$ only when $f = g = \rho^{-1/2}$ and $\sin\theta = 1$; that is, when a square coordinate grid in M maps onto a square grid in L (Fig. 2c). Any deviation from this square mapping makes a negative contribution to R, akin to a "surface distortion energy" cost term.

5 Magnification Factor

Now consider a number, N, of local regions of the embedding in L space (they need not be near each other). The kth such region has area ΔL_k in L space, ρ-value ρ_k, firing rate q_k per unit area in L space, and information rate $r_k \equiv r(M)$ per unit area in M space, where M is a node in region k. Assume that $f = g = \rho^{-1/2}$ and $\sin\theta = 1$ for each region, so that $\epsilon = 0$ as derived above. How should a fixed total area of M space (this area is $\Sigma_k \, \rho_k \Delta L_k$) be allocated among the N regions so as to maximize the total contribution, $\Sigma_k \, r_k \rho_k \Delta L_k$, to R from these regions?

The result (obtained using equation 4.1 for each r_k, and the Lagrange multiplier method) is that the ρ_k should be chosen such that the value of $(\rho_k + \rho_k^2 \beta/\alpha)/q_k$ is the same for all k. We thus obtain an "equation of state" relating ρ (the area of the M sheet that maps onto a unit area in L space) to the firing probability q of that region of the M sheet (measured per unit area in L space):

$$\rho = -(t/2) + [(t^2/4) + \lambda t q]^{1/2} \qquad (5.1)$$

where $t \equiv \alpha/\beta$, and λ is chosen so that the total area of M space being allocated has the desired value. Note that if the L space is two-dimensional and the mapping is bijective, $q \equiv P_L(L)$.

Our "equation of state" has two limiting regimes. (1) If $\rho\beta \ll \alpha$, then $\rho \propto q$ and $P_M(M)$ is constant. In this regime the lateral interaction g accounts for most of the spatial extent of the spread of activation within the M sheet (for given input L). (2) If $\rho\beta \gg \alpha$, then $\rho \propto q^{1/2}$. In this regime the feedforward function A accounts for most of the activation spread.

If M is a one-dimensional space, the corresponding limiting forms of the "equation of state" are, respectively, $\rho \propto q$ and $\rho \propto q^{1/3}$, where ρ is the linear magnification factor.

If one is not attempting to maximize the information rate, different mapping algorithms can be devised, which in general give rise to different magnification factors. For example, an earlier "feature map" algorithm (Kohonen 1982) tends to assign input vectors L to output nodes M so as to minimize the variance among the inputs assigned to the same node. Analysis of the magnification factor for that algorithm in the one-dimensional case (Ritter and Schulten 1986, Kohonen 1988) shows that, contrary to earlier supposition (Kohonen 1982), ρ is not proportional to q. By way of contrast, R-maximization yields a distribution of nodes for which (in the first limiting regime above) $\rho \propto q$ and the firing probability per node is uniform. This result is sometimes desired in practical classification applications, even apart from the issue of maximizing the information rate.

6 Information Content and Information Value

The leading bit and a lower order bit of a signal value have equal information content in the sense of Shannon. Yet the leading bit is often more important (to an animal's survival, for example). Since the proposed principle maximizes the information rate, how can it take any account of the relative importance of information? It does so in the present model by means of the function $A(L, M')$. If two inputs L_1, L_2 differ only in their low-order bits, then the overlap between $A(L_1, M')$ and $A(L_2, M')$ is large for any $x(M')$. Because of this, a given number of M nodes can more reliably (hence with greater information rate) discriminate the value of a leading bit than that of a low-order bit.

The function A can — but need not — represent a physical process (such as noise or spread of activation) that confounds sufficiently similar input signals. Even without regard to such a physical process, however, it may be desirable for a processing stage to ignore small differences in input signal values. How might one control the resolution below which such small differences are ignored? This type of control is useful in facilitating the formation of generalizations, and may be relevant to attentional mechanisms. Within the present information-theoretic framework one can control the desired resolution by maximizing, not the information that M conveys about L, but the information that M conveys about the coarse-grained value, $\hat{L}$, of L. (The introduction of $\hat{L}$ is a device for removing the informational value of discriminations among inputs that differ by less than a desired amount. It is not related to the derivation of the "coarse-grained" information rate in an earlier section.)

To outline how this quantity may be maximized, note that the inverse of the mapping $L \to \hat{L}$ is a mapping from each coarse-grained value $\hat{L}$ to a neighborhood of similar Ls. Define $A(\hat{L}, M')$ as the probability $\Pi(L \mid \hat{L})$ of $\hat{L}$ generating L via this inverse mapping, multiplied by the activation $a(L, M')$ of M' due to L, and integrated over L. [Given $\hat{L}$, assume $\Sigma_{M'} a(L, M')$ is constant over all L for which $\Pi(L \mid \hat{L})$ is nonnegligible.] Then equations 1.1, 2.1, and 2.2 all remain valid (with L replaced by $\hat{L}$), and we can use the methods described to maximize the average mutual information between $\hat{L}$ and M.

7 Conclusion

We started with a design principle: choose the parameters of a signal processing system so that the system's outputs optimally discriminate among an ensemble of inputs. We derived a learning rule that generates such a system, and found, moreover, that the rule combines elements of Hebb-like modification and cooperative and competitive learning to accomplish this task. Topographic mapping, map magnification factors, and other geometric properties emerge from an analysis of the optimization process. The approach described holds promise for the analysis of adaptation rules, information-theoretic optimization, and emergent structure in more complex and biologically realistic systems.

References

Kohonen, T. 1982. Analysis of a simple self-organizing process. *Biol. Cybernet.* **44**, 135–140.

Kohonen, T. 1988. Self-organization and associative memory, 2nd ed. Springer-Verlag, New York.

Linsker, R. 1988a. Self-organization in a perceptual network. *Computer* **21** (March), 105–117.

Linsker, R. 1988b. Towards an organizing principle for a layered perceptual network. In *Neural Information Processing Systems* (Denver, CO, 1987), D.Z. Anderson, ed., pp. 485–494. American Institute of Physics, New York.

Linsker, R. 1990. Perceptual neural organization: Some approaches based on network models and information theory. *Ann. Rev. Neurosci.* **13**, in press.

Ritter, H., and Schulten, K. 1986. On the stationary state of Kohonen's self-organizing sensory mapping. *Biol. Cybernet.* **54**, 99–106.

Shannon, C.E. 1949. In *The Mathematical Theory of Communication*, C.E. Shannon and W. Weaver, eds. University of Illinois Press, Urbana.

von der Malsburg, C., and Willshaw, D.J. 1977. How to label nerve cells so that they can interconnect in an ordered fashion. *Proc. Natl. Acad. Sci. U.S.A.* **74**, 5176–5178.

III

Models of Cortical Feature Maps

8

Models of Orientation and Ocular Dominance Columns in the Visual Cortex: A Critical Comparison

E. Erwin*
Beckman Institute, University of Illinois, Urbana, IL 61801 USA

K. Obermayer
The Rockefeller University, New York, NY 10021 USA and
Howard Hughes Medical Institute and Salk Institute, La Jolla, CA 92037 USA

K. Schulten
Beckman Institute, University of Illinois, Urbana, IL 61801 USA

Orientation and ocular dominance maps in the primary visual cortex of mammals are among the most thoroughly investigated of the patterns in the cerebral cortex. A considerable amount of work has been dedicated to unraveling both their detailed structure and the neural mechanisms that underlie their formation and development. Many schemes have been proposed, some of which are in competition. Some models focus on development of receptive fields while others focus on the structure of cortical maps, i.e., the arrangement of receptive field properties across the cortex. Each model used different means to determine its success at reproducing experimental map patterns, often relying principally on visual comparison. Experimental data are becoming available that allow a more careful evaluation of models. In this contribution more than 10 of the most prominent models of cortical map formation and structure are critically evaluated and compared with the most recent experimental findings from macaque striate cortex. Comparisons are based on properties of the predicted or measured cortical map patterns. We introduce several new measures for comparing experimental and model map data that reveal important differences between models. We expect that the use of these measures will improve current models by helping determine parameters to match model maps to experimental data now becoming available from a variety of species. Our study reveals that (1) despite apparent differences, many models are based on similar principles and consequently make similar predictions, (2) several models produce orientation map patterns that are not consistent with the experimental data from macaques, regardless of the plausibility of the models' suggested physiological implementations,

---

*Present address: Department of Physiology, Box 0444, University of California, San Francisco, San Francisco, CA 94143 USA.

and (3) no models have yet fully accounted for both the local and the global relationships between orientation and ocular dominance map patterns.

1 Introduction

Many cells in the mammalian primary visual cortex are binocular, responding better to stimulation of one eye over the other. They also usually respond more strongly to bars or gratings of one particular orientation (Hubel and Wiesel 1962, 1974). Early experiments with microelectrodes revealed a vertical organization, with columns of cells with similar properties running between pia and white matter, perpendicular to the cortical surface. These experiments also revealed a lateral organization characterized by mostly smooth changes in response properties with lateral distance. The results culminated in the proposal of two seemingly incompatible models of cortical organization—an "icecube" model (Hubel and Wiesel 1977) and a "pinwheel" model (Braitenberg and Braitenberg 1979; Götz 1987).

In recent years, imaging techniques (Blasdel 1992a,b; Blasdel and Salama 1986; Grinvald et al. 1986; Ts'o et al. 1990) have been developed that allow an increasingly improved characterization of striate cortex organization. A refined picture of map organization has emerged (Bartfeld and Grinvald 1992; Blasdel 1992a,b; Obermayer and Blasdel 1993; Obermayer et al. 1992c). We now know that some elements of organization from both the "icecube" and "pinwheel" models are present, but other elements had to be modified in light of the new data. We briefly review the recent findings in the macaque in Section 2.

Along with the study of cortical organization came a series of experiments suggesting that important elements of the organization of orientation and ocular dominance in macaque striate cortex are not prespecified but emerge during an activity-driven, self-organizing process. Occlusion of one eye, for example, leads to dramatic changes in the lateral organization of ocular dominance, which are to some extent reversible. Strabismus leads to changes in the degree of binocularity. Exposure to a restricted set of orientations causes changes in the distribution of cells with different preferred orientations (for reviews see, for example, Hubel et al. 1977; LeVay and Nelson 1991; Rauschecker 1991; Stryker et al. 1978). These findings as well as an even larger body of data obtained from other species (Goodman and Shatz 1993; Miller 1990) initiated considerable theoretical work in which the principles underlying the development of these patterns were explored. For a recent review see Miller (1990). Many different models have been proposed during the past two decades. However, the different approaches have rarely been thoroughly compared with each other, nor have many of them been tested against the recent experimental data.

Hence it seems timely to critically evaluate the most prominent and successful of the alternative modeling approaches. Such a study serves several purposes: first, it may help to exclude certain approaches; second, it may reveal that seemingly different models are actually related or based on similar principles; third, it may help determine which quantities can be computed to allow model comparisons; and, fourth, it may reveal which of these quantities are most useful for deciding between hypotheses.

In our contribution we make a first step in this direction. We extract principles of organization from recent data obtained from monkey striate cortex and develop numerical tests to demonstrate these properties. We apply these tests to the predictions of a large number of models for the formation of orientation and ocular dominance maps. Model predictions are also compared with available experimental data from the macaque. Several models were found to predict patterns that are inconsistent with the data, and thus are not sufficient models of macaque map structure or development, regardless of the plausibility of the proposed physiological mechanisms. As data become available from more species and under manipulated developmental conditions, the tests developed here will help compare model predictions with such data.

The paper is organized as follows. In Section 2 we briefly review the experimental facts on the patterns of orientation and ocular dominance. In Section 3 we critically evaluate some of the more prominent models, comparing their results with each other and with the experimental data. The discussion is organized around a set of principles we have found to underlie cortical organization. We begin with the two major organizing principles of continuity and diversity that are included in all modeling approaches and continue with less prominent, but equally important features of the map patterns, where differences between models appear. Section 4 summarizes the main results in a table and offers suggestions for future work.

2 Macaque Striate Cortex Orientation and Ocular Dominance Patterns

This section provides a summary of known experimental facts about the lateral organization of orientation and ocular dominance columns in macaque striate cortex. Most of the data being reviewed here were obtained with optical recordings (Blasdel and Salama 1986), since no other method can currently provide both high-resolution data of large surface areas and fairly unambiguous estimates of orientation preferences and ocular dominance in the same animal. Due to limitations of this method, however, data can be obtained only from the superficial layers. When comparing models, one must keep in mind that not all conclusions drawn from these data will necessarily carry over to deeper layers of cortex or be applicable in other species.

This section is included for completeness and cannot treat in depth all the issues involved. For a thorough and quantitative discussion we refer the reader to other sources (Blasdel 1992a,b; Obermayer and Blasdel 1993; Obermayer et al. 1992c; Swindale 1992). For experimental data on the cortical mapping of other features such as retinotopy, color sensitivity, and spatial frequency representation obtained by other methods, refer to other sources, e.g., LeVay and Nelson (1991) and Tootell et al. (1988), which also include large-scale maps of ocular dominance in all cortical layers (see also Florence and Kaas 1992; Swindale et al. 1987).

Figure 1 shows the lateral spatial pattern of orientation selectivity in the striate cortex of an adult macaque. Examples are shown of several elements of the lateral organization that have been termed linear zones, singularities, saddle points, and fractures. Linear zones are characterized by isoorientation contours that run in parallel for distances of 0.5–1.0 mm. Within these zones orientation preferences change linearly with lateral distance along a line. Singularities are point-like regions around which orientation preferences change by 180° along a closed path. Singularities come in two varieties: one where orientation preferences increase with clockwise motion around the center and one where they decrease. Saddle points occur in the centers of regions of almost constant orientation preference. Outward movement within two diagonally opposed quadrants, however, results in the same direction of rotation of orientation preference while outward movement within the remaining quadrants rotates orientation preference in the opposite sense. Finally, fractures are line-like regions across which orientation preferences change rapidly.

Fractures, saddle points, and singularities are grouped together in the recorded patterns (Swindale 1992). They are collectively called nonlinear regions to indicate the reversals and breaks in the pattern of change of orientation preference. Also note that the local direction of the isoorientation contours is independent of the local preferred orientations. This is true in both the linear and nonlinear zones.

Figure 2 shows the lateral spatial pattern of ocular dominance. This pattern was recorded from the same cortical region of the same macaque as in Figure 1. Regions of similar eye dominance are segregated in bands that run in parallel for a considerable distance, but sometimes branch and terminate.

Surprisingly the orientation preference and ocular dominance patterns are not independent as had once been believed (Hubel et al. 1978), but are correlated. For example, Figure 3a shows the Fourier transform of the map of orientation preference with an arrow indicating the direction perpendicular to the ocular dominance bands. At least for this region of cortex, the spectrum is characterized by a slightly elliptic band of modes with high amplitude centered around the origin. The minor axis is aligned approximately perpendicular to the ocular dominance band borders. Consequently, the map of orientation is stretched along this axis and it is stretched such that its wavelength along this direction nearly

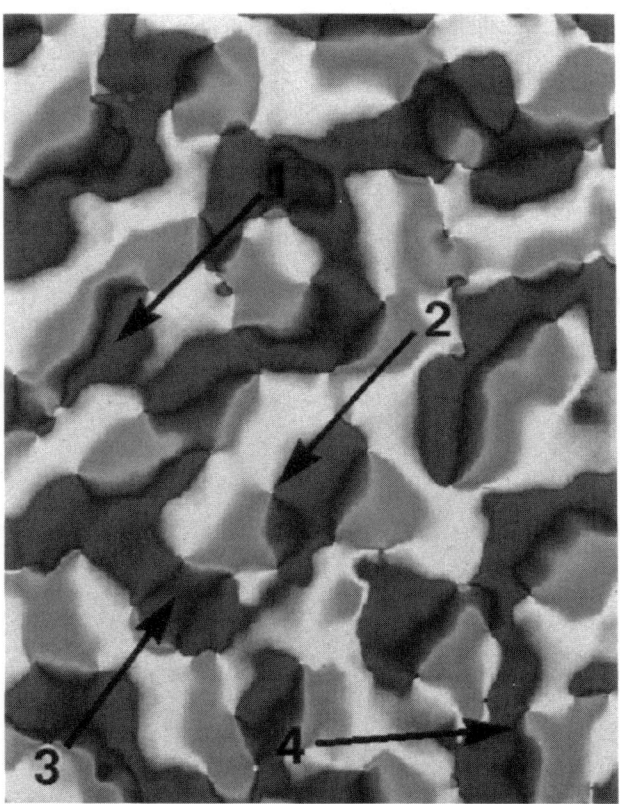

Figure 1: The lateral spatial pattern of orientation preference in the striate cortex of an adult macaque as revealed by optical imaging. The figure (Blasdel 1992a) shows a 4.1 × 3.0 mm surface region located near the border between cortical areas 17 and 18 and close to the midline [animal NM1 in Obermayer (1993)]. Local average orientation preference is indicated by color such that the interval of 180° is mapped onto a color circle. Arrows indicate (1) linear zones, (2) singularities, (3) saddle points, and (4) fractures.

matches the period of the ocular dominance pattern (Obermayer and Blasdel 1993). Additionally, ocular dominance and orientation preference slabs are each aligned with an individual common axis, and these axes—defined as the major axes of the corresponding power spectra—are orthogonal ("global orthogonality") (Obermayer 1993).

146   E. Erwin, K. Obermayer, and K. Schulten

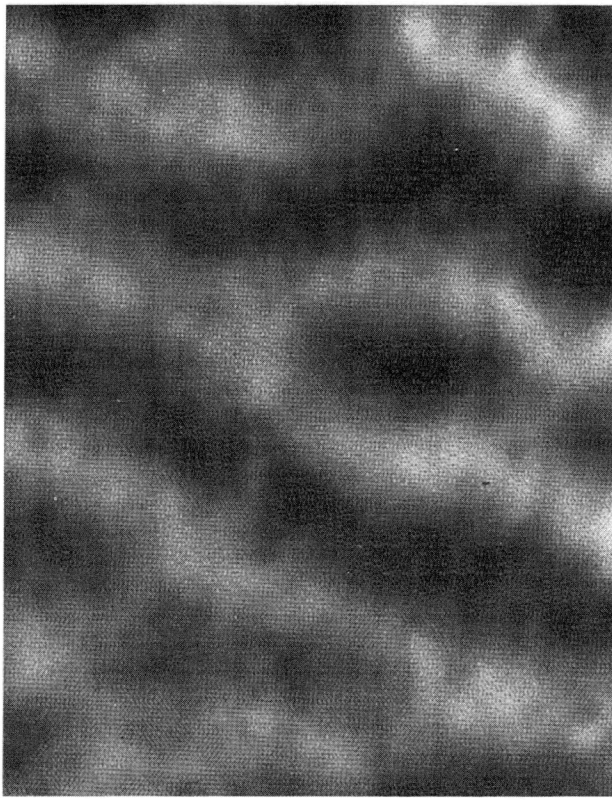

Figure 2: The lateral spatial pattern of ocular dominance in the macaque striate cortex (Blasdel 1992a). Dark and light regions are dominated by input from contralateral and ipsilateral eyes, respectively. Data were obtained from the same cortical region of the same animal (NM1) as in Figure 1.

Other correlations become apparent in a contour plot representation. Figure 4 displays a contour plot of the orientation map from Figure 1 overlaid with the borders of the ocular dominance bands from Figure 2. Three properties of this pattern are noteworthy: (1) singularities tend to align with the centers of ocular dominance bands; (2) saddle-points align, too; and (3) isoorientation contours intersect borders of ocular dominance bands at angles of approximately 90° locally, on a scale as fine as the small meanderings of the ocular dominance bands ("local orthogonality"). For a quantitative analysis, see Blasdel *et al.* (1994) and Obermayer and Blas-

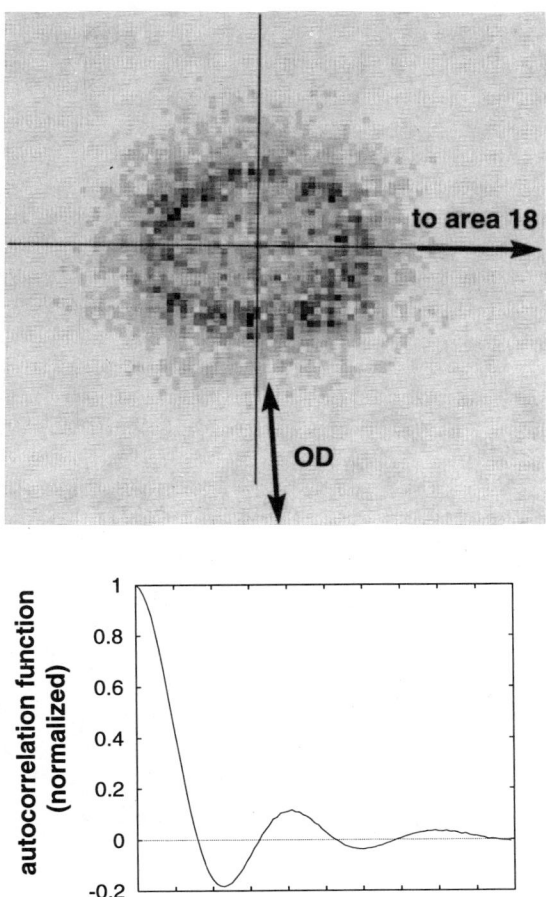

Figure 3: (a) The complex Fourier power spectrum of the spatial pattern of orientation preference $\|f(\mathbf{k})\|^2$, $f(\mathbf{k}) = \sum_{\mathbf{r}} \exp(i\mathbf{k}\mathbf{r})q(\mathbf{r})\{\sin[2\phi(\mathbf{r})] + i\cos[2\phi(\mathbf{r})]\}$ recorded from another macaque [NM4 in Obermayer (1993)]. The arrows indicate the direction perpendicular on average to the borders of the ocular dominance bands, and the direction perpendicular to the border to area 18. (b) Normalized autocorrelation function of preferred orientation as a function of distance. The figure shows the autocorrelation function for one of the Cartesian components of the orientation vector. One hundred units of cortical distance correspond to 1.252 mm.

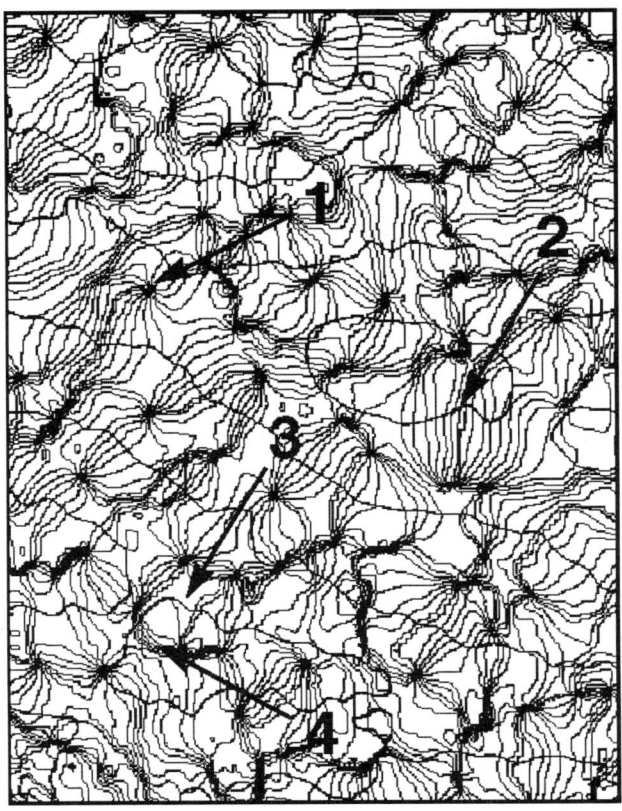

Figure 4: Macaque orientation and ocular dominance data combined (Obermayer *et al*. 1992c; Obermayer and Blasdel 1993). Black contours separate bands of opposite eye dominance. Light gray isoorientation contour lines indicate intervals of 11.25°. The medium gray contour represents the preferred orientation 0°. Arrows indicate (1) singularities, (2) linear zones, (3) saddle points, and (4) fractures.

del (1993). Correlations have also been reported for fractures, which tend either to align with the centers of ocular dominance bands or to run perpendicular to their borders (Blasdel and Salama 1986). Also, regions in the centers of ocular dominance bands tend to be less specifically tuned to their preferred orientation than regions that receive balanced input from both eyes (Blasdel 1992b; Livingstone and Hubel 1984).

Despite the correlations between them, both ocular dominance and orientation preference patterns exhibit irregularities and "global disorder." Such disorder is exhibited in the locally varying width of the ocular dominance bands as well as in their irregular termination and branching pattern. Figure 3b illustrates the presence of disorder in the orientation maps with an autocorrelation function along the Cartesian coordinates of orientation preference. The autocorrelation function takes a Mexican-hat shape with orientation preferences anticorrelated for distances around 300 μm. For neurons separated by longer distances, correlations decay to zero after a few oscillations indicating global disorder.

3 Common Properties of Cortical Map Models

Many models for the structure and formation of orientation and ocular dominance maps have been proposed. Although seemingly based on different assumptions, most produce maps that visually resemble the experimentally obtained maps. To sort through the conflicting models we extended and analyzed some of the more prominent of the previously proposed models and compared their predictions with the experimental data.

We found that models that appear to be based on different principles share many assumptions, and that these assumptions have a great impact on the developed patterns. The following discussion is organized around a list of these common assumptions, moving from the most generic to the most specific. Increasingly detailed comparisons between model and experimental data will be included along with each point.

To ease comparisons, we group models into categories based on similarities in goals or implementation (Table 1). Structural and spectral models attempt to characterize map patterns using schematic drawings or concise equations. In structural models this description is formulated in real space, while spectral models are formulated in Fourier space.

As model complexity increases, the pattern-generating equations are meant to correspond more closely to actual physiological processes, revealing more clearly the mechanisms underlying pattern formation. Correlation-based learning models involve Hebbian learning and linear intracortical interactions, while competitive Hebbian models are based on nonlinear lateral interactions. Several models do not fit well in these categories. The "generalized deformable" model of Yuille *et al.* (1991), for example, includes aspects of both competitive Hebbian and correlation-based learning models. Brief mathematical descriptions of some of the models discussed are included in the Appendix.

3.1 Basic Assumptions. Models of cortical map formation and structure include a collection of neural units in a model cortical array, usually on a two-dimensional grid. Usually each model neuron represents not

Table 1: Categories of Models of Visual Cortical Maps, and Their Abbreviations as Used in This Article.[a]

Class	Model	Reference
Structural models	Icecube	Hubel and Wiesel (1974)
	Pinwheel	Braitenberg and Braitenberg (1979)
	Götz	Götz (1987)
	Baxter and Dow	Baxter and Dow (1989)
Spectral models	Rojer and Schwartz	Rojer and Schwartz (1990)
	Niebur and Wörgötter	Niebur and Wörgötter (1993)
	Swindale	Swindale (1992a)
Correlation-based learning	Linsker	Linsker (1986c)
	Miller	Miller et al. (1989), Miller (1992, 1994)
Competitive Hebbian	SOM-h	Obermayer et al. (1990)
	SOM-l	Obermayer et al. (1992c)
	EN	Durbin and Mitchison (1990)
Other	Tanaka	Tanaka 1991b, Miyashita and Tanaka (1992)
	Yuille et al.	Yuille et al. (1991)

[a]Two versions of the self-organizing map model were investigated: SOM-h (high-dimensional weight vectors) and SOM-l (low-dimensional feature vectors).

one real neuron, but a collection of real neurons located in a cortical column or in a single layer of cortex. Each model neuron has a receptive field associated with it that defines how it responds to different types of simulated visual input.

Properties of receptive fields are often described through preferences for certain stimulus features, which in turn can be represented in various ways. The two most common ways to represent feature preferences are feature vectors and synaptic weight vectors.

In the feature vector representation, feature preferences are represented by a low-dimensional vector with independent components representing such features as ocular dominance, orientation preference, retinotopic position, or preferred direction in color space. In the weight vector representation a weight vector codes for the effective strength of the connections between a (simple) cortical cell and a set of receptor cells in an input layer. In these models, the weight vectors act as linear filters on the distribution of input activity. Receptive fields are defined by the strengths of the connections, and the locations and properties of the input cells.

It has been suggested that receptive fields be described not only as spatial filters but as spatiotemporal filters (e.g., Adelson and Bergen 1985; Emerson et al. 1992). Other suggestions aim at the inclusion of nonlinearities (Lehky et al. 1992) to account for complex cells, cells in higher brain areas, or intracortical feedback (Reggia et al. 1992; Sirosh and Miikkulainen 1994). These more realistic representations, however, have not yet been extensively used in models of cortical map structure and formation.

The method chosen to represent feature preferences will necessarily introduce assumptions about which features of visual input are important and hence influence model predictions. Abstract feature vectors allow one to generalize models to describe several phenomena within the same framework, but require that the types of features to be represented be fully determined in advance. Receptive fields represented with high-dimensional weight vectors can often be scrutinized for additional feature preferences beyond those for which the model was designed. High-dimensional models may also be explained with less abstracted physiological principles. However, they require greater computational resources and thus must generally be limited in other ways, such as through linear development rules, lower cortical resolution, and fewer simultaneous feature preferences.

3.2 Continuity and Diversity. It has long been recognized that two fundamental characteristics of orientation and ocular dominance organization are continuity and diversity (e.g., Baxter and Dow 1989; Obermayer *et al.* 1990; Swindale 1982).

Continuity stresses the fact that nearby columns of cells in striate cortex tend to prefer stimuli with similar features. Similarity between feature preferences is commonly defined as a small distance between their associated feature vectors calculated via a suitable norm. Models often enforce continuity by combining feature preferences of nearby cells through averaging or convolution operations, usually invoking a linear similarity measure by linearly averaging over each vector component individually. Other similarity measures are possible. The choice of similarity measure will affect the resulting map patterns (Yuille *et al.* 1991).

Diversity states that the space of all possible feature preferences should be filled as completely as possible, thus avoiding "perceptual scotomata" (Swindale 1991). Diversity is often enforced by bandpass filtering of the spatial pattern of feature preferences (Niebur and Wörgötter 1993; Rojer and Schwartz 1990), sometimes implemented using competitive networks (Durbin and Mitchison 1990; Obermayer *et al.* 1990, 1992c).

The two principles of continuity and diversity are partially contradictory and are balanced in visual maps. There are some regions where continuity is violated, such as the singularities and sharp fractures in the orientation preference map. Similarly there are regions where continuity is stressed over diversity. For example, the full range of orientation preferences is not represented near the saddle points.

The continuity and diversity principles have been the fundamental principles of almost all descriptive and developmental models of orientation or ocular dominance map patterns. They were already implemented in both Hubel and Wiesel's original icecube model (Hubel and Wiesel 1977) and in the early pinwheel models (Braitenberg and Brait-

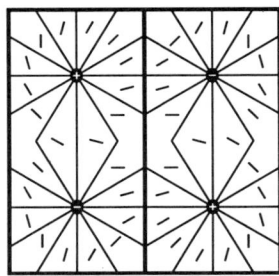

Figure 5: Schematic illustrations of two competing structural models. Heavy borders and shading define columns of cells with opposite eye preference; light borders separate columns of cells with similar preferred orientations, indicated by short lines. (a) The icecube model of cortical organization (Hubel and Wiesel 1974). (b) Götz' (1987) modified version of Braitenberg and Braitenberg's pinwheel model (1979). Positive and negative singularities are indicated by "+" and "−" where orientation preferences increase (decrease) with counterclockwise movement around the center of positive (negative) vortices.

enberg 1979; Götz 1987) (Fig. 5). However, maps from certain models that follow both of these principles may still differ in qualitative ways from experimental data. For example, the icecube model obeys the principles of continuity and diversity, but contains no singularities in the orientation preference map and no branching or termination of ocular dominance bands. Thus additional principles must be introduced. Some of these principles will be seen as modifications of the ideas of continuity and diversity.

3.3 Global Disorder. There are certain characteristic local features of cortical maps that recur in all regions of the maps. However, cortical maps do not consist of a crystal-like grid of exactly repeating units. Rather the maps are characterized by the liquid-like properties of local correlations and the absence of long-range order. These properties are reflected in the autocorrelation functions (Fig. 3b) of orientation and ocular dominance with respect to distance along the map surface.[1] Note that the principle of global disorder is distinct from the principle of diversity. Models with feature preferences arranged in a repeating patchwork

---

[1]The global disorder observed in cortical maps is the outcome of developmental processes and is not simply due to a folding of the cortical surface.

(Bauer and Dow 1991; Braitenberg 1985; Braitenberg and Braitenberg 1979; Dow and Bauer 1984; Götz 1987) meet both the continuity and diversity constraints, but do not show global disorder.[2]

Global disorder can be implemented in several ways. In some of the structural models it arises due to the explicit inclusion of noise (Niebur and Wörgötter 1993; Rojer and Schwartz 1990; Swindale 1982, 1992). The underlying assumption is that the map-organizing process is analogous to bandpass filtered white noise and the maps are consequently fully characterized by the filter parameters. Filtering is implemented either in the spatial domain by convolving arrays of randomly oriented vectors (Swindale 1982, 1992) with Mexican-hat type kernels or in the Fourier domain by multiplying white noise with a bandpass filter (Niebur and Wörgötter 1993; Rojer and Schwartz 1990). Continuity and diversity arise by suppressing both high- and low-frequency Fourier modes; global disorder results from applying the filter to white noise. The success of these models (Fig. 6) effectively suggests that the underlying principles of continuity, diversity, and global disorder are the most important principles of map structure.

Other models lead to a stationary state by an iterative process (Durbin and Mitchison 1990; Goodhill and Willshaw 1990; Miller 1992; Miller et al. 1989; Obermayer et al. 1992c; Swindale 1982, 1992). Usually there are many possible stationary states. The overwhelming majority of these tend to lack global order because of degeneracies due to translational symmetry[3] in the underlying pattern-generating equations or due to frustration (Swindale 1982, 1992). Random choice of initial conditions and/or randomly directed movement in the state space, e.g. in response to random inputs (Durbin and Mitchison 1990; Obermayer et al. 1990, 1992c), effectively cause a random choice of one of these stationary states. It is overwhelmingly probable that this stationary state will lack long-range order.

In competitive Hebbian models (Durbin and Mitchison 1990; Obermayer et al. 1990, 1992c), for example, an isotropic power spectrum and Fourier eigenmodes are generated since the pattern-generating equations are invariant under both translations and rotations. Similarity is enforced by modifying the feature vectors of cells only in groups of neighboring cells, moving them all closer to a presented input pattern. Diversity is the result of competition, implemented as a selection rule in the self-organizing map (Obermayer et al. 1990, 1992c), and by a softmax nonlinearity in the elastic net (Durbin and Mitchison 1990). Presenting the

---

[2]Models that introduce periodic boundary conditions as a convenience are not intended to imply that cortical patterns are periodic, and thus do not necessarily violate the principle of global disorder.

[3]If the equations governing development are invariant under translation in cortical and retinal coordinates, then Fourier transform leads to a set of independent equations, one for each Fourier mode. If each of those equations has more than one stationary state, the number of stationary states for the whole system is huge.

(a) Swindale's Model, $a \neq 0$

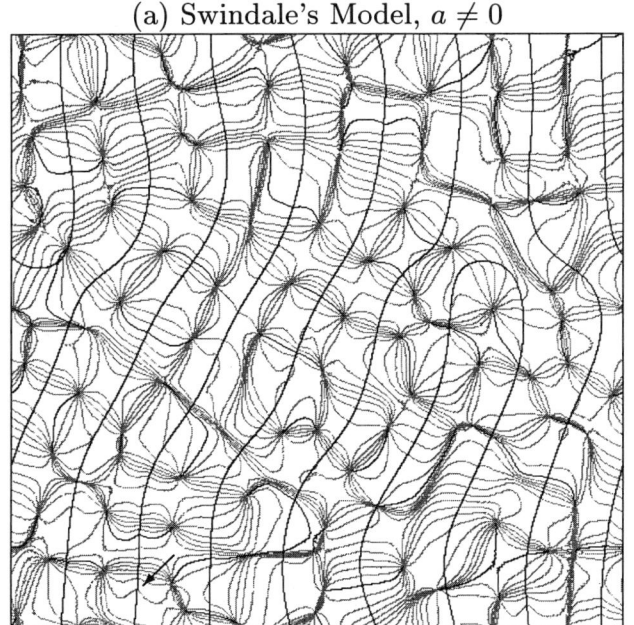

(b) Swindale's Model, $a = 0$

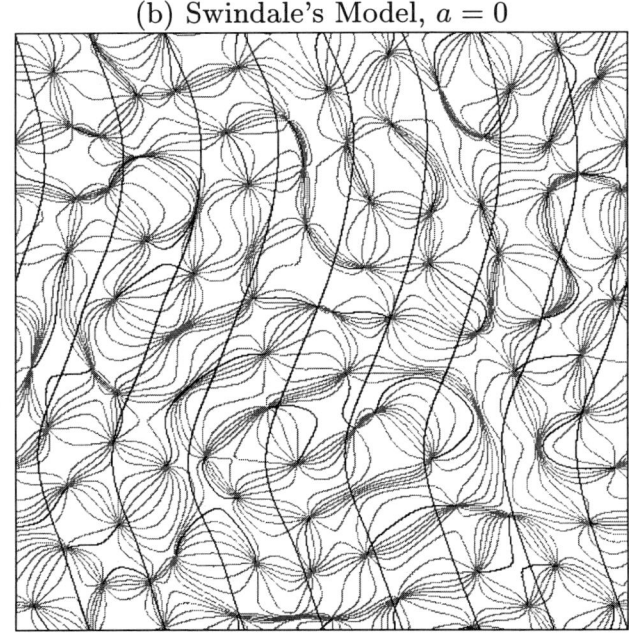

inputs in a random order causes a random choice among the possible stationary states and thus leads to global disorder.

3.4 Singularities and Linear Zones. Two features are prominent when visually inspecting the orientation map in Figure 1: singularities, points where all colors meet, and linear zones, regions with a rainbow appearance.

Singularities are point-like discontinuities in the orientation map, around which orientation preferences change by multiples of 180° along a closed loop. Macaque striate cortex contains only two types of singularities with vorticities[4] $+1/2$ and $-1/2$, respectively, with similar densities. All developmental models investigated so far generate maps that have this property. This is, however, not true for all of the structural models. Braitenberg's original proposal (Braitenberg 1985; Braitenberg and Braitenberg 1979), for example, included $+1$ singularities balanced by twice their density of $-1/2$ singularities, and the original icecube model (Hubel and Wiesel 1977) did not contain these features at all.

Linear zones are regions in the orientation map where isoorientation lines are (1) straight and run in parallel for a considerable distance, and where (2) isoorientation lines for similar intervals have similar spacing. With the help of a heuristic measure of "parallelness" that can be obtained by analyzing the gradients of orientation preference within small circular regions (see Obermayer 1993) it has been shown that linear zones are abundant in experimental maps. The existence of linear zones is related to the power spectrum. Linear zones are abundant only if the power spectrum has a strong bandpass characteristic, because linear zones are characterized by a periodic change of orientation preferences with distance. The ON/OFF competition model (Miller 1992, 1994) and the model of Tanaka (Miyashita and Tanaka 1992) generate maps with a power spectrum with significant energy in low-frequency modes, and lacking a significant bandpass characteristic. Linear zones thus appear less common

---

Figure 6: *Facing page.* (a) Model output from Swindale's (1992) spectral model in the same format as Figure 4. Model parameters (see Appendix): model size 512×512, $h_z = 1.32 \times 10^{-4} \exp[-(1.3r_1^2 + r_2^2)/1400] - 0.77 \times 10^{-4} \exp[-(r_1^2 + r_2^2)/2863]$, $h_\phi = 1.75 \times 10^{-4} \exp[-(r_1^2 + r_2^2)/823.0] - 1.06 \times 10^{-4} \exp[-(r_1^2 + r_2^2)/1646]$, $a = 20$. Initial values are normally distributed around 0 with variance 0.0025, map shown for $t = 500$ with $\alpha = 1.0$. The arrow indicates an area where an orientation column is distorted, or "kinked" at an ocular dominance band border. (b) Output from the same model with $a = 0$ (orientation and ocular dominance patterns not correlated); other parameters as in (a).

[4]Vorticity is defined as the factor of 360° by which orientation preferences increase (decrease) with counterclockwise movement around the center of positive (negative) vortices.

in these models than in macaque maps. Linear zones occur in all other models we studied, but are perhaps more prominent in the competitive Hebbian models than in macaque maps.

3.5 Anisotropies. Experimental patterns of orientation preference and ocular dominance are sometimes anisotropic, with elliptical, rather than circular, power spectra. In some species, such as macaque, the anisotropy in the ocular dominance pattern is strong enough to produce roughly parallel bands of ocular dominance across half of area 17 (Florence and Kaas 1992). In the cat the orientation preference patterns are anisotropic, while the ocular dominance bands are spotty and much less aligned (Andersen et al. 1988; Diao et al. 1990).

In models of cortical map formation anisotropies can emerge as a result of spontaneous symmetry breaking, pattern-generating equations that are not invariant under rotation, or through appropriately chosen boundary conditions. Models based on bandpass-filtered noise, for example, employ anisotropic kernels or filters (Niebur and Wörgötter 1993; Rojer and Schwartz 1990; Swindale 1980, 1992) (Fig. 6a,b). Feature maps (Durbin and Mitchison 1990; Goodhill and Willshaw 1990; Obermayer et al. 1990, 1992c) and some other models (Miller 1990; Miller et al. 1989) use anisotropic neighborhood or cortical-interaction functions (Fig. 7a). When the pattern-generating equations of a model are rotation invariant, anisotropic maps can still be produced using appropriate boundary conditions (Goodhill 1992) such as different shapes for the retina and cortex (Jones et al. 1991) (Fig. 7b) or perturbations of the model equations at the map edges, which can act as a seed leading to globally anisotropic maps (Swindale 1980; Tanaka 1991b). Interestingly, no models have yet been described that rely on spontaneous symmetry breaking to generate anisotropy.

3.6 Biases in Feature Preferences. The diversity principle, as stated above, must be modified to reflect that certain combinations of feature preferences are more common. For example, some experimenters have claimed that in certain or all layers of cortex more cells are responsive to a few particular orientations than to others (e.g., Bauer and Dow 1989). Other studies, including the optical imaging data from the superficial layers of V1 (Fig. 8) do not show any overrepresentation of a particular preferred orientation in the recorded areas (Finlay et al. 1976; Hubel and Wiesel 1968; Poggio et al. 1977). The optical imaging does, however, reveal a bias toward cells with high orientation specificity (Obermayer 1993).

While the experimental data are incomplete, it seems clear that all features are not represented equally. We find it instructive to consider how such biases can and have been introduced into existing models.

Orientation and Ocular Dominance

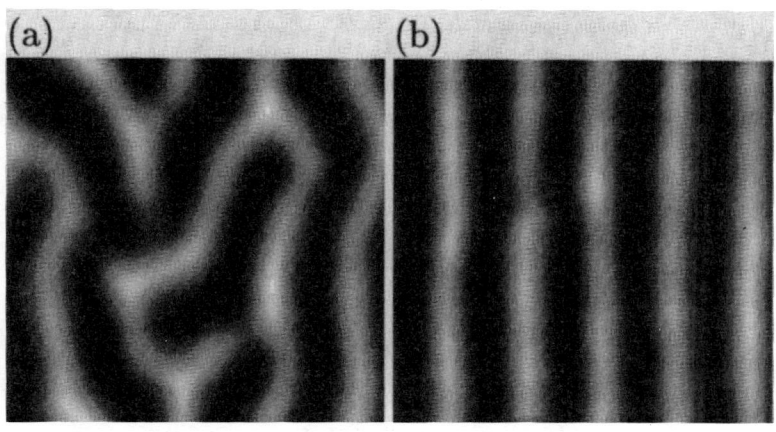

Figure 7: Anisotropic ocular dominance maps generated by the SOM-1 algorithm. In (a) an anisotropic neighborhood function was used: $h_{SOM}(\mathbf{r}, \mathbf{r}') = \exp\{-(r_1 - r'_1)^2/(2\sigma^2) - (r_2 - r'_2)^2/[2(1.3\sigma)^2]\}$, $\sigma = 16.97$. In (b) the effect of differing cortical and retinal shapes is simulated using a cortical sheet of size 512×512 and a retinal sheet of size 128×512. The initial values of $x(\mathbf{r})$ are amended to $x(\mathbf{r}) = 0.25r_1$ and training patterns are drawn from $0 \leq v_x < 128$, $0 \leq v_y < 512$, $q_{max} = 12.8$, $z_{max} = 14.08$. Other parameters in (a) and (b) as in Figure 10.

Several structural models build in biases in preferred orientations (Bauer and Dow 1991; Braitenberg 1985; Dow and Bauer 1984). Most other models could also be modified to favor certain features. In models where training patterns are used, sensory deprivation has been simulated by biases in the training set. Training biases lead to biases in feature preferences (Obermayer *et al.* 1992a), which may be consistent with experimental findings (Blakemore and van Sluyters 1975; Stryker *et al.* 1978).

Increased ability to control the distribution of specificities and feature preferences distinguishes iterative spectral models (Swindale 1982, 1992) from similar one-step models (Niebur and Wörgötter 1993; Rojer and Schwartz 1990). (See Appendix 5.2.1 and 5.2.2.) One-step models generate a single, fixed distribution of orientation specificities (taken as orientation vector length) (Fig. 9a). Although optical imaging tends to underestimate orientation specificities through spatial averaging, it still reveals a distribution favoring higher orientation specificity than the one-step spectral models predict (Fig. 9b).

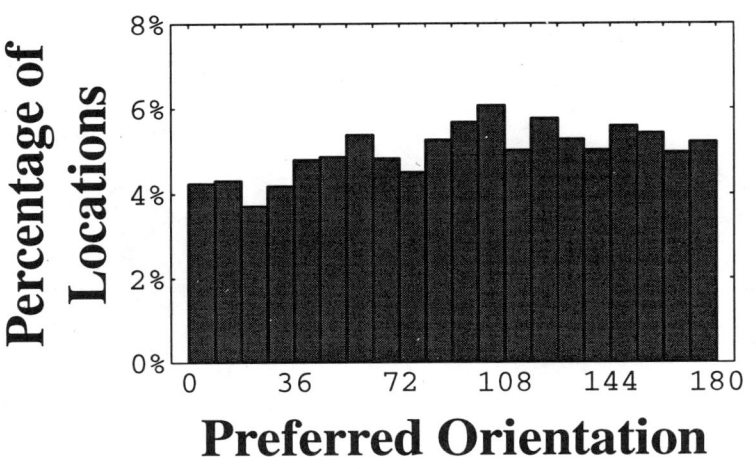

Figure 8: Histogram showing that preferred orientations in optical imaging data (animal NM1) are approximately evenly distributed. Each of 20 bins represents orientations in a 9° range.

Iterative spectral models allow the inclusion of functions linking development of distinct feature vector components and allow the possibility to reproduce any observed distribution of orientation specificities, preferred orientations, or ocularities, although so far no attempt has been made to precisely match experimental data. Linking functions can also be used to give correlations between otherwise independent feature components. Ultimately, however, the physiological basis of any linking function must be found if the model is to be used to predict map development.

3.7 Maps of Different Features Are Correlated. As explained in Section 2, the patterns of ocular dominance and orientation preference in macaque striate cortex are not independent. The two patterns are "globally orthogonal" such that the principal axes of the map patterns, measured on a length of about several ocular dominance bands, are not coincident, and may even be perpendicular. The two patterns also exhibit "local orthogonality" such that singularities and saddle points tend to align with the centers of ocular dominance bands, and isoorientation lines intersect ocular dominance band borders at approximately right angles.

Spectral models (Niebur and Wörgötter 1993; Rojer and Schwartz 1990; Swindale 1982, 1992) can be easily extended to include both ocular dominance and orientation preferences in three-dimensional feature

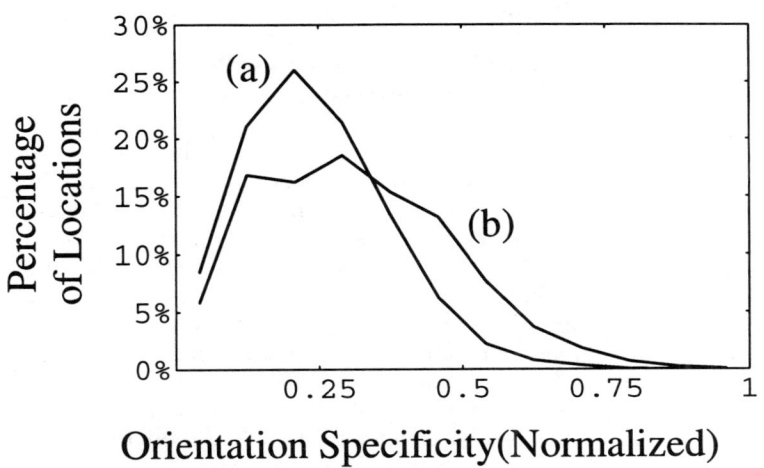

Figure 9: Histograms comparing the distribution of normalized orientation specificities q in maps from a one-step spectral model to experimental data. (a) One-step spectral models always generate a fixed distribution favoring low orientation specificities [data from the model of Niebur and Wörgötter (1993)]. (b) Optical imaging tends to underestimate orientation specificity compared to other experimental methods, yet still reveals a distribution favoring higher specificities than the one-step spectral models.

vectors. An array of these three-dimensional vectors can be component-wise convolved with a Mexican-hat kernel to generate ocular dominance and orientation preference patterns simultaneously. The two map patterns would not, however, be correlated unless the feature components were linked during pattern generation.

The Appendix (5.2.2) demonstrates two examples of linking functions that can be added to iterative spectral models. In a simple case, model cells are encouraged to develop (three-dimensional) feature vectors with approximately the same length. Thus cells with high monocularity will tend to have low orientation specificity and vice versa, which leads to the emergence of singularities in the centers of ocular dominance bands and to slabs of similar orientation preference intersecting ocular dominance borders preferentially at steep angles, i.e., local orthogonality.

A more physiologically interpretable linking function used by Swindale (1992) couples the separate feature components by reducing the speed at which orientation preference grows in regions where ocularity is high. Singularities with low orientation specificity will more likely develop in the centers of single-eye dominance bands where growth of orientation preference was slowed (Fig. 6a). Figure 6a and b compares maps with and without the linking function. With the linking function, the otherwise distinct feature maps are locally coupled such that a tendency toward local orthogonality between isoorientation and ocular dominance borders develops.

Close inspection reveals several instances where the orientation preference map is distorted such that orientation domain borders are "kinked" at the ocular dominance band borders (Fig. 6a, see arrow). Such kinks are not seen in present macaque maps. Kinks in the model result from the specific linking function used. This linking function also predicts a course of development in which strong orientation preference occurs first along the ocular dominance borders, and develops more slowly in the monocular regions. No other known model produces these kinks. Thus, observation of such a pattern in future experimental data from any species would support this model's developmental hypothesis.

A simple extension (see Appendix 5.2.1) to the model of Rojer and Schwartz (1990), whereby both ocular dominance and orientation preference are derived from a single filtered noise array, generates maps with complete local orthogonality. Yet global orthogonality cannot be achieved in this simple model. Using an anisotropic filter would result in anisotropic map patterns, but both patterns would necessarily be elongated along the same axis.

Since Swindale's (1992) model allows different filters for the orientation and ocular dominance components, the wavelengths and anisotropies of the two patterns may be separately specified to give global orthogonality while still maintaining the same degree of local orthogonality. Although local and global orthogonality appear to be distinct properties of macaque maps, no other model currently treats them independently.

In simulations of the simultaneous development of orientation and ocular dominance, competitive Hebbian models (Figs. 10 and 11) generate patterns that include all of the types of local correlations between these two patterns that have been observed in the macaque, but do not reproduce global orthogonality.[5] These correlations have been demonstrated for the self-organizing map (Obermayer et al. 1992b,c) and are also present when the elastic-net approach (Durbin and Mitchison 1990) is appropriately extended (see Appendix 5.4.2). The correlations trivially emerge when patterns with the undesired combinations, e.g., low orientation specificity combined with binocularity, are excluded from the training set. However, they also occur when the training set includes all possible combinations of feature preferences.

For the latter case, the emergence of correlations between features can best be explained in the dimension-reduction framework (Fig. 12). In this framework cortical maps are described as mappings between a high-

---

[5]Global orthogonality, however, can be heuristically introduced by allowing different neighborhood functions to act on different components of the feature vector.

Orientation and Ocular Dominance

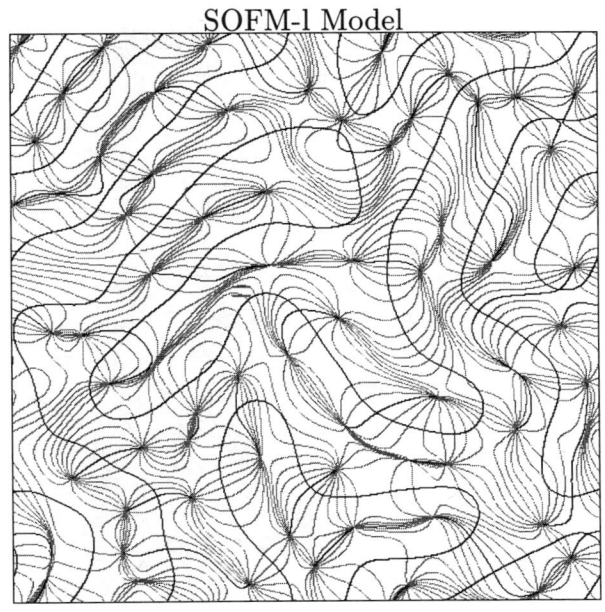

Figure 10: Model output from the self-organizing map (Obermayer et al. 1990, 1992c) in the format of Figure 4. Model size is 512 × 512 with periodic boundary conditions for the r_1 and r_2-axes. Training patterns $\mathbf{v} = \{v_x, v_y, v_q \sin(2v_\phi), v_q \cos(2v_\phi), v_z\}$ were chosen with uniform probability from $0 < v_x, v_y < 128$, $0 < v_\phi < \pi$, $0 < v_q < q_{max}$, $|v_z| < z_{max}$, $q_{max} = 51.2$, $z_{max} = 56.32$. Initial values: $x(\mathbf{r}) = r_1$, $y(\mathbf{r}) = r_2$, $q = 0.01 * q_{max}$, $z = 0$, with ϕ uniformly distributed over all angles. In the function $h_{SOM}(\cdot)$, $\sigma = 16.97$. Output is shown after 1,000,000 iterations with $\epsilon = 0.02$.

dimensional feature space and a two-dimensional cortical space that obey certain continuity and diversity constraints (Durbin and Mitchison 1990; Kohonen 1987; Obermayer et al. 1990). When training patterns are presented with equal probability out of an appropriate manifold in feature space, the magnification factor of the map between feature space and cortical coordinates will be approximately constant. Consequently, regions where one feature-vector component changes rapidly coincide with regions where other components change slowly. In regions where two feature components change fairly rapidly, they tend to do so along orthogonal axes in the cortex. If orientation selectivity and ocular dominance are represented by Cartesian coordinates as described in the Appendix,

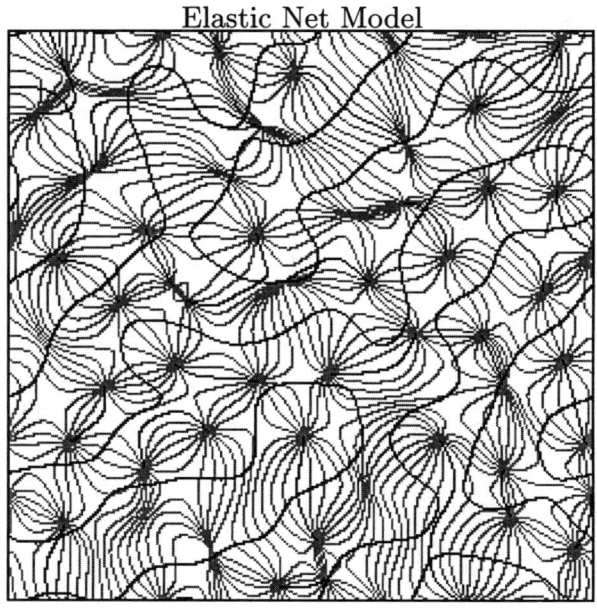

Figure 11: Model output from the elastic-net model (Durbin and Mitchison 1990) in the same format as Figure 4. Model size is 256 × 256 with periodic boundary conditions for r_1 and r_2. Initial values and training patterns as in Figure 10, with $q_{max} = 61.44$, $z_{max} = 46.08$. In the function $h_{EN}(\cdot)$, $\sigma = 2.771$. Output is shown after 2,000,000 iterations with $\alpha = 0.4$, $\beta = 0.0001$.

the model maps will then develop with local orthogonality between orientation and ocular dominance columns, similar to what has been found in the macaque maps.

The generalized deformable model of Yuille (Yuille *et al.* 1991) can be made to produce similar maps to the elastic-net model. Yet he points out that the model may be generalized by modifying the definition of the norm used to enforce similarity between neighboring neurons. Different norms could lead to other types of correlations that might occur in other species, such as coincident regions of rapid change in orientation and ocular dominance.

The magnitude of the correlations between orientation preference and ocularity cannot be adequately determined from the current experimental data, because noise and slight movements of cortex during recording tend to destroy such correlations. Thus while we note that the SOM,

Orientation and Ocular Dominance

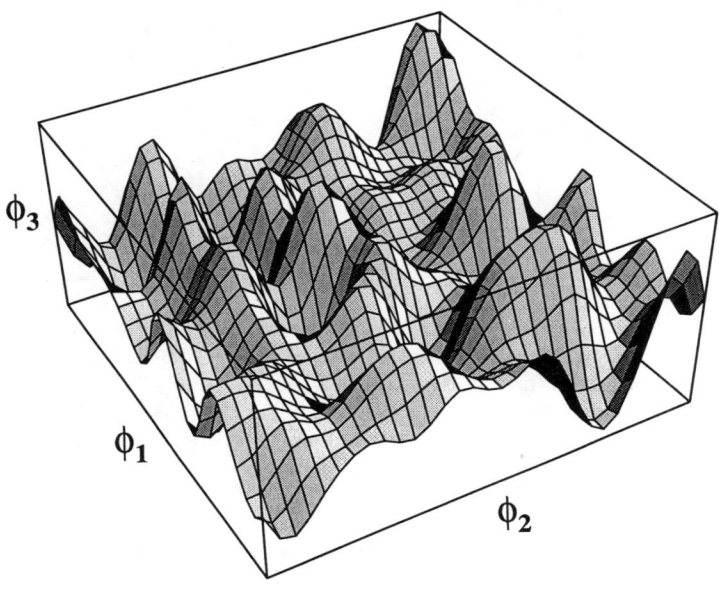

Figure 12: Dimension-reduction: This figure shows how points in a two-dimensional array might be mapped into a three-dimensional feature space with components ϕ_1, ϕ_2, and ϕ_3, representing such features as visual field location and ocular dominance. Dimension-reduction models often constrain the map to fill the input space with near-uniform density while maintaining continuity. This leads to maps where rapid changes in one feature vector component are correlated with slow changes in other vector components.

EN, and Rojer and Schwartz models predict stronger correlations than are observed experimentally, quantitative comparison is currently not recommended.

3.8 Correlations between Orientation Preference Coordinates and Cortical Coordinates. Several structural models imply particular relationships between the coordinate systems representing cortical location and orientation preference. For example, they may arrange cells preferring horizontal (or radial) stimuli in columns running in one direction across cortex while columns of cells preferring vertical (or concentric) stimuli run in the perpendicular direction (Bauer and Dow 1991; Dow and Bauer 1984).

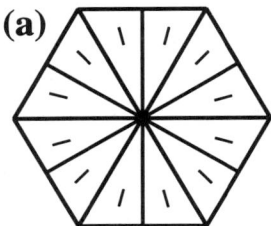 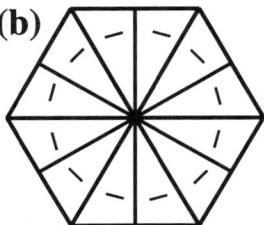

Figure 13: The pinwheel model (Braitenberg and Braitenberg 1979) tiles the plane with hexagonal hypercolumns each containing a +1 singularity. Six −1/2 singularities will be formed at the vertices where adjacent hypercolumns meet. Two versions of the model were suggested: (a) and (b). In each case, orientation preferences (short bars) are nearly perfectly correlated with the cortical orientation of the isoorientation lines (longer lines).

The implied link between coordinate systems is often visible if the maps are drawn using oriented line segments to directly represent preferred orientations of cells. Displaying maps from the pinwheel models (Braitenberg 1985; Braitenberg and Braitenberg 1979) in this way, line segments representing preferred orientations appear aligned along curves that either radiate out from, or circle around the +1 vortices (Fig. 13a and b). In this model, such an arrangement of the orientation selective cells arises from a simple, plausible scheme of synaptic connections. Although cortical maps are not as well ordered as this simplified model, this predicted link between cortical and retinal coordinates could be present to some degree.

A numerical test for such a link can be performed by comparing preferred orientations with the orientation of the isoorientation region contours. Alternatively the preferred orientations can be compared to the local orientation of the gradient vector of orientation preference with respect to cortical location, since this gradient vector is generally perpendicular to the isoorientation borders. In separate versions of the pinwheel model, the orientation preference vectors are either almost all perpendicular to (Fig. 13a) or almost all parallel to (Fig. 13b) the orientation gradient vectors. These trends are demonstrated in Figure 15g and h.

When analyzed in this way, the macaque optical imaging data show no preferred angle of intersection between orientation preference and its gradient vector (Fig. 15a) and thus no link between retinal and cortical coordinates.

Links between orientation preference and cortical coordinates are completely absent from models that treat orientation preference as an abstract

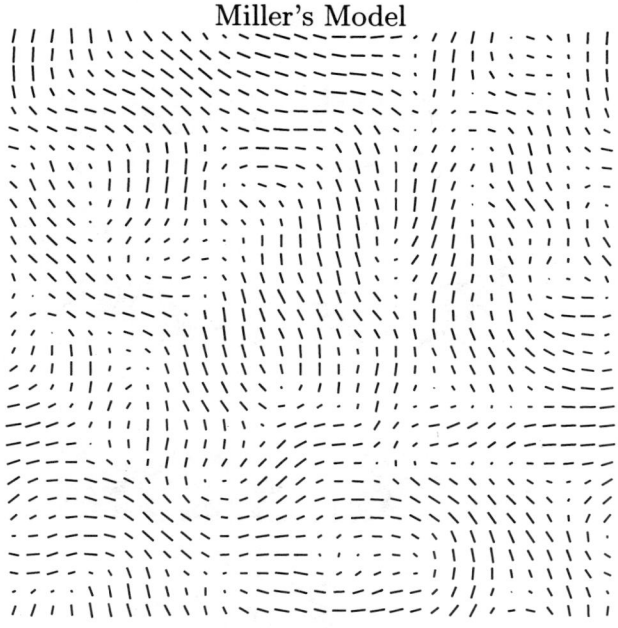

Figure 14: Orientation preference map from the correlation-based learning model of Miller (1992). Oriented lines represent the orientation preferences of an array of 32 × 32 cortical cells. Model parameters: $k_I = 1/9$, $\sigma_I = 3.0$, $C^{same}(\mathbf{x}, \mathbf{x}') = \exp(-\|\mathbf{x} - \mathbf{x}'\|/1.21) - (1/9)\exp(-\|\mathbf{x} - \mathbf{x}'\|/10.89)$, $C^{diff}(\mathbf{x}, \mathbf{x}') = (-1/2)C^{same}(\mathbf{x}, \mathbf{x}')$, arbor function $A(\mathbf{r}, \mathbf{x}) = \exp(-\|\mathbf{r} - \mathbf{x}\|/9.0)$. Initial synaptic weights were randomly distributed with uniform probability in the interval $1.6 < \Phi^i_{t=0}(\mathbf{r}, \mathbf{x}) < 2.4$. Map shown for $t = 900$ with $\alpha = 0.001$.

component of a feature vector, as in the spectral models (Fig. 15f) and the low-dimensional competitive Hebbian models (Fig. 15b). In models using the high-dimensional weight vector representation of receptive fields, a link often, but not necessarily, appears.

In one high-dimensional model (Miller 1992, 1994), cortical cells develop receptive fields with ON and OFF subfields, based on hypothetical correlations in the firing patterns of ON- and OFF-center geniculate cells (see Appendix 5.3). Orientation preferences result from alignment of the ON- and OFF-subfields, while intracortical interactions cause the orientation preferences of neighboring cells to be organized into a map across the cortical surface (Fig. 14). Although intended primarily as a model of development of single-cell orientation preferences, the model can ac-

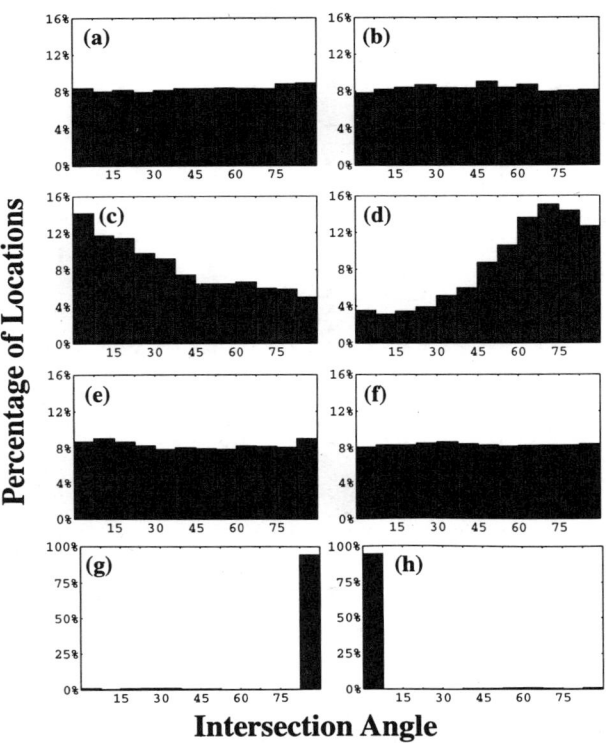

Figure 15: The histograms show the percentage of sites with a given difference angle $0 \leq I < 90°$ between preferred orientation $0 \leq \phi < 180°$ of a cortical cell and the orientation $0 \leq g < 180°$ on the cortical surface along which preferred orientation changes most rapidly. The difference angle is computed as $I = \min(|\phi - g|, 180° - |\phi - g|)$, where g is the angular component of the gradient $\mathbf{g} = [\nabla_{\mathbf{r}} \phi(\mathbf{r})] \mod 180°$, approximated as $g_1 = 0.5[(\phi_{r_1+1,r_2} - \phi_{r_1-1,r_2}) \mod 180°]$, $g_2 = 0.5[(\phi_{r_1,r_2+1} - \phi_{r_1,r_2-1}) \mod 180°]$. (a) In experimental data (Fig. 4), and in competitive Hebbian models such as (b) the self-organizing map (Fig. 10), the difference angle takes on all values with equal probability. (c)–(d) Two correlation-based models predict a bias in the difference angles: (c) bias toward low I for Miller's model (Fig. 14) and (d) bias toward high I for Linsker's (1986c) model. (e) Tanaka's correlation-based model (Miyashita and Tanaka 1992) and (f) spectral models such as Swindale's model (Fig. 6a) predict an even distribution. (g) The two variants of the pinwheel model predict near 100% correlations with $I = 0$ for Figure 13a, and (h) $I = 90°$ for Figure 13b. Data for (d) described in Figure 2 of Linsker (1986c). These data contained only 10 distinct ϕ values, and had to be smoothed by gaussian filtering to allow computation of gradients. Data for (e) provided by S. Tanaka.

count for many of the prominent features of lateral map organization, like singularities, and fractures.

Analyzing the maps generated by this model as above reveals that there can occur a strong correlation between a cell's orientation preference in retinal coordinates and the orientation of the isoorientation bands in cortical coordinates. This results in orientation preference vectors aligned with the local direction of the orientation gradient (Fig. 15c) similar to but weaker than the correlations seen for the pinwheel model (Fig. 13b). Although the relationship has not been well studied, the strength of the correlations does depend on model parameters, and there appear to be some parameter regimes where such correlations are not apparent.

A related model by Linsker (1986c) produces maps that show a similar type of correlations (Fig. 15d) although in this case resembling the alternate version of the pinwheel model (Fig. 13a). As Linsker (1986c) noted, when cortical cells have receptive fields containing parallel subfields of opposing types, such as excitatory and inhibitory (likewise for ON and OFF), the degree of similarity between receptive fields will depend not only on their orientation but also on their relative location and internal structure. Two cortical cells with identical receptive field structure that are in partially overlapping locations in the retina would have greater similarity if they were displaced along the axis of the subfield alignment than if they were displaced along the perpendicular axis. Thus if the growth of receptive fields is influenced by the degree of receptive field similarity, correlations can develop between orientation preference (receptive field alignment) and the direction of orientation column alignment in cortex.

Tanaka's model of correlation-based learning (Tanaka 1991a; Miyashita and Tanaka 1992), as well as the high-dimensional version of the self-organizing map (Obermayer et al. 1990), are both similar to Miller's model in that orientation preferences develop through alignment of subregions in the receptive fields and growth of columnar structure is related to the overlap of receptive fields. We have examined data from one sample map from Tanaka's model and found that it did not show any correlations between retinal and cortical coordinates (Fig. 15e). We have likewise not observed the high-dimensional self-organizing map to predict a link between coordinate systems (Fig. 15b). It is unknown whether such a correlation could develop for some other choices of parameters.

Correlations between retinal and cortical coordinates are not seen in macaque maps (Fig. 15a) although they could be present in maps from other species. Since the measure of correlations introduced here has not previously been used to test model and experimental data, additional study will be required to determine the effect of model parameters on such correlations, and whether they occur in differently organized maps from other species.

Differences between the models above suggest a few tentative hypotheses. First, comparing the self-organizing map model and the models of Linsker and Miller suggests that the presence of contrasting types of subfields (ON/OFF or $+/-$) increases the likelihood that correlations will develop. The phase of two receptive fields will have less impact on their degree of overlap if there is a single type of subfield, as in the self-organizing map model. Second, the self-organizing map and Tanaka's models indicate that the inclusion of some scatter in the topographic projection from retinal to cortical locations could cause any correlation that may develop between the direction of subfield alignment and receptive field location in retinal coordinates to not be visible in the cortical map. Third, correlations appear to be more likely in models that consider only linear development rules, omitting refinements that could be due to more complex nonlinear processes.

3.9 Orientation Maps Are Not a Linear Transformation of a Conservative Vector Field. A spectral model proposed by Rojer and Schwartz (1990) used the gradient of a bandpass-filtered noise pattern to characterize cortical orientation maps (see Appendix 5.2.1). The model does generate maps that superficially resemble experimentally observed maps (Fig. 16). However, since the model maps are derived through a linear mapping from a conservative vector field (in which vectors are always perpendicular to the field gradient) the model predicts a unique type of link between cortical and orientation preference coordinates (Erwin *et al.* 1993). This relationship restricts the range of patterns the model can produce, as is easily demonstrated visually near singularities (Fig. 17).

One way to numerically demonstrate these correlations, and show that they are not present in macaque data, is to multiply the preferred orientations (180° periodic) in the maps by two to give a vector field (360° periodic). Analyzing the resulting vector field in a manner similar to the method of Figure 15 reveals that the direction of these vectors is strongly correlated with the direction of their gradient vector field for the model map. Similar correlations do not appear in spectral models that do not involve conservative vector fields (e.g., Niebur and Wörgötter 1993; Swindale 1982). However, such correlations do also occur in Götz's (1987) version of the pinwheel model. Analyzing the macaque data in a similar manner reveals that it cannot be derived from a linear mapping to a conservative field.

This discussion helps illuminate the utility of models that attempt to characterize map patterns in simple equations. Without Rojer and Schwartz's model it is unlikely that we would have noted that macaque orientation maps are not a linear function of a conservative vector field. Knowing this property of experimental maps, new models should be tested to ensure that such a relationship has not been unintentionally included.

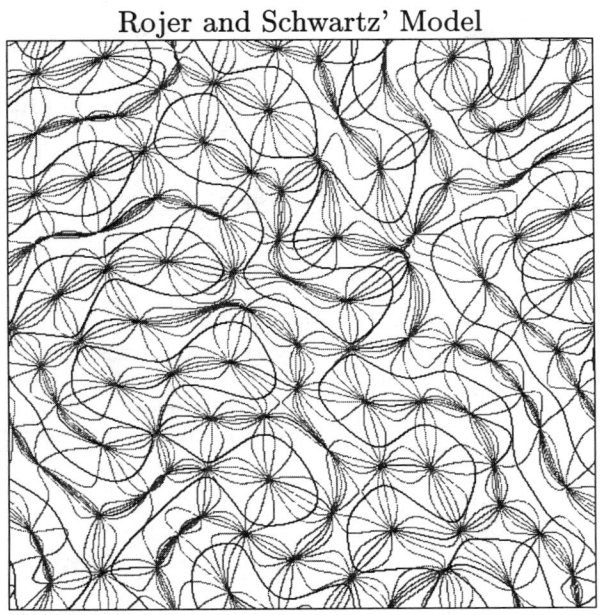

Figure 16: Orientation and ocular dominance map from a combined version of the models of Rojer and Schwartz (1990). Model size 512 × 512, $H(\mathbf{s}) = (1 + e^{-\alpha*(\rho_c - \delta/2 - \|\mathbf{s}\|)})^{-1} \times (1 + e^{-\alpha*(\|\mathbf{s}\| - \rho_c - \delta/2)})^{-1}$, $\rho_c = 4.96$, $\delta = 0.96$, $\alpha = 1.5625$. Noise array $n(\mathbf{r})$ values are normally distributed around 0 with variance 1.0. Note that the medium gray orientation contour, which indicates 0°, exits all of the +1/2 singularities (exactly one-half of the singularities) from the left or right side only. See Figure 17 for an explanation.

4 Discussion

In this contribution we have investigated several models for the structure and the formation of orientation and ocular dominance maps. The results of our comparison between model predictions and experimental data obtained from the upper layers of macaque striate cortex are summarized in Table 2. References to articles on each model are given in Table 1. Many of the models are also briefly described in the Appendix.

Data for our comparisons come primarily from implementations of selected models on computers at our site. Generally our implementation followed closely the published description of the models and parameters. However, we extended a few models to include simultaneous

Table 2: Summary Comparison of Model Predictions[a]

	General Properties
Global disorder	Included in all models except several structural models (icecube, Götz, pinwheel)
Power spectrum	Miller, Yuille *et al.*, and Tanaka maps often have low-pass, rather than bandpass power spectra
Anisotropies	All models here can produce anisotropic map patterns

	Orientation Maps
Singularities	Absent from icecube model Arise spontaneously in many models of map formation Several structural models (Pinwheel, one form of Baxter and Dow) suggested 360° periodic singularities Overall orientations of singularities are restricted in Rojer and Schwartz
Saddle points	Absent only in icecube model
Fractures	Structural models tend to omit fractures All others include fractures as loci of rapid, continuous orientation change Miller, Linsker may include actual discontinuities, but the map resolution is too low to allow a meaningful distinction between rapid change and discontinuity
Linear zones	Present to varying degrees in all models Less prominent in SOM-h, and correlation-based models
Linked coordinates	Pinwheel, Götz, and Baxter and Dow predict a link between a cell's preferred orientation and the direction of isoorientation columns For some parameters, Miller and Linsker suggest a similar link A link has not been observed in macaque data, nor in the remaining models
Conservative maps	Rojer and Schwartz, and Götz maps are a linear transformation of a conservative vector field Macaque maps, as well as other model maps, are not
Distribution of specificities	Most models that include a notion of feature specificity can be tuned to approximate experimentally observed distributions of specificity Among spectral models, the iterative approach (Swindale) allows finer control over the distribution of feature specificities than the one-step approach (Rojer and Schwartz, Niebur and Wörgötter)

[a]Model abbreviations are explained in Table 1.

Orientation and Ocular Dominance

Table 2: *Continued.*

Orientation deprivation and bias	Due to the method of learning by examples, competitive Hebbian models can easily simulate learning under exposure to a restricted or biased set of oriented visual features The other models here have not been applied to the same problem

Ocular Dominance

Monocular deprivation	All models that include ocular dominance can simulate development or appearance of maps in monocularly deprived animals
Strabismus	Miller, SOM, EN, and Tanaka models successfully reproduce development of maps in strabismic animals

Relationships between Ocular Dominance and Orientation Maps

Joint pattern development	Very few joint models of ocularity and orientation were proposed (SOM-h, SOM-l, Swindale) We have extended the EN and Rojer and Schwartz models to test their generalizability The model of Miller is currently being similarly extended, with no conclusive results at present
Orientation specificity and binocularity	All joint models correlate higher orientation specificity with binocularity and place singularities preferentially away from OD borders SOM-l, EN, and Rojer and Schwartz include a greater degree of correlation than observed in macaque
Local orthogonality	All joint models include some preference for ORI borders to be perpendicular to OD borders SOM-l, EN, and Rojer and Schwartz include a greater degree of correlation than observed in macaque Swindale's model makes a unique fine-scale prediction that has not been seen experimentally
Global orthogonality	Local and global orthogonality appear to be separate properties of experimental maps Only Swindale currently treats them separately in a model

development of orientation and ocular dominance so that we could compare them with the favorable results of the SOM models. We extended only several representative models where the extensions seemed to be a direct continuation of the model's principles and equations. Our extensions to the spectral model of Rojer and Schwartz, the correlation-based

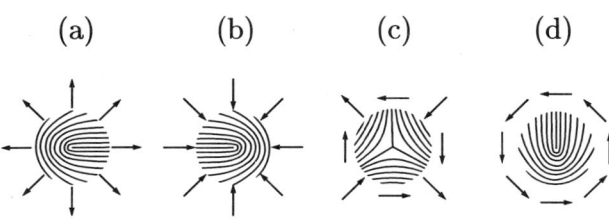

Figure 17: (a)–(d) Examples of vector fields (outside) and the associated orientation map (inside, local tangents to the curves) for typical singularities that can occur in the experimental data. The singularity (d) is an example of a feature not allowed by the model of Rojer and Schwartz (1990), because the curl of the associated vector field does not vanish at this location.

learning model of Miller, and the elastic-net model are described in Appendices 5.2.1, 5.3, and 5.4.2.

Among the pattern models, the spectral models perform better than the earlier structural models, mainly because they account for global disorder and for the coexistence of linear zones and singularities. The filtered noise approach for orientation selectivity (Niebur and Wörgötter 1993) and for ocular dominance (Rojer and Schwartz 1990) captures most of the important features of the individual maps, except for the high degree of feature selectivity that is observed in the macaque. Models by Swindale (1980, 1982, 1992) provide the currently best description of the individual orientation and ocular dominance patterns found in the macaque. Additionally, they can account for many correlations between the maps. Such a close match to experimental patterns has not yet been achieved in the more physiological high-dimensional models.

The particular form of the function used in Swindale's model to link development of orientation and ocular dominance leads to a prediction of occasional sudden changes in direction, or "kinks" in the isoorientation region borders at ocular dominance borders. This prediction is unique to Swindale's model. If such kinks are found in future high-resolution experimental images, it would support the model's prediction that orientation preference develops (or refines) first in binocular regions. Swindale's model is also unique in including separate mechanisms for generating local and global orthogonality. This extra freedom may be required to explain the structure of experimental maps.

Correlation-based learning models have led to valuable insight into the role of Hebbian learning in receptive field development (Linsker 1986a,b; Miller 1992; Yuille *et al.* 1989). They were not expected to predict the structure of cortical maps with as much precision. It is, however, instructive to note how the inclusion of realistic receptive field properties impacts on the cortical map patterns.

Correlation-based learning models perform well for ocular dominance (Miller et al. 1989). When applied to the formation of orientation maps (Linsker 1986c; Miller 1992), the ON/OFF-competition model underrepresents linear zones, and produces maps without a bandpass power spectrum. These points might be related to the low resolution of the maps necessitated by high computational demand.

Linsker's model always predicts a link between preferred orientation and direction of its vector gradient. Miller's model also predicts a link for some model parameters. Such a link is not present in the macaque data, thus constraining the range of parameters for which the model could apply to macaque data. If maps from different species are shown in the future to possess such a link, this would provide strong support for the correlation-based learning approach.

Competitive Hebbian models (Durbin and Mitchison 1990; Goodhill and Willshaw 1990; Obermayer et al. 1990, 1992c) lead to the currently best description of the observed patterns from a developmental perspective. These models attempt to describe the developmental process on a mesoscopic level, spatially as well as temporally, which has the advantage that the level of description matches the resolution of the experimental data. These models do not involve the microscopic concepts neuron, synapse, and spike, which makes it somewhat more difficult to relate model predictions to experimental data. Competitive Hebbian models make qualitatively correct predictions with respect to all the principles we have outlined above, except that they have not yet addressed the issue of global orthogonality as separate from local orthogonality. These models could be extended by, for example, including separate neighborhood functions for ocular dominance and orientation preference.

For correlations between orientation and ocular dominance maps, the competitive Hebbian models give the most realistic predictions. As expected, the predictions of the extended elastic-net model closely match the low-dimensional SOM algorithm. Since Yuille's generalized deformable model (Yuille et al. 1991) can be reduced to the elastic net, it should be equally capable of matching the experimental data if extended. Our extended version of the Rojer and Schwartz model failed to reproduce some of the experimentally observed correlations between orientation and ocularity. This observation is not intended to show a deficiency in their model as originally published. Rather, we wish to show how easily the property of local orthogonality and qualitatively correct correlations between singularities and ocularity emerge when the model is extended in a simple way. In our simulations with an extended version of the correlation-based learning model of Miller, maps with both well-organized orientation and ocular dominance failed to develop. We cannot, however, conclude that a more appropriate parameter regime does not exist. Further work on this joint model is in progress.

More stringent tests of the postulated mechanisms of activity-dependent neural development must rely on experiments that (1) monitor the actual timecourse of pattern formation and that (2) study pattern development under experimentally modified conditions (deprivation experiments). While progress has been made (Bonhoeffer *et al.* 1993; Löwel and Singer 1993; Hubel *et al.* 1977; Kim and Bonhoeffer 1993; Obermayer *et al.* 1994; Rauschecker 1991; Tanaka 1991b,c) there is currently not enough data on the spatial patterns available to constrain the present models. Unfortunately, no anatomical correlate has yet been found for orientation selectivity and binocularity in upper layers of monkey striate cortex. This quantity must be assessed physiologically and, therefore, after birth, which currently limits investigations to the final, refinement phase of orientation and ocular dominance development.

Further evidence to decide between proposed mechanisms might be derived from interspecies comparisons. The underlying assumption is that mechanisms of visual cortex development should be fairly universal and that any model of value should be able to account for interspecies variations. A few studies modeling cat and monkey patterns have been reported (Jones *et al.* 1991; Miller 1992; Obermayer *et al.* 1990; Rojer and Schwartz 1990; Swindale 1981). Yet, most studies focused on properties of the experimental patterns that arise from very basic assumptions like broken rotational symmetry, which leads to global map anisotropies. Consequently, most of the models were able to account for the observed interspecies variations. As more and better data become available (e.g., Blasdel *et al.* 1993), fewer of the existing models may continue to be useful.

Finally, one would like to have relatively simple models that make predictions about several aspects of cortical organization. Some current models do make predictions about features other than orientation preference and ocular dominance, such as receptive field location (Durbin and Mitchison 1990; Goodhill 1993; Jones *et al.* 1991; Obermayer *et al.* 1990, 1992c; Miyashita and Tanaka 1992; Yuille *et al.* 1991), color selectivity (Barrow and Bray 1992a), receptive field subfields, and spatial phase (Barrow and Bray 1992b; Berns *et al.* 1993; Linsker 1986c; Miller 1992, 1994; Miyashita and Tanaka 1992; Yuille *et al.* 1989), and correlations with locations of cytochrome-oxidase blobs (e.g., Götz 1988). Correlations between maps of different features are predicted by all of these models, and could be tested in suitably designed experiments.

5 Appendix: Model Descriptions

5.1 General Nomenclature. This Appendix gives brief formulations of several of the models included in this study. The model descriptions are intended to (1) ease comparison between different approaches by presenting models with common symbols, and (2) provide sufficient detail to allow interpretation of model parameters given in figure captions. By

Orientation and Ocular Dominance

necessity, the descriptions here reduce the complexity of some models. Refer to the original references for fuller descriptions and more general formulations.

Response properties of cortical cells or small cortical regions at each cortical location $\mathbf{r}$ are represented by a feature vector $\Phi(\mathbf{r})$. In the "low-dimensional" representation each component stands for a selected response property. Ocular dominance is represented by a scalar $z(\mathbf{r})$ where positive and negative numbers code for eye preferences and zero indicates binocularity. Preferred orientation $\phi(\mathbf{r})$ and degree of preference for that orientation $q(\mathbf{r})$ are denoted by more convenient Cartesian components $\phi(\mathbf{r}) = \{q(\mathbf{r})\sin[2\phi(\mathbf{r})], q(\mathbf{r})\cos[2\phi(\mathbf{r})]\}$ (Swindale 1982), where the factor of two enforces the assumption that the orientation maps code for the 180°-periodic orientation rather than the 360°-periodic direction of a stimulus.[6] Additional features, such as the retinal location $\{x(\mathbf{r}), y(\mathbf{r})\}$ of the receptive field or the preferred direction in color space, can be incorporated.

In the "high-dimensional" representation, the feature vector codes for the effective strength of the connections between a cortical cell and each of a set of N receptor cells in one or more input layers $\Phi(\mathbf{r}) = \{w_1(\mathbf{r}), w_2(\mathbf{r}), \ldots, w_N(\mathbf{r})\}$.

The subscript $\mathbf{r}$ for cortical location will be omitted in the equations below, except where necessary for clarity.

5.2 Spectral Models. Spectral models generate orientation and ocular dominance patterns by either convolving an array of random feature vectors with an appropriate kernel $h(\mathbf{r})$ in the space domain, or by filtering a noise array with an appropriate filter $H(\mathbf{s})$ in the Fourier domain. Convolution or filtering may be carried out either iteratively or in one step.

5.2.1 One-Step Spectral Models. The models of Rojer and Schwartz (1990). Let $n(\mathbf{r})$ be a white-noise pattern of independently chosen random numbers gaussian-distributed around 0 and let $h(\mathbf{r})$ be the space-domain representation of a bandpass filter $H(\mathbf{s})$. Then an ocular dominance-like pattern may be derived from

$$z = n * h \tag{5.1}$$

where $*$ denotes convolution.

An orientation map is derived through a similar process by taking the vector gradient with respect to the cortical coordinates r_1 and r_2 of the filtered noise array. The preferred orientation ϕ is then taken as the angular direction of this vector divided by two, and in a simple extension

---

[6]This assumption is based in part on the appearance of the singularities.

of the model, an orientation specificity q may be taken from the length of the vector

$$\phi = (1/2)\tan^{-1}(u_2/u_1), q = \|\mathbf{u}\|, \qquad \text{where } \mathbf{u} = \left\{\frac{\partial z}{\partial r_1}, \frac{\partial z}{\partial r_2}\right\} \qquad (5.2)$$

Due to the gradient operation, the orientation vector field is linearly related to a conservative field, and the model wrongly predicts correlations between orientation preferences and cortical locations such that

$$\oint q\sin(2\phi)dr_1 + q\cos(2\phi)dr_2 = 0 \qquad (5.3)$$

is fulfilled for every closed path (Erwin et al. 1993). Rojer and Schwartz proposed separate models for orientation preference and ocular dominance, and omitted orientation specificity. For comparing their predictions with other models, we extend their model by considering $z(r)$ to be simultaneously an ocular dominance and the precursor of an orientation array, and consider q to represent orientation specificity.

The model of Niebur and Wörgötter (1993). An orientation map is derived by applying a bandpass filter $H(\mathbf{s})$ and an inverse Fourier transform *IFT* to a white-noise array $N(\mathbf{s})$ of independent, uniformly distributed elements in the Fourier domain. The Cartesian coordinates of the orientation vector are given by the real and imaginary parts of the resulting array Γ:

$$\Gamma = IFT(H \cdot N) \qquad (5.4)$$
$$\{q\sin(2\phi), q\cos(2\phi)\} = \{Re(\Gamma), Im(\Gamma)\} \qquad (5.5)$$

5.2.2 Iterative Spectral Models. Iterative models begin with a random distribution of small feature preferences $\|\Phi_0\| \ll 1$. A feature map develops through iterative application of an update equation

$$\Phi_{t+1} = \Phi_t + \alpha(\Phi_t * h)f(\Phi_t), \qquad 0 < \alpha < 1 \qquad (5.6)$$

The function $f(\Phi)$ is chosen such that the components in Φ are appropriately coupled. A simple choice is

$$f(\Phi) = (1 - \|\Phi\|) \qquad (5.7)$$

which encourages all feature vectors to grow toward a common length. If $\Phi = \{q\sin(2\phi), q\cos(2\phi), z\}$ then equations 5.6 and 5.7 lead to correlations between orientation selectivity and ocular dominance, which are qualitatively similar to the correlations observed in the macaque.

The models of Swindale. Swindale (1992) chose to exert finer control over the map structure by using differently sized Mexican-hat kernels h_z and h_ϕ for the ocular dominance and orientation components of Φ, and a more complicated coupling function f. His update equations read

$$z_{t+1} = z_t + \alpha(z_t * h_z)(1 - z_t^2) \qquad (5.8)$$

Orientation and Ocular Dominance

$$\phi_{t+1} = \{q\sin(2\phi), q\cos(2\phi)\}$$
$$= \phi_t + \alpha(\phi_t * h_\phi)(1 - |z_t * h_z|)^a(1-q). \tag{5.9}$$

For $a = 0$, equations 5.8 and 5.9 one recovers Swindale's independent models for ocular dominance (Swindale 1980) and orientation columns (Swindale 1982).

5.3 Correlation-Based Learning Models. We present several models by Miller to illustrate the principles of correlation-based learning. Miller's ocular dominance development model (Miller et al. 1989) uses a "high-dimensional" feature vector $\Phi^i(\mathbf{r}, \mathbf{x})$ coding for the strength of connection from each cortical location $\mathbf{r}$ to each retinal location $\mathbf{x}$ in each of two eyes $i \in \{0, 1\}$. Activity patterns in the retina are described by their two-point correlation function within, $C^{\text{same}}(\mathbf{x}, \mathbf{x}')$, and between, $C^{\text{diff}}(\mathbf{x}, \mathbf{x}')$, eyes, assuming that the coordinate systems in each eye are in one-to-one correspondence. The feature vectors are initialized, and then develop through an update equation, which in its simplest form is

$$\Phi^i_{t+1} = \Phi^i_t + \alpha A(\mathbf{r}, \mathbf{x})[I * (C^{\text{same}} * \Phi^i_t) + I * (C^{\text{diff}} * \Phi^{1-i}_t)],$$
$$0 < \alpha < 1 \tag{5.10}$$

The arbor function $A(\mathbf{r}, \mathbf{x})$ determines the location and overall size of the receptive fields. The intracortical interaction function $I(\mathbf{r}, \mathbf{r}')$ represents the effect of interactions between nearby cortical cells. It is often defined as

$$I(\mathbf{r}, \mathbf{r}') = (0.5\delta(\|\mathbf{r} - \mathbf{r}'\|) + 0.5)[\exp(-\|\mathbf{r} - \mathbf{r}'\|^2/\sigma_I^2)$$
$$- k_I \exp(-\|\mathbf{r} - \mathbf{r}'\|^2/9\sigma_I^2)] \tag{5.11}$$

where $\delta(\cdot)$ is the Kronecker delta function.

Generally, nonlinearities will be added to equation 10 through additional terms, normalization of weight vectors, or limiting the maximum and minimum values of each synaptic weight value.

Miller's model for orientation preference (Miller 1992, 1994) is formally similar, with the two feature vectors Φ^{ON} and Φ^{OFF} now representing connections to separate populations of ON- and OFF-center cells in the LGN. The two correlation functions C^{same} and C^{diff} again represent the expected correlations between cells at a given distance in the retina and of either the same or opposite cell types. The preferred orientations and orientation specificities are determined from the scalar product of the weight vectors with sinusoidal grating patterns.

For some parameters, e.g., for large σ_I, the model implies a link between coordinate systems that has not been seen in experimental data.

We have extended the model equations to include orientation and ocular dominance maps at the same time by including four separate types of synapses—two eyes with two types of ganglion cells in each. So far we have not found any set of correlation functions for which simulations lead to the coordinated growth of orientation and ocular dominance maps.

5.4 Competitive Hebbian Models. Competitive Hebbian models are based on essentially the same set of assumptions as correlation-based learning, with one crucial difference: the weighted summation of time-averaged cortical cell outputs via the lateral interaction function I, equations 10 and 5.11, is replaced by a nonlinear lateral interaction in which competition enhances the activity of units already highly activated in response to individual stimuli. The most prominent competitive Hebbian models are based on the self-organizing map (Kohonen 1982a,b) and the elastic net (Durbin and Willshaw 1987). Yuille's generalized deformable model can also be reduced to a competitive Hebbian model (Yuille et al. 1991) by appropriate choice of parameters.

5.4.1 Self-Organizing Map Models. The self-organizing map model (Obermayer et al. 1992c) employs an iterative procedure, in which low-dimensional feature vectors $\Phi = \{x, y, q\sin(2\phi), q\cos(2\phi), z\}$ are changed according to

$$\Phi_{t+1}(\mathbf{r}) = \Phi_t(\mathbf{r}) + \alpha h_{\text{SOM}}(\mathbf{r}, \mathbf{r}')[\mathbf{v}_{t+1} - \Phi_t(\mathbf{r})], \qquad 0 < \alpha < 1 \quad (5.12)$$

At each iteration the stimulus $\mathbf{v}$ is chosen at random according to a given probability distribution $P(\mathbf{v})$. The function $h_{\text{SOM}}(\cdot)$ is given by

$$\begin{aligned} h_{\text{SOM}}(\mathbf{r}, \mathbf{r}') &= \exp(-\|\mathbf{r} - \mathbf{r}'\|^2 / 2\sigma^2), \\ \mathbf{r}'(\mathbf{v}, \{\Phi(\mathbf{r})\}) &= \min_{\mathbf{r}} d(\mathbf{v}, \Phi(\mathbf{r})) \end{aligned} \quad (5.13)$$

where $d(\cdot, \cdot)$ denotes the Euclidean distance.

A "high-dimensional" variant of the self-organizing map involves synaptic weights $\Phi(\mathbf{r}) = \{w_1(\mathbf{r}), w_2(\mathbf{r}), \ldots, w_N(\mathbf{r})\}$. In this model equation 5.12 is modified to

$$\Phi_{t+1}(\mathbf{r}) = \frac{\Phi_t(\mathbf{r}) + \alpha h_{\text{SOM}}(\mathbf{r}, \mathbf{r}') \mathbf{v}_{t+1}}{\|\Phi_t(\mathbf{r}) + \alpha h_{\text{SOM}}(\mathbf{r}, \mathbf{r}') \mathbf{v}_{t+1}\|}, \qquad 0 < \alpha < 1 \quad (5.14)$$

with the distance function in equation 5.13 replaced by $d(\mathbf{v}, \Phi) = 1 - \mathbf{v} \cdot \Phi$.

5.4.2 The Elastic-Net Model. The elastic-net algorithm (Durbin and Mitchison 1990; Durbin and Willshaw 1987) is an iterative procedure with the update rule:

$$\begin{aligned} \Phi_{t+1}(\mathbf{r}) &= \Phi_t(\mathbf{r}) + \alpha h_{\text{EN}}(\mathbf{r}, \mathbf{v}_{t+1})[\mathbf{v}_{t+1} - \Phi_t(\mathbf{r})] \\ &+ \sum_{\|\mathbf{r}'-\mathbf{r}\|=1} \beta [\Phi_t(\mathbf{r}') - \Phi_t(\mathbf{r})] \end{aligned} \quad (5.15)$$

with

$$h_{\text{EN}}(\mathbf{r}, \mathbf{v}_{t+1}) = \exp\{-d[\mathbf{v}_{t+1}, \Phi(\mathbf{r})]^2 / 2\sigma^2\} / \sum_{\mathbf{r}'} h_{\text{EN}}(\mathbf{r}, \mathbf{v}_{t+1}) \quad (5.16)$$

$d(\cdot, \cdot)$ is Euclidean distance. At each iteration, a stimulus **v** is chosen at random according to a given probability distribution $P(\mathbf{v})$.

We have extended previous modeling studies (Durbin and Mitchison 1990; Goodhill and Willshaw 1990) to include five-dimensional feature vectors $\Phi = \{x, y, q\sin(2\phi), q\cos(2\phi), z\}$. The extended model correctly predicts some of the correlations between the orientation and ocular dominance maps (Fig. 11).

Acknowledgments

This research has been supported by NSF (Grant 91-22522) and NIH (Grant P41RRO5969). Computer time on a CM-2 and a CM-5 was provided by the National Center for Supercomputing Applications, funded by NSF. Financial Support to E.E. by the Beckman Institute and to K.O. by ZiF (Universität Bielefeld) is gratefully acknowledged. We deeply appreciate model data supplied by R. Linsker, described in Linsker (1986c), and S. Tanaka (unpublished data). We thank K. Miller, E. Niebur, and A. Yuille for useful comments and discussions, and J. Malpeli for comments on the manuscript.

References

Adelson, E. H., and Bergen, J. R. 1985. Spatiotemporal energy models for the perception of motion. *J. Opt. Soc. Am. A* **2**, 284–299.

Andersen, P., Olavarria, J., and van Sluyters, R. C. 1988. The overall pattern of ocular dominance bands in cat visual cortex. *J. Neurosci.* **8**, 2183–2200.

Barrow, H. G., and Bray, A. J. 1992a. Activity-induced "colour blob" formation. In *Artificial Neural Networks II: Proceedings of the International Conference on Artificial Neural Networks*, I. Aleksander and J. Taylor, eds. Elsevier, Amsterdam.

Barrow, H. G., and Bray, A. J. 1992b. A model of adaptive development of complex cortical cells. In *Artificial Neural Networks II: Proceedings of the International Conference on Artificial Neural Networks*, I. Aleksander and J. Taylor, eds. Elsevier, Amsterdam.

Bartfeld, E., and Grinvald, A. 1992. Relationship between orientation-preference pinwheels, cytochrome oxidase blobs, and ocular dominance columns in primate striate cortex. *Proc. Natl. Acad. Sci. U.S.A.* **89**, 11905–11909.

Bauer, R., and Dow, B. M. 1989. Complementary global maps for orientation coding in upper and lower layers of the monkey's foveal striate cortex. *Exp. Brain Res.* **76**, 503–509.

Bauer, R., and Dow, B. M. 1991. Local and global principles of striate cortical organization: An advanced model. *Biol. Cybern.* **64**, 477–483.

Baxter, W. T., and Dow, B. M. 1989. Horizontal organization of orientation-sensitive cells in primate visual cortex. *Biol. Cybern.* **61**, 171–182.

Berns, G. S., Dayan, P., and Sejnowski, T. J. 1993. A correlational model for the development of disparity selectivity in visual cortex that depends on prenatal and postnatal phases. *Proc. Natl. Acad. Sci. U.S.A.* **90**, 8277–8281.

Blakemore, C., and van Sluyters, R. C. 1975. Innate and environmental factors in the development of the kitten's visual cortex. *J. Physiol. (London)* **248**, 663–716.

Blasdel, G. G. 1992a. Differential imaging of ocular dominance and orientation selectivity in monkey striate cortex. *J. Neurosci.* **12**(8), 3115–3138.

Blasdel, G. G. 1992b. Orientation selectivity, preference and continuity in monkey striate cortex. *J. Neurosci.* **12**(8), 3139–3161.

Blasdel, G. G., and Salama, G. 1986. Voltage sensitive dyes reveal a modular organization in monkey striate cortex. *Nature (London)* **321**, 579–585.

Blasdel, G. G., Livingstone, M., and Hubel, D. 1993. Optical imaging of orientation and binocularity in visual areas 1 and 2 of squirrel monkey (Samiri sciureus) cortex. *Soc. Neurosci. Abstr.* **19**, 1500.

Blasdel, G. G., Obermayer, K., and Kiorpes, L. 1994. Organization of ocular dominance and orientation columns in the striate cortex of neonatal macaque monkeys. *Vis. Neurosci.*, in press.

Bonhoeffer, T., Kim, D., and Singer, W. 1993. Optical imaging of the reverse suture effect in kitten visual cortex during the critical period. *Soc. Neurosci. Abstr.* **19**, 1800.

Braitenberg, V. 1985. An isotropic network which implicitly defines orientation columns: Discussion of an hypothesis. In *Models of the Visual Cortex*, D. Rose and V. G. Dobson, eds., pp. 479–484. John Wiley, New York.

Braitenberg, V., and Braitenberg, C. 1979. Geometry of orientation columns in the visual cortex. *Biol. Cybern.* **33**, 179–186.

Diao, Y.-C., Jia, W. G., Swindale, N. V., and Cynader, M. S. 1990. Functional organization of the cortical 17/18 border region in the cat. *Exp. Brain Res.* **79**, 271–282.

Dow, B. W., and Bauer, R. 1984. Retinotopy and orientation columns in the monkey: A new model. *Biol. Cybern.* **49**, 189–200.

Durbin, R., and Mitchison, G. 1990. A dimension reduction framework for understanding cortical maps. *Nature (London)* **343**, 341–344.

Durbin, R., and Willshaw, D. 1987. An analogue approach to the traveling salesman problem using an elastic net method. *Nature (London)* **326**, 689–691.

Emerson, R. C., Bergen, J. R., and Adelson, E. H. 1992. Directionally selective complex cells and the computation of motion energy in cat visual cortex. *Vision Res.* **32**(2), 203–218.

Erwin, E., Obermayer, K., and Schulten, K. 1993. A comparison of models of visual cortical map formation. In *Computation and Neural Systems*, F. H. Eeckman and J. M. Bower, eds., ch. 60, pp. 395–402. Kluwer Academic Publishers, Dordrecht.

Finlay, B. L., Schiller, P. H., and Volman, S. F. 1976. Meridional differences in orientation sensitivity in monkey striate cortex. *Brain Res.* **105**, 350–352.

Florence, S. L., and Kaas, J. H. 1992. Ocular dominance columns in area 17 of

Old World macaque and talapoin monkeys: Complete reconstructions and quantitative analyses. *Vis. Neurosci.* **8**, 449–462.

Goodhill, G. J. 1992. Correlations, competition, and optimality: Modelling the development of topography and ocular dominance. Ph.D. thesis, University of Sussex at Brighton.

Goodhill, G. J. 1993. Topography and ocular dominance: A model exploring positive correlations. *Biol. Cybern.* **69**, 109–118.

Goodhill, G. J., and Willshaw, D. J. 1990. Application of the elastic net algorithm to the formation of ocular dominance stripes. *Network* **1**, 41–59.

Goodman, C., and Shatz, C. 1993. Developmental mechanisms that generate precise patterns of neuronal connectivity. *Cell* **72**, 77–89.

Götz, K. G. 1987. Do "d-blob" and "l-blob" hypercolumns tessellate the monkey visual cortex? *Biol. Cybern.* **56**, 107–109.

Götz, K. G. 1988. Cortical templates for the self-organization of orientation-specific d- and l-hypercolumns in monkeys and cats. *Biol. Cybern.* **58**, 213–223.

Grinvald, A., Lieke, E., Frostig, R. P., Gilbert, C., and Wiesel, T. 1986. Functional architecture of cortex revealed by optical imaging of intrinsic signals. *Nature (London)* **324**, 351–354.

Hubel, D., and Wiesel, T. N. 1962. Receptive fields, binocular interaction and functional architecture in the cat's striate cortex. *J. Physiol. (London)* **160**, 106–154.

Hubel, D. H., and Wiesel, T. N. 1968. Receptive fields and functional architecture of monkey striate cortex. *J. Physiol.* **195**, 215–243.

Hubel, D., and Wiesel, T. N. 1974. Sequence regularity and geometry of orientation columns in monkey striate cortex. *J. Comp. Neurol.* **158**, 267–293.

Hubel, D., and Wiesel, T. N. 1977. Functional architecture of monkey striate cortex. *Proc. Roy. Soc. London B* **198**, 1–59.

Hubel, D., Wiesel, T. N., and LeVay, S. 1977. Plasticity of ocular dominance columns in monkey striate cortex. *Phil. Trans. Roy. Soc. Lond. B* **278**, 377–409.

Hubel, D., Wiesel, T. N., and Stryker, M. 1978. Anatomical demonstration of orientation columns in macaque monkey. *J. Comp. Neurol.* **177**, 361–380.

Jones, D. G., van Sluyters, R. C., and Murphy, K. M. 1991. A computational model for the overall pattern of ocular dominance. *J. Neurosci.* **11**(12), 3794–3808.

Kim, D., and Bonhoeffer, T. 1993. Chronical observation of the emergence of iso-orientation domains in kitten visual cortex. *Soc. Neurosci. Abstr.* **19**, 1800.

Kohonen, T. 1982a. Analysis of a simple self-organizing process. *Biol. Cybern.* **44**, 135–140.

Kohonen, T. 1982b. Self-organized formation of topologically correct feature maps. *Biol. Cybern.* **43**, 59–69.

Kohonen, T. 1987. *Self-Organization and Associative Memory.* Springer-Verlag, New York.

Lehky, S. R., Sejnowski, T. J., and Desimone, R. 1992. Predicting responses of nonlinear neurons in monkey striate cortex to complex patterns. *J. Neurosci.* **12**(9), 3568–3581.

LeVay, S., and Nelson, S. B. 1991. The columnar organization of visual cortex.

In *The Electrophysiology of Vision*, A. Leventhal, ed., pp. 15–34. Macmillan, London.

Linsker, R. 1986a. From basic network principles to neural architecture: Emergence of spatial opponent cells. *Proc. Natl. Acad. Sci. U.S.A.* **83**, 7508–7512.

Linsker, R. 1986b. From basic network principles to neural architecture: Emergence of orientation selective cells. *Proc. Natl. Acad. Sci. U.S.A.* **83**, 8390–8394.

Linsker, R. 1986c. From basic network principles to neural architecture: Emergence of orientation columns. *Proc. Natl. Acad. Sci. U.S.A.* **83**, 8779–8783.

Livingstone, M., and Hubel, D. 1984. Anatomy and physiology of a color system in the primate visual cortex. *J. Neurosci.* **4**, 309–356.

Löwel, S., and Singer, W. 1993. Strabismus changes the spacing of ocular dominance columns in the visual cortex of cats. *Soc. Neurosci. Abstr.* **19**, 359.2.

Miller, K. D. 1990. Correlation based models of neural development. In *Neuroscience and Connectionst Theory*, M. Gluck and D. Rumelhart, eds., pp. 267–354. Lawrence Erlbaum, Hillsdale, NJ.

Miller, K. D. 1992. Development of orientation columns via competition between on- and off-center inputs. *NeuroReport* **3**, 73–76.

Miller, K. D. 1994. A model for the development of simple cell receptive fields and the ordered arrangement of orientation columns through activity-dependent competition between on- and off-center inputs. *J. Neurosci.* **14**, 409–441.

Miller, K. D., Keller, J. B., and Stryker, M. P. 1989. Ocular dominance column development: Analysis and simulation. *Science* **245**, 605–615.

Miyashita, M., and Tanaka, S. 1992. A mathematical model for the self-organization of orientation columns in visual cortex. *NeuroReport* **3**(1), 69–72.

Niebur, E., and Wörgötter, F. 1993. Orientation columns from first principles. In *Computation and Neural Systems*, F. H. Eeckman and J. M. Bower, eds., ch. 62, pp. 409–413. Kluwer Academic Publishers, Dordrecht.

Obermayer, K. 1993. *Adaptive Neuronale Netze und ihre Anwendung als Modelle der Entwicklung Kortikaler Karten*. Infix–Verlag, St. Augustin.

Obermayer, K., and Blasdel, G. G. 1993. Geometry of orientation and ocular dominance columns in monkey striate cortex. *J. Neurosci.* **13**, 4114–4129.

Obermayer, K., Ritter, H., and Schulten, K. 1990. A principle for the formation of the spatial structure of cortical feature maps. *Proc. Natl. Acad. Sci. U.S.A.* **87**, 8345–8349.

Obermayer, K., Ritter, H., and Schulten, K. 1992a. A model for the development of the spatial structure of retinotopic maps and orientation columns. *IEICE Trans. Fund. Electr. Comm. Comp. Sci.* **E75-A**(5), 537–545.

Obermayer, K., Schulten, K., and Blasdel, G. G. 1992b. A comparison between a neural network model for the formation of brain maps and experimental data. In *Advances in Neural Information Processing Systems 4*, D. S. Touretzky and R. Lippman, eds., pp. 83–90. Morgan Kaufmann, San Mateo, CA.

Obermayer, K., Blasdel, G. G., and Schulten, K. 1992c. Statistical mechanical analysis of self-organization and pattern formation during the development of visual maps. *Phys. Rev. A* **45**(10), 7568–7589.

Obermayer, K., Kiorpes, L., and Blasdel, G. G. 1994. Development of orientation and ocular dominance columns in infant macaques. In *Advances in Neural Information Processing Systems 6*, J. D. Cowan, G. Tesauro, and J. Alspector, eds., pp. 543–550. Morgan Kaufmann, San Mateo, CA.

Poggio, G. F., Doty, R. W., Jr., and Talbot, W. H. 1977. Foveal striate cortex of behaving monkey single neuron responses to square wave gratings during fixation of gaze. *J. Neurophysiol.* **40**(6), 1369–1391.

Rauschecker, J. 1991. Mechanisms of visual plasticity: Hebb synapses, NMDA receptors, and beyond. *Physiol. Rev.* **71**, 587–615.

Reggia, J., D'Autrechy, C. L., Sutton, G., and Weinrich, M. 1992. A competitive distribution theory of neocortical dynamics. *Neural Comp.* **4**, 287–317.

Rojer, A. S., and Schwartz, E. L. 1990. Cat and monkey cortical columnar patterns modeled by bandpass-filtered 2d white noise. *Biol. Cybern.* **62**, 381–391.

Sirosh, J., and Miikkulainen, R. 1994. Cooperative self-organization of afferent and lateral connections in cortical maps. *Biol. Cybern.* **71**, 66–78.

Stryker, M. P., Sherk, H., Leventhal, A. G., and Hirsch, H. V. B. 1978. Physiological consequences for the cat's visual cortex of effectively restricting early visual experience with oriented contours. *J. Neurophysiol.* **41**, 896–909.

Swindale, N. V. 1980. A model for the formation of ocular dominance stripes. *Proc. Royal Soc. London B* **208**, 243–264.

Swindale, N. V. 1981. Rules for pattern formation in mammalian visual cortex. *Trends Neurosci.* **4**, 102–104.

Swindale, N. V. 1982. A model for the formation of orientation columns. *Proc. Royal Soc. London B* **215**, 211–230.

Swindale, N. V. 1991. Coverage and the design of striate cortex. *Biol. Cybern.* **65**, 415–424.

Swindale, N. V. 1992. A model for the coordinated development of columnar systems in primate striate cortex. *Biol. Cybern.* **66**, 217–230.

Swindale, N. V., Matsubara, J. A., and Cynader, M. S. 1987. Surface organization of orientation and direction selectivity in cat area 18. *J. Neurosci.* **7**, 1414–1427.

Tanaka, S. 1991a. Information among ocularity, retinotopy and on-/off-center pathways. In *Advances in Neural Information Processing Systems 3*, R. P. Lippman *et al.*, eds., pp. 18–25. Morgan Kaufmann, San Mateo, CA.

Tanaka, S. 1991b. Phase transition theory for abnormal ocular dominance column formation. *Biol. Cybern.* **65**, 91–98.

Tanaka, S. 1991c. Theory of ocular dominance column formation: Mathematical basis and computer simulation. *Biol. Cybern.* **64**, 263–272.

Tootell, R. B. H., *et al.* 1988. Functional-anatomy of macaque striate cortex. (series). *J. Neurosci.* **8**(5), 1500–1624.

Ts'o, D. Y., Frostig, R. D., Lieke, E. E., and Grinvald, A. 1990. Functional organization of primate visual cortex revealed by high resolution optical imaging. *Science* **249**, 417–420.

Yuille, A. L., Kammen, D. M., and Cohen, D. S. 1989. Quadrature and the development of orientation selective cortical cells by Hebb rules. *Biol. Cybern.* **61**, 183–194.

Yuille, A. L., Kolodny, J. A., and Lee, C. W. 1991. *Dimension reduction, generalized deformable models and the development of ocularity and orientation.* Tech. Rep. 91-3, Harvard Robotics Laboratory.

9

Development of Oriented Ocular Dominance Bands as a Consequence of Areal Geometry

H.-U. Bauer
Institut für Theoretische Physik and SFB "Nichtlineare Dynamik,"
Universität Frankfurt, Robert-Mayer-Str. 8-10,
60054 Frankfurt, Germany

It has been hypothesized that the different appearance of ocular dominance bands in the cat and the monkey is a consequence of the different mapping geometries in these species (LeVay *et al.* 1985; Anderson *et al.* 1988). Here I investigate the impact of areal geometries on the preferred direction of ocular dominance bands in two adaptive map formation models, the self-organizing feature map and the elastic net algorithm. In the case of the self-organizing feature map, the occurrence of instabilities that correspond to ocular dominance bands can be analytically investigated. The instabilities automatically yield stripes of correct orientation. These analytic results are complemented by simulations. In the case of the elastic net algorithm, simulations reveal two different parameter regimes of the algorithm, only one of which leads to stripes of correct orientation. The results suggest that neighborhood preservation in visual maps is enforced in the backward direction, such that neighboring cells in the cortex have neighboring receptive fields, and not vice versa.

1 Introduction

Maps constitute an important organizing principle in the brain. They can be generated or refined under the influence of external stimulation. As an example for the self-organization of maps, the formation of ocular dominance (OD) columns has often been investigated. A range of models has been developed in the last few years (von der Malsburg 1979; Swindale 1980; Miller *et al.* 1989; Goodhill 1993). Two more recent models are based on Kohonen's self-organizing feature map algorithm (Obermayer *et al.* 1992) and on the elastic net algorithm (Goodhill and Willshaw 1990).

To differentiate between all these models, and between parameter regimes within the models, it is helpful to consider additional features of the desired maps, beyond the occurrence of interleaved ocular dominance bands. Particularly interesting in this regard are qualitative features that do not require high precision quantitative fits. One example for such a qualitative feature is the different appearance of the ocular dominance systems in the striate cortex of the cat and the monkey. In the cat the OD stripes appear irregularly branched, and do not seem to have a preferred direction (Anderson *et al.* 1988). In the monkey the OD bands appear as a series of parallel stripes, which run perpendicular to the representation of the horizontal meridian (LeVay *et al.* 1985). The pattern is reminiscient of a zebra (Swindale 1980). The preferred orientation is parallel to the short semi-axis of the roughly elliptical striate cortex.

Noting that in the monkey the projection from the lateral geniculate nucleus (LGN) to the cortex can roughly be characterized as the map from two circles (for the two eyes) onto an ellipse elongated by a factor of 2:1, LeVay *et al.* hypothezised that the zebra-like pattern is simply a consequence of the geometric boundary conditions, and not of other anisotropies. This idea has been taken up by Jones *et al.* (1991), who investigated mappings from the LGN to the cortex in different animals. These authors contrasted the mentioned geometry in the monkey to that in the cat, which can roughly be described as a map from two ellipses in the LGN onto one ellipse in the cortex, and were able to reproduce the observed difference of the OD patterns by varying the geometric boundary conditions only.

The maps in the latter model were generated by systematic minimization of the cortical distance between the representations of points that are neighboring in the LGN. This procedure yields maps as a consequence of an optimization criterion, but not of a developmental model. It remains to be seen whether standard adaptive map formation algorithms lead to comparable results and if so under what circumstances. Complementing an independent study of this issue by Goodhill and Willshaw (1994) I here investigate the geometry effect on OD stripe formation in a slightly abstracted way. The central idea of the mentioned geometry hypothesis is that the elongation of the map along the different spatial dimensions is twice as long in the one direction as in the other. In comparison, the exact shape of the involved areas (circular, elliptic, etc.) is of minor importance for the hypothesis. Aiming at a model-independent corroboration of the hypothesis, I investigate the impact of different elongation ratios onto the layout of resulting stripe patterns in two standard map formation algorithms, the self-organizing feature map and the elastic net. The self-organizing feature map is interesting in this regard, because the occurrence of instabilities in this model has been analytically characterized (Ritter and Schulten 1988; Obermayer *et al.* 1992). As I will show in the next section and in the appendix, this analysis can be utilized to derive results in the present context, provided that the stable solutions are translationally invariant. We will therefore consider in the following squares and rectangles with periodic boundary conditions instead of the roughly circular or elliptic shapes of the LGN and the visual areas. Identical elongation ratios in both spatial directions will be called isotropic geometric boundary conditions, and differing elongation ratios will be called anisotropic boundary conditions.

The self-organizing feature map has just one intrinsic length scale, the width σ of the cortical neighborhood function. In contrast, the elastic net algorithm (Durbin and Willshaw 1987) has two length scales: the diameter of the receptive fields, k, and the width of a topology term, which is related to the cortical interaction. Depending on the relation between the two scales, qualitatively different solutions for the OD bands result, as will be shown in the third section. The consequences of these differences for the formation of ODC stripes under anisotropic conditions are described in the fourth section. A discussion of the results and their relation to other work concludes the paper.

2 Formation of OD Stripes in the Self-Organizing Feature Map

I will describe Kohonen's self-organizing feature map algorithm only very briefly and refer the reader to other publications for a more thorough treatment (Kohonen 1989; Ritter *et al.* 1990). Stimuli $\mathbf{v}$ in an input space V are mapped onto neurons located on the vertices $\mathbf{r}$ of a grid in an output space A. Each neuron has associated to it a receptive field in the input space, which is characterized by its receptive field center $\mathbf{w_r}(\in V)$. The stimulus $\mathbf{v}$ is mapped in a winner-take-all fashion onto that neuron $\mathbf{r}$ that has its receptive field center $\mathbf{w_r}$ closest to $\mathbf{v}$:

$$\mathbf{v} \to \mathbf{r}: \quad \|\mathbf{w_r} - \mathbf{v}\| = \min_{\mathbf{r}' \in A} \|\mathbf{w_{r'}} - \mathbf{v}\| \tag{2.1}$$

The map is adapted by successive application of stimuli $\mathbf{v}$, and by shifting the receptive field center of the winning neuron $\mathbf{r}$ as well as those of its neighbors $\mathbf{r}'$ toward the stimuli,

$$\delta \mathbf{w_{r'}} = \epsilon h_{\mathbf{r},\mathbf{r}'} (\mathbf{v} - \mathbf{w_r}) \tag{2.2}$$

The neighborhood function $h_{\mathbf{r},\mathbf{r}'}$ usually takes gaussian form and is characterized by a length scale σ,

$$h_{\mathbf{r},\mathbf{r}'} = \exp -\frac{(\mathbf{r} - \mathbf{r}')^2}{2\sigma^2} \tag{2.3}$$

No interesting structure emerges for maps from input to output spaces with equal dimensionality and matching dimensions, e.g., mapping a square onto a square. However, if the input space has an additional dimension, with a small width $2s$ (like a pizza box), then the map can exhibit nontrivial structure in the third dimension. For the map of stimuli in a $1 \times 1 \times 2s$ input space ($s \ll 1$) onto positions in an $N \times N$ output space, Ritter and Schulten derived a critical width s^* for the first occurrence of such structure (Ritter and Schulten 1988),

$$s^* = \frac{\sigma}{N}\sqrt{3e/2} \approx 2.02\frac{\sigma}{N} \tag{2.4}$$

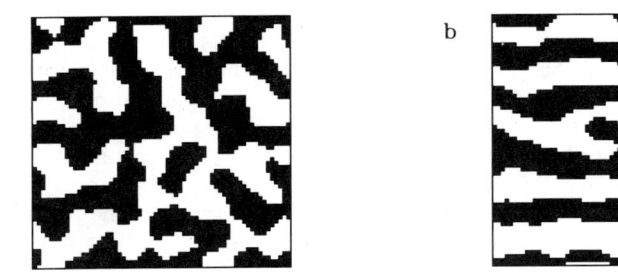

Figure 1: OD bands generated by the self-organizing feature map for the case of isotropic elongations (64 × 64, a), and anisotropic elongations (32 × 64, b). The stimuli (x, y, z) were evenly distributed in $0 < x, y < 1$, $-s < z < s$. In the above figures neurons with $w_z > 0$ are displayed in black, neurons with $w_z < 0$ in white. Simulations parameters were $\sigma = 2$, $s = 0.1$, $\epsilon = 0.2$, 10,000 steps, initialization retinotopic in x, y-direction, random in z-direction, periodic boundaries in x- and y-direction.

Identifying the two large dimensions with the retinal coordinates and the small dimensions with orientation, orientation specificity, and ocularity, this effect has been utilized by Obermayer *et al.* for the investigation of orientation columns and OD bands in cortical maps (Obermayer *et al.* 1990, 1992). Here, I do not consider orientation dimensions and restrict myself to maps with just a single additional dimension, which corresponds to ocular dominance. An example for OD bands which emerge under isotropic boundary conditions is displayed in Figure 1a. They have no preferred orientation, in agreement with the observations for the cat cortex.

Following Ritter and Schulten's derivation for the critical width one can also analyze the occurrence of instabilities in an elongated output space of dimensions $2N \times N$ (see appendix). The occurrence of the instability is finally characterized by the expectation value

$$\left\langle u_3(\mathbf{k})^2 \right\rangle = \frac{\epsilon \pi \sigma^2}{2} \frac{s^2 e^{-k^2 \sigma^2 / 2N^2}}{3 - s^2(4k_x^2 + k_y^2)e^{-k^2\sigma^2/2N^2}} \quad (2.5)$$

for the amplitude of Fourier modes of the map fluctuations (k_x, k_y denote the wave vectors of the relevant modes in the x- and y-direction). For increasing s, the mode amplitude diverges for the first time for a mode oriented purely along the x-direction, at a critical width

$$s_1^* = \frac{\sigma}{N}\sqrt{3e/8} = \frac{\sigma}{2N}\sqrt{3e/2} \approx 1.01\frac{\sigma}{N} \quad (2.6)$$

Ocular Dominance Bands

With increasing values of s, modes with $k_y \neq 0$ also become unstable. Modes that are oriented purely in the y-direction become unstable only at values of s above a value s_2^*, which is identical to the critical thickness of the $N \times N$-system,

$$s_2^* = \frac{\sigma}{N}\sqrt{3e/2} \approx 2.02\frac{\sigma}{N} \tag{2.7}$$

These results show that in the self-organizing feature map different elongation ratios of the map along different directions can indeed induce oriented stripes. For values of s that exceed the critical value s_1^* only slightly, the wave vectors of the unstable modes have only small components along the y-direction. Consequently the stripe patterns run roughly parallel to the shorter dimension, in agreement with the observations in the monkey cortex. Results of simulations that underline this analysis are shown in Figure 1b. Additional simulations with $s > s_2^*$ reveal that even in a parameter regime where modes in all directions are unstable the stripes are predominantly oriented parallel to the shorter dimension, analogous to Figure 1b. Thus I can conclude this section by noting that the self-organizing feature map exhibits geometry effects in the formation of OD bands that resemble closely the geometry effects hypothesized for the cat and the monkey.

3 Discretization Dependence of OD Stripes in the Elastic Net

The elastic net algorithm (Durbin and Willshaw 1987) is a different map formation algorithm that has been applied in the context of orientation (Durbin and Mitchison 1990) and ocular dominance column formation (Goodhill and Willshaw 1990). As in the self-organizing feature map, the algorithm involves neuron elements in an output space A, located at the vertices $\mathbf{r}$ of a grid, which have receptive field centers at positions $\mathbf{w_r}$ in the input space. Here the receptive fields have gaussian shape with width k. A stimulus $\mathbf{v}$ results in an excitation peak, where each neuron participates according to the value of its receptive field at $\mathbf{v}$, i.e., according to $\exp[-(\mathbf{w_r} - \mathbf{v})^2/2k^2]$, with the value of the overall excitation normalized to unity. This is in contrast to the self-organizing feature map, where only the best-matching neuron is excited, with no regard of receptive field forms. The receptive field centers are then adapted toward the stimulus and also toward the receptive field centers of the respective neighbors,

$$\delta\mathbf{w_r} = \alpha\frac{a_\mathbf{r}}{\sum_{\mathbf{r'} \in A} a_{\mathbf{r'}}}(\mathbf{v} - \mathbf{w_r}) + \beta k \sum_{\mathbf{r'} \in N_\mathbf{r}}(\mathbf{w'_r} - \mathbf{w_r}) \tag{3.1}$$

$$a_\mathbf{r} = e^{-((\mathbf{w_r}-\mathbf{v})^2/2k^2)} \tag{3.2}$$

where $N_\mathbf{r}$ is the set of the nearest neighbors of $\mathbf{r}$ in the output space.

In several contributions energy functions and optimization properties in the elastic net have been investigated (Simic 1990; Yuille 1990; Dayan 1993). Here I focus on a different issue. One length scale in the elastic net is given by the width of the receptive fields k. This length scale has no analog in the self-organizing feature map, where the winner-take-all mechanism could best be identified with the limit $k \to 0$. A second length scale is given in an indirect way via the discretization of the output space, which enters the second term, the topology term, on the right-hand side of equation 3.1. Considering the overall retinotopy of the map, the distance 1 between nearest neighbors in the cortex can be transformed into a corresponding distance $d \approx 1/N$ in the input space, where N denotes the discretization of the cortical area.

Let us now turn to the formation of ocular dominance bands. As in the simulations for the self-organizing feature map, and in analogy to the method used by Durbin and Mitchison (1990) I chose random stimuli $\mathbf{v}$ with $0 < v_x < 1$, $0 < v_y < 1$, $v_z = \pm s$, $s \ll 1$, and map these onto an $N \times N$ grid of neurons in the output space. To have control over the length scales involved in the problem, I keep k constant throughout the simulations. If k is chosen small enough, $k < k_{\text{crit}}(s)$, the resulting map exhibits structure in the third dimension. Analogously to the simulations by Goodhill and Willshaw (1990) for the one-dimensional case I find k_{crit} to vary linearly with s in a wide range; this allows us to choose k in a wide range by choosing s appropriately.

The two length scales k and d in the model allow us to investigate two different regimes. In the first regime $k \gg d$, the size and shape of the region of neurons reached by a stimulus through direct excitation plus the nearest neighbor interaction due to the topology term are dominated by the width of the receptive fields k (Fig. 2a). The results of simulated maps in this regime are displayed in Figure 3a–d. The maps differ in the discretization of the output space and, consequently, in the value of the parameter d (a: $d = 0.0156$, b: $d = 0.0312$, c: $d = 0.0625$). Since I expect k to be a decisive parameter in the model and want to compare results for different values of k later on, k was kept at a fixed value during the course of each simulation (here: $k = 0.1$ in all three cases). Comparison of Figure 3a,b,c shows that the discretization has no impact on the overall shape of the OD bands in this regime. This is also indicated by the maxima of the power spectra (Fig. 3d), which are subsequently shifted toward smaller values, with approximately a factor of 2 between successive maxima.

In the opposite case ($k \ll d$, Fig. 2b), the size and shape of the region effectively reached by the direct stimulation plus the neighborhood interaction should be dominated by d. Since d is proportional to the discretization of the cortical area, I now expect different discretizations to result in different OD stripes. Figure 3e–h shows simulations for this parameter regime. Indeed the resulting bands become finer if the dis-

Ocular Dominance Bands

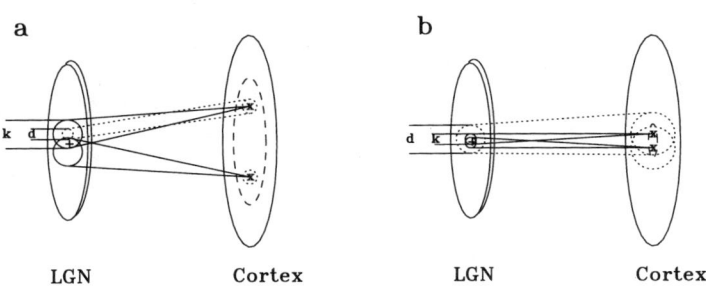

Figure 2: Illustrations for the relation between the width of receptive fields k and the width d resulting from the topology term. In both figures the cross (+) in the LGN denotes a stimulus, which is mapped onto two example neurons in the cortex (x-signs). The receptive fields of these neurons in the LGN are shown as cones with width k. The regions of all neurons in the cortex whose receptive fields contain the stimulus are indicated as dashed ellipses. The cortical interaction, manifest in the topology term of the elastic net rule, influences nearest neighbor neurons of the example neurons. The size of this nearest neighbor region is indicated by the dotted circles around the example neurons, and by the projection of this region back to the LGN (dotted circle in the LGN, diameter d). Depending on the size relation between k and d, two regimes can be identified. If the receptive field width k is large compared to d, many neurons in the cortex are directly excited by the stimulus. Including those nearest neighbor neurons that are reached by virtue of the topology term, the overall region of neurons effectively reached by the stimulus is only slightly changed as compared to the direct excitation region (a). If d is large compared to k, only a few neurons are directly excited by the stimulus. Addition of their nearest neighbors substantially alters the region of effective stimulation (b).

cretization is increased (i.e., the bands are of equal size with regard to the number of neurons across one band).

4 Anisotropic Geometry and OD Stripes in the Elastic Net

What are the consequences of the two parameter regimes for the formation of OD bands in an anisotropic geometry?

When the OD structure is independent of the discretization in the output space, different discretizations along the two directions do not alter the appearance of the stripe structure. Consequently, in an anisotropic

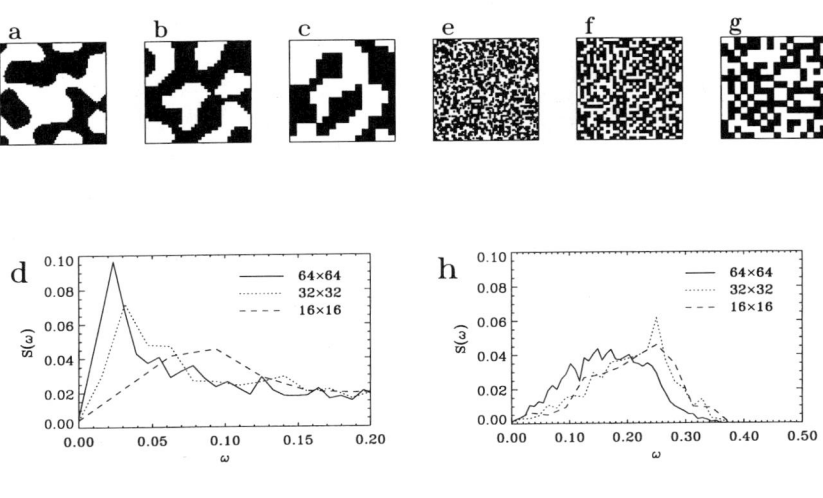

Figure 3: OD bands in elastic net maps of different discretization: 64×64 in a,e, 32×32 in b,f, 16×16 in c,g. d shows power spectra of the OD bands of a–c, averaged of five maps per spectrum, h the same for the maps of e–g. $\omega = 1/2$ corresponds to maximum frequency bands that alter the sign at every neuron across the output space. For all maps the stimuli **v** were randomly chosen with $0 < v_x, v_y < 1$, $v_z = \pm s$. a–d have $s = 0.2$ and $k = 0.1$, corresponding to the $k > d$ regime, e–h have $s = 0.025$ and $k = 0.01$, i.e., $k < d$. Other simulation parameters were $\alpha = 6.4$, $\beta = 0.001$ (a), $\alpha = 1.6$, $\beta = 0.001$ (b), $\alpha = 0.4$, $\beta = 0.001$ (c), $\alpha = 0.64$, $\beta = 0.001$ (e), $\alpha = 0.4$, $\beta = 0.001$ (f), $\alpha = 0.4$, $\beta = 0.001$ (g). Initialization is retinotopic in x, y-direction, random in z-direction, periodic boundary conditions: a–c, 4000 steps; e–g, 10,000 steps.

output space geometry with identical discretization length constants along the two directions, the OD bands appear elongated by the factor of the anisotropy along the longer dimension (Fig. 4a–d). Thus in this regime the elastic net produces OD bands with a preferred direction perpendicular to that observed in the monkey.

In the opposite case, with $d > k$, the simulations show stripes that have a preferred direction parallel to the shorter dimension (Fig. 4e–h). This case has already been described by Goodhill, using a different simulation procedure (Goodhill 1992; Goodhill and Willshaw 1994). In this latter regime, the stripe orientation coincides with that observed in the monkey and reproduced by the self-organizing feature map.

Ocular Dominance Bands

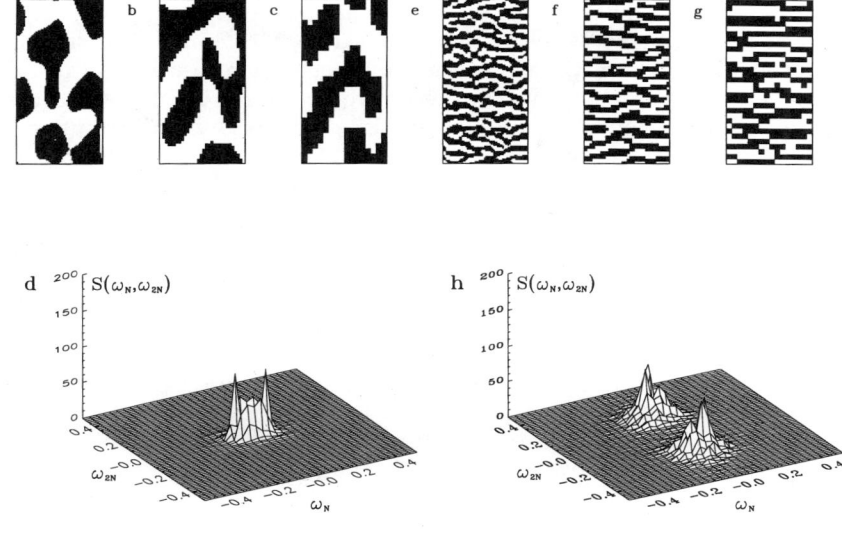

Figure 4: OD bands in elastic net maps from a square input space onto rectangular output spaces: 128×64 in a,e, 64×32 in b,f, 32×16 in c,g. a–c correspond to the $k > d$ regime ($s = 0.2$, $k = 0.1$), e–g to the $k < d$ regime ($s = 0.025$, $k = 0.01$). In the first case the stripes appear elongated along the longer dimension. In the second case they run parallel to the shorter dimension. The preferred orientation of the stripes for the respective cases is also manifest in the shape of the power spectra in d and h (d averaged over 5 nets with parameters as in b, h averaged over 5 nets as in f). Other simulation parameters were $\alpha = 6.4$, $\beta = 0.001$ (a), $\alpha = 1.6$, $\beta = 0.001$ (b), $\alpha = 0.4$, $\beta = 0.001$ (c), $\alpha = 0.64$, $\beta = 0.01$ (e), $\alpha = 0.4$, $\beta = 0.01$ (f), $\alpha = 0.4$, $\beta = 0.01$ (g); a–c, 4000 steps; e–g, 50,000 steps.

5 Discussion

Complementing previous results by Jones *et al.* (1991) and Goodhill *et al.* (1994) about the impact of geometry on the layout of OD stripes, my results show that not only the elastic net algorithm, but also the self-organizing feature map is able to generate oriented OD bands as a consequence of anisotropic geometric boundary conditions. For the self-organizing feature map, this effect is analytically substantiated. In contrast, my simulations for the elastic net revealed two parameter regimes for this algorithm, only one of which yields bands oriented in the correct direction. In this latter regime the width d of a topology term in the update rule exceeds the width k of receptive fields. The topology term reflects the consequences of an intracortical interaction. If the length scales k and d are to be compared with length scales of the self-organizing feature map, one has to note that here a stimulus excites only one output node in a winner-take-all fashion. Even though receptive field sizes do not explicitly occur, the winner-take-all mechanism can be regarded as implementing the limit of small receptive field sizes k. The intracortical interaction is assumed to yield a gaussian-shaped activity distribution of width σ around the best-matching neuron. Therefore, the self-organizing feature map automatically operates in a regime analogous to the $k < d$ regime of the elastic net. Thus it is no surprise that the stripe orientations in these two cases coincide.

In the present contribution I regarded the geometry hypothesis as essentially an assertion that the elongation ratios in the two spatial directions differ. Formulated in this way, the hypothesis does not depend on the particular shapes of the areas involved. A model using square or rectangular layout as well as periodic boundary conditions suffices to analytically or numerically test this hypothesis. In such a model, the target area must not necessarily represent the whole cortical area, but can represent just a fraction of it. My results show that differing elongation ratios suffice to produce the oriented stripes. Possible effects of secondary geometry effects, like open boundary conditions, are not considered here. Even though an interaction between the boundary and OD stripes close to the boundary is conceivable, these surface effects would not dominate the overall appearance of the stripes in the interior of the area. Instead, consideration of both boundary effects as well as elongation effects in the rather small systems accessible to computer simulations could pose problems in assigning particular OD stripe arrangements to one or the other origin. For similar reasons, to keep causes and effects separate, I also did not try to reproduce further details of observed OD band systems.

Finally, to conclude the paper, I would like to point out a different aspect of my results. On a more abstract level, the mapping situations considered here can simply be regarded as neighborhood preserving mappings from some m-dimensional input space onto an n-dimensional output space. Neighborhood preservation can be enforced in the forward as well as the backward direction. For the example of retinotopy, neighborhood preservation in the forward direction amounts to having neighboring points on the retina project onto neighboring points in a visual area. In the backward direction it means that neighboring cells in the visual area have neighboring receptive fields in the retina. If the input and output spaces of a map do not coincide in the number of dimensions and in the extensions along them, violations of neighborhood preservation can occur. Using a topographic product, these violations can quantitatively be evaluated (Bauer and Pawelzik 1992). Depending on whether a map formation algorithm enforces neighborhood preservation in the forward or the backward direction, the violations can have a different appearance, even when the mapping geometry is identical.

In the case of OD maps, as considered in the present paper, a violation is induced by the differing input and output space dimensions: $m = 3$, $n = 2$. The self-organizing feature map, which can be regarded as the archetypical algorithm enforcing neighborhood preservation in the backward direction since its only lateral interaction takes place in the target area, correctly reproduces the stripe layout. In the elastic net, the correct orientation of the OD bands in elongated areas depends crucially on the intracortical interaction ($d > k$ regime) that enforces neighboring elements to align their receptive fields in the input space, i.e., which preserves neighborhoods in the backward direction. Thus my results are compatible with the hypothesis put forward already by Durbin and Mitchison (1990) and by Swindale (1982) in the context of the formation of orientation columns, that neighborhood preservation in cortical maps operates in a backward direction. To be not just compatible, but to support this hypothesis, one also has to consider the OD stripe layout resulting from maps that preserve neighborhoods in the forward direction. The elastic net in the $k > d$-regime, where the size of regions of excitation evoked by neighboring points in the LGN exceeds the width of the intracortical interaction, can roughly be identified with such a mapping algorithm. Since my numerical results show wrongly oriented stripes in this regime, I can conclude that the alternative hypothesis of forward preservation is incompatible with the observed stripe layout.

To further clarify this issue, two tracks can be followed. First, one could develop further map formation algorithms that treat neighborhood preservation in a forward and backward direction on an equal footing. With such algorithms one could compare the two alternatives in a simpler way than by interpreting the parameter regimes of the elastic net. Second, one can search for more examples of neighborhood violations in cortical maps. One such example, field discontinuities in the extrastriate areas of cat and monkey visual cortex (Tusa *et al.* 1979; Albus and Beckmann 1980; Allman and Kaas 1974), have recently been reproduced using the self-organizing feature map (Wolf *et al.* 1993, 1994). This example is particularly striking, because here neighborhood violations occur in the forward direction only, not in the backward direction.

Appendix: Instability Condition in an Elongated Output Space

The analysis of instabilities in self-organizing feature maps used in the present paper rests on the availability of the Fokker-Planck equation (Ritter and Schulten 1988),

$$\frac{1}{\epsilon}\partial_t S(\mathbf{u}, t) = \sum_{rmr'n} \frac{\partial}{\partial \mathbf{u}_{rm}} \mathbf{B}_{rmr'n} \mathbf{u}_{r'n} S(\mathbf{u}, t) + \frac{\epsilon}{2} \sum_{rmr'n} \mathbf{D}_{rmr'n} \frac{\partial^2 S(\mathbf{u}, t)}{\partial \mathbf{u}_{rm} \mathbf{u}_{r'n}} \quad (A.1)$$

for the distribution $S(\mathbf{u}, t)$ of states of the map. $\mathbf{u} = \mathbf{w} - \bar{\mathbf{w}}$ denotes the deviation of the overall weight vector $\mathbf{w}$ from its equilibrium value $\bar{w}$, m, n denote the dimensions of the input space, $\mathbf{r}, \mathbf{r}'$ denote positions in the output space. $\mathbf{B}_{rmr'n}$ and $\mathbf{D}_{rmr'n}$ are successively defined as

$$\mathbf{B}_{rmr'n} = \left[\frac{\partial \mathbf{V}_{rm}(\mathbf{w})}{\partial \mathbf{w}_{r'n}}\right]_{\mathbf{w}=\bar{\mathbf{w}}} \quad (A.2)$$

$$\mathbf{V}_{rm}(\mathbf{w}) = \sum_s (\mathbf{w}_{rm} - \bar{\mathbf{v}}_{sm}) h_{rs} \hat{P}_s(\mathbf{w}) \quad (A.3)$$

$$\bar{\mathbf{v}}_r = \frac{1}{\hat{P}_r(\mathbf{w})} \int_{F_r(\mathbf{w})} d\mathbf{v} P(\mathbf{v}) \mathbf{v} \quad (A.4)$$

$$\hat{P}_r(\mathbf{w}) = \int_{F_r(\mathbf{w})} d\mathbf{v} P(\mathbf{v}) \quad (A.5)$$

$$\mathbf{D}_{rmr'n}(\mathbf{w}) = \sum_s h_{rs} h_{r's} \left[(\mathbf{w}_{rm} - \bar{\mathbf{v}}_{sm})(\mathbf{w}_{r'n} - \bar{\mathbf{v}}_{sn})\hat{P}_s(\mathbf{w}) \right.$$
$$\left. + \int_{F_s(\mathbf{w})} d\mathbf{v} P(\mathbf{v})(\mathbf{v}_m \mathbf{v}_n - \bar{\mathbf{v}}_{sm}\bar{\mathbf{v}}_{sn})\right] \quad (A.6)$$

$F_r(\mathbf{w})$ denotes that region of the input space, which has neuron $\mathbf{r}$ as its best-matching neuron. $\hat{P}_r(\mathbf{w})$ is the probability of a stimulus falling into $F_r(\mathbf{w})$, and $\bar{\mathbf{v}}_r$ is the mean of the stimuli in this region. $\mathbf{V}_{rm}(\mathbf{w})$ and $\mathbf{D}_{rmr'n}(\mathbf{w})$ denote the expectation value of a synaptic change in a single learning step $\delta \mathbf{w}_{rm}$ and its correlation $\delta \mathbf{w}_{rm} \delta \mathbf{w}_{r'n}$, respectively.

Assuming translational invariance of the equilibrium solution, the modes of equation A.1 decouple after Fourier transformation. The stability of the individual modes can be discussed in terms of the eigenvalues of two matrices $\hat{\mathbf{B}}$ and $\hat{\mathbf{D}}$ that replace the matrices $\mathbf{B}$ and $\mathbf{D}$ of equation A.1. To compute these eigenvalues, the geometry-dependent variables

$$\mathbf{M} = \frac{1}{2s} \int_{F_r(\bar{\mathbf{w}})} d\mathbf{v} \left(\mathbf{v}\mathbf{v}^T - \bar{\mathbf{v}}_r\bar{\mathbf{v}}_r^T\right) \quad (A.7)$$

$$\mathbf{a}_{rr'} = \frac{\partial \bar{\mathbf{v}}_r(\mathbf{w})}{\partial \mathbf{w}_{r'}} \bigg|_{\bar{\mathbf{w}}} \quad (A.8)$$

$$\mathbf{b}_{rr'} = \frac{1}{\hat{P}_r} \frac{\partial \hat{P}_r(\mathbf{w})}{\partial \mathbf{w}_{r'}} \bigg|_{\bar{\mathbf{w}}} \quad (A.9)$$

have to be evaluated. At this point of the derivation, specifics of the particular mapping problem at hand enter through equations A.7, A.8, and A.9.

In the present geometry, with an input space of dimensions $1 \times 1 \times 2s$ mapping onto an output space of dimensions $2N \times N$, the equilibrium excitation region $F_r(\bar{\mathbf{w}})$ of an output neuron at $\mathbf{r} = (i, j)$ is bounded by

$i/2 < x < (i+1)/2, j < y < j+1, -s < z < s$. Such an excitation region leads to

$$M = \frac{1}{2N} \begin{pmatrix} 1/96 & 0 & 0 \\ 0 & 1/24 & 0 \\ 0 & 0 & s^2/6 \end{pmatrix} \quad \text{(A.10)}$$

$$\mathbf{a_{rr'}} = \frac{1}{N} \begin{pmatrix} 13/24 & 0 & 0 \\ 0 & 5/3 & 0 \\ 0 & 0 & 10s^2/3 \end{pmatrix} \delta_{rr'}$$

$$- \frac{1}{N} \begin{pmatrix} -1/4 & 0 & 0 \\ 0 & 1/3 & 0 \\ 0 & 0 & 4s^2/3 \end{pmatrix} (\delta_{r+e_x,r'} + \delta_{r-e_x,r'})$$

$$- \frac{1}{N} \begin{pmatrix} 1/48 & 0 & 0 \\ 0 & -1/4 & 0 \\ 0 & 0 & s^2/3 \end{pmatrix} (\delta_{r+e_y,r'} + \delta_{r-e_y,r'}) \quad \text{(A.11)}$$

and

$$\mathbf{b_{rr'}} = \sum_{n=\pm e_x} \mathbf{n}(\delta_{r+n,r'} - \delta_{rr'}) + \frac{1}{2} \sum_{n=\pm e_y} \mathbf{n}(\delta_{r+n,r'} - \delta_{rr'}) \quad \text{(A.12)}$$

Using these new terms, we can proceed along Ritter and Schulten's lines and arrive at an expectation value

$$\langle u_3(\mathbf{k})^2 \rangle = \frac{\epsilon \lambda_3^D}{2\lambda_3^B} = \frac{\epsilon \pi \sigma^2}{2} \frac{s^2 e^{-k^2\sigma^2/2N^2}}{3 - s^2(4k_x^2 + k_y^2)e^{-k^2\sigma^2/2N^2}} \quad \text{(A.13)}$$

for modes in the z-direction. As long as $\langle u_3(\mathbf{k})^2 \rangle$ remains positive the mode is stable. However, with increasing s this condition can be violated, and the mode can turn unstable. Equation (A.13) indicates that this happens first for a mode purely in x-direction, at

$$s_1^* = \frac{\sigma}{N}\sqrt{\frac{3e}{8}} = \frac{1}{2}\frac{\sigma}{2N}\sqrt{\frac{3e}{2}} \quad \text{(A.14)}$$

With increasing s, modes with $k_y \neq 0$ also become unstable. However, at any such $s > s_1^*$ the fastest growing mode is the one in x-direction.

Acknowledgments

Helpful discussions with Klaus Pawelzik, Fred Wolf, and Ken Miller are gratefully acknowledged. This work has been supported by the Deutsche Forschungsgemeinschaft through Sonderforschungsbereich 185 "Nichtlineare Dynamik," TP E3.

References

Albus, K., and Beckmann, R. 1980. Second and third visual areas of the cat: Interindividual variability in retinotopic arrangement and cortical location. *J. Physiol.* **299**, 247–276.

Allman, J. M., and Kaas, J. H. 1974. The organization of the second visual area (V2) of the owl monkey: A second order transformation of the visual hemifield. *Brain Res.* **76**, 247–265.

Anderson, P. A., Olavarria, J., and Van Sluyters, R. C. 1988. The overall pattern of ocular dominance bands in cat visual cortex. *J. Neurosci.* **8**, 2183–2200.

Bauer, H.-U., and Pawelzik, K. 1992. Quantifying the neighborhood preservation of self-organizing feature maps. *IEEE Trans. Neural Networks* **3**, 570–580.

Dayan, P. 1993. Arbitrary elastic topologies and ocular dominance. *Neural Comp.* **5**, 392–401.

Durbin, R., and Mitchison, G. 1990. A dimension reduction framework for understanding cortical maps. *Nature (London)* **343**, 644–647.

Durbin, R., and Willshaw, D. 1987. An analogue approach to the travelling salesman problem using an elastic net method. *Nature (London)* **326**, 689–691.

Goodhill, G. 1992. *Correlations, competition and optimality: Modelling the development of topography and ocular dominance.* CSRP 226, University of Sussex, Great Britain.

Goodhill, G. 1993. Topography and ocular dominance: A model exploring positive correlations. *Biol. Cybern.* **69**, 109–118.

Goodhill, G. J., and Willshaw, D. J. 1990. Application of the elastic net algorithm to the formation of ocular dominance stripes. *Network* **1**, 41–59.

Goodhill, G. J., and Willshaw, D. J. 1994. Elastic net model of ocular dominance: Overall stripe pattern and monocular deprivation. *Neural Comp.* **6**, 615–621.

Jones, D. G., Van Sluyters, R. C., and Murphy, K. M. 1991. A computational model for the overall pattern of ocular dominance. *J. Neurosci.* **11**, 3794–3808.

Kohonen, T. 1989. *Self-Organization and Associative Memory.* Springer-Verlag, Berlin.

LeVay, S., Connolly, M., Houde, J., and Van Essen, D. C. 1985. The complete pattern of ocular dominance stripes in the striate cortex and visual field of the macaque monkey. *J. Neurosci.* **5**, 486–501.

Miller, K. D., Keller, J. B., and Stryker, M. P. 1989. Ocular dominance column development: Analysis and computation. *Science* **245**, 605–615.

Obermayer, K., Ritter, H., and Schulten, K. 1990. A principle for the formation of the spatial structure of cortical feature maps. *Proc. Natl. Acad. Sci. U.S.A.* **87**, 8345–8349.

Obermayer, K., Blasdel, G. G., and Schulten, K. 1992. Statistical-mechanical analysis of self-organization and pattern formation during the development of visual maps. *Phys. Rev A* **45**, 7568–7589.

Ritter, H., and Schulten, K. 1988. Convergence properties of Kohonen's topology conserving maps: Fluctuations, stability and dimension selection. *Biol. Cybern.* **60**, 59–71.

Ritter, H., Martinetz, T., and Schulten, K. 1990. *Neuronale Netze*. Addison-Wesley, Reading, MA.

Simic, P. D. 1990. Statistical mechanics as the underlying theory of 'elastic' and 'neural' optimizations. *Network* **1**, 89–103.

Swindale, N. V. 1980. A model for the formation of ocular dominance stripes. *Proc. R. Soc. London* **B 208**, 243–264.

Swindale, N. V. 1982. A model for the formation of orientation columns. *Proc. R. Soc. London* **B 215**, 211–230.

Tusa, R. J., Rosenquist, A. C., and Palmer, L. A. 1979. Retinotopic organization of areas 18 and 19 in the cat. *J. Comp. Neur.* **185**, 657–678.

von der Malsburg, C. 1979. Development of ocularity domains and growth behaviour of axon terminals. *Biol. Cybern.* **32**, 49–62.

Wolf, F., Bauer, H.-U., and Geisel, T. 1993. Field discontinuities and islands in a model of cortical map formation. In *Computation and Neural Systems*, F. Eeckman and J. Bower, eds., pp. 403–408. Kluwer Academic, Boston, Dordrecht, London.

Wolf, F., Bauer, H.-U., and Geisel, T. 1994. Formation of Field discontinuities and islands in visual cortical maps. *Biol. Cybern.* **70**, 525–531.

Yuille, A. L. 1990. Generalized deformable models, statistical physics, and matching problems. *Neural Comp.* **2**, 1–24.

10

The Joint Development of Orientation and Ocular Dominance: Role of Constraints

Christian Piepenbrock
Department of Computer Science, Technical University of Berlin, Berlin, Germany

Helge Ritter
Faculty of Technology, University of Bielefeld, Bielefeld, Germany

Klaus Obermayer
Department of Computer Science, Technical University of Berlin, Berlin, Germany

Correlation-based learning (CBL) has been suggested as the mechanism that underlies the development of simple-cell receptive fields in the primary visual cortex of cats, including orientation preference (OR) and ocular dominance (OD) (Linsker, 1986; Miller, Keller, & Stryker, 1989). CBL has been applied successfully to the development of OR and OD individually (Miller, Keller, & Stryker, 1989; Miller, 1994; Miyashita & Tanaka, 1991; Erwin, Obermayer, & Schulten, 1995), but the conditions for their joint development have not been studied (but see Erwin & Miller, 1995, for independent work on the same question) in contrast to competitive Hebbian models (Obermayer, Blasdel, & Schulten, 1992). In this article, we provide insight into why this has been the case: OR and OD decouple in symmetric CBL models, and a joint development of OR and OD is possible only in a parameter regime that depends on nonlinear mechanisms.

1 The Correlation-Based Learning Model

Following the CBL-approach (Linsker, 1986; Miller, 1990), we consider four populations $i = 1, 2, 3, 4$ of geniculate "input" cells, which we call left-eye-ON, left-eye-OFF, right-eye-ON, and right-eye-OFF, respectively, and one type of cortical cells receiving the afferents. Cells are modeled as connectionist-type neurons and are arranged in two-dimensional layers, where $\vec{\alpha}, \vec{\beta}$ denote geniculate locations and $\vec{x}, \vec{y}$ specify cortical positions (in the same coordinate system). The geniculo-cortical projection is described by synaptic strengths $S^i_{\vec{\alpha},\vec{x}}$ for the connections between geniculate cells $(i, \vec{\alpha})$ and cortical cells $\vec{x}$. The activity-driven development of $S^i_{\vec{\alpha},\vec{x}}$ is generally described by a Hebbian model (Miller, 1990),

$$\frac{d}{dt} S^i_{\vec{\alpha},\vec{x}}(t) = A_{\vec{\alpha},\vec{x}} \sum_{j,\vec{\beta},\vec{y}} I_{\vec{x},\vec{y}} C^{ij}_{\vec{\alpha},\vec{\beta}} S^j_{\vec{\beta},\vec{y}}(t) - \gamma S^i_{\vec{\alpha},\vec{x}}(t) - \epsilon A_{\vec{\alpha},\vec{x}}, \tag{1.1}$$

where:

- $A_{\vec{\alpha},\vec{x}}$ is the localized arbor function, which ensures topography and is established by an intrinsic process before activity-driven processes set in. $A_{\vec{\alpha},\vec{x}}$ represents the synaptic density between a geniculate neuron at $\vec{\alpha}$ (independent of layer i) and a cortical neuron at $\vec{x}$.

- $I_{\vec{x},\vec{y}}$ denotes the effective intracortical interactions between neurons at locations $\vec{x}$ and $\vec{y}$. This function couples the receptive field development of cortical neurons and thus induces correlations between the receptive field properties of neighboring cells (i.e., cortical map development).

- $C^{ij}_{\vec{\alpha},\vec{\beta}}$ are the two point correlation functions of geniculate activities at $(i, \vec{\alpha})$ and $(j, \vec{\beta})$. These functions determine the structural properties of the developing receptive fields—whether ON/OFF subfields or eye dominance emerge.

- The last two terms are necessary to constrain the growth of synaptic weights in Hebbian models. Weights may be normalized by multiplicatively scaling them or by subtracting a constant. Multiplicative (M) constraints are implemented by a nonzero time-dependent γ; subtractive (S) constraints require a nonzero time-dependent ϵ (Miller & MacKay, 1994).

2 Analysis of the Model

We make two biologically motivated assumptions to characterize the conditions analytically under which OR and OD develop in this model framework. The first generally used assumption is symmetry of the activity correlation of ON and OFF cells and left and right eye. Symmetry leads to only four independent components of the correlation matrix $\{C^{ij}\}$:

$$\begin{aligned}
C^1 &\equiv C^{11} = C^{22} = C^{33} = C^{44} \text{ same eye, same cell type} \\
C^2 &\equiv C^{12} = C^{21} = C^{34} = C^{43} \text{ same eye, different cell type} \\
C^3 &\equiv C^{13} = C^{24} = C^{31} = C^{42} \text{ opposite eye, same cell type} \\
C^4 &\equiv C^{14} = C^{23} = C^{32} = C^{41} \text{ opposite eye, different cell type .}
\end{aligned} \quad (2.1)$$

Under this assumption, equation 2.1 decouples into four independent differential equations for the development of the modes, as shown in Table 1.

We conclude that if development proceeds purely linearly without bound, the ratio of OR and OD becomes arbitrarily large or small. Thus, either ON/OFF segregation or OD segregation ultimately dominates. Erwin and Miller (1995) independently obtained this linear system decomposition.

Table 1: Modes of Development

	Left ON	Left OFF	Right ON	Right OFF	Competition	Property	Left eye	Right* eye
$S^{SUM}_{\vec{\alpha}\vec{x}}=$	$(S^1_{\vec{\alpha}\vec{x}}$	$+S^2_{\vec{\alpha}\vec{x}}$	$+S^3_{\vec{\alpha}\vec{x}}$	$+S^4_{\vec{\alpha}\vec{x}})$	No competition	unspecific		
$S^{OD}_{\vec{\alpha}\vec{x}}=$	$(S^1_{\vec{\alpha}\vec{x}}$	$+S^2_{\vec{\alpha}\vec{x}}$	$-S^3_{\vec{\alpha}\vec{x}}$	$-S^4_{\vec{\alpha}\vec{x}})$	Left eye/right eye	OD		
$S^{OR^+}_{\vec{\alpha}\vec{x}}=$	$(S^1_{\vec{\alpha}\vec{x}}$	$-S^2_{\vec{\alpha}\vec{x}}$	$+S^3_{\vec{\alpha}\vec{x}}$	$-S^4_{\vec{\alpha}\vec{x}})$	ON/OFF	OR^+		
$S^{OR^-}_{\vec{\alpha}\vec{x}}=$	$(S^1_{\vec{\alpha}\vec{x}}$	$-S^2_{\vec{\alpha}\vec{x}}$	$-S^3_{\vec{\alpha}\vec{x}}$	$+S^4_{\vec{\alpha}\vec{x}})$	ON/OFF	OR^-		

*The images show typical cortical receptive fields (arbor diameter $A_\oslash = 13$ grid points) for each mode. For *unspecific* and *OD*, the sum of the ON and OFF afferents is shown, whereas for OR^+ and OR^- their difference is shown (gray = 0).

The second assumption is translation invariance due to the locally homogeneous structure of the neuronal layers:

$$A_{\vec{\alpha},\vec{x}} = A_{(\vec{\alpha}-\vec{x})}, \quad I_{\vec{x},\vec{y}} = I_{(\vec{x}-\vec{y})}, \quad C^{ij}_{\vec{\alpha},\vec{\beta}} = C^{ij}_{(\vec{\alpha}-\vec{\beta})}. \quad (2.2)$$

Fourier transformation of equation 1.1 then yields

$$\frac{d}{dt}\hat{S}^i_{\vec{w},\vec{k}}(t) = \hat{A}_{\vec{w},\vec{k}} * \sum_j \hat{I}_{\vec{k}}\hat{C}^{ij}_{\vec{w}}\hat{S}^j_{\vec{w},\vec{k}}(t) - \gamma \hat{S}^i_{\vec{w},\vec{k}}(t) - \epsilon \hat{A}_{\vec{w},\vec{k}}, \quad (2.3)$$

where ˆ denotes the Fourier transform of the corresponding quantity and $*$ is the convolution operator. Diagonalization of $\hat{I}\hat{C}^{ij}$ yields a system that can easily be solved for its modes in the case of infinite arbors ($A_{\vec{\alpha},\vec{x}} = 1$). We obtain eigenvalues $\lambda^{SUM}_{\vec{w},\vec{k}}$, $\lambda^{OD}_{\vec{w},\vec{k}}$, $\lambda^{OR^+}_{\vec{w},\vec{k}}$, and $\lambda^{OR^-}_{\vec{w},\vec{k}}$, one corresponding to each mode in the table (Erwin & Miller, 1995; Piepenbrock, Ritter, & Obermayer, 1996). These eigenvalues depend on the input correlation functions $\hat{C}^{ij}_{\vec{w},\vec{k}}$ and the cortical interaction function $\hat{I}_{\vec{k}}$. The modes with the strongest eigenvalues will dominate the development process. The eigenvalue analysis for $A_{\vec{\alpha},\vec{x}} = 1$ gives a good approximation of a realistic system's behavior since a synaptic density function A with a finite radius mainly results in a smoothing in the spatial frequency domain due to the convolution but does not basically alter the principal mode.

Based on these two assumptions, we can now derive conditions on the eigenvalues and (thereby indirectly) on the geniculate correlation functions and activity patterns. Most cortical receptive fields show ocular dominance, but they are unstructured with respect to input signals from the left and right eye (they have no left or right eye subfields). Consequently, for OD development $\lambda^{OD}_{\vec{w},\vec{k}}$ must have its maximum at spatial frequency $\vec{w} = 0$ (Miller et al., 1989). Orientation selectivity in simple cells, on the other hand, is based on ON and OFF subfields that alternate at a typical spatial frequency within the receptive field (Miller, 1994). Therefore we require $\lambda^{OR^+}_{\vec{w},\vec{k}}$ to have its peak at this typical spatial frequency $|\vec{w}|$. Hence, we make the ansatz:

$$C^{OD}_{\vec{\alpha}} = C^1_{\vec{\alpha}} + C^2_{\vec{\alpha}} - C^3_{\vec{\alpha}} - C^4_{\vec{\alpha}} = \frac{1}{\varphi^2} e^{-\vec{\alpha}^2/\varphi^2}$$

$$C^{OR^+}_{\vec{\alpha}} = C^1_{\vec{\alpha}} - C^2_{\vec{\alpha}} + C^3_{\vec{\alpha}} - C^4_{\vec{\alpha}} = \left(\frac{1}{\sigma^2} e^{-\vec{\alpha}^2/\sigma^2} - \frac{1}{\sigma^2 \nu^2} e^{-\vec{\alpha}^2/(\nu\sigma)^2} \right) c\xi \quad (2.4)$$

$$C^1_{\vec{\alpha}} = -C^4_{\vec{\alpha}} \ ; \qquad C^2_{\vec{\alpha}} = -C^3_{\vec{\alpha}}$$

and we obtain

$$\lambda^{OD}_{\vec{w},\vec{k}} = \hat{I}_{\vec{k}} \hat{C}^{OD}_{\vec{w}} \ ; \qquad \lambda^{OR^+}_{\vec{w},\vec{k}} = \hat{I}_{\vec{k}} \hat{C}^{OR^+}_{\vec{w}} \ ; \qquad \lambda^{SUM}_{\vec{w},\vec{k}} = \lambda^{OR^-}_{\vec{w},\vec{k}} = 0. \quad (2.5)$$

The parameters φ, σ, and ν denote the widths of the activity correlation functions, ξ denotes the ratio of λ^{OR^+} and λ^{OD}, and c is a normalization constant. The choice for $\lambda^{OR^+}_{\vec{w},\vec{k}}$ has a maximum at spatial ON/OFF wavelength $\pi\sigma\sqrt{(\nu^2-1)/(2\ln\nu)}$ of any orientation. Preference for a particular orientation is then a result of symmetry breaking due to the localized arbor function. OR may develop in our model framework driven by either the OR^+ or the OR^- mode. For OR^- the receptive fields of binocular cortical cells have ON and OFF subfields exchanged in the left and right eye (see Table 1), but the resulting orientation maps are equivalent in both cases. Thus we consider only $\lambda^{OR^+}_{\vec{w},\vec{k}}$ development.

In a linear symmetric CBL model, OR and OD develop independent of each other. Equally strong development of OR and OD is not possible except at the infinitely sharp phase boundary. The structure of the phase boundary changes, however, as soon as nonlinearities are incorporated. Erwin and Miller (1995) recently presented simulations using appropriate nonlinearities and showed that a finite parameter regime emerges in which OR and OD codevelop. Let us investigate how this parameter regime varies with the choice of nonlinearities. In the purely linear case, the OR/OD phase transition can be expected for equally strong modes $\lambda^{OD}_{\vec{w},\vec{k}}$, and $\lambda^{OR^+}_{\vec{w},\vec{k}}$, and we choose the parameters $c\xi$ in equation 2.4 such that both eigenvalues have equal maxima for $\xi = 1$. This is the case for $c = \nu^{2/(\nu^2-1)}/(1-\nu^{-2})$; that is, ξ represents the ratio of the maxima of $\lambda^{OR^+}_{\vec{w},\vec{k}}$ and $\lambda^{OD}_{\vec{w},\vec{k}}$. This type of correlation structure allows us to analyze the mode mixing of OR and OD in a simple setting. For $\xi \ll 1$ all neurons become monocular, and we expect the phase boundary at $\xi = 1$; for $\xi \gg 1$, binocular orientation selective receptive fields develop.

We may biologically interpret the meaning of this eigenvalue structure. The development of OD requires positive activity correlations C^{OD} between neurons (averaged over ON and OFF) that decrease with distance within one eye (Miller et al., 1989). OR, however, can develop only if the activities of ON and OFF neurons differ and $C^{OR+} \propto C^1 - C^2$ forms a Mexican hat–like correlation structure (Miller, 1994). Our assumption of λ^{SUM} and λ^{OR-} to be equal to zero is biologically not very realistic. It means that the activity correlations within the eye ($C_{\vec{\alpha}}^1$ and $C_{\vec{\alpha}}^2$) have to be of the opposite sign as the correlations between the eyes ($C_{\vec{\alpha}}^4$ and $C_{\vec{\alpha}}^3$) (see equation 2.5). Such correlation functions may be introduced by inhibitory connections between the geniculate layers but are unlikely after birth and eye opening when the left and right eye activities should be correlated. The assumption is not essential for a realistic development of receptive fields, however. Even for nonzero λ^{SUM} and λ^{OR-}, the outcome of the development is basically unchanged as long as these modes do not become the leading modes and govern the development process (Erwin & MIller, 1995; Piepenbrock et al., 1996).

3 Simulations

To study the transition zone between OD and OR development, we start with a reduced model setup and add mechanisms one by one to analyze the effects of different nonlinearities separately. We systematically vary the following components of the model:

- Geniculate (lateral geniculate nucleus, LGN) neurons project to the cortex in a topographic order. This projection is enforced by the synaptic density function $A_{\vec{\alpha},\vec{x}}$. In our implementation, it is simply chosen as 1 for $|\vec{x} - \vec{\alpha}| < \frac{1}{2}A_\oslash$ and 0 else. To verify the approximation from equation 2.3, we also simulated a fully connected $A_{\vec{\alpha},\vec{x}} = 1$ network.

- Cortical neurons interact with each other. When they effectively excite each other at short distances and inhibit each other at larger distances, typical cortical maps develop for OD (with OD bands) and OR (with pinwheels). I is given by

$$I_{\vec{x},\vec{y}} = e^{-(\vec{x}-\vec{y})^2/\mu^2} - \frac{1}{\zeta^2} e^{-(\vec{x}-\vec{y})^2/(\zeta\mu)^2} + \delta_{\vec{x},\vec{y}}. \tag{3.1}$$

We compared this with simple independent cortical neurons ($I_{\vec{x},\vec{y}} = \delta_{\vec{x},\vec{y}}$) to study the influence of cortical interaction on orientation selectivity.

- Synaptic weights should be positive or negative. Weights that become zero in our model have to be clipped by a hard nonlinear constraint. To study the behavior of the linear model, we also consider synaptic weights that can change their sign during development.

- Hebbian learning models require synaptic weight normalization. We use hard constraints that normalize the total weight at every time step and do not consider constraints over the projective field of LGN neurons. Subtractive and multiplicative constraints that keep the total synaptic weight constant are called S1 and M1, respectively. A multiplicative M2 constraint limits the total squared synaptic weight (Miller & MacKay, 1994). We consider two normalization approaches: total synaptic strength is constrained (1) for each cortical neuron separately or (2) over the whole cortex, a biologically less realistic model that (together with a multiplicative constraint) uniformly scales all synaptic weights but does not qualitatively alter the behavior of the unconstrained model.

All simulations of cortical OR and OD development are run with cortical neurons arranged on a 32×32 grid with periodic boundary conditions. The random initial weights are identical for all simulations ($A_{\vec{\alpha},\vec{x}} \pm 20$ percent uniformly distributed noise), and parameters are $A_\oslash = 13$, $\varphi = 7.1$, $\sigma = 2.1$, $\nu = 3$, $\mu = 2$, and $\zeta = 3$. At each iteration step we (1) compute the unconstrained derivatives and (2) apply an S1 constraint (if desired); then we (3) add the derivatives to the synaptic weights $S^i_{\vec{\alpha},\vec{x}}$, (4) clip the weights (if desired), and (5) normalize the weights multiplicatively (using M1 or M2 constraints). The S1 constraint applies only to unclipped synapses and keeps the total synaptic weight constant. Nevertheless, some weights might get clipped in step 4, and a multiplicative M1 renormalization (step 5) becomes necessary (this is the update scheme from Miller, 1994). The update step size is chosen at the first iteration to change the initial weights by 1 percent on average. The simulations run for 1000 update steps, or until 95 percent of the synaptic weights reach the limits. The receptive fields are usually fully developed after 100 to 200 steps (average weight change less than 1/1000 percent relative to initial weights), and test simulations with up to 5000 steps near the phase boundaries did not show any further change in the synaptic strengths.

For each map we computed three different values: OD, OR, and OS. The OD value is the root mean square (r.m.s.) eye dominance (Erwin & Miller, 1995), and the OR value is the r.m.s ON/OFF subfield segregation value of the cortical neurons. Orientation-selective neurons need not only segregated ON and OFF subfields (high OR value) but also an arrangement of those subfields that yields orientation-specific responses (high OS value). The degree of orientation tuning is measured by the mean cortical orientation specificity OS (in the spirit of Miller, 1994):

$$\text{OD} = \frac{1}{N}\sqrt{\sum_{\vec{x}}\left(\frac{\sum_{\vec{\alpha}} S^{OD}_{\vec{\alpha},\vec{x}}}{\sum_{\vec{\alpha}} |S^{SUM}_{\vec{\alpha},\vec{x}}|}\right)^2} \qquad (3.2)$$

$$\text{OR} = \frac{1}{N}\sqrt{\sum_{\vec{x}}\left(\frac{\sum_{\vec{\alpha}} S^{OR+}_{\vec{\alpha},\vec{x}}}{\sum_{\vec{\alpha}} |S^{SUM}_{\vec{\alpha},\vec{x}}|}\right)^2} \qquad (3.3)$$

$$\text{OS} = \sum_{\vec{x}} \frac{\sqrt{\left(\sum_{\vec{w}\neq 0} |\hat{S}^{OR+}_{\vec{w},\vec{x}}| \sin 2\varphi_{\vec{w}}\right)^2 + \left(\sum_{\vec{w}\neq 0} |\hat{S}^{OR+}_{\vec{w},\vec{x}}| \cos 2\varphi_{\vec{w}}\right)^2}}{N \sum_{\vec{w}\neq 0} |\hat{S}^{OR+}_{\vec{w},\vec{x}}|}. \qquad (3.4)$$

The OS value represents the sharpness of the neurons' orientation tuning curves where each neuron is stimulated with wave patterns of different orientations $\varphi_{\vec{w}}$ at different spatial frequencies ω (which results in wave vectors $\vec{w} = \omega[\cos\varphi_{\vec{w}}, \sin\varphi_{\vec{w}}]^T$). The response to different wave patterns $\vec{w}$ in the linear model is given by the power spectrum of $\hat{S}^{OR+}_{\vec{w},\vec{x}}$ Fourier transformed along the LGN dimensions. OS values may range from 0 for cortical maps without any orientation preference up to OS = 1 for neurons that respond to exactly one orientation. Realistic values are generally 0.05 for no OS and about 0.1 to 0.3 for well-orientation-tuned neurons.

The OS value alone is not sufficient as a measure for cortical orientation selectivity because it measures the width of the orientation tuning curve irrespective of its amplitude. For our simulation data, the orientation selectivity may be computed even if the cell orientation response rate (OR value) is almost zero. This is biologically unrealistic, and therefore we report the OS values only to show that the simulation results with high OR value actually yield orientation-selective cells.

In a biologically more realistic definition, OR and OS would have to be determined for each eye separately weighted by the neurons' eye dominance values. This, however, is not necessary in our simulations because our model yields only cortical maps with identical orientation patterns in both eyes.

4 Results

In our simulations we begin with a biologically unrealistic simple linear setup of the model and then add nonlinearities and constraints. The results of the simulations are shown in Figure 1. In the simplest case (top left), we assume full connectivity between the LGN and the cortex, synaptic weights that may be negative or positive, and no cortical interaction. Synaptic growth is limited by an M2 constraint. The system is completely linear, and we find a sharp OD/OR phase boundary for $\xi = 1$ as predicted by the linear system analysis. A joint development of OD and OR is possible only

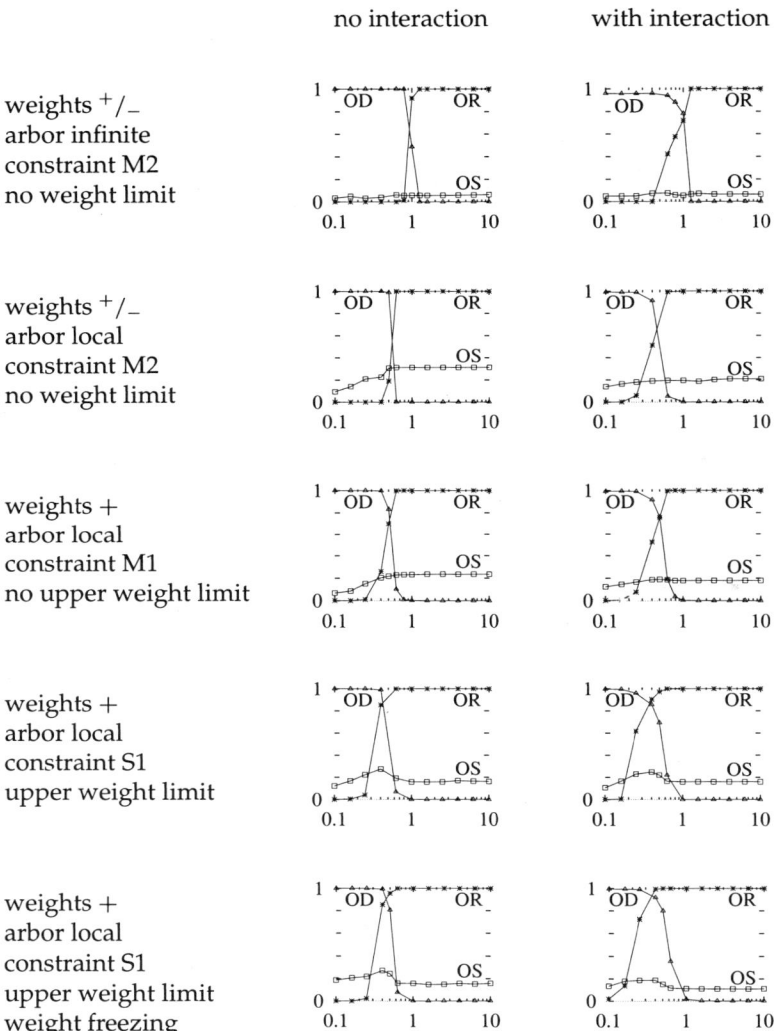

Figure 1: Phase diagrams of cortical OR and OD development. Parameter on the abscissa is ξ (i.e., the ratio of the maxima of $\lambda^{OR+}_{\vec{w},k}$ and $\lambda^{OD}_{\vec{w},k}$). For infinite arbors the OD/OR phase transition is at $\xi = 1$. Convolving the localized $\hat{A}$ with λ^{OR+} and λ^{OD} results in a predicted phase transition at $\xi = 0.73$. The left column represents simulation results where neurons develop independent of each other (no cortical interaction), whereas results with cortical interaction (and the constraint enforced separately for each neuron) are shown on the right side.

if ξ is *exactly* one. In this fully connected network, however, neurons may develop ocular dominance and ON/OFF receptive subfields, but the cells do not become orientation selective (low OS value) because the receptive fields have a large number of ON and OFF subfields in a random pattern. Orientation selectivity requires a certain ratio between arbor diameter and the strongest-growing spatial frequency mode. In our case, the arbor function localizes synaptic growth and thus smooths the growing modes in the spatial frequency domain. This results in a shift of the phase boundary from $\xi = 1$ to a lower value. The system is still linear, and a joint development of OD and OR does not occur.

Now we introduce nonlinear mechanisms to study conditions for coupled OR and OD development. When we couple the development of neighboring neurons by introducing a cortical interaction function, we do not necessarily make the system nonlinear. If we enforce the constraint over the whole cortex (biologically not very realistic), the system remains linear, and we obtain graphs very similar to the ones shown in the left column (data not shown). Their orientation specificity, however, is slightly lower than in the case of independent cortical neurons (as has been noted by Miller, 1994) because the interactions force some cells to develop receptive fields that are not ideally tuned for orientation (e.g., around pinwheels). An M1 constraint simply scales all the weights, but if we apply it separately over each cortical receptive field (as for all results shown in Figure 1), then introducing an interaction function makes the system nonlinear. As a result we obtain a finite parameter domain in which OR and OD may develop concurrently.

Synaptic weights should not change their sign in a biologically realistic model. Therefore we have studied models where we clip the weights at zero. We compare the results for zero weight clipping with M1 (a scheme we have used in Piepenbrock et al., 1996) to zero and upper weight clipping with S1 constraints (used in Erwin & Miller, 1995). The two growing modes S^{OD} and S^{OR^+} are both zero-sum modes; their growth does not alter the summed synaptic weight over each receptive field. Thus, under both M1 and S1 constraints, synaptic growth is initially unconstrained. Only when some synapses have reached their clipping values does the constraint begin to limit growth (Miller & MacKay, 1994). The only non-zero-sum modes are modes of S^{SUM}, so only if S^{SUM} modes had nonzero eigenvalues would the constraint influence the development process from the beginning.

The graphs in the third row show simulation results for only positive synaptic weights. We use an M1 constraint that simply scales the weights (like an M2 constraint). The only significant difference between the second and the third row is the clipping of weights at zero. In the absence of intracortical connections (left column), this creates a finite parameter domain for joint OD/OR development. If the weights are allowed to change their sign, an M2 constraint is necessary to limit synaptic growth (second row). For weight clipping, however, an M1 (third row, left) and an M2 (data not shown) constraint yield virtually identical results in the case of independent cortical neurons. Both constraints scale the synaptic weights but do not qualitatively alter the outcome of the unconstrained development, and the only nonlinearity is the weight clipping.

The last two rows present the simulation results for subtractive constraints. In this case the weights have to be clipped at zero as well as at some maximum value (Miller & MacKay, 1994). Without maximum weight clipping, all but one synaptic weight within the receptive field would decay to zero. The size of the final receptive fields can be influenced by the choice of the maximum value, and we chose eight times the mean initial synaptic weight, as in Miller (1994). The difference between the last two rows is the treatment of synaptic weights that have saturated at zero or at the maximum value. If we limit the synaptic weights but allow them to change again later in the development process, we obtain the graph in the second-last row. The last row results if weights are frozen as soon as they reach the minimum or maximum value, as in Erwin and Miller (1995).

OR and OD develop about equally strong near the phase boundary, and the amount of "randomness" in the initial synaptic weights determines how long it takes until the stronger mode begins to dominate the development process. If the weights are frozen at their limit values before this happens, we observe a joint development of OR and OD. On the other hand, if they are only clipped at the limits, the weights may change again later, and the influence of the initial conditions is reduced. This effect yields a slightly larger joint development parameter domain for the frozen synaptic weights in the bottom graphs.

The simulations in the bottom-right graph use the same mechanisms as Erwin and Miller (1995) and almost identical parameters.[1] It is not surprising that the last graph exhibits the largest parameter domain for joint OR and OD development since the simulation includes several nonlinear mechanisms—a minimum and a maximum synaptic weight value, as well as freezing of the weights that reach the limits.

In the results shown in Figure 1, we varied the nonlinear mechanism but did not systematically change all the other model parameters. Our simulations (including simulations using the parameters from Erwin & Miller, 1995), however, indicate that the effects of the nonlinear mechanisms are robust against changes in $\varphi, \sigma, \xi, \zeta$, and μ, and the parameter domains of joint OR and OD development remain qualitatively unchanged (i.e., the sharp phase transition of the purely linear CBL model changes into a parameter region of joint OR/OD development in a nonlinear model). This region is enlarged when more nonlinear mechanisms are added (as in Figure 1).

---

[1] They report better orientation selectivity for smaller parameters σ and for a tapered arbor function $A_{\vec{\alpha},\vec{x}}$. The effects of changes in the correlation functions on OR development are discussed in Miller (1994).

5 Summary

The main result of this note is that OR and OD decouple in the linear symmetric model and a sharp phase boundary divides the parameter domains of OR and OD. Nonlinear mechanisms may create a transition region near the phase boundary where a joint development of OR and OD is possible. We have identified three such mechanisms: (1) normalizing synaptic weights separately for each cortical neuron with M1/M2 constraints, (2) clipping of synaptic weights, and (3) freezing of synaptic weights. The size of the transition region depends on the nonlinearities present in the model, and the transition zone is broadest if the mechanisms are applied simultaneously.

The basic assumption underlying CBL is that the modeled receptive field features develop early, when the developments of S^{OD}, S^{OR^-}, and S^{OR^+} are essentially linear. This is true for $\xi \ll 1$ or $\xi \gg 1$, and all our simulations yield almost identical OD or OR maps. Close to the phase boundary, however, where OD and OR develop concurrently, the nonlinear mechanisms we have studied (M constraints, weight clipping, weight freezing) lead to different outcomes for identical initial conditions. Hence, the final receptive field properties are determined late at a time when the nonlinearities set in to stabilize the receptive fields.

When discussing the biological significance of a model, it is very important to investigate carefully the effects of the different mechanisms involved. CBL models require constraints to limit synaptic growth, and for this reason we tested different types of constraints in our simulations. These constraints are only clumsy approximations for the real biological mechanisms, but the simulations give hints on which aspect of the constraining mechanism may be most important for the joint development of OR and OD. Multiplicative constraints implement synaptic decay that is proportional to the synaptic strength, whereas under subtractive constraints, all synapses decay at the same rate, irrespective of their strength. Furthermore, subtractive constraints require weight clipping not only at zero but also for some maximum value (Miller & MacKay, 1994). It is plausible that such constraints exist in biological neurons (Miller & MacKay, 1994), but their underlying mechanisms have not been identified yet. The simulation results show that the size of the parameter domain for joint OD/OR development depends more on weight clipping or freezing and on separate constraints for each neuron than on the choice of M1 or S1 constraints. Furthermore, this parameter domain is enlarged if different nonlinear mechanisms act together.

Note

After part of this work was completed, we learned that Erwin and Miller (1995) independently derived the diagonalization of equation 1.1. We thank Ken Miller for his review and discussions that helped to improve this paper.

Acknowledgments

This research was funded in part by DFG (grant Ob 102/2-1) and a scholarship from the Boehringer Ingelheim Fonds to C. P. Computing time (CM5) was made available by NCSA and HLRZ Jülich.

References

Erwin, E., & Miller, K. D. (1995). Modeling joint development of ocular dominance and orientation in primary visual cortex. In *Proc. of the CNS-95*.

Erwin, E., Obermayer, K., & Schulten, K. (1995). Models of orientation and ocular dominance columns in the visual cortex: A critical comparison. *Neural Computation* 7:425–468.

Linsker, R. (1986). From basic network principles to neural architecture: Emergence of orientation selective cells. *Proc. Natl. Acad. Sci. USA* 83:8390–8394.

Miller, K. D. (1990). Derivation of linear Hebbian equations from a nonlinear Hebbian model of synaptic plasticity. *Neural Computation* 2:321–333.

Miller, K. D. (1994). A model for the development of simple cell receptive fields and the ordered arrangements of orientation columns through activity-dependent competition between ON- and OFF-center inputs. *Journal of Neuroscience* 14:409–441.

Miller, K. D., Keller, J. B., & Stryker, M. P. (1989). Ocular dominance column development: Analysis and simulation. *Science* 245:605–615.

Miller, K. D., & MacKay, D. J. C. (1994). The role of constraints in Hebbian learning. *Neural Comp.* 6:100–126.

Miyashita, M., & Tanaka, S. (1991). A mathematical model for the self-organization of orientation columns in visual cortex. *Neuroreport* 3:69–72.

Obermayer, K., Blasdel, G. G., & Schulten, K. (1992). A statistical mechanical analysis of self-organization and pattern formation during the development of visual maps. *Phys. Rev. A* 45:7568–7589.

Piepenbrock, C., Ritter, H., & Obermayer, K. (1996). Cortical map development driven by spontaneous retinal activity waves. In *Artificial Neural Networks—ICANN 96*. New York: Springer-Verlag.

11

A Self-Organizing Model of "Color Blob" Formation

Harry G. Barrow
Alistair J. Bray
Julian M. L. Budd
School of Cognitive and Computing Sciences,
University of Sussex, Falmer, Brighton, East Sussex BN1 9QH, UK

This paper explores the possibility that the formation of color blobs in primate striate cortex can be partly explained through the process of activity-based self-organization. We present a simulation of a highly simplified model of visual processing along the parvocellular pathway, that combines precortical color processing, excitatory and inhibitory cortical interactions, and Hebbian learning. The model self-organizes in response to natural color images and develops islands of unoriented, color-selective cells within a sea of contrast-sensitive, orientation-selective cells. By way of understanding this topography, a principal component analysis of the color inputs presented to the network reveals that the optimal linear coding of these inputs keeps color information and contrast information separate.

1 Introduction

Cytochrome oxidase (CO), an endogenous metabolic marker (see Wong-Riley 1994), produces a characteristic patchy or "blob-like" pattern of staining in the deep and especially the superficial layers of primate area V1 (Wong-Riley 1979; Carroll and Wong-Riley 1982; Horton and Hubel 1981; Hendrickson *et al.* 1981; Horton 1984; Livingstone and Hubel 1984). The CO blobs mark an important type of functional segregation in the monkey primary visual cortex. Cells within CO blobs tend to have concentric, monocular, low spatial frequency, color-selective receptive field properties, but cells outside ("interblob" region) generally have complex or hypercomplex, oriented, binocular, high spatial frequency, broadband-selective responses (Livingstone and Hubel 1984; Ts'o and Gilbert 1988). At the blob–interblob boundaries, however, neurons appear to have mixed responses with complex, oriented, *and* color-selective receptive fields (Ts'o and Gilbert 1988). Together with the observed smooth variation in the density of cytochrome oxidase staining (Trusk *et al.* 1990) and the uniformity of dendritic field size in blob and interblob regions (Malach 1992), this mixed response suggests a continuum of receptive field properties rather than a discrete segregation of function. The CO blobs, similar in size to physiologically identified "color columns" (Hubel and Wiesel 1968; Gouras 1974; Michael 1981), therefore represent vertically aligned groups of cells with color-selective receptive field properties.

The precise nature of CO blob cell receptive fields is, however, much less clear. First, cells within a single CO blob may code for only one color contrast, that is, red-green (R-G), blue-yellow (B-Y), broad-band opponency (e.g., Ts'o and Gilbert 1988), or have only mixed color opponency, for example, some cells R-G and others are B-Y opponent (e.g., Livingstone and Hubel 1984). Second, many CO blobs cells were originally thought to have "double opponent" properties, cells with center-surround spatial structure but with color opponency in each subfield (Livingstone and Hubel 1984). It is now believed that double opponent cells are rare as most cells initially classified as double opponent have broad-band surrounds, so-called "modified Type II cells" (for a discussion see Ts'o and Gilbert 1988). In fact, most of the cells within CO blobs have receptive field types similar to those present in the geniculate (cf. Livingstone and Hubel 1984; Wiesel and Hubel 1966).

How do CO blobs develop? Current evidence supports the view that the formation of CO blobs is, to some degree, genetically predetermined. First, in the macaque monkey, CO blobs appear many weeks before birth (Horton 1984). Second, there appear to be differences in the type of geniculate input terminating in CO blob compared to interblob regions (Lachica et al. 1992; Nealy and Maunsell 1994). Third, normal CO blob development in the macaque monkey is apparently unaffected by the absence of visual stimulation when both eyes are removed prenatally (Kuljis and Rakic 1990). Last, the mean size of a CO blob (relative to the growing cortex) during maturation changes little (Purves and Lamantia 1993). The size of CO blobs, however, can be altered by the level of neural activity postnatally. The removal or blockade of the retinal impulses from one eye in the adult macaque monkey, for example, leads to a considerable shrinkage in CO blob size in the deprived-eye column (Horton 1984; Wong-Riley and Carroll 1984; Trusk et al. 1990). So while the CO blobs may form without visual stimulation, their postnatal plasticity suggests that the maintenance of CO blobs may depend, at least partly, on activity-based mechanisms. But even if one assumes that CO blobs are genetically predetermined, it is far from clear if the receptive field properties within and between the CO blobs can develop without visual stimulation. So far, no empirical work has compared the codevelopment of CO blobs with the functional properties of neurons.

The possibility therefore exists that, like other forms of functional segregation in the central nervous system, activity-dependent self-organizing mechanisms may play some part in the development of color columns. In this paper, we explore this possibility by training an unsupervised neural network model of the early visual pathway on inputs from natural color images. We find that color-selective, blob-like formations develop without any initial bias, through self-organization alone. Some understanding of the behavior of this network is achieved though analysis of the statistics of natural images. A preliminary account of this work has been presented elsewhere (Barrow and Bray 1992).

2 A Network Model

In this section we outline a simple network model of processing in the early visual pathway. In combining excitatory and inhibitory cortical interactions with Hebbian-type learning to generate a topographic mapping, the model falls within an approach that has yielded a degree of success. Early work by von der Malsburg demonstrated such a combination was sufficient for learning orientation selectivity with simple stimuli (von der Malsburg 1973). More recently, works by others such as Miller et al. (1989), Miller (1990, 1994), and Goodhill (1993), have demonstrated that such models can provide an explanation of the formation of retinal topography, orientation, and ocular dominance columns, and the separation of the "on" and "off" signals. Linsker (1990) and more recently Miller (1994) have demonstrated that these correlation-based models can be partly understood through examination of the correlations in their inputs. Erwin et al. (1995) have lately provided an excellent critique of such models.

All the above work deals with black and white imagery; none considers color inputs, and the separate correlations they entail. In this work, we examine whether a similar-styled explanation to that provided by such models for various types of functional segregation in the cortex can also be given for the development of color blobs. Because the output of such an activity-based model is determined by the correlations within the inputs (Miller 1994), it is essential that both the statistics of the color inputs presented and precortical processing on these inputs are realistic. Accordingly, we use input from natural color images, and model preprocessing at the retina and lateral geniculate nucleus (LGN), similar to that for the parvochannel in macaque monkeys. However, we recognize that an accurate model of color processing in primates (in line with detailed, known neurophysiology) would have to be considerably more detailed than that described here, involving a more complicated architecture. Our model attempts to maintain the simplicity of the similar models mentioned above, while accommodating essential biological constraints, to show that Hebbian development on visual scenes can lead to structures similar to those found in actual cortex; we do not pretend to model such biological structures precisely. The simple architecture of our model is shown in Figure 1.

2.1 Precortical Processing. Inputs are presented from color images, represented as arrays in the red, green, and blue spectral bands. We model responses of on-center and off-center cells for the broad-band and

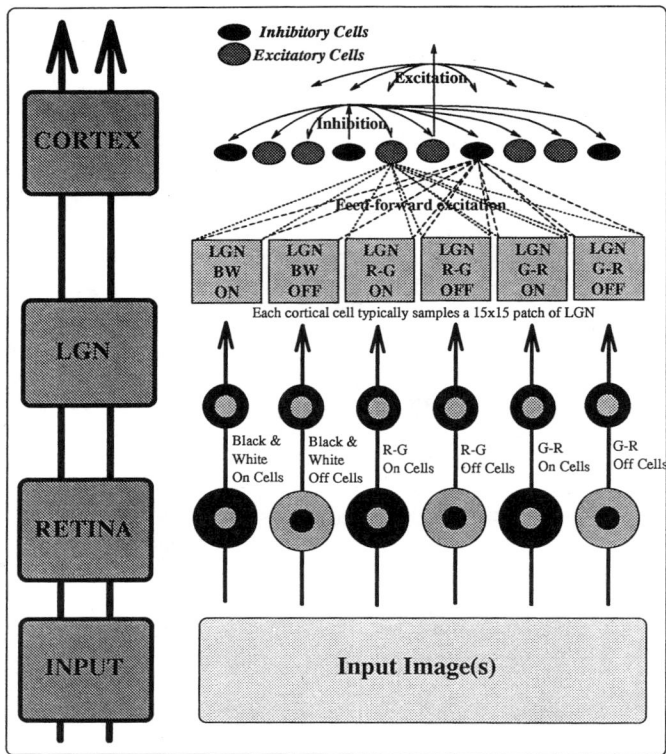

Figure 1: **Architecture of the network model**. The model consists of three stages: the retina, LGN, and striate cortex. We model the on- and off-center cells for the broad-band channel and for the red/green color-opponent channels so that six types of retinal ganglion cell project from the retina to the LGN. Lateral inhibition is applied to the channels independently in the LGN, and the corresponding six types of geniculate cells project to cells in the cortex. We model the cortex using a dual-population model that simulates short-range lateral excitation and longer-range inhibition. When the network activity is stable, the synaptic weights between geniculate and cortical cells adapt according to a Hebbian-type rule.

red/green channels.[1] There are therefore six types of retinal and six types of LGN cells (Table 1). On- and off-center channels at the retina

---

[1]We ignore the blue-yellow channel since it involves only about 6% of all ganglion cells.

Model of "Color Blob" Formation

Table 1: Retinal and LGN Cells

On-channel	Retina	LGN	Off-channel	Retina	LGN
Broad-band	R_w^+	L_w^+	Broad-band	R_w^-	L_w^-
Red-green	R_{rg}^+	L_{rg}^+	Red-green	R_{rg}^-	L_{rg}^-
Green-red	R_{gr}^+	L_{gr}^+	Green-red	R_{gr}^-	L_{gr}^-

Table 2: Outputs of the Retinal Cells

	Linear	Nonlinear
On-channel		
Broad-band	$r_w^+ = G_{rc} * I_w - k \cdot G_{rs} * I_w$	$R_w^+ = \max(r_w^+ + b, 0)$
Red-green	$r_{rg}^+ = G_{rc} * I_r - k \cdot G_{rs} * I_g$	$R_{rg}^+ = \max(r_{rg}^+ + b, 0)$
Green-red	$r_{gr}^+ = G_{rc} * I_g - k \cdot G_{rs} * I_r$	$R_{gr}^+ = \max(r_{gr}^+ + b, 0)$
Off-channel		
Broad-band	$r_w^- = G_{rs} * I_w - k \cdot G_{rc} * I_w$	$R_w^- = \max(r_w^- + b, 0)$
Red-green	$r_{rg}^- = G_{rs} * I_g - k \cdot G_{rc} * I_r$	$R_{rg}^- = \max(r_{rg}^- + b, 0)$
Green-red	$r_{gr}^- = G_{rs} * I_r - k \cdot G_{rc} * I_g$	$R_{gr}^- = \max(r_{gr}^- + b, 0)$

are modeled using a difference of gaussians, where each gaussian kernel is applied to a particular spectral band. For example, the output of a red-green opponent cell is a function of the difference between a small red sensitive gaussian center and a larger green-sensitive gaussian surround. Assuming a small retinal gaussian G_{rc} and a larger one G_{rs} we define nonlinear outputs R of the retinal cells as thresholded versions of linear difference-of-gaussian signals r (Table 2) where I_r, I_g, I_w are the red, green, and gray-level intensity images (i.e., outputs of the retinal cones) and $*$ is the convolution operator. Each gaussian is normalized to have unit integral, and k determines the relative weighting of center and surround. To obtain the nonlinear output R we superimpose r on a background firing rate b and clip the negative component of the new signal to zero. In line with Wehmeier et al. (1989), the gaussians have standard deviations in the ratio of 1:3; in line with Robson (1983) $k = 0.88$. These six signals are carried (by the retinal ganglion cells) to the LGN. The broad-band channel carries mainly luminance contrast information, whereas the red/green channels carry color information. In Figure 2a the output of the red-green on-center ganglion cells is shown when the picture in Figure 6a is presented as input.

We use difference-of-gaussian processing again at the LGN to simulate local inhibition. We assume a central gaussian the same size as the retinal one $\sigma_{lc} = \sigma_{rc}$, and a larger surround such that $\sigma_{ls} = 2\sigma_{lc}$. We also assume

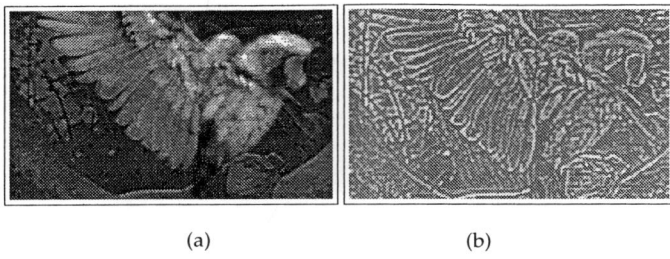

(a) (b)

Figure 2: **Output of retinal and geniculate cells.** (a) On the left, the output R_{rg}^+ of the red-green on-center retinal cells is shown when the image in Figure 6(a) is presented. While broad-band cells carry spatial contrast information alone, it can be seen that the color-opponent cells also code the difference between red and green spectral input. Hence cells in the red body of the parrot are highly active. (b) The output of the geniculate cells L_{rg}^+, given the same input, is shown (histogram equalization has been used to aid display). Lateral inhibition at this stage enhances spatial contrast and removes the DC color signal. As a result, color information is transmitted only where there is also spatial contrast, i.e., at boundaries.

Table 3: Output of the Six Cell Types

	Linear	Nonlinear
On-channel		
Broad-band	$l_w^+ = G_{lc} * R_w^+ - G_{ls} * R_w^+$	$L_w^+ = \max(l_w^+ + b', 0)$
Red-green	$l_{rg}^+ = G_{lc} * R_{rg}^+ - G_{ls} * R_{rg}^+$	$L_{rg}^+ = \max(l_{rg}^+ + b', 0)$
Green-red	$l_{gr}^+ = G_{lc} * R_{gr}^+ - G_{ls} * R_{gr}^+$	$L_{gr}^+ = \max(l_{gr}^+ + b', 0)$
Off-channel		
Broad-band	$l_w^- = G_{lc} * R_w^- - G_{ls} * R_w^-$	$L_w^- = \max(l_w^- + b', 0)$
Red-green	$l_{rg}^- = G_{lc} * R_{rg}^- - G_{ls} * R_{rg}^-$	$L_{rg}^- = \max(l_{rg}^- + b', 0)$
Green-red	$l_{gr}^- = G_{lc} * R_{gr}^- - G_{ls} * R_{gr}^-$	$L_{gr}^- = \max(l_{gr}^- + b', 0)$

equal weighting of the center and surround so that, within image regions of uniform color and intensity, the LGN response will be zero. Again, we superimpose a linear signal l against a background firing rate b' to provide the output L of the six cell types (Table 3).

In Figure 2b the output of the red-green on-center geniculate cells is shown when the picture in Figure 6a is presented; the color information carried by the retinal cells now remains only where there is also a luminance contrast.

Model of "Color Blob" Formation

2.2 Cortical Processing. Our model of simple cell connectivity and self-organization is based on that first proposed by von der Malsburg (1973) and Miller (1990). It consists of two types of unit representing the two broad categories of cells in the primate striate cortex. The excitatory units represent spiny cells and the inhibitory ones represent smooth cells. Their numbers are in the ratio of 4:1 to reflect observed cell counts. Both types of cells receive excitatory feedforward input from the LGN. Excitatory cells excite all neighboring cells within a short radius, and the inhibitory cells inhibit all neighbors within a larger radius.

The cortical units receive feedforward input through their connections to geniculate cells. The recurrent network settles into a stable state where intracortical feedback is no longer changing. All units then adapt their connections to the geniculate cells using a Hebbian-type learning-rule. This process of presenting inputs, settling, and adapting continues until the feedforward connections themselves settle to stable values.

2.2.1 Unit Model. Cortical cells are modeled with a membrane potential equation:

$$C\frac{dv}{dt} = (v^+ - v)g^+ + (v^- - v)g^- + (v^r - v)g^r$$

where C is the cell membrane capacitance, v is the membrane potential, v^+ and v^- are the reversal potentials for sodium and potassium, respectively, and v^r is the resting potential. Conductances g^+, g^-, g^r are for sodium, potassium, and leakage, respectively, and we assume that g^+ and g^- depend linearly upon summed excitatory and inhibitory input, respectively. The equation can be rewritten as

$$\tau\frac{dv}{dt} = v^\infty - v \quad \text{where} \quad v^\infty = \frac{v^+g^+ + v^-g^- + v^rg^r}{(g^+ + g^- + g^r)}$$

and

$$\tau = \frac{C}{(g^+ + g^- + g^r)}$$

v^∞ is an attractor to which the ambient voltage is drawn exponentially if conductances remain constant, and τ is the cell time constant. Cells are treated as simple fixed-threshold relaxation oscillators that fire when the membrane potential reaches a threshold value v^θ and then reset their potential to v^0. The firing rate f is given by

$$f = \frac{1}{t^\theta + \tau^r} \quad \text{where} \quad t^\theta = \tau \ln(\frac{v^\infty - v^0}{v^\infty - v^\theta})$$

where τ^r is an absolute refractory period and t^θ is the time taken for the voltage to rise from v^0 to v^θ. The output f is plotted against g^+ and g^-, as shown in Figure 3; it has a fixed threshold determined by $v^\infty \geq v^\theta$, approximates linearity when just above threshold, and saturates with a value $1/\tau^r$ if $g^+ \gg g^-$. Excitatory and inhibitory conductances, g_j^+ and

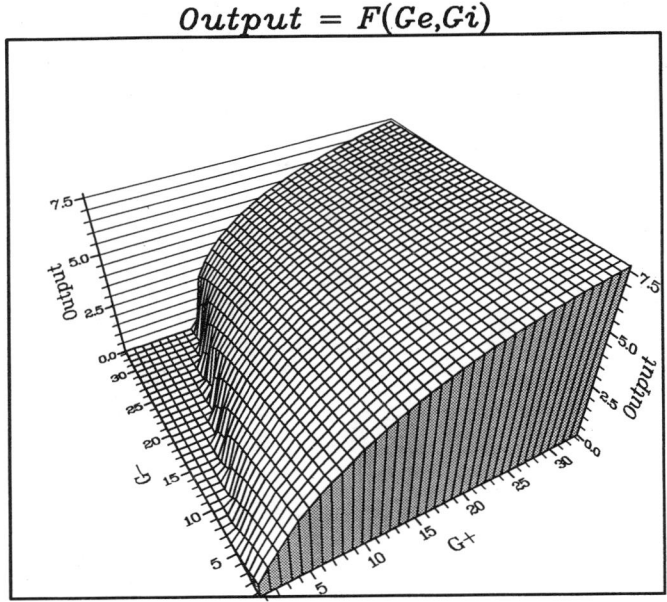

Figure 3: Unit output as a function of g^+ and g^-. The firing rate f of a unit is given by $f = 1/\left(\tau^r + \tau \log\left[(v^\infty - v^0)/(v^\infty - v^\theta)\right]\right)$ where $v^\infty = (v^+ g^+ + v^- g^- + v^r g^r)/(g^+ + g^- + g^r)$, $\tau = C/(g^+ + g^- + g^r)$, and τ^r is an absolute refractory time. Here f is plotted against g^+ and g^-. It shows a well-defined threshold, approximate linearity above the threshold, and saturation when the ratio $g^+:g^-$ is large.

g_j^-, are weighted sums of stimulation from connecting LGN and cortical cells:

$$g_j^+ \propto \sum_k u_{jk} y_k + \sum_i w_{ji} x_i \quad \text{and} \quad g_j^- \propto \sum_l u_{jl} y_l$$

where y_k is the output of excitatory cortical cell k, y_l is the output of inhibitory cell l, x_i is the output of LGN cell i, and u_{jk}, u_{jl}, and w_{ji} are connection strengths between cortical cell j and excitatory cortical, inhibitory cortical and LGN cells, respectively. In our simulations we set $C = 4.15$, $g^r = 0.01$, $v^+ = 55.0$, $v^- = -85.0$, $v^r = -70.0$, $v^0 = -85.0$, $v^\theta = -55.0$, and $\tau^r = 0.1$.

2.2.2 Adaptation.

Intracortical connections have a fixed gaussian distribution, inhibition extending further than excitation. The adaptive feed-

Model of "Color Blob" Formation 221

forward connections between cortical and geniculate cells are initialized with random positive values (from the uniform distribution 0.0...1.0), modulated by a gaussian function of distance, and normalized such that the sum of weights from the 6 types of geniculate cell connecting to any cortical cell is 6.0. Small fragments of image are presented to the model, network activity settles, and then the connections w_{ci} are adapted using a variant of the Hebbian learning rule:

$$\frac{dw_{ci}}{dt} = \alpha y_c (p_{ci} x_i - w_{ci})$$

where α is a small learning constant ($\alpha = 0.001$), c is an index over both excitatory and inhibitory cortical cells, and p_{ci} is a probability function maintaining a gaussian distribution of connection strength.

2.3 Simulations. Inputs were sampled from the two color images (resolution 320 × 200) in Figure 6. For computational efficiency, we applied retinal and LGN processing once throughout each image at the start of the simulation, storing the six arrays of LGN output. The free parameter G_{rs} that determines spatial scale was set at 2 pixels.[2]

Subsequently, for each input presentation we extracted six 15 × 15 subarrays from the stored arrays. This "window" was centered on a random location in the image, providing the output of 1350 LGN cells in total. The outputs of these cells were normalized so that the total amount of activity, summed over all channels, was constant (= 6.0). The cortex was modelled with an array of 30 × 30 excitatory units and a spatially coextensive array of 15 × 15 inhibitory units. All 1125 cortical units received feedforward input from the 1350 geniculate cells, each unit having its own connection weight to each geniculate input.[3] The strength of intracortical feedback connections was a gaussian function of separation: the excitatory and inhibitory gaussians had standard deviations equal to 5 and 23% of the cortical space, respectively.[4]

2.4 Results.

2.4.1 Geniculocortical Connections. It can be seen from Figure 4 that most excitatory units develop similar connections in the broad-band, redgreen and green-red channels. The profiles of these connection strengths show two-dimensional (2D) orientation preference, with many of the pro-

---

[2]The ratios are such that $G_{rs}/3 = G_{rc} = G_{lc} = G_{ls}/2$.
[3]The gaussian probability function p that maintains an envelope on geniculocortical weights had a standard deviation of 3.5.
[4]There were no wrap-around effects, but the sum of each unit's excitatory and inhibitory connections was independently normalized to have a set value.

files resembling 2D Gabor functions (Daugman 1985). This is to be expected from the work of Linsker (1990), Miller (1990), and Barrow (1987). It is striking, however, that there are small clusters of cells embedded within this sea of oriented fields that are different. These cells code color

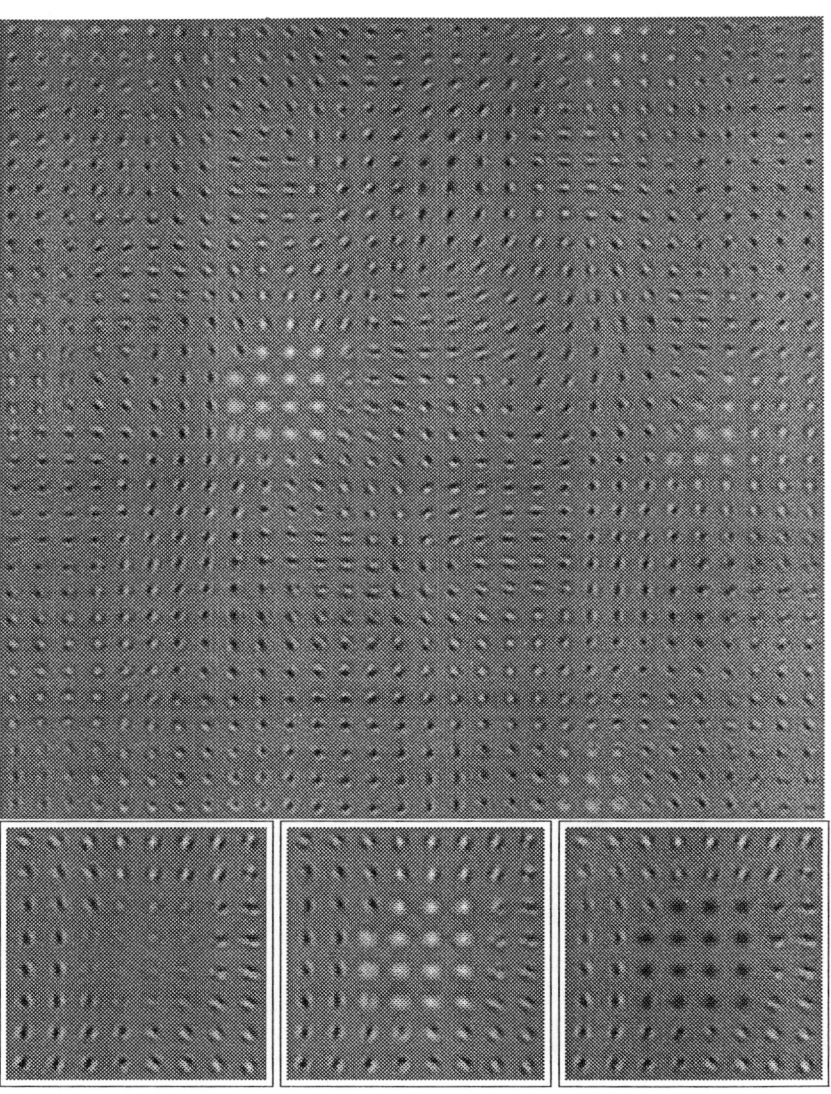

Model of "Color Blob" Formation

information and their connections to the red-green and green-red geniculate cells appear to be center-only (though occasionally there appears to be an added center-surround component). Note particularly that their connections to the broad-band cells have almost zero strength. For the most part, these color-selective cells seem to be responsive to *red-ness*, although there is at least one region that appears to encode *green-ness*. The red-sensitive cells make strong connections to both the on-center red-green and the off-center green-red geniculate cells (the green-sensitive cells connecting strongly to the other two types of color-opponent geniculate cells).

Figure 5 shows the weight patterns for a small sample of the excitatory units (which develop weight patterns very similar to inhibitory units at the same cortical location). In this sample it is easy to distinguish between the cells that are coding for orientation and the nonoriented cells that are coding color. We also show some cells (more unusual) that exhibit less obvious profiles, and appear to combine both color- and orientation-selective properties.

2.4.2 Average Receptive Fields. To analyze the receptive field properties of the units in the network it is necessary to go beyond studying the connections between geniculate and cortical cells in isolation. The receptive field of a cortical unit is a function of preprocessing in the retina and LGN, as well as intracortical feedback. Studying the adaptive weights gives insight into the average geniculate output that stimulates a cortical cell (since the weights tend toward a weighted average of the patterns to

---

Figure 4: *Facing page*. **Connections between geniculate and excitatory cortical units.** In the large display, connections between red-green geniculate cells and the excitatory cortical cells are shown. Connection strengths to the off-cells L_{rg}^- have been subtracted from those to the on-cells L_{rg}^+ for each cortical unit. For most cells, connections display selectivity to orientation, and preferred orientation varies smoothly across the cortical area. Connections for such cells are similar in the broad-band and green-red channels to those shown here for the red-green. However, there are clusters of cells that tend to display no orientation preference. In the three smaller displays beneath we show connections for one such cluster in all three broad-band, red-green, and green-red channels (left to right). These cells tend to have very weak connections to all broad-band geniculate cells, while their connections to either "green-sensitive" or "red-sensitive" geniculate cells tend to be strong (with zero connections to cells of the opposing color), and have a center-surround profile. We suggest that such cells respond to "red-ness" or "green-ness," and receive little information from the broad-band channel.

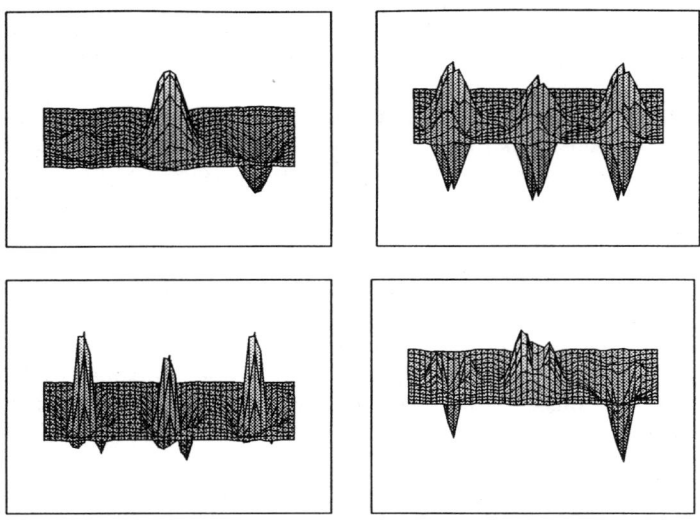

Figure 5: **Profiles of excitatory/geniculate connections.** Four profiles are shown for the connections of units in Figure 4. The left side of the profile shows the difference between broad-band on- and off-center connections; the middle shows a similar difference for the red-green channel, and the right for the green-red. Top left shows unit (11,15) (whenever indexing into displays we use raster notation where the origin is top-left, the first number indexes right and the second indexes downwards) — a typical color-sensitive cell with nonoriented connections to red-green on-center and green-red off-center cells, and very weak connections to broad-band cells. Top right shows unit (10,6) — a typical orientation-selective cell; profiles in the three color channels are similar and resemble 2D Gabor-functions. Bottom left shows cell (18,26) — it has similar center-surround profiles in all three color channels, suggesting it codes contrast regardless of orientation. Finally, the bottom right shows cell (25,17) — this appears to have combined properties of color-selective cells (strong connections to red-green on-center and green-red off-center) and contrast-sensitive cells (off-center center-surround profiles). It seems from examination that although most cells fall easily into one of the two categories for color or orientation selectivity, there are a small number that have more complex profiles. These complexities highlight a need for different methods for determining their receptive fields.

which a unit responds). However, it does not tell us directly the retinal input that will make the cell active.

To discover the sort of patterns to which different cortical units were responding (once the network's cortical connections were stable) we com-

Model of "Color Blob" Formation

puted the average visual input that activated each unit. That is, we computed a weighted average of visual input for each cortical unit, where the weighting was determined by the output of the unit, after settling. Hence, if a unit responded strongly to a pattern then this pattern contributed a proportionately large amount to the average, whereas if it did not respond at all then it contributed nothing.

Figure 6b displays weighted averages for the inhibitory units[5] (behavior of the inhibitory units is almost identical to that of the excitatory ones, but since there are fewer of them patterns are easier to display). It is apparent that units are generally responding to either edges and bars regardless of color, chromatic boundaries, or orientation. In this example such color selection is strongly biased toward red stimuli.[6] In another experiment, identical except that visual input was taken from a wider variety of images, an equal representation of red and green was found.

2.4.3 Artificial Stimuli. As a final means of determining what sort of visual pattern activated the different cortical units we performed some limited "neurophysiological" experiments with artificial visual stimuli. We hypothesized that units outside the "blobs" would respond maximally to a luminance edge or bar of the optimal orientation, regardless of its color, whereas those units within blobs would respond maximally to a center-surround stimulus of the correct color contrast. Accordingly, we chose a few of the units illustrated in Figure 6b and attempted to find optimal stimuli for them.

First, we created a visual stimulus, corresponding to a circular colored spot against a different colored background. We parameterized this stimulus by spot color, spot size, and background color. We then selected a unit we expected to be selective to color contrast only. We varied the visual stimulus until we found those values of the parameters that elicited the greatest response from that unit (in context of the whole network). [7] We then created stimuli with the same radius while altering the spot and foreground colors. We found that the unit typically responded to these stimuli only if there was an appropriately colored center. That is to say, if the unit was from a red blob then a red component to the spot color was usually necessary; if from a green blob, a green center was required. Figure 7a and 7b shows the results of this process for two color-selective units, (1,12) and (11,14) in Figure 6.

Second, we created a visual stimulus, corresponding to a black/white step-edge, parameterized by phase and orientation. We then selected a unit we expected to be selective for orientation only. We varied the visual stimulus until we found those values of phase and orientation that elicited the greatest response from that unit (in context of the whole

---
[5]To display these, we computed a single average color over all units and subtracted this color from the profile for each unit.
[6]The eigenvector analysis of the images used (in the next section) reflects this bias.
[7]This was done using a simple hill-climbing algorithm for optimization.

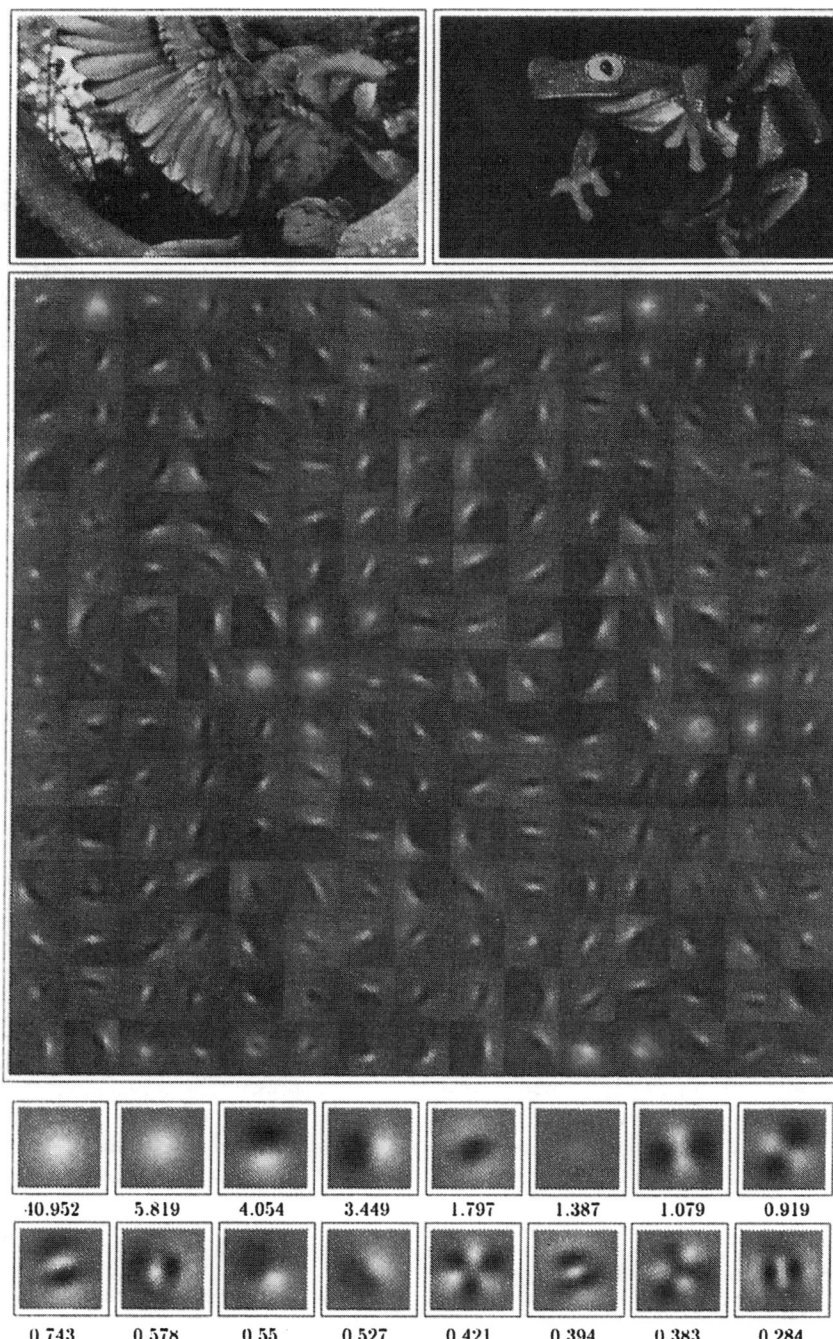

Model of "Color Blob" Formation

network). We then created stimuli with the same orientation and phase, while altering the color of the edge. We found that, regardless of edge-color, these stimuli normally elicited a strong response from the unit. Figure 7c shows results for orientation-selective unit (4,1) in Figure 6.

3 A Linear Analysis

The model that we have presented reflects some of the details and non-linearities of the primate visual system: retinal ganglion cells code for color contrast and luminance contrast, also separating information into on- and off-channels; LGN cells similarly have thresholds, and excitatory and inhibitory inputs may affect cell firing rates nonlinearly. However, it has been argued that the cortical cells we model do have a quasilinear response in their dynamic range (e.g., Stafstrom *et al.* 1984). It has also been argued that the goal that early visual processing is attempting to satisfy is to recode the input using a set of orthogonal, approximately linear basis functions, so compressing the input in a near-optimal manner (see Linsker 1990). In light of this, it is interesting to ask what is the optimal linear coding of the inputs that we present to our network. If the inputs, which are high-dimensional vectors, occupy only a subspace of the whole space, then we expect that the "features" a quasilinear network such as ours learns will lie within this subspace, and be a function of its structure.

3.1 Determining the Principal Components.
We computed the principal components for the set of inputs taken from the two images in Figure 6. We split the images into their three spectral bands, and generated the set of inputs to our network by extracting three 20×20 patches, one from each of the spectral images, for every position in the image (each position constituting an input). Each patch was modulated with

---

Figure 6: *Facing page.* **Images, Receptive Fields and Eigenvectors.** (top) Two color images (resolution 320×200). (center) For each inhibitory cell in the cortical array a weighted average over many visual patterns is shown: the weighting is proportional to the response of the unit to that pattern. It is apparent that units are either selective to oriented edges or bars without preference for color, or selective for "red" input without preference for orientation. (bottom) The first sixteen principal components of all small patches (20×20) taken from these two images are shown, with their eigenvalues beneath. Most of the eigenvectors have very similar spectral components. However, there are some noticeable exceptions: the second eigenvector is unoriented and "red" and the sixth is unoriented and "green." Later eigenvectors with smaller eigenvalues also show oriented red-cyan edges. For a color reproduction of this figure, see <http://mitpress.mit.edu/Obermayer>.

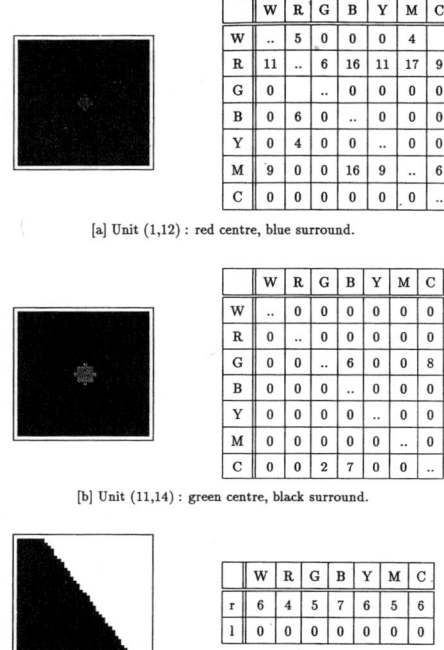

	W	R	G	B	Y	M	C
W	..	5	0	0	0	4	
R	11	..	6	16	11	17	9
G	0		..	0	0	0	0
B	0	6	0	..	0	0	0
Y	0	4	0	0	..	0	0
M	9	0	0	16	9	..	6
C	0	0	0	0	0	0	..

[a] Unit (1,12) : red centre, blue surround.

	W	R	G	B	Y	M	C
W	..	0	0	0	0	0	0
R	0	..	0	0	0	0	0
G	0	0	..	6	0	0	8
B	0	0	0	..	0	0	0
Y	0	0	0	0	..	0	0
M	0	0	0	0	0	..	0
C	0	0	2	7	0	0	..

[b] Unit (11,14) : green centre, black surround.

	W	R	G	B	Y	M	C
r	6	4	5	7	6	5	6
l	0	0	0	0	0	0	0

[c] Unit (1,14) : an oriented edge.

Figure 7: **Cell responses to artificial stimuli.** (a, b) The colored center-surround stimuli that elicit maximal responses from the two inhibitory units (1,12) and (11,14) (see Figure 6) are shown on the left. Unit (1,12) strongly prefers red/magenta against a blue background, whereas unit (11,14) prefers green against a black background. In the tables on the right are shown the unit's responses to stimuli with the optimal geometry, but with spot and background being any combination of white (W), red (R), green (G), blue (B), yellow (Y), magenta (M), or cyan (C) (rows determining center-color, and columns the surround-color). Precise interpretation is difficult, but it is apparent that unit (1,12) has a general preference for a red component in its center (i.e. red, yellow, or magenta) and unit (11,14) responds only if the central region has a green component (i.e. green or cyan). (c) The black/white step-edge that elicited maximal response from the inhibitory unit (1,14) (see Figure 6) is shown on the left; the stimulus is parameterized by phase and orientation. The table on the right shows the unit's response to stimuli of optimal orientation and phase, but with either the left (l) or right (r) side of the edge being black and the other being one of W, R, G, B, Y, M, or C. The responses to the 14 stimuli are shown: in cases where the direction of luminance contrast was correct, the unit was responsive regardless of color.

Model of "Color Blob" Formation

a gaussian of $\sigma = 5.0$ pixels to remove directional bias and possible edge effects, and the three patches were composed to give a vector of 1200($= 3 \times 20 \times 20$) elements. The two images of resolution 320 × 200 yield 108,962 such vectors and we found the principal components of this set by computing the eigenvectors of the corresponding covariance matrix (a matrix of 1200 × 1200). Finally, we took the 16 eigenvectors with largest eigenvalues[8] and reconstructed the color image patches that they represent.

3.2 Results. These 16 color eigenvectors, with their corresponding eigenvalues, are shown in Figure 6c.[9] The first component is a DC luminance component; the second is unoriented, and has a strong positive red DC component;[10] the third to fifth are low spatial-frequency contrast components without spectral differentiation; the sixth is unoriented, and has a strong positive green component; the remainder reflect higher spatial-frequency components, and generally show little spectral differentiation except for the eleventh and twelfth components, which are orthogonal red-cyan edges. From this we make the following conclusions:

- Luminance: The largest variation in the data by far is that of general luminance, which is reflected in the first eigenvector.

- Contrast: A large amount of the variation in the data can be accounted for as variation along a small number of vectors having similar profiles in the three spectral subspaces. These eigenvectors seem to code luminance contrast independently of color and resemble oriented bars and edges, although higher spatial frequency contrasts are reflected in the many eigenvectors with small eigenvalues. A very small amount of variation can be accounted for as variation along vectors having different profiles in the spectral subspaces; these seem to code color contrast.

- Color: A major variation in the data can be accounted for by two vectors for which the variation depends upon general color but not spatial structure.

- General: It seems that the optimal linear code keeps color and contrast apart, bringing them together only to account for subtle variations in the data. The noncolor part of the code reflects the known power spectrum of natural images (Field 1987)

---

[8]The sum of the first 16 eigenvalues is over 90% of the sum of all eigenvalues.
[9]For display, $g_i = 127.5 + (e_i * 127.5/e_{max})$ where i indexes into eigenvector e, g ($0 < g \leq 255$) is the spectral intensity, and e_{max} is the maximum absolute value in e.
[10]It should be borne in mind that all eigenvectors are orthogonal to one another; therefore, this vector with a positive red component must also have a negative cyan component (dominated by the red in the display) to maintain orthogonality to the first eigenvector.

We carried out similar analyses for different images and smaller window sizes and found that window size made no significant difference to the eigenvectors and values. Different images yielded some small variation in eigenvectors, and the ordering of the vectors, reflecting different statistics. However, they supported the same general conclusions.

3.3 Interpretation. It is interesting to compare the differences between the linear code and what is known of the biological code, with reference to the network described above, and speculate upon reasons for the differences.

First, the eigenvector analysis suggests that color coding, and some general luminance coding, should be DC, ignoring spatial contrast. However, in reality both color and luminance contrast are implemented at the earliest retinal stages in the mammalian visual system. For this reason we are particularly bad at judging either absolute luminance, or color in the absence of boundaries (see Land 1964). We suggest two possible speculative explanations why the biological design may have evolved to be as it is. One reason is that the principle of optimality guiding evolution may be different to that of maximizing information: an evolving organism is not interested in *all* information but in that information that maximizes its survival chances. It may be that it is color and luminance contrast that is most useful for survival, and the DC component, if not filtered out early, would dominate and reduce fitness. Another reason might be that to code the DC component would require neurons to be accurate over such a huge range that their resolution would be poor; by ignoring the DC they can have an adaptive dynamic range with much higher resolution (this would be similar to the strategy adopted by foveal sampling of the image).

Second, examination of the receptive fields in Figure 6 and Figure 7 seems to suggest many color-selective cells are interested in the overall color of their input, regardless of luminance or color contrast. This would be expected from the eigenvector analysis; however, it is not the same as the properties of cells in color blobs that exhibit both color and luminance contrast selectivity, and would be surprising since we modeled both types of contrast at the retina. However, in our model cortical cells can respond *only* to input patterns containing luminance or color contrast[11]; these cells therefore respond not to "red-ness" per se but to red color borders, regardless of the orientation of the border or the color making up its other side.[12] As such, they must be classified as red-center, broad-band-surround in line with Figure 7a. We predict that a larger model, with cells having a larger inhibitory range, would result in increased response selectivity; for instance, cells might respond only to red-green borders at all orientations, and so become red-center green-surround.

---

[11] Otherwise geniculate cells will have zero output.

[12] It is this generality of response that leads to the cell's high metabolic rate.

4 Discussion

In the research reported here, we have been able to demonstrate that it is *possible* for color-blob type structures to develop in an artificial neural network purely through activity-induced adaptation in reponse to natural color images. Moreover, a single mechanism simultaneously develops unoriented color-selective cells and orientation-selective achromatic cells, with smooth variation of receptive fields across the cortical array. The key components of the model that are responsible for this behavior include the following:

- Input from natural color images. The local statistics of images determine the types of receptive field developed by cortical units.
- Multichannel preprocessing of image data. The center-surround receptive fields of retinal and geniculate cells accentuate the importance of contrast and color contrast at boundaries in the image.
- Hebbian-type unsupervised adaptation of cortical units. This results in units with weight patterns related to the principal components of preprocessed image fragments.
- Lateral excitatory and inhibitory interaction within the cortex. The long-range inhibition implements competition among units, so that they do not all develop the same pattern of weights. The short-range excitation causes neighboring units to develop similar weight patterns, so that receptive field properties vary smoothly across the array.

The combination of these components results in several of the characteristics of primate striate cortex. Moreover, related research suggests that the same mechanisms may also be responsible for ocular dominance stripes and retinotopic mapping (Miller *et al.* 1989; Miller 1990, 1994; Goodhill 1993). The apparent complexity and sophistication of cortical organization might be due primarily to the interaction of a basic set of mechanisms and architecture with the implicit structure of the sensory data.

We should state firmly, however, that we do not claim that activity-induced adaptation is solely responsible for cortical organization. There is evidence, for example, that tropic mechanisms play a part in development of retinotopic maps (see Constantine-Paton *et al.* 1990).

Even if cortical organization were discovered to be *largely* specified in detail genetically, there would still be the question of how the specification might have evolved. Our experiments hint at a possible answer. Suppose that at an early evolutionary stage the primary mechanism of organization of some characteristic was activity-induced adaptation. While the final result might confer an advantage on a mature individual, an immature one would be more vulnerable. If evolution could discover a process that would accelerate development, the species would become fitter. It is interesting to speculate that in some cases the plasticity of the nervous system might be the driving force in breaking new ground for a species, with genetic specification an optimization process following behind, rather than the other way round (see Hinton and Nowlan 1987).

Acknowledgments

Thanks to Jim Stone for various suggestions relating to this work, and detailed comments on the paper. This work has been supported by a grant from the UK Science and Engineering Research Council and the Ministry of Defence.

References

Barrow, H. G. 1987. Learning receptive fields. *IEEE First International Conference on Neural Nets*, IV, 115–121.

Barrow, H. G., and Bray, A. J. 1992. Activity-induced "colour blob" formation. In *Artificial Neural Networks II: Proceedings of the International Conference on Artificial Neural Networks*, I. Aleksander and J. Taylor, eds., Elsevier, Amsterdam.

Carroll, E., and Wong-Riley, M. T. T. 1982. Light and e.m. analysis of cytochrome oxidase-rich zones in the striate cortex of squirrel monkeys. *Soc. for Neurosc. Abstr.* **8**, 706.

Constantine-Paton, M., Cline, H. T., and Debski, E. 1990. Patterned activity, synaptic convergence, and the NMDA receptor in developing visual pathways. *Annu. Rev. Neurosci.* **13**, 129–154.

Daugman, J. G. 1985. Uncertainty relation for resolution in space, spatial frequency, and orientation optimised by two-dimensional visual cortical filters. *J. Opt. Soc. Am.* **2**, 1160–1169.

Erwin, E., Obermayer, K., and Schulten, K. 1995. Models of orientation and ocular dominance columns in the visual cortex: A critical comparison. *Neural Comp.* **7**, 425–468.

Field, D. J. 1987. Relations between the statistics of natural images and the response properties of cortical cells. *J, Opt. Soc. Am.* **4**, 2379–2394.

Goodhill, G. J. 1993. Topography and ocular dominance: A model exploring positive correlations. *Biol. Cybern.* **69**, 109–118.

Gouras, P. 1974. Opponent-colour cells in different layers of foveal striate cortex. *J. Physiol. (London)* **238**, 583–602.

Hendrickson, A. E., Hunt, S. P., and Wu, J. Y. 1981. Immunocytochemical localization of glutamic acid decarboxylase in monkey striate cortex. *Nature (London)* **292**, 605.

Hinton, G. E., and Nowlan, S. J. 1987. How learning can guide evolution. *Complex Syst.* **1**, 495–502.

Horton, J. C. 1984. Cytochrome oxidase patches: A new cytoarchitectonic feature of monkey visual cortex. *Phil. Transact. Royal Soc. London (Biol.)* **304**, 199–253.

Horton, J. C., and Hubel, D. H. 1981. Regular patchy distribution of cytochrome oxidase staining in primary visual cortex of macaque monkey. *Nature (London)* **292**, 762–764.

Hubel, D. H., and Wiesel, T. N. 1968. Receptive fields and functional architecture of monkey striate cortex. *J. Physiol.* **195**, 215–243.

Kuljis, R. O., and Rakic, P. 1990. Hypercolumns in primate visual cortex can develop in the absence of cues from photoreceptors. *Proc. Natl. Acad. Sci. U.S.A.* **87**, 5303–5306.

Lachica, E. A., Beck, P. D., and Casagrande, V. A. 1992. Parallel pathways in macaque striate cortex: Anatomically defined columns in layer III. *Proc. Natl. Acad. Sci. U.S.A.* **89**, 3566–3570.

Land, E. H. 1964. The retinex. *Sci. Am.* **52**, 247–264.

Linsker, R. 1990. Self-organization in a perceptual system: How network models and information theory may shed light on neural organization. In *Connectionist Modeling and Brain Function: The Developing Interface*, S. J. Hanson and C. R. Olson, eds., pp. 351–392. MIT Press, Cambridge, MA.

Livingstone, M. S., and Hubel, D. H. 1984. Anatomy and physiology of a color system in the primate visual cortex. *J. Neurosci.* **4**, 309–356.

Malach, R. 1992. Dendritic sampling across processing streams in monkey striate cortex. *J. Comp. Neurol.* **315**, 303–312.

Michael, C. R. 1981. Columnar organization of color cells in monkey's striate cortex. *J. Neurophysiol.* **46**, 587–604.

Miller, K. D. 1990. Correlation-based models of neural development. In *Neuroscience and Connectionist Theory*, M. A. Gluck and D. E. Rumelhart, eds., pp. 267–353. Lawrence Erlbaum Associates, Hillsdale, NJ.

Miller, K. D. 1994. A model for the development of simple cell receptive fields and the ordered arrangement of orientation columns through activity-dependent competition between ON- and OFF-center inputs. *J. Neurosci.* **14**, 409–441.

Miller, K. D., Keller, J. B., and Stryker, M. P. 1989. Ocular dominance column development: Analysis and simulation. *Science* **245**, 605–615.

Nealy, T. A., and Maunsell, J. H. R. 1994. Magnocellular and parvocellular contributions to the responses of neurons in macaque striate cortex. *J. Neurosci.* **14**, 2069–2079.

Purves, D., and Lamantia, A. 1993. Development of blobs in the visual cortex of macaques. *J. Comp. Neurol.* **334**, 169–175.

Robson, J. G. 1983. Frequency domain visual processing. In *Physical and Biological Processing of Images*, O. J. Braddick and A. C. Sleigh, eds. Springer-Verlag, New York.

Stafstrom, C. E., Schwindt, P. C., and Crill, W. E. 1984. Repetitive firing in layer V neurons from cat neocortex in vitro. *J. Neurophysiol.* **52**, 264–277.

Trusk, T. C., Kaboord, W. S., and Wong-Riley, M. T. T. 1990. Effects of monocular enucleation, tetrodotoxin, and lid suture on cytochrome oxidase reactivity in supragranular puffs of adult macaque striate cortex. *Visual Neurosci.* **4**, 185–204.

Ts'o, D. Y., and Gilbert, C. D. 1988. The organization of chromatic and spatial interactions in the primate striate cortex. *J. Neurosci.* **8**, 1712–1727.

Malsburg, C. von der 1973. Self-organisation of orientation sensitive cells in the striata cortex. *Kybernetik* **14**, 85–100.

Wehmeier, U., Dong, D., Koch, C., and Van Essen, D. 1989. Modelling the mammalian visual system. In *Methods in Neuronal Modelling*, C. Koch and I. Segev, eds. MIT Press, Cambridge, MA.

Wiesel, T. N., and Hubel, D. H. 1966. Spatial and chromatic interactions in the lateral geniculate body of the rhesus monkey. *J. Neurophysiol.* **29**, 1115–1156.

Wong-Riley, M. T. T. 1979. Changes in the visual system of monocularly sutured or enucleated cats demonstrable with cytochrome oxidase histochemistry. *Brain Res.* **171**, 11–28.

Wong-Riley, M. T. T. 1994. Primate visual cortex: Dynamic metabolic organization and plasticity revealed by cytochrome oxidase. In *Cerebral Cortex Vol. 10, Primary Visual Cortex in Primates*, A. Peters and K. S. Rockland, eds., pp. 141–200. Plenum Press, New York.

Wong-Riley, M. T. T., and Carroll, E. W. 1984. The effect of impulse blockage on cytochrome oxidase activity in the monkey visual system. *Nature (London)* **307**, 262–264.

12

A Type of Duality between Self-Organizing Maps and Minimal Wiring

Graeme Mitchison
The Laboratory of Molecular Biology, Hills Road, Cambridge, CB2 2QH, U.K.

I show here that two interpretations of neural maps are closely related. The first, due to Kohonen, sees these maps as forming by an adaptive process in response to stimuli. The second—the minimal wiring or dimension-reduction perspective—interprets the maps as the solution of a minimization problem, where the goal is to keep the "wiring" between neurons with similar receptive fields as short as possible. Recent work by Luttrell provides a bridging concept, by showing that Kohonen's algorithm can be regarded as an approximation to gradient descent on a certain functional. I show how this functional can be generalized in a way that allows it to be interpreted as a measure of wirelength.

1 Introduction

Self-organizing algorithms have been widely used to model the formation of neural maps (von der Malsburg 1973; Willshaw and von der Malsburg 1976; Swindale 1980; Kohonen 1984; Miller *et al.* 1989; Obermayer *et al.* 1990). The maps produced by these algorithms tend to place neurons with similar receptive field properties close together. If connections were made mostly between neurons with similar receptive fields, this arrangement would allow the connections to be short. This suggests that maps produced by a wirelength constraint may be related to those made by self-organizing algorithms (Durbin and Mitchison 1990). I show here that Kohonen's algorithm and minimal wiring are indeed closely related mathematically.

2 Self-Organization and Dimension Reduction

Kohonen's algorithm (Kohonen 1984) defines a map $f: X \to Y$, where X can be interpreted as a neural structure (e.g., visual cortex), Y as a parameter space of variables describing the stimuli that neurons respond to (e.g., oriented light bars), and the image $f(x)$ as the stimulus to which a neuron x responds most strongly. The algorithm describes how f changes in response to a stimulus $y \in Y$:

$$\Delta f(x) \sim A[x - n_f(y)][y - f(x)] \qquad (2.1)$$

where A is a weighting function, a gaussian for instance, and $n_f(y)$ is the point x' in X that minimizes $|y - f(x')|$.

In the case of visual cortex X could be taken to be a 2D sheet (a surface view of the cortex), and Y would encode retinotopic position, orientation, ocular dominance, and perhaps other variables, and would therefore be of a higher dimension. To picture the behavior of such maps, it is helpful to consider a very simplified case, where X is a line and Y a square. One can then see how the algorithm leads to a folded map of X into Y (e.g., Fig. 4a).

An alternative conceptual framework was proposed by Durbin and Mitchison (1990), who suggested that one should look at one-to-one functions g from Y to X that map points that lie close in Y as close as possible on X. Because the dimension of Y is generally greater than X they referred to g as a "dimension reducing" map. The idea is that g maps receptive fields onto the units in X in such a way that operations that are local in the parameter space take place in a spatially localized region of the neural structure. Thus connections between neurons with similar receptive fields can be kept short; in fact, one can make this the defining property of these maps and look for maps from Y to X that minimize some measure of wirelength.

An example of this problem (Mitchison and Durbin 1986) arises in the simplified case considered above, where Y is a square, treated as a discrete $k \times k$ array, and X is a line, treated as the discrete set of points $1, 2, \ldots, k^2$. One seeks 1-1 maps g that minimize the wirelength measure defined by

$$C = \sum_{i,j} |g(i,j) - g(i+1,j)|^p + |g(i,j) - g(i,j+1)|^p \qquad (2.2)$$

with $p > 0$. When $p = 1$, C just sums the distance in X between the images of a point (i, j) in Y and those of its four nearest neighbors in Y. The minimizing map is shown in Figure 1; it is qualitatively different from the type of map produced by the Kohonen algorithm. Something more like the latter is produced when $p < 1$, for then longer connections are relatively less heavily penalized and the map tends to become folded in a way that allows many short connections to be made at the cost of occasional longer ones (of the same type as Fig. 4c).

3 Interpretations of Kohonen's Algorithm in Terms of Functionals

Consider two maps $f : X \to Y$ and $g : Y \to X$. The functional

$$D = \int A(\xi) |y - f[g(y) + \xi]|^2 \, d\xi \, dy \qquad (3.1)$$

Self-Organizing Maps and Minimal Wiring

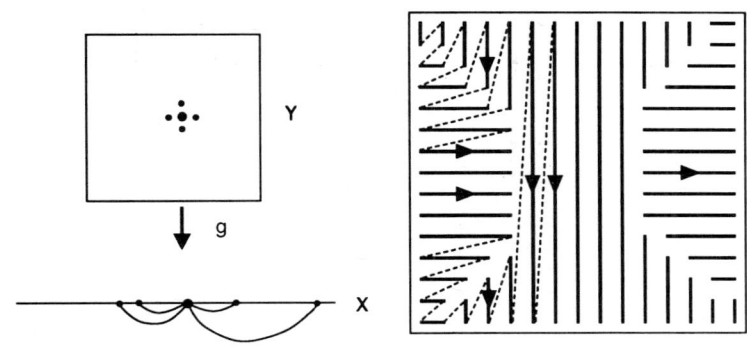

Figure 1: An example of a wirelength measure. The parameter space Y is a square, represented discretely as a $k \times k$ array, and the neural tissue X is a line segment, represented by the integers $1, 2 \ldots, k^2$. The map $g : Y \to X$ is assumed to be one-to-one. Each point x in X is therefore the image under g of some y in Y; we can think of this as assigning the receptive field characterized by y. If y is the point (i,j), the four nearest neighbors in Y are mapped to four points in X, and the requirement is that these be connected by neural "wiring." (At the boundaries, the number of these connections is reduced to those that lie within the square; there is no wrap-around.) The cost C given by 2.2 measures the lengths of these connections, each link being counted once only. The minimal cost map for $p = 1$ is also shown. It is represented by joining up points in Y that map to successive values in X, i.e., by sketching the inverse image of X in Y. The arrows indicate the direction on the line X, and the dotted lines mark jumps in Y between consecutive points in X.

measures the mean squared error in encoding by the function g and decoding by the function f, given that noise ξ with distribution A is added to the encoded message $g(y)$. Gradient descent on f gives the rule $\Delta f(x) \sim -\delta D/\delta f(x) = \int [y - f(x)]A[x - g(y)]\,dy$. Instead of choosing x and integrating over y, one can pick a y and change all x according to $\Delta f(x) \sim [y - f(x)]A[x - g(y)]$, which is like Kohonen's rule with $g(y)$ replacing $n_f(y)$. In fact, in the case where A is a δ-function, it is clear that D is minimized by choosing $g(y)$ to be the point in X that maps closest to y under f, since then $D = \int |y - f[g(y)]|^2\,dy$. Thus, if we ignore the noise for the purpose of calculating g, we obtain 2.1. This is Luttrell's interpretation of Kohonen's algorithm (Luttrell 1989, 1990); the intuition behind it is illustrated in Figure 2. Following Luttrell, we refer to 3.1 as a minimal distortion (MD) functional.

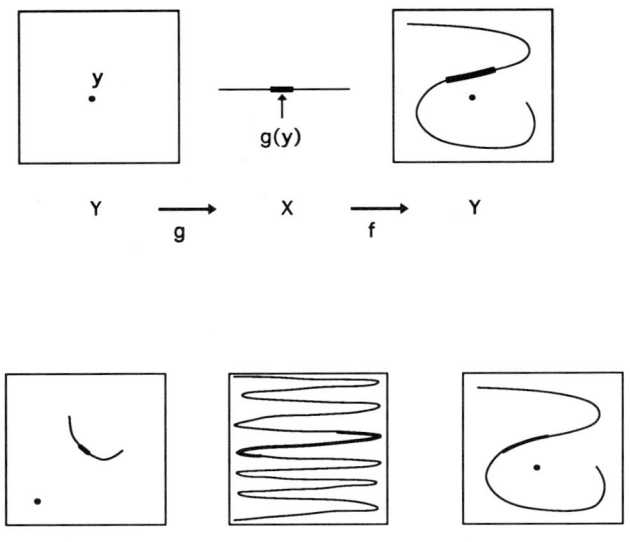

Figure 2: Luttrell's interpretation of Kohonen's algorithm envisages two maps, an encoding map g, here shown mapping from the square Y to the line X, and a decoding map f. Noise is added to the image of a point under g—the thickened line segment around $g(y)$—and the aim is to find maps f and g that minimize the error: the average distance from points in Y to the distribution of decoded points (shown, for the point y, as the thickened arc). One can get some feeling for how this works by supposing that g is the nearest neighbor map n_f, and imagining two fairly extreme types of map f. In the first, f maps to a short segment in Y, which means that the spread due to noise is small. The error is small for a point y that lies close to this segment, but is large for a point that lies far from it (leftmost figure below). In the second case f tries to map close to every point in Y by making lots of wiggles. For every y in Y there is therefore a point in the image set that comes close, but the fact that the curve is stretched out means that the image points are widely spread out by the noise (center below), and this gives rise to a large overall error. The best solution (right below) requires the kind of compromise between length and the space-filling property that is characteristic of self-organizing maps.

When A is not a δ-function, n_f gives only an approximation to g. One might hope to obtain a more accurate energy function for Kohonen's algorithm by replacing g by n_f, and defining

$$E = \int A(\xi)|y - f[n_f(y) + \xi]|^2 \, d\xi \, dy \qquad (3.2)$$

Self-Organizing Maps and Minimal Wiring

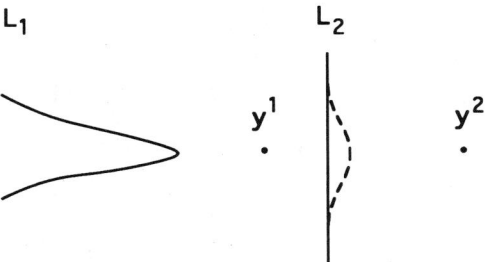

Figure 3: A situation in which the NN functional increases when the Kohonen algorithm is applied. We take the standard dimension-increasing case, and consider the functional $\int P(y)A(\xi)|y - f[n_f(y) + \xi]|^2 d\xi dy$ (Ritter and Schulten 1988). This, except for the term $P(y)$ that allows a nonuniform distribution of stimuli—elsewhere in the paper assumed to be constant—is the analogue of 3.2. We consider a distribution P where there are only two stimuli, y^1 and y^2. Two segments, L_1 and L_2 of a line mapped into a 2D space are shown. Initially, the nearest point to both y^1 and y^2 lies on L_2, and since y^2 is farther from L_2, the effect of a cycle during which both stimuli are applied is to pull L_2 a little toward y^2 (final position shown by dotted line). We can arrange that, after this round, the nearest point to y^1 lies on L_1. By making the curvature of L_1 large, the increased contribution from $\int A(\xi)|y^1 - f[n_f(y^1) + \xi]|^2 d\xi$ can be made sufficiently large to ensure that the functional increases.

(Ritter and Schulten 1988; we use the integral notation as shorthand for the discrete sum used to compute such functionals). In fact, E cannot be an exact energy function, as shown by the situation in Figure 3 (see also Erwin *et al.* 1992). However, we shall see that E often gives a good approximation to an energy function. We refer to E as the nearest-neighbor (NN) functional.

4 Wirelength Interpreted as a Functional

Suppose we reverse the order of the maps used in the previous section to define the MD functional, so f does the "encoding" and g the "decoding," with the noise acting on the parameter space. The MD functional analogous to 3.1 is then

$$D = \int B(v)|x - g[f(x) + v]|^2 dx\, dv \qquad (4.1)$$

and the corresponding NN functional is

$$E = \int B(v)|x - g[n_g(x) + v]|^2 \, dx \, dv \tag{4.2}$$

Comparing 4.2 with 2.2 suggests that one can interpret 4.2 as a wirelength functional. In 2.2, g can be regarded as allocating receptive fields to points on the 1D cortex X. In 4.2, the map n_g acts as an inverse to g, associating to each x in X the receptive field $n_g(x)$. The functional 4.2 then measures the average result of picking an x in X, taking its receptive field $n_g(x)$, perturbing this by v, then taking the squared distance in X from x to the point that has this perturbed receptive field.

It is natural to generalize both 4.1 and 4.2 so as to allow other measures of wirelength. For example, one might replace $|x - g[f(x) + v]|^2$ by $|x - g[f(x) + v)]|^p$, as in 2.2, or by a gaussian, as proposed by Yuille et al. (1991). A generalized functional of the MD type is $D(f, g; A, B) = \int A[x - g(f(x) + v)]B(v) \, dx \, dv$, where A and B are arbitrary functions (we shall often leave out A and B from the notation). Its NN analogue is $D(n_g, g; A, B) = \int A[x - g(n_g(x) + v)]B(v) \, dx \, dv$. One might hope that these functionals would be minimized by similar maps. Further, comparing $D(n_g, g; A, B)$ with 3.2 suggests that one may be able to minimize this functional, approximately at least, by a generalized Kohonen-type self-organizing algorithm operating in the dimension-reducing direction

$$\Delta g(y) \sim A'[x - g(y)]B[y - n_g(x)] \tag{4.3}$$

One can rewrite $D(f, g)$ in a way that shows a type of duality between self-organizing mapping algorithms and minimal wiring. Substituting $y = f(x) + v$ we have $D(f, g) = \int A[x - g(y)]B[y - f(x)] \, dx \, dy$, and putting $\xi = x - g(y)$ gives $D(f, g) = \int A(\xi)B[y - f(g(y) + \xi)] \, d\xi \, dy$. Again, one might hope that similar maps minimize this functional and $D(f, n_f)$, and that a good approximation to the f that minimizes $D(f, n_f)$ can be found by a Kohonen-type algorithm

$$\Delta f(x) \sim A[x - n_f(y)]B'[y - f(x)] \tag{4.4}$$

One can think of this as defining a self-organizing map of the "cortex," i.e., in the standard dimension-increasing direction $X \to Y$. The situation can be summed up by the following schema:

dimension-increasing Kohonen map 4.4 $\leftrightarrow$ *minimal* $D(f, n_f)$ $\leftrightarrow$ *minimal* $D(f, g)$ $\leftrightarrow$ *minimal wiring functional* $D(n_g, g)$ $\leftrightarrow$ *dimension-reducing Kohonen map* 4.3

where $\leftrightarrow$ indicates an approximation whose quality has to be ascertained.

5 The Gaussian Case

As mentioned above, 2.2 produces the most biologically plausible-looking maps when $p < 1$ (Durbin and Mitchison 1990). Unfortunately, the algorithms using $|x - x_0|^p$ as a wirelength measure behave badly near $x = x_0$

Self-Organizing Maps and Minimal Wiring   241

when $p < 1$. Yuille *et al.* (1991), in the context of a dimension-reducing model using the elastic net (Durbin and Willshaw 1987), suggested using the cost function $-A$, where A is a gaussian. This behaves well at $x = x_0$, and might be expected to allow fractal-type maps since, like 2.2 with $p < 1$, it does not penalize long distances too highly. We now examine this case, assuming that both A and B in $D(f,g;A,B)$ are gaussians, with standard deviations σ_A and σ_B, respectively, and *maximizing* the corresponding MD and NN functionals (which is equivalent to minimizing these functionals with $-A$ in place of A).

The self-organizing cortical mapping algorithm 4.4 then becomes

$$\Delta f(x) \sim [y-f(x)] \exp\{-[x-n_f(y)]^2/2\sigma_A^2\} \exp\{-[y-f(x)]^2/2\sigma_B^2\} \quad (5.1)$$

This amounts to a standard form of Kohonen's algorithm—compare with 2.1—except for the factor $\exp\{-[y - f(x)]^2/2\sigma_B^2\}$, which implies that a point in X must map sufficiently close to the stimulus y for $f(x)$ to be appreciably changed by the algorithm. In neural language, this amounts to the entirely plausible condition that a neuron's response characteristics can be altered by a stimulus only if the neuron is sufficiently strongly activated by that stimulus.

Figure 4a shows a map computed by 5.1 for the case $X =$ line, $Y =$ square, with $\sigma_A = 0.005$ (the 1D variance) and $\sigma_B = 0.2$. The self-organizing algorithm in the dimension-reducing direction 4.3 has a similar form to 5.1; Figure 4b shows the computed map g, and 4c its "inverse" n_g. MD maps, i.e., maps f and g that maximize $D(f,g)$, were obtained by gradient ascent on f and g, writing $D(f,g)$ in the form $\int A[x - g(y)]B[y - f(x)]\,dx\,dy$ and functionally differentiating with respect to f and g. This gives the *bidirectional* algorithm:

$$\Delta f(x) \sim A[g(y) - x]B'[f(x) - y]$$
$$\Delta g(y) \sim A'[g(y) - x]B[f(x) - y] \quad (5.2)$$

Figure 4d shows the map f computed in this way. Although its overall shape is different from the NN map in 4a, the periodicity and "wiggliness" are similar. This is reflected in the similar values of the functionals $D(f, n_f)$ for 4a and $D(f,g)$ for 4d (Table 1); the NN map f does a good job of maximizing $D(f,g)$. Thus the Kohonen-type algorithm 4.4 seems to find near-maximal maps, even though $D(f, n_f)$ is not an exact energy function; in fact, one can apply 4.4 with the constraint that only steps that increase $D(f, n_f)$ are accepted, and this gives final maps very similar to their unconstrained counterparts (this is also true in the dimension-reducing direction). The $\leftrightarrow$ steps in the first line of our schema therefore represent good approximations, and this is true for a range of values of σ_A and σ_B (Table 1).

The map n_g in Figure 4c looks different from either 4a or 4d, but this is largely due to the discrete nature of the lattice used for the computations (see legend to Fig. 4); suitably smoothed, the generic resemblance

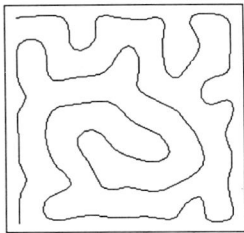
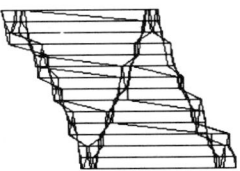

Figure 4: (a) was obtained by the NN map 4.4 from an initial random map. The unit interval $X = [0,1]$ was subdivided into 225 points, and Y treated as the square $[0,1] \times [0,1]$. With the standard Kohonen algorithm, "annealing," or gradually decreasing the size of the neighborhood of points that are moved by the algorithm, often gives the best maps (Kohonen 1984). Similar procedures worked for all the algorithms used here (i.e., 4.3, 4.4, and 5.2). The variances σ_A and σ_B were intially set to 0.2, a large enough value to give a smooth map, and then decreased every 100 iterations so as to attain their final values in 10 steps. The rate constant for the update equation 4.4 was 0.1. (b,c) Dimension-reducing map defined by the NN algorithm 4.3 for A and B gaussian with $\sigma_A = 0.01$, $\sigma_B = 0.2$. Y was represented as the 15×15 discrete lattice, and X as the unit interval $[0,1]$. The map was initially random, and the annealing procedure and rate constant were the same as for (a). The map g is shown in (b) by mapping each lattice point (i,j) onto the point $[g(i,j),j]$; one can informally describe this representation as sliding every point of the square lattice horizontally so that it lies over its image value (under g) in the line. The map n_g is shown in (c) by tracing the map n_g on the lattice while moving continuously along the unit interval X. *Continued facing page.*

becomes evident. In fact, the value of $D(n_g, g)$ from the maps in 4b and 4c is not far from the computed maximal value of $D(f,g)$ (Table 1). Thus the $\leftrightarrow$ steps in the second line of our schema amount to good approximations when $\sigma_A = 0.005$, $\sigma_B = 0.2$. When σ_A is larger, e.g., for the other values of σ_A and σ_B shown in Table 1, the situation is more subtle. Given maps f and g that maximize $D(f,g)$, we have seen that f gives a good approximation to the NN map from 4.4; Table 1 also shows that the map g, together with n_g derived from it, comes close to maximizing the wiring functional: compare the values of $D(n_g, g)$ from 4.3 and 5.2 in Table 1 for all σ_A, σ_B. Yet when $\sigma_A = 0.2$ and 0.5, $D(f,g)$ and $D(n_g, g)$ are no longer so close in value, and this reflects the fact that the map f differs substantially from n_g for larger values of σ_A. This means we can regard the associated $\leftrightarrow$ steps as good approximations, but must relinquish the intuitive notion that $f(x)$ and $n_g(x)$ serve the same role of defining the "receptive field at x."

Self-Organizing Maps and Minimal Wiring

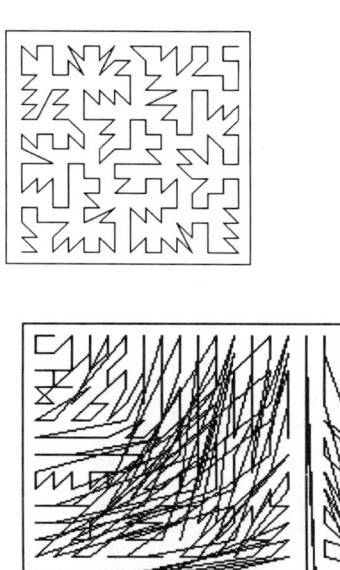
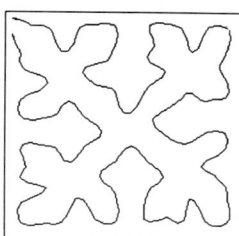
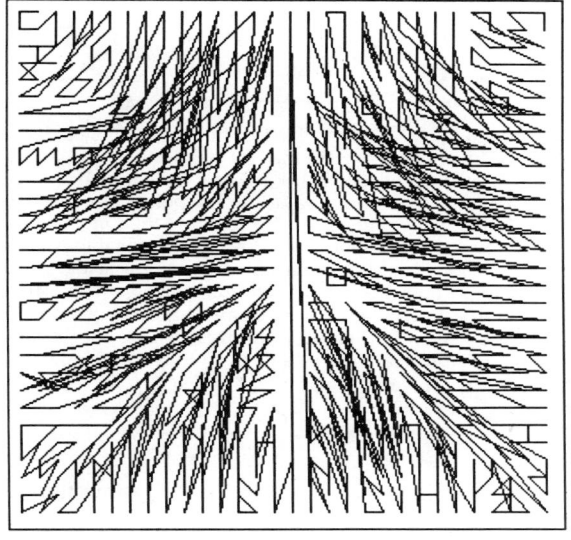

Figure 4: (d) The MD map obtained by 5.2 from a random initial map, with annealing procedure as above and a rate constant of 0.03. The source space for each of the maps, f and g, was treated as discrete—a 15×15 lattice for Y and 225 points for X—and its image space as continuous. The program cycled through a random ordering of all point pairs (x, y), where each of x, y was chosen from the corresponding discrete set. (e) The map n_g obtained from 4.3 when $A(x) = |x|$ and $B(y - y_0) = 0$ unless y is y_0 or one of its four nearest neighbors, when $B(y - y_0) = 1$. The algorithm becomes $\Delta g(y) \sim B[y - n_g(x)]$ if $x > g(y)$ and $\Delta g(y) \sim -B[y - n_g(x)]$ if $x \leq g(y)$. A small rate constant (0.001) gave the best results, and no annealing was necessary, the map sorting itself out from a random starting configuration. Note that the map is similar to, but not identical to, the theoretical best solution for 2.2 with $p = 1$ (Fig. 1), the central region of stripes in the latter being reduced to a single stripe in n_g. This probably reflects the fact that the map obtained from 4.3 is not constrained to spread its image points uniformly on the line, whereas the image points defined by 2.2 are equally spaced (the points $1, 2, \ldots, k^2$).

Table 1: Values of MD and NN Functionals[a]

	$\sigma_A = 0.005$ $\sigma_B = 0.2$	$\sigma_A = 0.5$ $\sigma_B = 0.05$	$\sigma_A = 0.2$ $\sigma_B = 0.2$
$D(f, n_f)$ f from 4.4	2.69	3.45	36.4
$D(n_g, g)$ g from 4.3	2.66	3.15	29.6
$D(f, g)$	2.69	3.49	38.6
$D(f, n_f)$	2.69	3.47	36.8
$D(n_g, g)$ f, g from 5.2	2.65	3.23	28.7

[a]This shows the values of MD and NN functionals calculated for various maps. Comparisons of these functionals, for the case of quadratic B (equations 3.1 and 3.2), have also been made by Luttrell (1992). Each map, computed as described in the legend to Figure 4, assigned continuous values to the points of a discrete source space (a 15 × 15 lattice for Y and 225 points for X). To compute the functional, the continuous image space was sampled progressively more finely until a stable value was achieved. Typically, a 30×30 lattice for Y and 1000 points for X gave satisfactory results. In the case of the Kohonen-like algorithms 4.3 and 4.4, the functionals whose values are given—$D(n_g, g)$ and $D(f, n_f)$ respectively—are those that are (approximately) maximized by the algorithm. The bidirectional algorithm 5.2 maximizes $D(f, g)$, but the values of $D(n_g, g)$ and $D(f, n_f)$ are also given (calculating n_f and n_g from the maximizing maps f and g, respectively), for comparison with 4.3 and 4.4.

6 Conclusions

The duality between minimal wiring and self-organizing maps rests on the fact that the functionals defined by $\int A[x - g(f(x) + v)]B(v)\,dx\,dv$ and $\int A(\xi)B[y - f(g(y) + \xi)]\,d\xi\,dy$ are equivalent, even though the direction of the underlying maps has been reversed (and the roles of the noise and wirelength functions, A and B, have been swapped). We could *define* these to be our wirelength and self-organizing functionals, respectively. But if we wish to stick closer to the concept of a Kohonen-type self-organizing map, and of a wirelength measure like 2.2, then certain approximations have to be checked: the ↔ steps in our schema. These turn out to be quite accurate for gaussian functions A and B, though only the case where the variance of A is small is realistic from the point of view of generating cortex-like maps. Some further exploration of the range of validity of these approximations is called for. Other, nongaussian, wiring measures might also be investigated. For example, Figure 4e shows the dimension-reducing NN map obtained with an absolute value wirelength. This is modeled on the cost function 2.2 with $p = 1$, and the resemblance to the theoretical best solution for this cost function is striking (Fig. 1).

Acknowledgments

I thank David MacKay for stimulating discussions, and Geoffrey Goodhill, Stephen Luttrell, Martin Simmen, and David Willshaw for helpful comments on this paper.

References

Durbin, R. M., and Mitchison, G. J. 1990. A dimension reduction framework for cortical maps. *Nature (London)* **343**, 644–647.

Durbin, R. M., and Willshaw, D. 1987. An analog approach to the travelling salesman problem using an elastic net method. *Nature (London)* **326**, 689–691.

Erwin, E., Obermayer, K., and Schulten, D. 1992. Self-organizing maps: Ordering, convergence properties and energy functionals. *Biol. Cybern.* **67**, 47–55.

Kohonen, T. 1984. *Self-Organization and Associative Memory*. Springer-Verlag, Berlin.

Luttrell, S. P. 1989. Self-organization: A derivation from first principles of a class of learning algorithms. *Proc. 3rd IEEE IJCNN*, Washington **2**, 495–498.

Luttrell, S. P. 1990. Derivation of a class of training algorithms. *IEEE Transact. Neural Networks* **1**, 229–232.

Luttrell, S. P. 1992. Self-supervised adaptive networks. *IEE Proc.-F* **139**, 371–377.

Miller, K. D., Keller, J. B., and Stryker, M. P. 1989. Ocular dominance column development: Analysis and simulation. *Science* **245**, 605–615.

Mitchison, G. J., and Durbin R. 1986. Optimal numberings of an $N \times N$ array. *S.I.A.M. J. Alg. Disc. Meth.* **7**, 571–582.

Obermayer, K., Ritter, H., and Schulten, K. 1990. A principle for the formation of the spatial structure of cortical feature maps. *Proc. Natl. Acad. Sci. U.S.A.* **87**, 8345–8349.

Ritter, H., and Schulten, K. 1988. Kohonen's self-organizing maps: Exploring their computational capabilities. In *IEEE International Conference on Neural Networks* (San Diego 1988), Vol. 1, pp. 109–116. IEEE, New York.

Swindale, N. V. 1980. A model for the formation of ocular dominance stripes. *Proc. R. Soc. London B* **208**, 243–264.

von der Malsburg, C. 1973. Self-organization of orientation sensitive cells in the striate cortex. *Kybernetik* **14**, 85–100.

Willshaw, D. J., and von der Malsburg, C. 1976. How patterned neural connections can be set up by self-organization. *Proc. R. Soc. London B* **194**, 431–445.

Yuille, A. L., Kolodny, J. A., and Lee, C. W. 1991. Dimension reduction, generalized deformable models and the development of ocularity and orientation. *Proc. IJCNN*, Seattle **2**, 597–602.

IV

Self-Organizing Maps for Unsupervised Data Analysis

13

A Bayesian Analysis of Self-Organizing Maps

Stephen P. Luttrell
Adaptive Systems Theory Section, Defence Research Agency,
St. Andrews Rd., Malvern, Worcestershire, WR14 3PS, United Kingdom

In this paper Bayesian methods are used to analyze some of the properties of a special type of Markov chain. The forward transitions through the chain are followed by inverse transitions (using Bayes' theorem) backward through a copy of the same chain; this will be called a folded Markov chain. If an appropriately defined Euclidean error (between the original input and its "reconstruction" via Bayes' theorem) is minimized with respect to the choice of Markov chain transition probabilities, then the familiar theories of both vector quantizers and self-organizing maps emerge. This approach is also used to derive the theory of self-supervision, in which the higher layers of a multilayer network supervise the lower layers, even though overall there is no external teacher.

1 Introduction

A self-organizing map (SOM) is an adaptive function that transforms (or maps) from an input vector space to an output vector space, where the adaptation is driven entirely by signals derived from the input space. In the context of neural networks an SOM would therefore be realized as an unsupervised network whose training algorithm acts to minimize a suitably defined error function in the network's input space. The aim of this paper is to develop a theoretical framework that unifies several different strands of unsupervised network theory, and for this purpose it is best to develop the theory anew, rather than to build a hybrid theory out of an assortment of existing theories.

1.1 Variational Formulation of SOM Optimization. In order to create a theoretically clean framework it is necessary to express the optimization of an SOM in terms of a variational principle. Thus define a scalar functional D as follows

$$D \equiv \int dx\, P(x)\, d[x, \mathbf{y}(x), \mathbf{x}'(\mathbf{y})] \tag{1.1}$$

where the vectors x and $\mathbf{y}$ sit in the input and output spaces, respectively, and the functions $\mathbf{y}(x)$ and $\mathbf{x}'(\mathbf{y})$ transform from x-space to $\mathbf{y}$-space and vice versa, respectively. These are the functions that must be optimized so as to minimize the value of D. The scalar function $d[x, y(x), x'(y)]$ contributes to the functional D an amount that depends on the currently selected input vector x, and on the functions $y(x)$ and $x'(y)$. $P(x)$ is a probability density (or measure) that weights the x integral nonuniformly. In practice $P(x)$ might be used to represent the relative frequency of occurrence of each input vector x in a representative set of input vectors, in which case D would be the average of $d[x, y(x), x'(y)]$ over that set of vectors.

In equation 1.1 the functional dependence of $d[x, y(x), x'(y)]$ can be simplified to $d\{x, x'[y(x)]\}$, so D simplifies to

$$D = \int dx\, P(x)\, d\{x, x'[y(x)]\} \tag{1.2}$$

This is possible because in $d[x, y(x), x'(y)]$ the vector y in the function $x'(y)$ is a placeholder that receives the output of the function $y(x)$. The variational problem is then to find functions $y(x)$ and $x'(y)$ that minimize D as defined in equation 1.2.

Equation 1.2 can readily be extended to include the effects of an additive noise process acting in y-space. Thus D becomes

$$D = \int dx\, P(x) \int d\mathbf{n}\, \pi(\mathbf{n})\, d\{x, x'[y(x) + \mathbf{n}]\} \tag{1.3}$$

where $\pi(\mathbf{n})$ is the probability density of the noise vector $\mathbf{n}$. The variational problem is then to find functions $y(x)$ and $x'(y)$ that minimize this augmented expression for D. A side effect of including the noise process is that the information that is stored in the output vector y [produced by the action of $y(x)$ transforming the input vector x] is represented in such a way that it is robust with respect to the damaging effects of the noise process.

1.2 Variational Principle versus Unsupervised Network Notation. By making the replacement $d(x, x') = \|x - x'\|^2$ (i.e., a Euclidean distance) in equation 1.3 this variational formulation can be shown to lead to a type of SOM that is similar to, but not precisely the same as, the unsupervised network that is known as the Kohonen map (see Kohonen 1984) with the noise probability density $\pi(\mathbf{n})$ playing the role of the SOM neighborhood function. This type of analysis was also introduced in a nonneural context to design an optimal vector quantizer (VQ) codebook for encoding data for transmission along a noisy channel (Kumazawa et al. 1984; Favardin 1990; Favardin and Vaishampayan 1991).

The above variational principle can be related to a corresponding unsupervised network as shown in Table 1.

Note that in practice the output y of an unsupervised network is usually the index of the "winning node," which is a discrete-valued quantity.

Table 1: Variational Principle and Unsupervised Networks.

Term	Variational principle	Unsupervised network
x	Input vector	Training/test vector
$\mathbf{y}(x)$	Input to output transformation	Encoding prescription
$x'(\mathbf{y})$	Output to input transformation	Reference vector
$d[x, \mathbf{y}(x), x'(\mathbf{y})]$	Function	Error function
$P(x)$	Integration measure	Probability density of training/test vectors
D	Functional	Average error over the training/test set

Whether the output is continuous or discrete is unimportant to the variational approach, but in this paper a continuum notation is used because it is more compact.

The basic derivations of the variational formulation are in Luttrell (1989a,c, 1990), a simple application to time series compression is in Luttrell (1989b), the compression of synthetic aperture radar images is in Luttrell (1989d), an analysis of the density of reference vectors is in Luttrell (1991a), and an extension of unsupervised networks to multilayer networks in which higher layers supervise lower layers (self-supervised networks) is in Luttrell (1991b, 1992).

1.3 Encoding Prescriptions. It has been noted (Luttrell 1989a,c, 1990; Favardin and Vaishampayan 1991) that the above Euclidean error function is not minimized when the nearest neighbor encoding prescription is used. Exact minimization requires a new type of winner-take-all encoding prescription to be used; the nearest neighbor prescription must be replaced by the so-called minimum distortion prescription, in which the choice of winner is influenced by the reference vectors to which it is connected by the SOM neighborhood function. Figure 1 shows graphically how nearest neighbor and minimum distortion encoding are related.

The minimum distortion prescription was used in Luttrell (1991a) to study the equilibrium density of reference vectors in a one-dimensional input space, where it was reported that the result was insensitive to the choice of neighborhood function used in the SOM, provided that it was a monotonically decreasing symmetric function. The corresponding results using a standard SOM with the nearest neighbor prescription appeared in Ritter (1991), where it was shown that a neighborhood-sensitive density of reference vectors emerged.

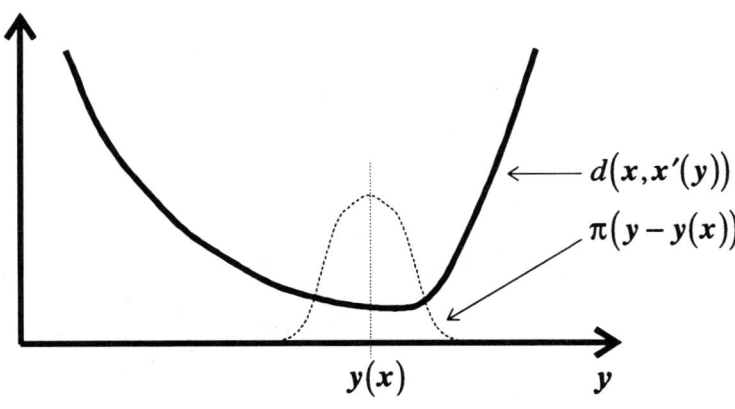

Figure 1: Assume that the input vector x and the function $x'(y)$ are such that the error function $d[x, x'(y)]$ has the y dependence shown above by the solid curve. There is a well-defined minimum, and the shape of the minimum is skewed so that $d[x, x'(y)]$ increases more rapidly to the right than to the left of the minimum. Assume that the SOM neighborhood function $\pi[y - y(x)]$ is the symmetric function denoted by the dashed curve. The error function must be averaged over y (weighted by the SOM neighborhood function) to determine the expected error for the particular choice of x, $x'(y)$, and $y(x)$. In effect, $d[x, x'(y)]$ is convolved with $\pi(y)$ to produce a smeared error function. The encoding prescription is one's choice of $y(x)$, and the optimum choice is not the position of the minimum of the original error function with respect to y (nearest neighbor encoding), but rather the position of the minimum of the smeared error function with respect to y (minimum distortion encoding). Because of the skewed $d[x, x'(y)]$ the minimum distortion encoding of x is thus displaced a little to the left of the nearest neighbor encoding.

1.4 Self-Supervised Multilayer SOMs. Hierarchical multilayer SOMs were studied in Luttrell (1991b, 1992). For instance, a 2-layer version of this type of network splits the input space into a number of lower dimensional subspaces, and trains a SOM in each subspace. Simultaneously, another SOM is trained on the outputs of the above SOMs to produce the final network output. This approach can be cascaded to more stages if required. This type of multilayer SOM can be refined by introducing an error function that measures the average Euclidean error between the input vector and a reference vector that is constructed from the final network output (Luttrell 1991b, 1992). This forces the optimization of the layers to be tied together in such a way that they have to be trained cooperatively. For instance, in a 2-layer network the outputs

A Bayesian Analysis of Self-Organizing Maps

from the SOMs in the first layer have to be matched to the capabilities of the SOM in the second layer; this is achieved by sending backpropagation signals from the second layer to the first layer. However, these backpropagation signals are not derived from an external supervisor, so this type of training algorithm is called "self-supervised."

1.5 Purpose of This Paper. The purpose of this paper is to embed the above variational formulation of SOMs in a more general framework in which the transformations $\mathbf{y}(x)$ and $x'(\mathbf{y})$ are replaced by probabilistic transformations $P_1(\mathbf{y} \mid x)$ and $P_2(x' \mid \mathbf{y})$. Equation 1.2 then becomes

$$D = \int dx\, P(x) \int d\mathbf{y}\, dx'\, P_2(x' \mid \mathbf{y})\, P_1(\mathbf{y} \mid x)\, d(x, x') \tag{1.4}$$

The integration over $\mathbf{y}$ and x' performs a weighted average of $d\{x, x'[\mathbf{y}(x)]\}$ over a variety of alternative transformations $\mathbf{y}(x)$ and $x'(\mathbf{y})$, rather than just a single pair of transformations as would have been the case in the basic variational formulation. Similarly equation 1.3 becomes

$$D = \int dx\, P(x) \int d\mathbf{n}\, \pi(\mathbf{n}) \int d\mathbf{y}\, dx'\, P_2(x' \mid \mathbf{y} + \mathbf{n})\, P_1(\mathbf{y} \mid x)\, d(x, x') \tag{1.5}$$

This "sum over alternatives" is useful for a number of reasons.

1. Theoretical manipulations are easier to perform on "soft" probabilities than on "hard" deterministic functions.

2. The probabilistic approach lends itself well to a simulated annealing approach in numerical simulations.

3. Contact with standard results can be made by making the replacement $d(x, x') = \|x - x'\|^2$ (i.e., a Euclidean distance) in equation 1.5. This leads to a probabilistic generalization of standard SOM theory.

4. If a single pair of transformations $\mathbf{y}(x)$ and $x'(\mathbf{y})$ was being used, but one was uncertain about which particular pair, then a probabilistic formulation would be necessary.

1.6 Structure of This Paper. The principal new result in this paper is a Bayesian derivation of the properties of SOMs starting from a generalization of equation 1.4. Thus a Markov chain of probabilistic transformations of the input vector is inverted by sending the (probabilistic) output of the chain back through the inverse probabilistic transformations (derived from Bayes' theorem) to eventually reemerge as a (probabilistic) reconstructed version of the input vector. This type of structure will be called a folded Markov chain (FMC). This FMC is then optimized by minimizing the average Euclidean error between the input vector and its reconstruction. Various constraints can be placed on this optimization. For instance, if a 2-stage FMC (i.e., 2 stages of probabilistic transformation) is considered, and only its first stage is optimized, then the theory of SOMs emerges (as in Luttrell 1989a,c, 1990). Alternatively, if the state space of each stage of a 2-stage FMC is split into two (or more) lower dimensional subspaces, then the theory of self-supervision emerges (as in Luttrell 1991b, 1992).

The structure of this paper is as follows. In Section 2 the idea of an FMC is introduced, where Bayes' theorem is used to invert a Markov chain of probabilistic transformations. In Section 3 the relationship between FMCs and VQs and SOMs is derived, and it is shown how a 1-stage (or 2-stage) FMC contains a VQ (or SOM) as a special case. In Section 4 these results are extended to the case of a pair of coupled FMCs, and it is shown how self-supervision emerges naturally. In the Appendix the relationship between the continuum notation that is used in this paper and the more usual discrete notation is explained (Section 6.1) and a more complete and technically rigorous derivation of the results of Section 3 is presented (Section 6.2). The main new results are contained in Sections 3 and 4.

2 Basic Theory

The notation that is used for probabilities is very carefully chosen so as to avoid ambiguities that could arise if the notation $P(\cdots)$ were used blindly to denote "the probability density of ...." However, occasional use of the ambiguous $P(\cdots)$ notation is made where there is no possibility of an ambiguity arising. Also, a careful distinction is drawn between the notation that is used for inverse probabilities (obtained from Bayes' theorem) and the notation that is used for forward probabilities; the former always appear with a tilde over the P, which thus appears as $\tilde{P}$. Also the state space(s) will be assumed to be continuous, except where otherwise noted. This is because the corresponding discrete space results can be written down by inspection of the continuum results, and because the meaning of a continuum calculation is usually more transparent than its discrete counterpart.

The type of Markov chain that will be considered is shown in Figure 2. This is a folded Markov chain (FMC) which performs an L-stage transformation of an input vector x_0 to an output vector x_L (via $L-1$ intermediate vectors $x_1, x_2, \ldots, x_{L-1}$), and then performs the Bayes inverse transformation to arrive eventually at a reconstructed input vector x'_0. The delta function $\delta(x'_L - x_L)$ is used to ensure that $x'_L = x_L$. The conditional probabilities are related by Bayes' theorem as follows

$$\tilde{P}_{k,k+1}(x_k \mid x_{k+1}) P_{k+1}(x_{k+1}) = P_{k+1,k}(x_{k+1} \mid x_k) P_k(x_k) \tag{2.1}$$

where $P_k(x_k)$ denotes the marginal probability (density) of x_k. To construct any joint probability in the FMC system it is both necessary and

A Bayesian Analysis of Self-Organizing Maps

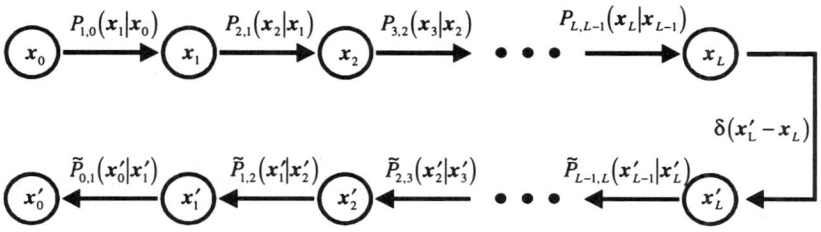

Figure 2: A folded Markov chain (i.e., both the forward and backward directions are represented). The top (bottom) half of the diagram represents the forward (backward) pass through the chain. The conditional probability $P_{k+1,k}(x_{k+1} \mid x_k)$ is used as a probabilistic transformation that generates the probable states of layer $k+1$ from the state of layer k, and the conditional probability $\tilde{P}_{k,k+1}(x'_k \mid x'_{k+1})$ is similarly used to generate the probable states of layer k from the state of layer $k+1$; this is also referred to generically as stage k of the FMC. These two conditional probabilities are related by Bayes' theorem.

sufficient to specify $P_0(x_0)$ and the L transformations $P_{1,0}(x_1 \mid x_0), P_{2,1}(x_2 \mid x_1), \ldots, P_{L,L-1}(x_L \mid x_{L-1})$. Thus

$$\begin{aligned}P(x_0, x_1, \ldots, x_L; x'_L, \ldots, x'_1, x'_0) &= P_0(x_0)\, P_{1,0}(x_1 \mid x_0)\, P_{2,1}(x_2 \mid x_1) \cdots \\ &\quad \times P_{L,L-1}(x_L \mid x_{L-1})\delta(x'_L - x_L) \\ &\quad \times \tilde{P}_{L-1,L}(x'_{L-1} \mid x'_L) \cdots \\ &\quad \times \tilde{P}_{1,2}(x'_1 \mid x'_2)\, \tilde{P}_{0,1}(x'_0 \mid x'_1) \end{aligned} \quad (2.2)$$

The marginal probability $P_k(x_k)$ is obtained by integrating over all variables other than x_k, which yields

$$P_k(x_k) = \int dx_0\, dx_1 \ldots dx_{k-1}\, P_0(x_0)\, P_{1,0}(x_1 \mid x_0)\, P_{2,1}(x_2 \mid x_1) \cdots \\ \times P_{k,k-1}(x_k \mid x_{k-1}) \quad (2.3)$$

Note that Bayes' theorem guarantees that the marginal probabilities of x_k and x'_k are the same. In this paper our attention will be restricted to FMCs with 1 or 2 stages only (i.e. $L = 1$ or 2). Furthermore, whenever an FMC is to be optimized, only its first stage will be optimized.

3 1- and 2-Stage Folded Markov Chains

FMCs are especially interesting in adaptive network design theory, because they turn out to contain some well-known systems as special cases: a VQ is a special case of a 1-stage FMC, and an SOM is a special case of

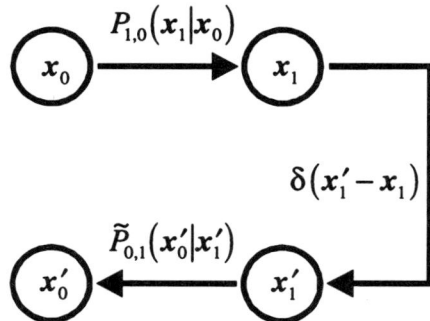

Figure 3: A 1-stage folded Markov chain. When $P_{1,0}(x_1 \mid x_0) = \delta[x_1 - x_1(x_0)]$, and D is minimized with respect to $x_1(x_0)$, this reduces to a vector quantizer with an infinite number of reference vectors (i.e., continuum limit). See the Appendix for a detailed discussion of the relationship between the continuum and discrete cases. Bayes' theorem ensures that $\tilde{P}_{1,0}(x_1' \mid x_0')$ cannot be varied independently of $P_{1,0}(x_1 \mid x_0)$.

a 2-stage FMC. The success of these derivations relies on the similarities that exist between the following two situations:

1. Direct/inverse probabilities occur in Bayes' theorem as applied to a Markov chain, which might be used in the analysis of scattering problems in layered media, for instance. The sequence of processing operations is source→scattering→inverse scattering→reconstruction.

2. Encoding/decoding operations occur in VQs and SOMs, which might be used in the analysis of information transmission down a noisy communication channel, for instance. The sequence of processing operations is source→encode→decode→reconstruction.

3.1 1-Stage Folded Markov Chain: Vector Quantizer. A 1-stage FMC is shown in Figure 3. The derivation starts from the definition of the average Euclidean error D between x_0 and x_0' in a 1-stage FMC.

$$\begin{aligned} D &= \int dx_0 \, dx_1 \, dx_0' \, dx_1' \, P_0(x_0) \, P_{1,0}(x_1 \mid x_0) \, \delta(x_1' - x_1) \\ &\quad \times \tilde{P}_{0,1}(x_0' \mid x_1') \, \|x_0' - x_0\|^2 \end{aligned} \tag{3.1}$$

After integrating out the (irrelevant) x_1' using the delta function $\delta(x_1' - x_1)$, using Bayes' theorem in the form $\tilde{P}_{0,1}(x_0 \mid x_1)P_1(x_1) = P_{1,0}(x_1 \mid x_0)P_0(x_0)$

A Bayesian Analysis of Self-Organizing Maps

(i.e., equation 2.1 with $k = 0$), and rearranging the order of the integrations, this reduces to

$$D = \int dx_1 \, P_1(x_1) \int dx_0 \, dx'_0 \, \tilde{P}_{0,1}(x_0 \mid x_1) \, \tilde{P}_{0,1}(x'_0 \mid x_1) \, \|x'_0 - x_0\|^2 \quad (3.2)$$

The next step is to expand the norm as $\|x_0\|^2 + \|x'_0\|^2 - 2x_0.x'_0$ and to perform the integrations where possible to obtain

$$D = 2 \int dx_1 \, P_1(x_1) \left[\int dx_0 \, \tilde{P}_{0,1}(x_0 \mid x_1) \, \|x_0\|^2 - \left\| \int dx_0 \, \tilde{P}_{0,1}(x_0 \mid x_1) \, x_0 \right\|^2 \right] \quad (3.3)$$

which may be rewritten as

$$D = 2 \int dx_1 \, P_1(x_1) \int dx_0 \, \tilde{P}_{0,1}(x_0 \mid x_1) \left\| x_0 - \int du_0 \, \tilde{P}_{0,1}(u_0 \mid x_1) \, u_0 \right\|^2 \quad (3.4)$$

The derivation of equation 3.4 from equation 3.2 is well-known; it says that the average Euclidean error between pairs of vectors drawn independently from $\tilde{P}_{0,1}(x_0 \mid x_1)$ is twice the variance of vectors drawn from $\tilde{P}_{0,1}(x_0 \mid x_1)$. Finally, Bayes' theorem (i.e., equation 2.1 with $k = 0$) can be used to obtain the required result.

$$D = 2 \int dx_0 \, P_0(x_0) \int dx_1 \, P_{1,0}(x_1 \mid x_0) \left\| x_0 - \int du_0 \, \tilde{P}_{0,1}(u_0 \mid x_1) \, u_0 \right\|^2 \quad (3.5)$$

Equation 3.5 has all of the right structure to relate FMCs to VQs. It has a source of input vectors $P_0(x_0)$, a "soft" encoder $P_{1,0}(x_1 \mid x_0)$, and a reference vector $\int du_0 \, \tilde{P}_{0,1}(u_0 \mid x_1) \, u_0$ attached to each x_1 with which to compare the input vector x_0 to compute a Euclidean distortion. The only differences between this FMC and a standard VQ are:

1. $P_{1,0}(x_1 \mid x_0)$ is not a winner-take-all encoder. Each input vector x_0 is transformed into each possible output vector x_1 with probability $P_{1,0}(x_1 \mid x_0)$. In the language of neural networks, it is as if each possible output vector had an "activity" specified by $P_{1,0}(x_1 \mid x_0)$. A winner-take-all would result if $P_{1,0}(x_1 \mid x_0)$ were replaced by a probability whose mass was concentrated all at one point; this would be a delta function $\delta[x_1 - x_1(x_0)]$.

2. The reference vector $\int du_0 \, \tilde{P}_{0,1}(u_0 \mid x_1) \, u_0$ is dependent on the encoder $P_{1,0}(x_1 \mid x_0)$; they are related by Bayes' theorem (i.e., equation 2.1 with $k = 0$). In a VQ the reference vector and the encoder are also related because the encoder is usually a nearest neighbor prescription, which in turn depends on the location of the reference vectors. It is not at all obvious that these two pictures (the FMC and the VQ) are related in a simple way.

Now consider a modified form of equation 3.5 in which D becomes

$$D = 2 \int dx_0 \, P_0(x_0) \int dx_1 \, P_{1,0}(x_1 \mid x_0) \, \|x_0 - x'_0(x_1)\|^2 \tag{3.6}$$

where $\int du_0 \, \tilde{P}_{0,1}(u_0 \mid x_1) \, u_0$ has been replaced by the function $x'_0(x_1)$. Functionally differentiate this expression for D with respect to $x'_0(x_1)$ to obtain

$$\frac{\delta D}{\delta x'_0(x_1)} = -4 \int dx_0 \, P_0(x_0) \, P_{1,0}(x_1 \mid x_0) \, [x_0 - x'_0(x_1)] \tag{3.7}$$

The stationary point $\delta D / \delta x'_0(x_1) = 0$ is obtained when $x'_0(x_1)$ satisfies

$$x'_0(x_1) = \frac{\int dx_0 \, P_0(x_0) \, P_{1,0}(x_1 \mid x_0) \, x_0}{\int dx_0 \, P_0(x_0) \, P_{1,0}(x_1 \mid x_0)} \tag{3.8}$$

By using Bayes' theorem (i.e., equation 2.1 with $k = 0$) this stationarity condition reduces to

$$x'_0(x_1) = \int dx_0 \, \tilde{P}_{0,1}(x_0 \mid x_1) \, x_0 \tag{3.9}$$

So the modified expression for D in equation 3.6 reduces to the original expression for D in equation 3.5 provided that $x'_0(x_1)$ is chosen to minimize D. This is a major simplification, because the coupling (via Bayes' theorem) between $P_{1,0}(x_1 \mid x_0)$ and $\int du_0 \, \tilde{P}_{0,1}(u_0 \mid x_1) \, u_0$ that appeared in equation 3.5 can now safely be ignored by the simple trick of using equation 3.6 instead [with the proviso that $x'_0(x_1)$ should always be optimized so as to minimize D].

At this point the minimization of D (as written in equation 3.6) with respect to $P_{1,0}(x_1 \mid x_0)$ should be considered. However, this derivation is messy, so it is presented in the Appendix. Instead, a simplified (and strictly incomplete) version of this derivation is presented below.

Make the following replacement in equation 3.6

$$P_{1,0}(x_1 \mid x_0) \to \delta[x_1 - x_1(x_0)] \tag{3.10}$$

which converts $P_{1,0}(x_1 \mid x_0)$ into a winner-take-all encoder. A winner-take-all encoder might appear intuitively to be the obvious solution to the problem of minimizing D with respect to $P_{1,0}(x_1 \mid x_0)$. However, other solutions may also be possible in general. A detailed derivation is given in the Appendix to show how this result emerges in the case of a Euclidean error function. Also a couple of simple counterexamples are presented in the Appendix to show how non-winner-take-all encoders can also be valid solutions.

With these replacements D becomes

$$D = 2 \int dx_0 \, P_0(x_0) \, \|x_0 - x'_0[x_1(x_0)]\|^2 \tag{3.11}$$

A Bayesian Analysis of Self-Organizing Maps

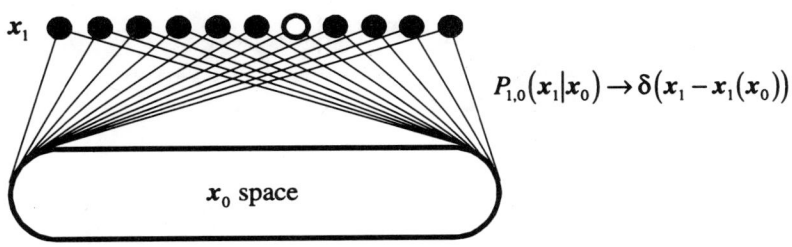

Figure 4: A discrete VQ represented as a network. The bottom layer is the input space (or x_0), the top layer is the output space (or x_1), and the connections between the two represent a soft encoding operation $P_{1,0}(x_1 \mid x_0)$, akin to that used in Yair et al. (1992). A winner-take-all VQ uses an encoder of the form $P_{1,0}(x_1 \mid x_0) = \delta[x_1 - x_1(x_0)]$. The input and output layers of this network are represented in different ways: the input layer is the vector x_0 represented as in Figure 3, whereas each node of the the output layer corresponds to exactly one possible state of the vector x_1. Note also that the connections are not to be interpreted as weights in the conventional sense, rather they merely indicate the functional interdependence of the various parts of the network. An example of a winner in the output layer is represented by the open circle.

which is exactly what would be written for the continuum version of a VQ (apart from the trivial overall factor of 2). The network representation of a VQ is shown in Figure 4 for a discrete-valued output, which should be compared with the FMC representation shown in Figure 3.

The gradient of D with respect to $x'_0(x_1)$ is given by the functional derivative

$$\frac{\delta D}{\delta x'_0(x_1)} = -4 \int dx_0 \, P_0(x_0) \, \delta[x_1 - x_1(x_0)] \, [x_0 - x'_0(x_1)] \qquad (3.12)$$

By inspecting the dependence of Equation 3.11 on $x_1(x_0)$, and by setting $\delta D/\delta x'_0(x_1)$ in Equation 3.12 to zero, the following batch training prescription for minimizing D can be obtained

$$x_1(x_0) = \arg\min_{x_1} \|x_0 - x'_0(x_1)\|^2$$

$$x'_0(x_1) = \frac{\int dx_0 \, P_0(x_0) \, \delta[x_1 - x_1(x_0)] \, x_0}{\int dx_0 \, P_0(x_0) \, \delta[x_1 - x_1(x_0)]} \qquad (3.13)$$

These results merit the following remarks:

1. The function $x'_0(x_1)$ can be interpreted as the continuum version of a VQ codebook, where x_1 is the (continuum) code index and $x'_0(x_1)$ is the code vector (or reference vector) associated with that index.

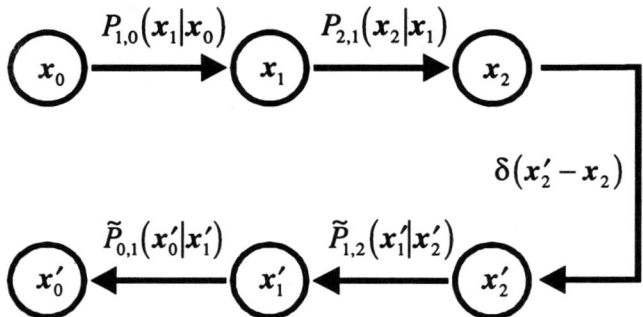

Figure 5: A 2-stage folded Markov chain. This is basically the same as Figure 3, except that $P_{2,1}(x_2 \mid x_1)$ causes the information that flows through the folded Markov chain to be further corrupted before it can begin its return journey.

2. The result for $x'_0(x_1)$ corresponds to equation 3.6 with $P_{1,0}(x_1 \mid x_0) \to \delta[x_1 - x_1(x_0)]$, and it is the "centroiding" prescription for updating the code vectors after a batch of training data has been presented to a VQ, as used in the LBG algorithm (Linde et al. 1980).

3. The result for $x_1(x_0)$ is the "nearest neighbor" encoding prescription for encoding the input of a VQ.

An on-line training prescription can also be obtained to implement updates to $x'_0(x_1)$ after each input vector x_0 is selected at random from $P_0(x_0)$. The on-line prescription is

$$x'_0(x_1) \to x'_0(x_1) + \epsilon \, \delta[x_1 - x_1(x_0)] \, [x_0 - x'_0(x_1)] \tag{3.14}$$

Note that the delta function permits nonzero updates only for $x_1 = x_1(x_0)$; this is the continuum version of updating the nearest neighbor code vector toward the input vector. The relationship between this continuum result and the corresponding discrete result is discussed in the Appendix.

This completes the demonstration that an optimal 1-stage FMC is a VQ. Note that the use of a Euclidean error is sufficient (but not necessary) for this result to emerge. There are choices of error function for which this result does not emerge.

3.2 2-Stage Folded Markov Chain: Self-Organizing Map.

The above derivation may be extended to a 2-stage FMC, as shown in Figure 5. Because the derivation is so similar to the case of a 1-stage FMC, only an abbreviated derivation will be given. For simplicity, the following

A Bayesian Analysis of Self-Organizing Maps

notation will be used

$$P_{2,0}(x_2 \mid x_0) = \int dx_1 \, P_{2,1}(x_2 \mid x_1) \, P_{1,0}(x_1 \mid x_0)$$
$$\tilde{P}_{0,2}(x_0 \mid x_2) \, P_2(x_2) = P_{2,0}(x_2 \mid x_0) \, P_0(x_0) \tag{3.15}$$

$P_{2,0}(x_2 \mid x_0)$ is the probability (density) that x_2 will be generated by x_0, taking into account all of the possible values that the intermediate state x_1 might take. $\tilde{P}_{0,2}(x_0 \mid x_2)$ is the corresponding inverse probability that is obtained from Bayes' theorem.

Using this notation the expression for D becomes (compare equation 3.1)

$$D = \int dx_0 \, dx_1 \, dx_2 \, dx_0' \, dx_1' \, dx_2'$$
$$P_0(x_0) \, P_{1,0}(x_1 \mid x_0) \, P_{2,1}(x_2 \mid x_1) \, \delta(x_2' - x_2)$$
$$\tilde{P}_{1,2}(x_1' \mid x_2') \, \tilde{P}_{0,1}(x_0' \mid x_1') \, \|x_0' - x_0\|^2 \tag{3.16}$$

which simplifies to (compare equation 3.5)

$$D = 2 \int dx_0 \, P_0(x_0) \int dx_2 \, P_{2,0}(x_2 \mid x_0) \left\| x_0 - \int du_0 \, \tilde{P}_{0,2}(u_0 \mid x_2) \, u_0 \right\|^2 \tag{3.17}$$

Consider a modified form of D (compare equation 3.6)

$$D = \int dx_0 \, P_0(x_0) \int dx_2 \, P_{2,0}(x_2 \mid x_0) \, \|x_0 - x_0'(x_2)\|^2 \tag{3.18}$$

Set $\delta D / \delta x_0'(x_2) = 0$ to obtain (compare equation 3.8 and equation 3.9)

$$x_0'(x_2) = \frac{\int dx_0 \, P_0(x_0) \, P_{2,0}(x_2 \mid x_0) \, x_0}{\int dx_0 \, P_0(x_0) \, P_{2,0}(x_2 \mid x_0)} = \int dx_0 \, \tilde{P}_{0,2}(x_0 \mid x_2) \, x_0 \tag{3.19}$$

The modified expression for D in Equation 3.18 reduces to the original expression in equation 3.17 provided that $x_0'(x_2)$ is chosen to minimize D, so equation 3.18 will be used in preference to equation 3.17 [with the proviso that $x_0'(x_2)$ should always be chosen to minimize D].

Make the replacement $P_{1,0}(x_1 \mid x_0) \to \delta[x_1 - x_1(x_0)]$, which converts $P_{1,0}(x_1 \mid x_0)$ into a winner-take-all encoder (see the discussion following equation 3.10, and the Appendix for more details), and note that $P_{2,0}(x_2 \mid x_0) = \int dx_1 \, P_{2,1}(x_2 \mid x_1) \, P_{1,0}(x_1 \mid x_0)$, to obtain D as (compare equation 3.11)

$$D = 2 \int dx_0 \, P_0(x_0) \int dx_2 \, P_{2,1}[x_2 \mid x_1(x_0)] \, \|x_0 - x_0'(x_2)\|^2 \tag{3.20}$$

The functional derivative $\delta D / \delta x_0'(x_2)$ is thus (compare equation 3.12)

$$\frac{\delta D}{\delta x_0'(x_2)} = -4 \int dx_0 \, P_0(x_0) \, P_{2,1}[x_2 \mid x_1(x_0)] \, [x_0 - x_0'(x_2)] \tag{3.21}$$

which leads to the following batch training prescription for minimizing D (compare equation 3.13)

$$x_1(x_0) = \arg\min_{x_1} \int dx_2 \, P_{2,1}(x_2 \mid x_1) \, \|x_0 - x_0'(x_2)\|^2$$
$$x_0'(x_2) = \frac{\int dx_0 \, P_0(x_0) \, P_{2,1}[x_2 \mid x_1(x_0)] \, x_0}{\int dx_0 \, P_0(x_0) \, P_{2,1}[x_2 \mid x_1(x_0)]} \qquad (3.22)$$

and the following on-line training prescription (compare equation 3.14)

$$x_0'(x_2) \to x_0'(x_2) + \epsilon \, P_{2,1}[x_2 \mid x_1(x_0)] \, [x_0 - x_0'(x_2)] \qquad (3.23)$$

These results correspond to the results that were reported in Luttrell (1989a,c, 1990). They can be interpreted as the generalization of the VQ results in the previous section to the case where the output of the VQ is corrupted by the action of $P_{2,1}(x_2 \mid x_1)$ before Bayes' theorem is then used in an attempt to reconstruct the input vector.

This winner-take-all version of a 2-stage FMC turns out to be an SOM whose network representation is shown in Figure 6 for a discrete-valued output, which should be compared with the FMC representation that is shown in Figure 5.

The SOM interpretation of these results for optimizing a 2-stage FMC is as follows:

1. The function $x_0'(x_2)$ can be interpreted as the continuum version of the SOM reference vectors, where x_2 is the (continuum) index and $x_0'(x_2)$ is the reference vector associated with that index. The batch update prescription for $x_0'(x_2)$ is a generalization of the LBG "centroiding" prescription (Linde 1980) that accounts for the effect of $P_{2,1}(x_2 \mid x_1)$.

2. The result for $x_1(x_0)$ is not a "nearest neighbor" encoding prescription. Rather, it says that $x_1(x_0)$ is the value that x_1 must take in order to ensure that the distortion D is minimized after taking into account the effect of $P_{2,1}(x_2 \mid x_1)$. Thus the nearest neighbor encoding prescription has become a minimum distortion encoding prescription. This reduces to the nearest neighbor encoding prescription when $P_{2,1}(x_2 \mid x_1) \to \delta(x_2 - x_1)$, as expected.

3. The on-line training prescription is the continuum version of the standard SOM training prescription, where $P_{2,1}(x_2 \mid x_1)$ plays the role of the SOM neighborhood function. $P_{2,1}(x_2 \mid x_1)$ also has this interpretation in the batch training prescription.

This completes the demonstration that an optimal 2-stage FMC is an SOM. Note that minimum distortion encoding is used, rather than nearest neighbor encoding, so this type of SOM is only an approximation to the standard SOM that was discussed in Kohonen (1984).

A Bayesian Analysis of Self-Organizing Maps

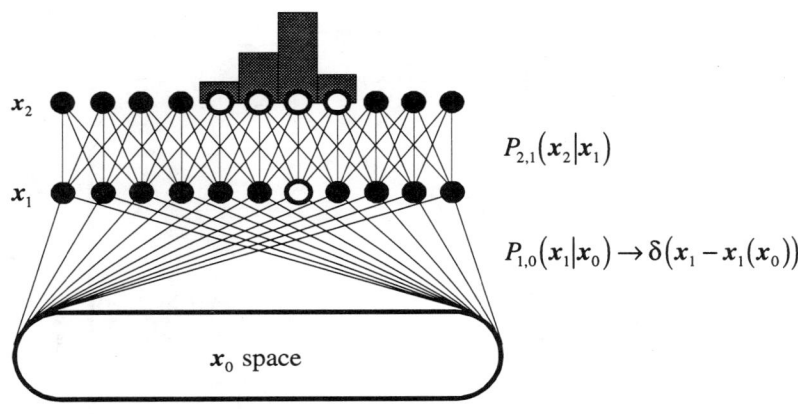

Figure 6: A discrete SOM represented as a network. This is the same as the VQ network in Figure 4 with an additional stage of processing applied to its output layer. Each node in the hidden and output layer of this SOM network corresponds to exactly one possible state of the vector x_1 and x_2, respectively. $P_{2,1}(x_2 \mid x_1)$ serves as the SOM neighborhood function by connecting together states of x_1 so that they become ordered (across the page in this case). Note that the VQ network in Figure 4 does not have this ordering property, although the states of x_1 (or nodes) are still drawn in an ordered fashion, for convenience. An example of a winner in the hidden layer is drawn as an open circle, as are each of the corresponding soft winners in the output layer. An example of the degree to which each node in the output layer is activated is indicated by a histogram, which records $P_{2,1}(x_2 \mid x_1)$ for each possible state that x_2 might take.

4 Coupled 2-Stage Folded Markov Chains

In Luttrell (1991b, 1992) some interesting results were reported where the behavior of a multilayer SOM could be interpreted as if the higher network layers were supervising the lower layers, and the term "self-supervision" was introduced to describe this effect. The purpose of this section is to show how these results can be derived from the theory of FMCs.

4.1 Splitting the Markov Chain State Spaces. The derivation starts by splitting each state of a 2-stage FMC into two lower dimensional pieces, as shown in Figure 7.

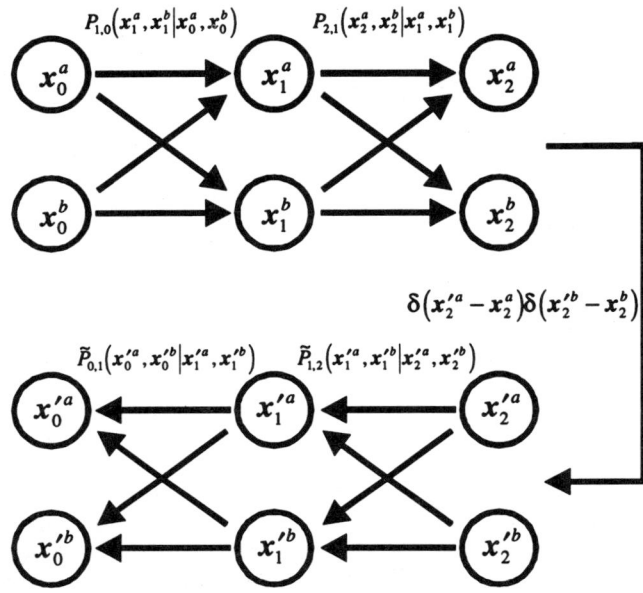

Figure 7: A 2-stage folded Markov chain with each state split into two lower dimensional pieces. This is basically the same as Figure 5, except that the states have been exploded to reveal their internal structure.

Figure 7 can be obtained by making the following changes to the notation in Figure 5

$$\begin{aligned} x_0 &\to (x_0^a, x_0^b) & x_0' &\to (x_0'^a, x_0'^b) \\ x_1 &\to (x_1^a, x_1^b) & x_1' &\to (x_1'^a, x_1'^b) \\ x_2 &\to (x_2^a, x_2^b) & x_2' &\to (x_2'^a, x_2'^b) \end{aligned} \quad (4.1)$$

so the FMC in Figure 7 is the same as the FMC in Figure 5, apart from the notation that is used to describe its state spaces. This tautology is motivated by the need to break up high dimensional spaces, such as might occur in image processing problems, into a number of coupled lower dimensional spaces. For instance, if the coupling between the FMCs is weak, then a series expansion about zero coupling strength could be attempted. The lowest order term in this expansion would correspond to a pair of uncoupled FMCs, and the higher order terms would correspond to interactions between the FMCs.

A Bayesian Analysis of Self-Organizing Maps

If the new notation in equation 4.1 is used together with the generalization of equation 3.10

$$P_{1,0}(x_1^a, x_1^b \mid x_0^a, x_0^b) \rightarrow \delta[x_1^a - x_1^a(x_0^a, x_0^b)] \, \delta[x_1^b - x_1^b(x_0^a, x_0^b)] \tag{4.2}$$

in the expression for the distortion D in a 2-stage FMC (see equation 3.17), and noting that $P_{2,0}(x_2 \mid x_0) = \int dx_1 \, P_{2,1}(x_2 \mid x_1) \, P_{1,0}(x_1 \mid x_0)$, then D reduces to

$$\begin{aligned}
D = {} & 2 \int dx_0^a \, dx_0^b \, P_0(x_0^a, x_0^b) \int dx_2^a \, dx_2^b \, P_{2,1}[x_2^a, x_2^b \mid x_1^a(x_0^a, x_0^b), x_1^b(x_0^a, x_0^b)] \\
& \times \left(\left\| x_0^a - \int du_0^a \, \tilde{P}_{0,2}(u_0^a \mid x_2^a, x_2^b) \, u_0^a \right\|^2 \right. \\
& \left. + \left\| x_0^b - \int du_0^b \, \tilde{P}_{0,2}(u_0^b \mid x_2^a, x_2^b) \, u_0^b \right\|^2 \right)
\end{aligned} \tag{4.3}$$

where the Euclidean error has been split into a sum of contributions from the a and the b subspaces of x_0. The Euclidean error terms have an interesting structure. For instance, in FMC a the Euclidean distance between x_0^a and $\int du_0^a \, \tilde{P}_{0,2}(u_0^a \mid x_2^a, x_2^b) \, u_0^a$ is computed, which explicitly depends via $\tilde{P}_{0,2}(u_0^a \mid x_2^a, x_2^b)$ on the outputs (x_2^a, x_2^b) of both FMC a and FMC b. In the previous section terms like $\int du_0 \, \tilde{P}_{0,2}(u_0 \mid x_2) \, u_0$ turned out to correspond to SOM reference vectors, so by analogy it is expected that $\int du_0^k \, \tilde{P}_{0,2}(u_0^k \mid x_2^a, x_2^b) \, u_0^k$ ($k = a, b$) will also turn out to be the reference vectors for a pair of coupled SOMs corresponding to FMC a and FMC b.

Unfortunately, because of the coupling between FMC a and FMC b, $\int du_0^k \, \tilde{P}_{0,2}(u_0^k \mid x_2^a, x_2^b) \, u_0^k$ ($k = a, b$) depend on both x_2^a and x_2^b. The purpose of the following derivation is to find an approximate way of optimizing D that does not involve these simultaneous dependencies on both x_2^a and x_2^b, but uses quantities like $\int du_0^k \, \tilde{P}_{0,2}(u_0^k \mid x_2^k) \, u_0^k$ rather than $\int du_0^k \, \tilde{P}_{0,2}(u_0^k \mid x_2^a, x_2^b) \, u_0^k$ for $k = a, b$.

Thus each term can be split in the following manner for $k = a, b$

$$\begin{aligned}
\left\| x_0^k - \int du_0^k \, \tilde{P}_{0,2}(u_0^k \mid x_2^a, x_2^b) \, u_0^k \right\|^2 = {} & \left\| \left(x_0^k - \int du_0^k \, \tilde{P}_{0,2}(u_0^k \mid x_2^k) \, u_0^k \right) \right. \\
& + \left(\int du_0^k \, \tilde{P}_{0,2}(u_0^k \mid x_2^k) \, u_0^k \right. \\
& \left. \left. - \int du_0^k \, \tilde{P}_{0,2}(u_0^k \mid x_2^a, x_2^b) \, u_0^k \right) \right\|^2
\end{aligned} \tag{4.4}$$

where the distinction between $\int du_0^k \, \tilde{P}_{0,2}(u_0^k \mid x_2^a, x_2^b) \, u_0^k$ and $\int du_0^k \, \tilde{P}_{0,2}(u_0^k \mid x_2^k) \, u_0^k$ has been carefully used to separate the x_0^k and $\int du_0^k \, \tilde{P}_{0,2}(u_0^k \mid x_2^a, x_2^b) \, u_0^k$ terms. The following two definitions are introduced for $k = a, b$

$$\begin{aligned}
D_0(k) \equiv {} & 2 \int dx_0^a \, dx_0^b \, P_0(x_0^a, x_0^b) \\
& \times \int dx_2^k \, P_{2,1}[x_2^k \mid x_1^a(x_0^a, x_0^b), x_1^b(x_0^a, x_0^b)]
\end{aligned}$$

$$D_1(k) \equiv 2 \int dx_2^a \, dx_2^b \, P_2(x_2^a, x_2^b) \\
\times \left\| x_0^k - \int du_0^k \, \tilde{P}_{0,2}(u_0^k \mid x_2^k) \, u_0^k \right\|^2 \\
\times \left\| \int du_0^k \, \tilde{P}_{0,2}(u_0^k \mid x_2^k) \, u_0^k - \int du_0^k \, \tilde{P}_{0,2}(u_0^k \mid x_2^a, x_2^b) \, u_0^k \right\|^2 \quad (4.5)$$

and used together with Bayes' theorem in the form

$$P_0(x_0^a, x_0^b) \, P_{2,1}[x_2^a, x_2^b \mid x_1^a(x_0^a, x_0^b), x_1^b(x_0^a, x_0^b)] \\
= \tilde{P}_{0,2}(x_0^a, x_0^b \mid x_2^a, x_2^b) \, P_2(x_2^a, x_2^b) \quad (4.6)$$

to obtain D in the form

$$D = D_0(a) + D_0(b) - D_1(a) - D_1(b) \quad (4.7)$$

The first two terms in equation 4.7 have a structure that is simpler than in equation 4.3. For instance, $D_0(a)$ depends on the Euclidean distance between x_0^a and $\int du_0^a \, \tilde{P}_{0,2}(u_0^a \mid x_2^a) \, u_0^a$, which depends only on the output of FMC a and not on the output of FMC b. An analogous remark applies to $D_0(b)$.

The last two terms in equation 4.7 contain the undesirable terms such as $\int du_0^a \, \tilde{P}_{0,2}(u_0^a \mid x_2^a, x_2^b) \, u_0^a$. In the following derivation these terms will be discarded to obtain an approximate scheme for minimizing D.

4.2 Least Upper Bound Optimization Scheme. Note that the following inequalities hold

$$D_0(a) \geq 0 \quad D_0(b) \geq 0 \quad D_1(a) \geq 0 \quad D_1(b) \geq 0 \quad D \geq 0 \quad (4.8)$$

These lead to the following constraint on D

$$0 \leq D \leq D_0(a) + D_0(b) \quad (4.9)$$

Although ideally D itself should be minimized, it turns out to be much simpler to minimize its upper bound $D_0(a) + D_0(b)$. This least upper bound prescription achieves what is required, namely the elimination of the undesirable $D_1(a)$ and $D_1(b)$ terms that depend on $\int du_0^k \, \tilde{P}_{0,2}(u_0^k \mid x_2^a, x_2^b) \, u_0^k$ for $k = a, b$. This approximate prescription becomes exact in the limit where the coupling between the FMCs in Figure 7 tends to zero.

This approximate approach to optimizing the FMC is shown in Figure 8.

At this point it is appropriate to introduce a modified form of $D_0(k)$ in which $\int du_0^k \, \tilde{P}_{0,2}(u_0^k \mid x_2^k) \, u_0^k$ in equation 4.5 is replaced by the function $x_0^{\prime k}(x_2^k)$ for $k = a, b$

$$D_0(k) = 2 \int dx_0^a \, dx_0^b \, P_0(x_0^a, x_0^b) \\
\times \int dx_2^k \, P_{2,1}[x_2^k \mid x_1^a(x_0^a, x_0^b), x_1^b(x_0^a, x_0^b)] \, \left\| x_0^k - x_0^{\prime k}(x_2^k) \right\|^2 \quad (4.10)$$

A Bayesian Analysis of Self-Organizing Maps

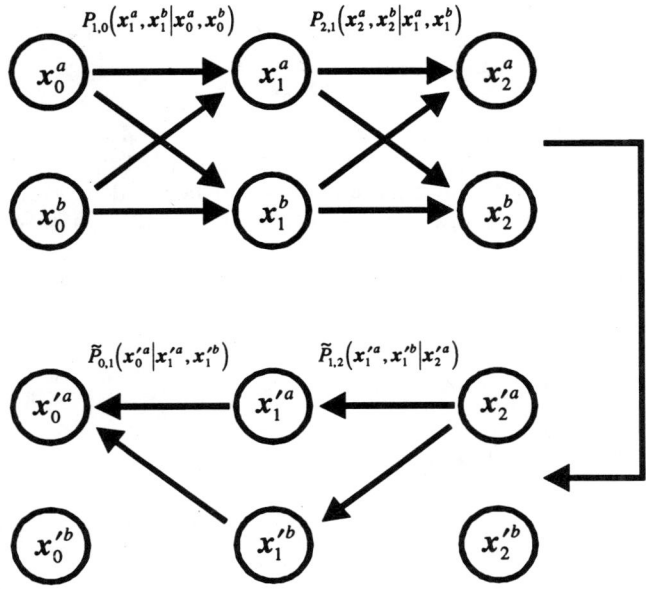

Figure 8: An approximation to a 2-stage folded Markov chain with each state split into two lower dimensional pieces. Only the $\tilde{P}_{0,2}(x_0^a \mid x_2^a)$ part is indicated on the reverse part of the chain. The approximation arises because x_2^a, rather than (x_2^a, x_2^b), is used as the initial state on the reverse part of the chain. An analogous discussion holds for $\tilde{P}_{0,2}(x_0^b \mid x_2^b)$.

The functional derivative $\delta D_0(k)/\delta x_0'^k(x_2^k)$ then becomes for $k = a, b$

$$\frac{\delta D_0(k)}{\delta x_0'^k(x_2^k)} = -4 \int dx_0^a\, dx_0^b\, P_0(x_0^a, x_0^b)$$
$$\times P_{2,1}[x_2^k \mid x_1^a(x_0^a, x_0^b), x_1^b(x_0^a, x_0^b)]\,[x_0^k - x_0'^k(x_2^k)] \quad (4.11)$$

and the cross derivatives $\delta D_0(a)/\delta x_0'^b(x_2^b)$ and $\delta D_0(b)/\delta x_0'^a(x_2^a)$ are zero. The stationary point $\delta D_0(k)/\delta x_0'^k(x_2^k) = 0$ is obtained when $x_0'^k(x_2^k)$ satisfies for $k = a, b$

$$x_0'^k(x_2^k) = \frac{\int dx_0^a\, dx_0^b\, P_0(x_0^a, x_0^b)\, P_{2,1}[x_2^k \mid x_1^a(x_0^a, x_0^b), x_1^b(x_0^a, x_0^b)]\, x_0^k}{\int dx_0^a\, dx_0^b\, P_0(x_0^a, x_0^b)\, P_{2,1}[x_2^k \mid x_1^a(x_0^a, x_0^b), x_1^b(x_0^a, x_0^b)]} \quad (4.12)$$

Note that this result can readily be generalized to an arbitrary choice of $P_{1,0}(x_1^a, x_1^b \mid x_0^a, x_0^b)$ (i.e., not assuming equation 4.2).

By using Bayes' theorem in the form shown in Equation 4.6 this reduces to

$$x_0'^k(x_2^k) = \int dx_0^k \, \tilde{P}_{0,2}(x_0^k \mid x_2^k) \, x_0^k \qquad k = a, b \qquad (4.13)$$

Thus the modified expression for $D_0(k)$ in equation 4.10 reduces to the original expression for $D_0(k)$ in equation 4.5 provided that $x_0'^k(x_2^k)$ is chosen to minimize $D_0(k)$, so equation 4.10 will be used in preference to equation 4.5 [with the proviso that $x_0'^k(x_2^k)$ should always be chosen to minimize $D_0(k)$].

When the upper bound of D in equation 4.9 is minimized with respect to $x_1^k(x_0^a, x_0^b)$ using equation 4.10 it yields for $k = a, b$

$$x_1^k(x_0^a, x_0^b) = \arg_{x_1^k} \min \left[\begin{array}{l} \int dx_2^a \, P_{2,1}(x_2^a \mid x_1^a, x_1^b) \, \|x_0^a - x_0'^a(x_2^a)\|^2 \\ + \int dx_2^b \, P_{2,1}(x_2^b \mid x_1^a, x_1^b) \, \|x_0^b - x_0'^b(x_2^b)\|^2 \end{array} \right] \qquad (4.14)$$

and the following on-line training prescription for $k = a, b$

$$x_0'^k(x_2^k) \rightarrow x_0'^k(x_2^k) + \epsilon \, P_{2,1}[x_2^k \mid x_1^a(x_0^a, x_0^b), x_1^b(x_0^a, x_0^b)] \, [x_0^k - x_0'^k(x_2^k)] \qquad (4.15)$$

These results correspond to the self-supervised training scheme that was proposed in Luttrell (1991b, 1992), which was the result of a detailed study of the problem of designing an encoder/decoder for a pair of communication channels whose transmitted information was degraded by a noise process (both external noise and noisy coupling between the channels). The improvement in performance when channel coupling is taken into account was shown to be significant, so the least upper bound approximation is justified in hindsight for this type of system.

The following remarks can be made about these results:

1. The functions $x_0'^a(x_2^a)$ and $x_0'^b(x_2^b)$ are the continuum versions of the reference vectors of a pair of SOMs corresponding to FMC a and FMC b, respectively.

2. The results for $x_1^a(x_0^a, x_0^b)$ and $x_1^b(x_0^a, x_0^b)$ are modified forms of the minimum distortion encoding prescription, in which the coupling between the FMC a and FMC b manifests itself through $P_{2,1}(x_2^a \mid x_1^a, x_1^b)$ and $P_{2,1}(x_2^b \mid x_1^a, x_1^b)$.

3. In both the batch and the on-line training prescription $P_{2,1}(x_2^a \mid x_1^a, x_1^b)$ and $P_{2,1}(x_2^b \mid x_1^a, x_1^b)$ play the role of neighborhood functions for SOM a and SOM b, respectively. However, the coupling between the SOMs causes these neighborhood functions to be dependent on the input data, as will be discussed in more detail below.

A Bayesian Analysis of Self-Organizing Maps

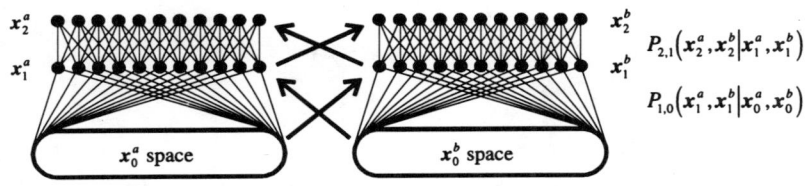

Figure 9: A pair of coupled discrete SOMs represented as a pair of coupled networks of the type shown in Figure 6. As derived above, the coupling $P_{2,1}(x_2^a, x_2^b \mid x_1^a, x_1^b)$ between networks a and b expresses itself as a pair of data dependent neighborhood functions $P_{2,1}(x_2^a \mid x_1^a, x_1^b)$ and $P_{2,1}(x_2^b \mid x_1^a, x_1^b)$. When the first stage of each of these coupled SOMs is optimized, taking account of $P_{2,1}(x_2^a \mid x_1^a, x_1^b)$ and $P_{2,1}(x_2^b \mid x_1^a, x_1^b)$, the encoding functions $x_1^a(x_0^a, x_0^b)$ and $x_1^b(x_0^a, x_0^b)$ become mutually coupled.

4.3 Network Representation of Self-Supervision. In Figure 9 the network representation of the pair of coupled SOMs is shown for a discrete-valued output. The detailed interpretation of equation 4.14 and equation 4.15 is shown in Figure 10.

The marginal probabilities $P_{2,1}(x_2^a \mid x_1^a, x_1^b)$ and $P_{2,1}(x_2^b \mid x_1^a, x_1^b)$ are obtained by projecting $P_{2,1}(x_2^a, x_2^b \mid x_1^a, x_1^b)$ onto x_2^a and x_2^b, respectively. The data dependence of $P_{2,1}(x_2^a, x_2^b \mid x_1^a, x_1^b)$ causes these marginal probabilities to be data dependent. In particular, they can be biased as shown in Figure 10, which causes the neighborhood functions (in the SOM interpretation) in x_2^a and x_2^b space to be biased.

The data dependence has another subtle side effect in Figure 10. The input transformations $x_1^a(x_0^a, x_0^b)$ and $x_1^b(x_0^a, x_0^b)$ depend on the marginal probabilities $P_{2,1}(x_2^a \mid x_1^a, x_1^b)$ and $P_{2,1}(x_2^b \mid x_1^a, x_1^b)$, because the input transformations satisfy a minimum distortion criterion which depends on these marginal probabilities (see equation 4.14). However, the marginal probabilities themselves are data dependent, because they depend on x_1^a and x_1^b, which in turn depend on the input transformations. Overall, the marginal probabilities and the input transformations are mutually dependent, which makes the minimum distortion encoding prescription quite subtle to implement in this case.

Further details on self-supervision can be found in Luttrell (1991b, 1992), where a detailed discussion and numerical simulation of the consequences of using a particular type of $P_{2,1}(x_2^a, x_2^b \mid x_1^a, x_1^b)$ are presented, a comparison is made between nearest neighbor and minimum distortion encoding, and a comparison is made between using mutually depen-

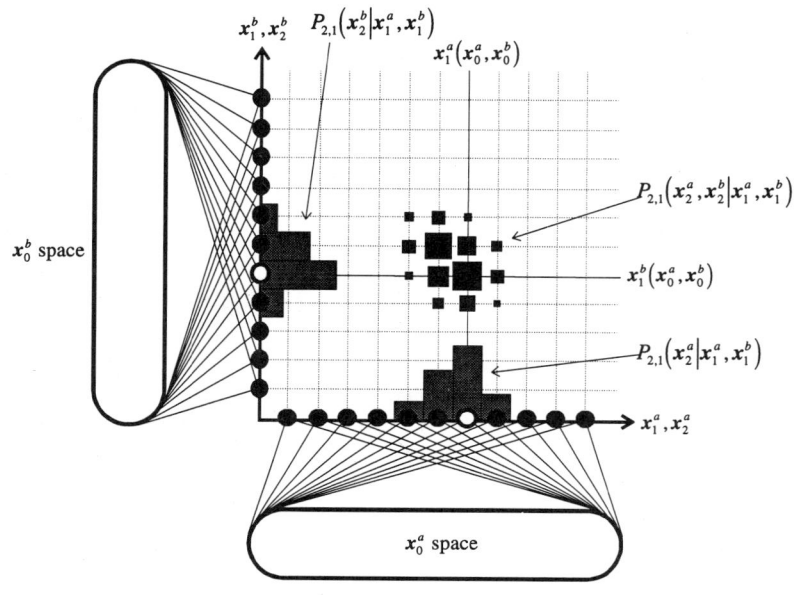

Figure 10: Diagram showing the detailed operation of a pair of coupled FMCs. For simplicity, (x_2^a, x_2^b) is assumed to sit in the same vector space as (x_1^a, x_1^b). Examples of the winners $x_1^a(x_0^a, x_0^b)$ and $x_1^b(x_0^a, x_0^b)$ are indicated by the open circles. These are then jointly smeared into the distribution $P_{2,1}(x_2^a, x_2^b \mid x_1^a, x_1^b)$, which is drawn as a 2-dimensional histogram. As derived above, the optimization depends on a pair of neighborhood functions $P_{2,1}(x_2^a \mid x_1^a, x_1^b)$ and $P_{2,1}(x_2^b \mid x_1^a, x_1^b)$, which are the marginal probabilities of $P_{2,1}(x_2^a, x_2^b \mid x_1^a, x_1^b)$, and which are drawn as one-dimensional histograms in the diagram. These data-dependent neighborhood functions not only influence the optimization of the FMC, but also determine the winners that should have been used in the first place.

dent neighborhood functions $P_{2,1}(x_2^k \mid x_1^a, x_1^b)$ ($k = a, b$) and independent neighborhood functions $P_{2,1}(x_2^a \mid x_1^a)$ and $P_{2,1}(x_2^b \mid x_1^b)$.

5 Conclusions

In this paper it has been demonstrated that VQ theory, SOM theory, and the theory of self-supervision all emerge naturally when an FMC is optimized so as to minimize the expected Euclidean error between an input vector and its attempted reconstruction (using Bayes' theorem).

A Bayesian Analysis of Self-Organizing Maps   271

FMC theory can be used to facilitate many computations that would otherwise be theoretically and/or numerically intractable. The "soft" probabilities that are used in the FMC are easier to compute with than the "hard" delta functions in the corresponding winner-take-all VQs and SOMs. The results contained in this paper guarantee that these "soft" computations reduce to the required "hard" computations when the first stage of the FMC is optimized.

6 Appendix

6.1 Relationship between Continuum and Discrete Vector Quantizers.

Throughout this paper continuum notation is used. In the case of a VQ this has the effect that the index that is used to select the winning reference vector is assumed to be a continuous-valued quantity, rather than a discrete-valued quantity. The purpose of this appendix is to relate the continuum case to the discrete case.

It is sufficient to discuss the meaning of the on-line training prescription in equation 3.13 and equation 3.14, which is presented again here for convenience.

$$\begin{aligned} x_1(x_0) &= \arg\min_{x_1} \|x_0 - x_0'(x_1)\|^2 \\ x_0'(x_1) &\to x_0'(x_1) + \epsilon \delta[x_1 - x_1(x_0)] [x_0 - x_0'(x_1)] \end{aligned} \tag{6.1}$$

where x_1 is assumed to lie in the unit N-dimensional hypercube. The discrete counterpart of this on-line prescription is

$$\begin{aligned} k_1(x_0) &= \arg\min_{k_1} \|x_0 - x_{0,k_1}'\|^2 \\ x_{0,k_1}' &\to x_{0,k_1}' + \epsilon \delta_{k_1,k_1(x_0)} (x_0 - x_{0,k_1}') \end{aligned} \tag{6.2}$$

where k_1 is a point on an N-dimensional cubic lattice.

The relationship between the nearest neighbor encoding prescriptions $x_1(x_0)$ and $k_1(x_0)$ is simple to understand, so no further comment is required. On the other hand, the interpretation of the update prescription for $x_0'(x_1)$ is quite subtle, so it will now be discussed in some detail.

In order to interpret the continuum prescription correctly it is necessary to integrate over a small region S with volume δV that encloses the point $x_1 = x_1(x_0)$, and to assume that $x_0'(x_1)$ is a smooth function of x_1 (for a justification of this assumption, see the last paragraph of this appendix). This leads to the result

$$x_0'(x_1) \to x_0'(x_1) + \frac{\epsilon}{\delta V} [x_0 - x_0'(x_1)] \text{ where } x_1 \in S \text{ and } x_1(x_0) \in S \tag{6.3}$$

which can be compared directly with the update prescription for x_{0,k_1}'. Note that $\epsilon/\delta V$, rather than ϵ, determines the size of the updates of the reference vectors that are attached to points x_1 inside S. The smaller the volume δV is, the smaller ϵ has to be to keep the updates the same size. The most natural prescription is to impose a lower bound δL on the length scale of x_1 of interest, which then imposes a natural size on the volume of S such that $\delta V = \delta L^N$. Since x_1 is assumed to lie in the unit hypercube, this prescription leads to a finite effective number of reference vectors given by δL^{-N}, which would correspond to an N-dimensional cubic lattice whose size was $1/\delta L$ lattice spacings in each dimension.

An interesting side effect of introducing this inner length scale δL (which is effectively a regularization constant) is that it automatically generates an SOM on-line training prescription. To see this, note that in equation 6.3 a whole volume δV of reference vectors x_1 in the neighborhood S of the point $x_1 = x_1(x_0)$ is updated. This is precisely the type of update prescription that creates an SOM. Furthermore, this justifies with hindsight the assumption made earlier that $x'_0(x_1)$ is a smooth function of x_1.

6.2 Full Optimization of 2-Stage Folded Markov Chains. In this appendix it will be shown that if a 2-stage FMC with a Euclidean error function is optimized with respect to $P_{1,0}(x_1 \mid x_0)$, then it reduces to $P_{1,0}(x_1 \mid x_0) = \delta[x_1 - x_1(x_0)]$. Because a 2-stage FMC contains a 1-stage FMC as a special case, it is necessary to present the derivation only for a 2-stage FMC. The result that is obtained depends on certain properties of the Euclidean error function; it is not a general property of FMCs.

There are two constraints that must be respected during the optimization of $P_{1,0}(x_1 \mid x_0)$. Total probability must be conserved

$$\int dx_1 \, P_{1,0}(x_1 \mid x_0) = 1 \quad \text{for all } x_0 \tag{6.4}$$

and $\tilde{P}_{0,1}(x_0 \mid x_1)$ must vary in response to variations of $P_{1,0}(x_1 \mid x_0)$ in such a way that Bayes' theorem is respected (i.e., equation 2.1 with $k = 0$)

$$\tilde{P}_{0,1}(x_0 \mid x_1) \left[\int du_0 \, P_{1,0}(x_1 \mid u_0) P_0(u_0) \right] = P_{1,0}(x_1 \mid x_0) P_0(x_0)$$

$$\text{for all } x_0, x_1 \tag{6.5}$$

The first constraint will be imposed for all x_0 by using a Lagrange multiplier function $\lambda(x_0)$, whereas the second constraint will be imposed by using Bayes' theorem to eliminate $\tilde{P}_{0,1}(x_0 \mid x_1)$ from D.

The overall quantity $\bar{D}$ to be minimized is therefore

$$\begin{aligned}\bar{D} = & \int dx_0 \, dx_1 \, dx_2 \, dx'_0 \, dx'_1 \, dx'_2 \\ & \times P_0(x_0) P_{1,0}(x_1 \mid x_0) P_{2,1}(x_2 \mid x_1) \delta(x'_2 - x_2) \\ & \times \tilde{P}_{1,2}(x'_1 \mid x'_2) \tilde{P}_{0,1}(x'_0 \mid x'_1) \, \|x'_0 - x_0\|^2 \\ & - \int dx_0 \, \lambda(x_0) \int dx_1 \, P_{1,0}(x_1 \mid x_0)\end{aligned} \tag{6.6}$$

A Bayesian Analysis of Self-Organizing Maps

Integration over x_2 and use of Bayes' theorem on both $\tilde{P}_{1,2}(x_1' \mid x_2')$ and $\tilde{P}_{0,1}(x_0' \mid x_1')$ transforms $\bar{D}$ into a form that is suitable for differentiation with respect to the sought after quantity $P_{1,0}(x_1 \mid x_0)$

$$\begin{aligned}
\bar{D} &= \int dx_0 \, dx_1 \, dx_0' \, dx_1' \, dx_2' \, P_0(x_0) \, P_{1,0}(x_1 \mid x_0) \, P_{1,0}(x_1' \mid x_0') \, P_0(x_0') \\
&\quad \times \frac{P_{2,1}(x_2' \mid x_1) \, P_{2,1}(x_2' \mid x_1')}{(\int du_0 \, du_1 \, P_{2,1}(x_2' \mid u_1) \, P_{1,0}(u_1 \mid u_0) \, P_0(u_0))} \, \|x_0' - x_0\|^2 \\
&\quad - \int dx_0 \, \lambda(x_0) \int dx_1 \, P_{1,0}(x_1 \mid x_0)
\end{aligned} \tag{6.7}$$

Functional differentiation of $\bar{D}$ with respect to $P_{1,0}(z_1 \mid z_0)$, and using the symmetry of $\bar{D}$ under interchange of x_0 and x_0', then leads to

$$\begin{aligned}
\frac{\delta \bar{D}}{\delta P_{1,0}(z_1 \mid z_0)} &= 2 \int dx_0 \, dx_1 \, dx_0' \, dx_1' \, dx_2' \, \delta(x_0 - z_0) \, \delta(x_1 - z_1) \\
&\quad \times P_0(x_0) \, P_{1,0}(x_1' \mid x_0') \, P_0(x_0') \\
&\quad \times \frac{P_{2,1}(x_2' \mid x_1) \, P_{2,1}(x_2' \mid x_1')}{(\int du_0 \, du_1 \, P_{2,1}(x_2' \mid u_1) \, P_{1,0}(u_1 \mid u_0) \, P_0(u_0))} \, \|x_0' - x_0\|^2 \\
&\quad - \int dx_0 \, dx_1 \, dx_0' \, dx_1' \, dx_2' \, P_0(x_0) \, P_{1,0}(x_1 \mid x_0) \, P_{1,0}(x_1' \mid x_0') \, P_0(x_0') \\
&\quad \times \frac{P_{2,1}(x_2' \mid x_1) \, P_{2,1}(x_2' \mid x_1')}{[\int du_0 \, du_1 \, P_{2,1}(x_2' \mid u_1) \, P_{1,0}(u_1 \mid u_0) \, P_0(u_0)]^2} \\
&\quad \times \left[\int dv_0 \, dv_1 \, \delta(v_0 - z_0) \, \delta(v_1 - z_1) \, P_{2,1}(x_2' \mid v_1) \, P_0(v_0) \right] \\
&\quad \times \|x_0' - x_0\|^2 \\
&\quad - \int dx_0 \, \lambda(x_0) \int dx_1 \, \delta(x_0 - z_0) \, \delta(x_1 - z_1)
\end{aligned} \tag{6.8}$$

Using Bayes' theorem this simplifies to

$$\begin{aligned}
\frac{\delta \bar{D}}{\delta P_{1,0}(z_1 \mid z_0)} &= 2 P_0(z_0) \int dx_2' \, P_{2,1}(x_2' \mid z_1) \int dx_1' \, \tilde{P}_{1,2}(x_1' \mid x_2') \\
&\quad \times \int dx_0' \, \tilde{P}_{0,1}(x_0' \mid x_1') \, \|x_0' - z_0\|^2 \\
&\quad - P_0(z_0) \int dx_2' \, P_{2,1}(x_2' \mid z_1) \int dx_1 \, \tilde{P}_{1,2}(x_1 \mid x_2') \\
&\quad \times \int dx_1' \, \tilde{P}_{1,2}(x_1' \mid x_2') \\
&\quad \times \int dx_0 \, dx_0' \, \tilde{P}_{0,1}(x_0 \mid x_1) \, \tilde{P}_{0,1}(x_0' \mid x_1') \, \|x_0' - x_0\|^2 \\
&\quad - \lambda(z_0)
\end{aligned} \tag{6.9}$$

Expansion and factorization eventually lead to the result

$$\frac{\delta \bar{D}}{\delta P_{1,0}(z_1 \mid z_0)} = 2 P_0(z_0) \int dx'_2 \, P_{2,1}(x'_2 \mid z_1)$$

$$\times \left\| \int dx'_0 \, dx'_1 \, \tilde{P}_{0,1}(x'_0 \mid x'_1) \, \tilde{P}_{1,2}(x'_1 \mid x'_2) \, x'_0 - z_0 \right\|^2$$

$$- \lambda(z_0) \tag{6.10}$$

The stationarity condition $\delta \bar{D}/\delta P_{1,0}(x_1 \mid x_0) = 0$ is therefore

$$2 P_0(x_0) \int dx'_2 \, P_{2,1}(x'_2 \mid x_1) \left\| \int dx'_0 \, \tilde{P}_{0,2}(x'_0 \mid x'_2) \, x'_0 - x_0 \right\|^2 = \lambda(x_0) \tag{6.11}$$

The right-hand side of equation 6.11 is a function only of x_0, whereas the left-hand side is a function of both x_0 and x_1, where x_1 appears only in the $P_{2,1}(x'_2 \mid x_1)$ factor. Because x_1 appears only on the left-hand side of this equation, its effect must somehow vanish.

There are two types of solution in which the dependence on x_1 vanishes:

1. $P_0(x_0) = 0$. The dependence of the left-hand side of equation 6.11 is suppressed by the zero-valued $P_0(x_0)$ factor. Any legal probability $P_{1,0}(x_1 \mid x_0)$ is thus permitted for values of x_0 that have $P_0(x_0) = 0$. This solution may be eliminated because for those x_0 that have $P_0(x_0) = 0$ where there is no need to define $P_{1,0}(x_1 \mid x_0)$ anyway.

2. $P_0(x_0) > 0$. Note that the variance-like factor

$$\left\| \int dx'_0 \, \tilde{P}_{0,2}(x'_0 \mid x'_2) \, x'_0 - x_0 \right\|^2 \geq 0,$$

so there are two situations to consider:

 a. $\| \cdots \|^2 > 0$. In order to suppress the x_1 dependence of the left-hand side of equation 6.11 x_1 must be uniquely determined by the value of x_0. So $x_1 = x_1(x_0)$ and $P_{1,0}(x_1 \mid x_0) = \delta[x_1 - x_1(x_0)]$.
 b. $\| \cdots \|^2 = 0$. Apparently, any legal probability $P_{1,0}(x_1 \mid x_0)$ is permitted. However, any $P_{1,0}(x_1 \mid x_0) \neq \delta[x_1 - x_1(x_0)]$ will guarantee that the variance-like factor $\| \cdots \|^2 > 0$, so the only $P_{1,0}(x_1 \mid x_0)$ that can possibly survive are $P_{1,0}(x_1 \mid x_0) = \delta[x_1 - x_1(x_0)]$. Note that with $P_{1,0}(x_1 \mid x_0) = \delta[x_1 - x_1(x_0)]$ it is still possible that $\| \cdots \|^2 > 0$, in which case this solution can be eliminated.

The only solution that remains is $P_{1,0}(x_1 \mid x_0) = \delta[x_1 - x_1(x_0)]$. This result establishes the fact that the replacement of $P_{1,0}(x_1 \mid x_0)$ by $\delta[x_1 - x_1(x_0)]$ used in equation 3.10 (and in equation 4.2, in the case of coupled FMCs) emerges naturally from minimizing D in the function space of probabilities $P_{1,0}(x_1 \mid x_0)$.

A Bayesian Analysis of Self-Organizing Maps

It is important to note that the choice of a Euclidean error function is sufficient (but not necessary) for $P_{1,0}(x_1 \mid x_0) = \delta[x_1 - x_1(x_0)]$ to emerge. Also, note that it is not true in general that optimization of $P_{1,0}(x_1 \mid x_0)$ leads to $P_{1,0}(x_1 \mid x_0) = \delta[x_1 - x_1(x_0)]$. For instance, this is the case when $\|x_0 - x_0'\|^2$ is replaced by either of the following two functional forms

$$\|x_0 - x_0'\|^2 \rightarrow \begin{cases} A(x_0) + B(x_0') & \text{counterexample 1} \\ A(x_0)B(x_0') & \text{counterexample 2} \end{cases} \quad (6.12)$$

Although these might not be considered to be sensible error functions, the fact that counterexamples exist is in itself important.

These counterexamples may be described briefly as follows:

1. Counterexample 1 leads to a D that has no dependence on $P_{1,0}(x_1 \mid x_0)$. Optimization of $P_{1,0}(x_1 \mid x_0)$ will allow any legal probability, so $P_{1,0}(x_1 \mid x_0) \neq \delta[x_1 - x_1(x_0)]$ is permitted.

2. Counterexample 2 is more complicated to analyze. However, it is possible to show that $P_{1,0}(x_1 \mid x_0)$, when viewed as a matrix, has a block diagonal structure. This type of $P_{1,0}(x_1 \mid x_0)$ does not imply a deterministic relationship between x_0 and x_1, so $P_{1,0}(x_1 \mid x_0) \neq \delta[x_1 - x_1(x_0)]$ is permitted.

Acknowledgments

The author is indebted to the following people for critically reading this paper: Eric Jakeman, David Lowe, and Graeme Mitchison.

References

Farvardin, N. 1990. A study of vector quantisation for noisy channels. *IEEE Trans. IT* **36**, 799–809.

Farvardin, N., and Vaishampayan, V. 1991. On the performance and complexity of channel-optimised vector quantisers. *IEEE Trans. IT* **37**, 155–160.

Kohonen, T. 1984. *Self Organisation and Associative Memory*. Springer-Verlag, Berlin.

Kumazawa, H., Kasahara, M., and Namekawa, T. 1984. A construction of vector quantisers for noisy channels. *Elect. Eng. Jpn.* **67B**, 39–47.

Linde, Y., Buzo, A., and Gray, R. M. 1980. An algorithm for vector quantiser design. *IEEE Trans. COM* **28**, 84–95.

Luttrell, S. P. 1989a. Self-organisation: A derivation from first principles of a class of learning algorithms. *Proc. 3rd IEEE Int. Joint Conf. Neural Networks*, Washington, DC, **2**, 495–498.

Luttrell, S. P. 1989b. Hierarchical vector quantisation. *Proc. IEE Part I*, **136**, 405–413.

Luttrell, S. P. 1989c. Hierarchical self-organising networks. *Proc. 1st IEE Conf. Artificial Neural Networks*, London, 2–6.

Luttrell, S. P. 1989d. Image compression using a multilayer neural network. *Patt. Recog. Lett.* **10**, 1–7.

Luttrell, S. P. 1990. Derivation of a class of training algorithms. *IEEE Trans. NN* **1**, 229–232.

Luttrell, S. P. 1991a. Code vector density in topographic mappings: Scalar case. *IEEE Trans. NN* **2**, 427–436.

Luttrell, S. P. 1991b. Self-supervised training of hierarchical vector quantisers. *Proc. 2nd IEE Conf. Artificial Neural Networks*, Bournemouth, 5–9.

Luttrell, S. P. 1992. Self-supervision in multilayer adaptive networks. *Proc. IEE Part F* **139(6)**, 371–377.

Ritter, H. 1991. Asymptotic level density for a class of vector quantisation processes. *IEEE Trans. NN* **2**, 173–175.

Yair, E., Zeger, K., and Gersho, A. 1992. Competitive learning and soft competition for vector quantiser design. *IEEE Trans. SP* **40**, 294–309.

14

Hyperparameter Selection for Self-Organizing Maps

Akio Utsugi
*National Institute of Bioscience and Human Technology,
Higashi Tsukuba Ibaraki 305, Japan*

The self-organizing map (SOM) algorithm for finite data is derived as an approximate maximum a posteriori estimation algorithm for a gaussian mixture model with a gaussian smoothing prior, which is equivalent to a generalized deformable model (GDM). For this model, objective criteria for selecting hyperparameters are obtained on the basis of empirical Bayesian estimation and cross-validation, which are representative model selection methods. The properties of these criteria are compared by simulation experiments. These experiments show that the cross-validation methods favor more complex structures than the expected log likelihood supports, which is a measure of compatibility between a model and data distribution. On the other hand, the empirical Bayesian methods have the opposite bias.

1 Introduction

Several standard learning methods for neural networks are being reconstructed as an estimation algorithm of a stochastic model. Such statistical treatment of learning enables inference at a higher level than a simple parameter estimation level, such as the evaluation of model reliability and automatic model selection. For example, MacKay (1992) studied backpropagation learning in a unifying Bayesian framework and presented a selection method of hyperparameters and model structure.

Among many learning methods, the self-organizing map (SOM) (Kohonen 1988, 1990) is unique from the viewpoint of data analysis because of its ability to extract topological structure hidden in data. However, since this learning was originally defined only at an algorithmic level, its development to higher-level inference is difficult.

Statistical models behaving in a similar manner as SOM are also studied. The elastic net (Durbin et al. 1989), which is one of the generalized deformable models (GDM) (Yuille 1990), learns a topology-preserving map as maximum a posteriori (MAP) estimates for the parameters of a Bayesian stochastic model. Although this model was studied originally in the context of an optimization problem such as the traveling salesman problem, it can be used for smoothing data along a specified topology. However, this requires the determination of two hyperparameters: the size of noise and the smoothness of route. The selection of these hyperparameters was attempted by an empirical Bayesian method similar to that of MacKay for backpropagation learning (Utsugi 1993).

This article first reviews the hyperparameter selection method. Next, the SOM algorithm for finite data is derived as an approximate MAP estimation algorithm for GDM. Thus, SOM and GDM can be considered equivalent at a stochastic model level. Finally, cross-validation, another representative model selection method, is applied to hyperparameter selection for our model and compared with the empirical Bayesian method by simulation experiments.

2 Empirical Bayesian Hyperparameter Selection for GDM

2.1 Construction of GDM as Stochastic Model.

Initially, we regard the simplest type of gaussian mixture model as a stochastic model for competitive learning (Nowlan 1990). For a data set X consisting of m-dimensional data points $x_i = (x_{i1}, \ldots, x_{im})'$ ($i = 1, \ldots, n$), the likelihood function of the model with r components is given by

$$f(X|w, \beta) = \prod_{i=1}^{n} \sum_{s=1}^{r} \frac{1}{r} f(x_i|w_s, \beta), \tag{2.1}$$

where

$$f(x_i|w_s, \beta) = \left(\frac{\beta}{2\pi}\right)^{m/2} \exp\left(-\frac{\beta}{2}\|x_i - w_s\|^2\right) \tag{2.2}$$

is a component gaussian density with the centroid $w_s = (w_{s1}, \ldots, w_{sm})'$ and the variance $1/\beta$, and $w = (w_1', \ldots, w_r')'$.

Furthermore, we consider a gaussian smoothing prior to express smooth variation of the centroids along a topological space. Using a discretized differential operator matrix D on the topological space, the density of this smoothing prior is defined by

$$g(w|\alpha) = \prod_{j=1}^{m} \left(\frac{\alpha}{2\pi}\right)^{l/2} (\det{}^+ D'D)^{1/2} \exp\left(-\frac{\alpha}{2}\|Dw_{(j)}\|^2\right), \tag{2.3}$$

where $w_{(j)} = (w_{1j}, \ldots, w_{rj})'$, $l = \operatorname{rank} D'D$, and $\det{}^+ D'D$ denotes the product of positive eigenvalues of $D'D$. The hyperparameter α represents the strength of smooth constraint. Although the elastic net uses the first-order differential operator on a one-dimensional closed-loop topology, we can use various kinds of differential operators and topologies.

From the likelihood (cf. equation 2.1) and the prior (cf. equation 2.3), we obtain the log posterior by Bayes' theorem:

$$\log g(w|X, \alpha, \beta) = \log f(X|w, \beta) + \log g(w|\alpha) + const.$$

$$= \sum_{i=1}^{n} \log \sum_{s=1}^{r} \exp\left(-\frac{\beta}{2} \|x_i - w_s\|^2\right)$$

$$- \frac{\alpha}{2} \sum_{j=1}^{m} \|Dw_{(j)}\|^2 + const. \quad (2.4)$$

This corresponds to the negative energy function of an elastic net, whose maximizer gives the MAP estimates of centroids. The elastic net algorithm is a MAP estimation algorithm using the gradient ascent method. We can also use the expectation-maximization (EM) algorithm (Yuille et al., 1994; Utsugi 1994), which is explained in section 3.

2.2 Selection of Hyperparameters by Empirical Bayesian Method. Next, we obtain the marginal likelihood of hyperparameters α and β:

$$f(X|\alpha, \beta) = \int f(X|w, \beta) g(w|\alpha) dw \propto \int g(w|X, \alpha, \beta) dw$$

$$= \int f(w, X|\alpha, \beta) dw. \quad (2.5)$$

This is also called the evidence of the hyperparameters. Although we desire to obtain the optimal values of hyperparameters by maximizing the evidence, we have difficulty calculating the integral in equation 2.5 exactly. Here, we use a gaussian approximation (MacKay 1992), where the logarithm of the integrand is substituted by its quadratic approximation at the maximizer.

In this case, using the MAP estimate $\hat{w}$ and the negative Hesse matrix of the log posterior,

$$H(w) = -\frac{\partial^2}{\partial w \partial w'} \log g(w|X, \alpha, \beta), \quad (2.6)$$

the integrand is approximated as

$$f(w, X|\alpha, \beta) \simeq f(\hat{w}, X|\alpha, \beta) \exp\left(-\frac{1}{2} w' H(\hat{w}) w\right). \quad (2.7)$$

Then the evidence is approximated as

$$f(X, S_{\hat{w}}|\alpha, \beta) = \int_{S_{\hat{w}}} f(w, X|\alpha, \beta) g(w|\alpha) dw$$

$$= \int_{S_{\hat{w}}} g(w|X, \alpha, \beta) dw$$

$$\simeq (2\pi)^{rm/2} (\det H(\hat{w}))^{-1/2} f(\hat{w}, X|\alpha, \beta) \quad (2.8)$$

where $S_{\hat{w}}$ is a region dominated by $\hat{w}$ in the parameter space. This evidence consists of probability mass on only $S_{\hat{w}}$, and thus it should be called local evidence. We use the local evidence to select the values of hyperparameters, like MacKay's manner for backpropagation learning.

Now, the log evidence is calculated by

$$\log f(X, S_{\hat{w}} | \alpha, \beta) \simeq \frac{nm}{2} \log \beta + \sum_{i=1}^{n} \log \sum_{s=1}^{r} \exp\left(-\frac{\beta}{2} \|x_i - \hat{w}_s\|^2\right)$$

$$+ \frac{lm}{2} \log \alpha$$

$$- \frac{\alpha}{2} \sum_{j=1}^{m} \|D\hat{w}_{(j)}\|^2$$

$$- \frac{1}{2} \log \det H(\hat{w}) + const. \tag{2.9}$$

The matrix $H(\hat{w})$ is the sum of negative Hesse matrices of the log likelihood and the log prior, which are denoted by $H_f(\hat{w})$ and H_g, respectively. The matrix $H_f(\hat{w})$ consists of submatrices,

$$H_{st}(\hat{w}) = -\frac{\partial^2}{\partial w_s \partial w'_t} \log f(X | \hat{w}, \beta)$$

$$= \begin{cases} \beta^2 \sum_{i}^{n} p_{si}(p_{si} - 1)(x_i - \hat{w}_s)(x_i - \hat{w}_s)' + \beta n_s I_m, & s = t \\ \beta^2 \sum_{i}^{n} p_{si} p_{ti}(x_i - \hat{w}_s)(x_i - \hat{w}_t)', & s \neq t \end{cases}$$

$$(s, t = 1, \ldots, r), \tag{2.10}$$

where I_m is an identity matrix with size m. The quantity p_{si} is defined by

$$p_{si} = \frac{f(x_i | \hat{w}_s, \beta)}{\sum_{s=1}^{r} f(x_i | \hat{w}_s, \beta)}, \tag{2.11}$$

which is called the fuzzy membership of the ith data to the sth component, and $n_s = \sum_{i=1}^{n} p_{si}$ is the estimated number of data points belonging to the sth component. The matrix H_g is given by

$$H_g = \alpha D'D \otimes I_m, \tag{2.12}$$

where $\otimes$ denotes the Kronecker product.

By maximizing the evidence, we obtain estimates of α and β. Simulation experiments showed that this method gives good solutions (Utsugi 1993).[1]

---

[1] This evidence is improved from the previously presented one, for which r was used instead of l in equation 2.9. In a wide range of α, these are almost the same. However, the old evidence grows infinitely as $\alpha \to \infty$, while the new one stays finite.

3 Derivation of SOM Algorithm

In this section, the original SOM algorithm for finite data is derived as an approximate MAP estimation algorithm for the GDM.

Initially, we showed that the EM algorithm of GDM is an alternate iteration of smoothing and soft classification. Now we define binary membership variables $Y = (y_{si})$, where y_{si} denotes the membership of the ith data point to the sth component. Regarding these variables as missing data, we obtain a complete likelihood,

$$f(X, Y|w, \beta) = \prod_{i=1}^{n}\prod_{s=1}^{r}\left(\frac{1}{r}f(x_i|w_s, \beta)\right)^{y_{si}}, \tag{3.1}$$

which would be an exact likelihood if the missing data were acquired. In the EM algorithm, the following function is maximized instead of the genuine log posterior (cf. equation 2.4),

$$Q(w) = E_Y(\log f(X, Y|w, \beta)|X, \hat{w}, \beta) + \log g(w|\alpha), \tag{3.2}$$

where $\hat{w}$ is a temporary estimate and $E_Y(\cdot|\cdot)$ denotes conditional expectation with respect to Y. The maximizer of Q is used as $\hat{w}$ at the next step. This procedure is iterated until convergence. By calculating Q, we obtain

$$Q(w) = -\frac{\beta}{2}\sum_{i=1}^{n}\sum_{s=1}^{r}p_{si}\|x_i - w_s\|^2 - \frac{\alpha}{2}\sum_{j=1}^{m}\|Dw_{(j)}\|^2 + const., \tag{3.3}$$

where p_{si} is the fuzzy membership (cf. equation 2.11) using the temporary estimate $\hat{w}$. This maximization of Q is equivalent to the independent minimizations of

$$H_j(w_{(j)}) = \sum_{s=1}^{r}n_s(\bar{x}_{sj} - w_{sj})^2 + \gamma\|Dw_{(j)}\|^2, \quad (j = 1,\ldots,m), \tag{3.4}$$

where $\bar{x}_{sj}$ is the mean of data weighted by the fuzzy membership,

$$\bar{x}_{sj} = \frac{1}{n_s}\sum_{i=1}^{n}p_{si}x_{ij}, \tag{3.5}$$

and $\gamma = \alpha/\beta$. Each function H_j can be regarded as a discretized Laplacian smoothing criterion (O'Sullivan 1991) for the observations $\{\bar{x}_{sj} : s = 1, \ldots, r\}$ with confidence weights $\{n_s\}$, which are obtained through the soft competition process (cf. equation 2.11). A smooth curve minimizing this criterion is used as the next temporary estimate and is given by

$$\tilde{w}_{(j)} = KN\bar{x}_{(j)}, \tag{3.6}$$

where N is a diagonal matrix consisting of $\{n_s\}$, $\bar{x}_{(j)} = (\bar{x}_{1j}, \ldots, \bar{x}_{rj})'$ and

$$K = (N + \gamma D'D)^{-1}. \tag{3.7}$$

From the above explanation, the EM algorithm of GDM can be regarded as an alternate iteration of discretized Laplacian smoothing and soft classification.

On the other hand, Mulier and Cherkassky (1995) interpreted the batch SOM algorithm as an alternate iteration of kernel smoothing and hard classification. Using n_t and $\bar{x}_t = (\bar{x}_{t1}, \ldots, \bar{x}_{tm})'$, which are the number and the mean of data points in the Voronoi region of the weight point of the tth inner unit, they expressed the weight update rule of SOM as

$$\tilde{w}_{sj} = \sum_{t=1}^{r} \kappa(s, t) n_t \bar{x}_{tj} \Big/ \sum_{t=1}^{r} \kappa(s, t) n_t, \qquad (j = 1, \ldots, m), \tag{3.8}$$

where $\kappa(s, t)$ is a kernel function, for example, a gaussian density function with respect to $s - t$ for the normal one-dimensional topology. This is regarded as extended Nadaraya-Watson kernel smoothing (Härdle 1990) of the observations $\{\bar{x}_{tj}\}$ with confidence weights $\{n_t\}$.

In this point, the difference between GDM and SOM is summarized as follows: (1) soft classification versus hard classification, (2) discretized Laplacian smoothing versus kernel smoothing, and (3) in the original SOM, incremental learning is used rather than batch learning. Each method used in SOM can be regarded as an approximation of the associated method used in GDM, as explained below.

The soft competition process (cf. equation 2.11) turns hard as $\beta \to \infty$, and thus hard classification gives a good approximation for soft classification if β is large.[2]

The discretized Laplacian smoothing can also be approximated by kernel smoothing. As shown in the appendix, a curve smoothed by discretized Laplacian smoothing (cf. equation 3.6) is expressed by the kernel smoothing form (cf. equation 3.8) using the entries of K as the values of kernel function $\kappa(s, t)$. In reality, this kernel function is variable according to the variation of N, unlike SOM. In many cases, however, N is nearly proportional to I_r at the last stage of learning, since the expectation of N is proportional to I_r. In particular, for the second-order differential operator on a one-dimensional

---

[2] Also, hard competition can be derived from a MAP estimation algorithm of GDM with a classification likelihood rather than the mixture likelihood (cf. equation 2.1). The classification likelihood has the same form as the complete likelihood (cf. equation 3.1), though Y is regarded as a parameter rather than missing data. In general, classification likelihood approaches lead to poorer results than mixture likelihood approaches (McLachlan & Basford 1988).

line-segment topology, whose entries are

$$d_{ij} = \begin{cases} -2 & |i-j+1| = 0 \\ 1 & |i-j+1| = 1 \quad (i=1,\ldots,r-2; j=1,\ldots,r) \\ 0 & \text{otherwise,} \end{cases} \quad (3.9)$$

we can obtain an explicit form of the kernel function using Silverman's (1984) equivalent kernel of spline smoothing (Utsugi 1994). This kernel function has a Mexican-hat shape with a width proportional to $\gamma^{1/4}$.

Finally, we can also use a generalized EM algorithm (Dempster et al. 1977), where we use

$$w = (1-c)\hat{w} + c\tilde{w} \qquad (0 < c \leq 1) \quad (3.10)$$

as the next temporary estimate instead of $\tilde{w}$. Using small c, we can make the variation of the parameter in one leaning step arbitrarily small, where batch and incremental leaning are similar.

4 Comparison of Hyperparameter Selection Methods

4.1 Hyperparameter Selection by Cross-Validation. In section 2, an empirical Bayesian method for hyperparameter selection was studied. Another commonly used method for such problems is cross-validation. In this section, we apply cross-validation to our problem and compare the results with those of the empirical Bayesian method through simulation experiments.

Generally the rationale of cross-validation is as follows. The expected log likelihood (ELL) by a true data distribution is a good measure of model adequacy. In reality, we cannot calculate this value because of the unknown true data distribution. Instead, we use a cross-validation score as an unbiased estimate of ELL. However, this estimated criterion has considerable variance for small data, and its maximizer is not an unbiased estimate for the peak position of ELL. In the next simulation, we will calculate ELL, in addition to cross-validation scores and evidence, to observe the bias and variance of these criteria.

4.2 Simulation Experiments. We apply a GDM with 20 components and the differential operator (cf. equation 3.9) to two types of artificial data sets: low and high noise condition (see Figure 1). By using the values of hyperparameters at rectangular grid points in the hyperparameter space, we obtain the graph of each criterion. The landscapes and contour maps in Figures 2 and 3 are obtained by averaging each criterion for 20 different data sets. The histograms of peak positions for individual data sets also are shown in the figures. Figure 4 illustrates the configurations of estimated centroid parameters under several values of (α, β) in the low-noise condition. From these figures, we can conclude the following.

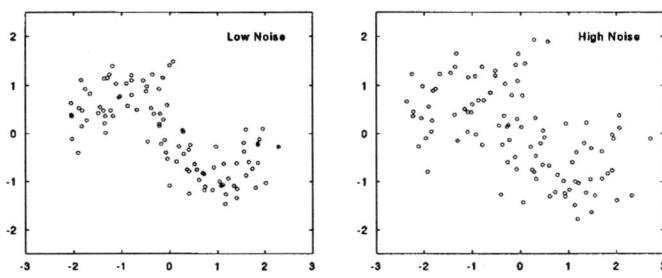

Figure 1: Scatter plots for samples of data sets. Artificial data $x_i = (x_{i1}, x_{i2})'$, ($i = 1, \ldots, 100$) are generated from two independent standard gaussian random series $\{e_{i1}\}$ and $\{e_{i2}\}$ by $x_{i1} = 4(i-1)/n - 2 + \sigma e_{i1}$, $x_{i2} = \sin[2\pi(i-1)/n] + \sigma e_{i2}$. Two conditions of noise level are used: low noise ($\sigma = 0.3$) and high noise ($\sigma = 0.5$). For each condition, 20 data sets are used in the simulation.

In the case of low noise (see Figure 2), peak positions of all criteria are close to each other except for a few peaks of cross-validation scores. In the area where the majority of the peaks are gathering, the configurations of centroid parameters have good appearances (see Figure 4, $\log_{10} \alpha = 2$, $\log_{10} \beta = 1$). Thus, we can say that both methods succeed for the most part. However, cross-validation scores have two peaks with much lower α than the other peaks, which lead to configurations that are too complicated. This is probably due to the flatness of the averaged landscape in its low α area and large variance of cross-validation scores. Because of this instability, the cross-validation method is inferior to the other method in this case, though its averaged landscape is similar to that of ELL.

Figure 2: *Facing page*. Landscapes and contour maps of averaged criteria and peak-position histograms for 20 data sets in the low-noise condition. For each data set, the MAP estimates of centroids are obtained by the EM algorithm of GDM ($r = 20$). The values of hyperparameters are taken from the grid points in the hyperparameter space. For each fixed β, α is decremented in the grid, and the MAP estimates in the preceding α are used as initial values of centroids. Log evidence is calculated by equation 2.9. Cross-validation scores are obtained in the following manner. A data set is divided randomly into 10 groups of the same size. For each group, centroids are reestimated using the data in all but the group, where the MAP estimates from all data are used as initial values. For the reestimated centroids, their log likelihood is calculated using the data in the group. A cross-validation score is given as the mean of the log likelihoods. ELL is approximated by the mean log likelihood of the MAP estimates evaluated by 1000 newly generated data.

Hyperparameter Selection for Self-Organizing Maps

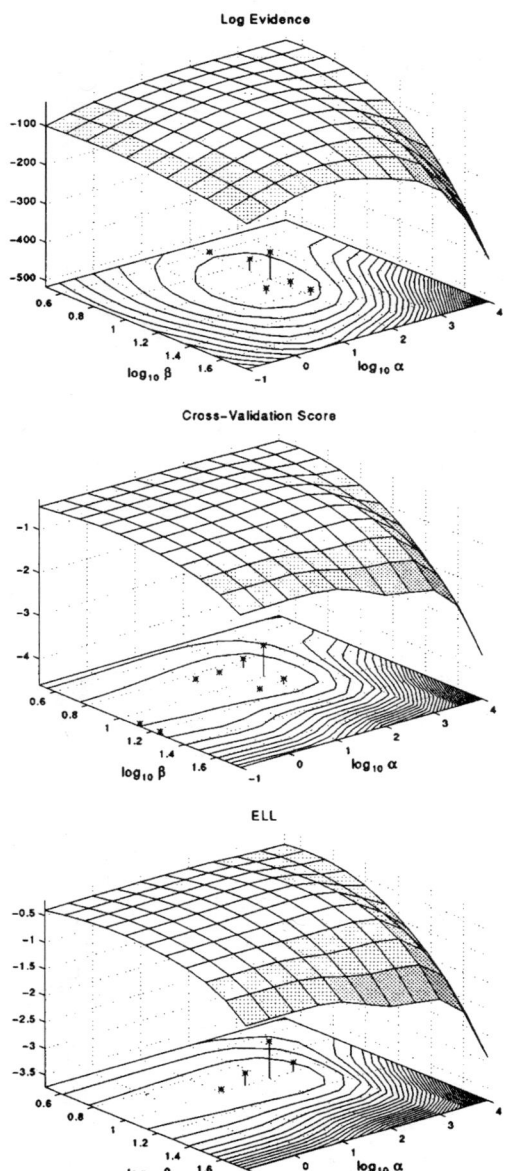

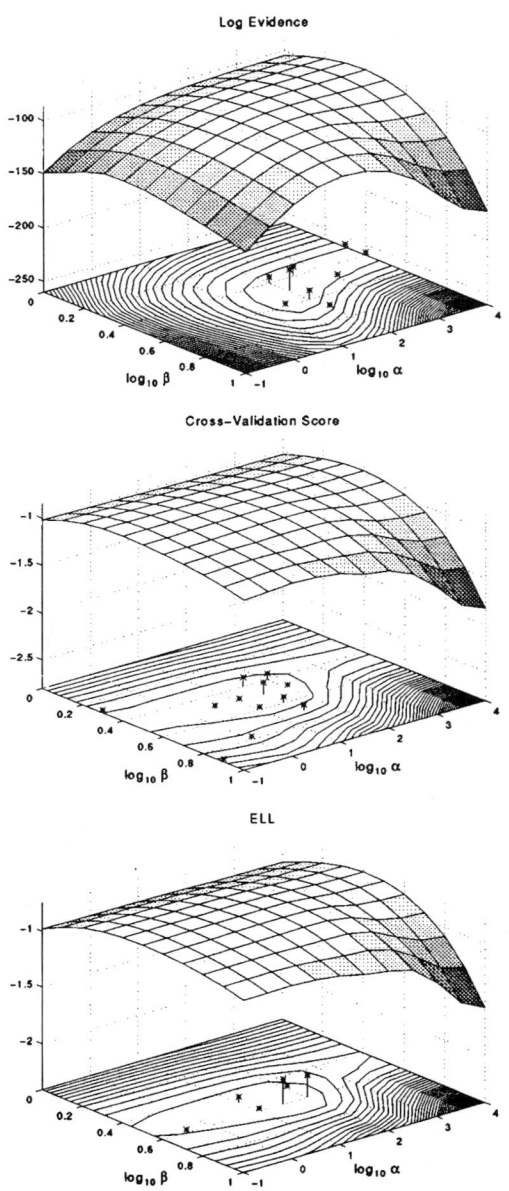

Figure 3: Landscapes and contour maps for averaged criteria and peak position histograms in the high-noise condition.

Hyperparameter Selection for Self-Organizing Maps

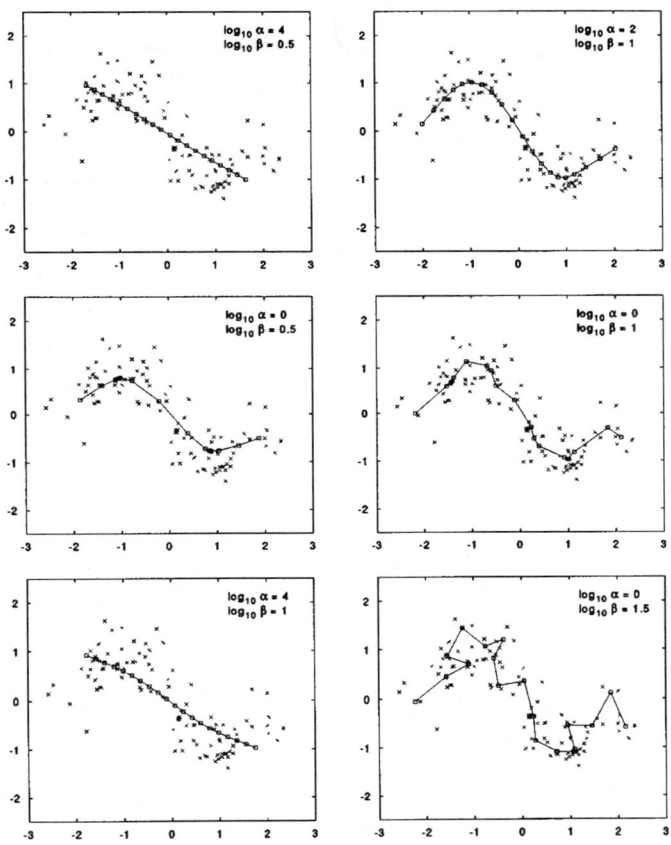

Figure 4: Samples of centroid configurations for several hyperparameter values in the low-noise condition.

In the case of high noise (see Figure 3), the discrepancies among the criteria increase. While cross-validation has a bias toward low α again, evidence comes to have the opposite bias. In this case, we have difficulty choosing between the methods. However, the property that evidence leads to the simplest model unless sufficient data for structure determination are given may be desirable because it agrees with a general strategy of data analysis that linear models rather than nonlinear ones should be used for very noisy data.

5 Conclusion

We derived the SOM algorithm as an approximate MAP estimation algorithm for a GDM. Several methods to evaluate the quality of hyperparameters for this model were developed by empirical Bayesian estimation and cross-validation. These methods were compared through simulation studies. It was found that the cross-validation methods favor complex structures, while the empirical Bayesian methods favor simple ones. Because of these properties and the long calculation time for cross-validation, the empirical Bayesian methods are recommended for this model.

Appendix

In this appendix, we consider the relation between kernel smoothing and discretized Laplacian smoothing.

Initially, we show

$$KN1_r = 1_r, \tag{A.1}$$

where 1_r is an r-dimensional column vector with all ones. In general, $D1_r = 0$ since D is a differential operator. Thus, using equation 3.7,

$$(KN)^{-1}1_r = (I_r + \gamma N^{-1}D'D)1_r = 1_r. \tag{A.2}$$

This means that $(KN)^{-1}$ has 1_r as an eigenvector with the eigenvalue one; thus KN also have the same property. This leads to equation A.1.

From equations 3.6 and A.1, a curve smoothed by discretized Laplacian smoothing is expressed by the kernel smoothing form (cf. equation 3.8) using the entries of K as the values of kernel function $\kappa(s, t)$.

References

Dempster, A. P., Laird, N. M., & Rubin, D. B. (1977). Maximum likelihood from incomplete data via the EM algorithm. *J. Roy. Statist. Soc., Ser. B, 39,* 1–38.

Durbin, R., Szeliski, R., & Yuille, A. (1989). An analysis of the elastic net approach to the traveling salesman problem. *Neural Computation, 1,* 348–358.

Härdle, W. (1990). *Smoothing techniques with implementation in S.* Berlin: Springer-Verlag.

Kohonen, T. (1988). *Self-organization and associative memory* (2nd ed.). Berlin: Springer-Verlag.

Kohonen, T. (1990). The self-organizing map. *Proc. IEEE, 78,* 1464–1480.

MacKay, D. J. C. (1992). A practical Bayesian framework for backprop networks. *Neural Computation, 4,* 448–472.

McLachlan, G. J., & Basford, K. E. (1988). *Mixture models: Inference and applications to clustering.* New York: Marcel Dekker.

Mulier, F., & Cherkassky, V. (1995). Self-organization as an iterative kernel smoothing process. *Neural Computation, 7,* 1141–1153.

Nowlan, S. J. (1990). Maximum likelihood competitive learning. In *Advances in neural information processing systems 2* (pp. 574–582). San Mateo, CA: Morgan Kaufmann.

O'Sullivan, F. (1991). Discretized Laplacian smoothing by Fourier methods. *J. Amer. Statist. Assoc., 86,* 634–642.

Silverman, B. W. (1984). Spline smoothing: The equivalent variable kernel method. *Ann. Statist., 12,* 898–916.

Utsugi, A. (1993). A Bayesian model of topology-preserving map learning (in Japanese). *Trans. IEICE D-II,* J76-D-II, 1232–1239.

Utsugi, A. (1994). Lateral interaction in Bayesian self-organizing maps (in Japanese). *Trans. IEICE D-II,* J77-D-II, 1329–1336.

Yuille, A. L. (1990). Generalized deformable models, statistical physics, and matching problems. *Neural Computation, 2,* 1–24.

Yuille, A. L., Stolorz, P., & Utans, J. (1994). Statistical physics, mixture of distributions and the EM algorithm. *Neural Computation, 6,* 334–340.

15

GTM: The Generative Topographic Mapping

Christopher M. Bishop
Markus Svensén
Christopher K. I. Williams
*Neural Computing Research Group, Department of Computer Science
and Applied Mathematics, Aston University, Birmingham B4 7ET, U.K.*

Latent variable models represent the probability density of data in a space of several dimensions in terms of a smaller number of latent, or hidden, variables. A familiar example is factor analysis, which is based on a linear transformation between the latent space and the data space. In this article, we introduce a form of nonlinear latent variable model called the generative topographic mapping, for which the parameters of the model can be determined using the expectation-maximization algorithm. GTM provides a principled alternative to the widely used self-organizing map (SOM) of Kohonen (1982) and overcomes most of the significant limitations of the SOM. We demonstrate the performance of the GTM algorithm on a toy problem and on simulated data from flow diagnostics for a multiphase oil pipeline.

1 Introduction

Many data sets exhibit significant correlations between the variables. One way to capture such structure is to model the distribution of the data in terms of latent, or hidden, variables. A familiar example of this approach is factor analysis, which is based on a linear transformation from latent space to data space. In this article, we show how the latent variable framework can be extended to allow nonlinear transformations while remaining computationally tractable. This leads to the GTM (generative topographic mapping) algorithm, which is based on a constrained mixture of gaussians whose parameters can be optimized using the EM (expectation-maximization) algorithm.

One of the motivations for this work is to provide a principled alternative to the widely used self-organizing map (SOM) algorithm (Kohonen, 1982) in which a set of unlabeled data vectors t_n ($n = 1, \ldots, N$) in a D-dimensional data space is summarized in terms of a set of reference vectors having a spatial organization corresponding to a (generally) two-dimensional sheet. Although this algorithm has achieved many successes in practical applications, it also suffers from some significant deficiencies, many of which are highlighted in Kohonen (1995). They include the absence of a cost function, the lack of a theoretical basis for choosing learning rate parameter schedules and neighborhood parameters to ensure topographic ordering, the absence of any general proofs of convergence, and the fact that the model does not define a probability density. These problems can all be traced to the heuristic origins of the SOM algorithm.[1] We show that the GTM algorithm overcomes most of the limitations of the SOM while introducing no significant disadvantages.

An important application of latent variable models is to data visualization. Many of the models used in visualization are regarded as defining a projection from the D-dimensional data space onto a two-dimensional visualization space. We shall see that, by contrast, the GTM model is defined in terms of a mapping *from* the latent space *into* the data space. For the purposes of data visualization, the mapping is then inverted using Bayes' theorem, giving rise to a posterior distribution in latent space.

2 Latent Variables

The goal of a latent variable model is to find a representation for the distribution $p(\mathbf{t})$ of data in a D-dimensional space $\mathbf{t} = (t_1, \ldots, t_D)$ in terms of a number L of latent variables $\mathbf{x} = (x_1, \ldots, x_L)$. This is achieved by first considering a function $\mathbf{y}(\mathbf{x}; \mathbf{W})$, which maps points $\mathbf{x}$ in the latent space into corresponding points $\mathbf{y}(\mathbf{x}; \mathbf{W})$ in the data space. The mapping is governed by a set of parameters $\mathbf{W}$ and could consist, for example, of a feedforward neural network, in which case, $\mathbf{W}$ would represent the weights and biases. We are interested in the situation in which the dimensionality L of the latent variable space is less than the dimensionality D of the data space, since we wish to capture the fact that the data set itself has an intrinsic dimensionality that is less than D. The transformation $\mathbf{y}(\mathbf{x}; \mathbf{W})$ then maps the latent variable space into an L-dimensional non-Euclidean manifold $\mathcal{S}$ embedded within the data space.[2] This is illustrated schematically for the case of $L = 2$ and $D = 3$ in Figure 1.

If we define a probability distribution $p(\mathbf{x})$ on the latent variable space, this will induce a corresponding distribution $p(\mathbf{y}|\mathbf{W})$ in the data space. We shall refer to $p(\mathbf{x})$ as the prior distribution of $\mathbf{x}$, for reasons that will become clear shortly. Since $L < D$, the distribution in $\mathbf{t}$-space would be confined to the L-dimensional manifold and hence would be singular. Since in reality the data will only approximately live on a lower-dimensional manifold, it is appropriate to include a noise model for the $\mathbf{t}$ vector. We choose the distribution of $\mathbf{t}$, for given $\mathbf{x}$ and $\mathbf{W}$, to be a radially symmetric gaussian

---

[1] Biological metaphor is sometimes invoked when motivating the SOM procedure. It should be stressed that our goal here is not neurobiological modeling, but rather the development of effective algorithms for data analysis, for which biological realism need not be considered.

[2] We assume that the matrix of partial derivatives $\partial y_k / \partial x_i$ has full column rank.

Generative Topographic Mapping

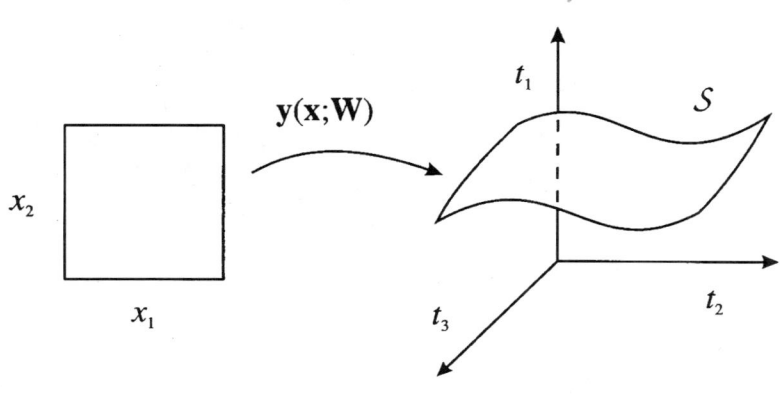

Figure 1: The nonlinear function y(x; W) defines a manifold S embedded in data space given by the image of the latent variable space under the mapping x → y.

centered on y(x; W) having variance β^{-1} so that

$$p(t|x, W, \beta) = \left(\frac{\beta}{2\pi}\right)^{D/2} \exp\left\{-\frac{\beta}{2}\|y(x; W) - t\|^2\right\}. \tag{2.1}$$

Note that other models for $p(t|x)$ might also be appropriate, such as a Bernoulli for binary variables (with a sigmoid transformation of y) or a multinomial for mutually exclusive classes (with a softmax, or normalized exponential transformation of y [Bishop, 1995]), or even combinations of these. The distribution in t-space, for a given value of W, is then obtained by integration over the x-distribution,

$$p(t|W, \beta) = \int p(t|x, W, \beta) p(x)\, dx. \tag{2.2}$$

For a given a data set $\mathcal{D} = (t_1, \ldots, t_N)$ of N data points, we can determine the parameter matrix W, and the inverse variance β, using maximum likelihood. In practice it is convenient to maximize the log likelihood, given by

$$\mathcal{L}(W, \beta) = \ln \prod_{n=1}^{N} p(t_n|W, \beta). \tag{2.3}$$

Once we have specified the prior distribution $p(x)$ and the functional form of the mapping y(x; W), we can in principle determine W and β by maximiz-

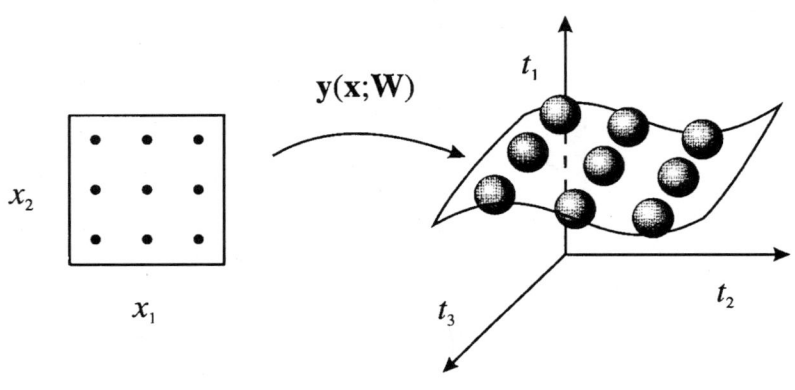

Figure 2: In order to formulate a latent variable model similar in spirit to the SOM, we consider a prior distribution $p(\mathbf{x})$ consisting of a superposition of delta functions, located at the nodes of a regular grid in latent space. Each node $\mathbf{x}_i$ is mapped to a corresponding point $\mathbf{y}(\mathbf{x}_i; \mathbf{W})$ in data space and forms the center of a corresponding gaussian distribution.

ing $\mathcal{L}(\mathbf{W}, \beta)$. However, the integral over $\mathbf{x}$ in equation 2.2 will, in general, be analytically intractable. If we choose $\mathbf{y}(\mathbf{x}; \mathbf{W})$ to be a linear function of $\mathbf{W}$, and we choose $p(\mathbf{x})$ to be gaussian, then the integral becomes a convolution of two gaussians, which is itself a gaussian. For a noise distribution $p(\mathbf{t}|\mathbf{x})$ that is gaussian with a diagonal covariance matrix, we obtain the standard factor analysis model. In the case of the radially symmetric gaussian given by equation 2.1, the model is closely related to principal component analysis since the maximum likelihood solution for $\mathbf{W}$ has columns given by the scaled principal eigenvectors (Tipping & Bishop, 1997). Here we wish to extend this formalism to nonlinear functions $\mathbf{y}(\mathbf{x}; \mathbf{W})$, and in particular to develop a model similar in spirit to the SOM algorithm. We therefore consider a specific form for $p(\mathbf{x})$ given by a sum of delta functions centered on the nodes of a regular grid in latent space,

$$p(\mathbf{x}) = \frac{1}{K} \sum_{i=1}^{K} \delta(\mathbf{x} - \mathbf{x}_i), \tag{2.4}$$

in which case the integral in equation 2.2 can again be performed analytically. Each point $\mathbf{x}_i$ is then mapped to a corresponding point $\mathbf{y}(\mathbf{x}_i; \mathbf{W})$ in data space, which forms the center of a gaussian density function, as illustrated in Figure 2. From equations 2.2 and 2.4, we see that the distribution function in data space then takes the form

$$p(\mathbf{t}|\mathbf{W}, \beta) = \frac{1}{K} \sum_{i=1}^{K} p(\mathbf{t}|\mathbf{x}_i, \mathbf{W}, \beta), \qquad (2.5)$$

and the log likelihood function becomes

$$\mathcal{L}(\mathbf{W}, \beta) = \sum_{n=1}^{N} \ln \left\{ \frac{1}{K} \sum_{i=1}^{K} p(\mathbf{t}_n|\mathbf{x}_i, \mathbf{W}, \beta) \right\}. \qquad (2.6)$$

For the particular noise model $p(\mathbf{t}|\mathbf{x}, \mathbf{W}, \beta)$ given by equation 2.1, the distribution $p(\mathbf{t}|\mathbf{W}, \beta)$ corresponds to a constrained gaussian mixture model (Hinton, Williams, & Revow, 1992) since the centers of the gaussians, given by $\mathbf{y}(\mathbf{x}_i; \mathbf{W})$, cannot move independently but are related through the function $\mathbf{y}(\mathbf{x}; \mathbf{W})$. Note that, provided the mapping function $\mathbf{y}(\mathbf{x}; \mathbf{W})$ is smooth and continuous, the projected points $\mathbf{y}(\mathbf{x}_i; \mathbf{W})$ will necessarily have a topographic ordering in the sense that any two points $\mathbf{x}_A$ and $\mathbf{x}_B$ that are close in latent space will map to points $\mathbf{y}(\mathbf{x}_A; \mathbf{W})$ and $\mathbf{y}(\mathbf{x}_B; \mathbf{W})$, which are close in data space.

2.1 The EM Algorithm. If we now choose a particular parameterized form for $\mathbf{y}(\mathbf{x}; \mathbf{W})$, which is a differentiable function of $\mathbf{W}$ (for example, a feedforward network with sigmoidal hidden units), then we can use standard techniques for nonlinear optimization, such as conjugate gradients or quasi-Newton methods, to find a weight matrix $\mathbf{W}^*$, and an inverse variance β^*, which maximize $L(\mathbf{W}, \beta)$.

However, our model consists of a mixture distribution which suggests that we might seek an EM algorithm (Dempster, Laird, & Rubin, 1977; Bishop, 1995). By making a suitable choice of model $\mathbf{y}(\mathbf{x}; \mathbf{W})$ we will see that the M-step corresponds to the solution of a set of linear equations. In particular we shall choose $\mathbf{y}(\mathbf{x}; \mathbf{W})$ to be given by a generalized linear regression model of the form

$$\mathbf{y}(\mathbf{x}; \mathbf{W}) = \mathbf{W}\phi(\mathbf{x}), \qquad (2.7)$$

where the elements of $\phi(\mathbf{x})$ consist of M fixed basis functions $\phi_j(\mathbf{x})$, and $\mathbf{W}$ is a $D \times M$ matrix. Generalized linear regression models possess the same universal approximation capabilities as multilayer adaptive networks, provided the basis functions $\phi_j(\mathbf{x})$ are chosen appropriately. The usual limitation of such models, however, is that the number of basis functions must typically grow exponentially with the dimensionality L of the input space (Bishop, 1995). In out context, this is not a significant problem since the dimensionality is governed by the number of latent variable variables, which will typically be small. In fact, for data visualization applications, we generally use $L = 2$.

The maximization of $L(\mathbf{W}, \beta)$ given by equation 2.6 can be regarded as a missing-data problem in which the identity i of the component that generated each data point $\mathbf{t}_n$ is unknown. We can formulate the EM algorithm for this model as follows. First, suppose that, at some point in the algorithm, the current weight matrix is given by $\mathbf{W}_{\text{old}}$, and the current inverse noise variance is given by β_{old}. In the E-step we use $\mathbf{W}_{\text{old}}$ and β_{old} to evaluate the posterior probabilities, or responsibilities, of each gaussian component i for every data point $\mathbf{t}_n$ using Bayes' theorem in the form

$$R_{in}(\mathbf{W}_{\text{old}}, \beta_{\text{old}}) = p(\mathbf{x}_i | \mathbf{t}_n, \mathbf{W}_{\text{old}}, \beta_{\text{old}}) \qquad (2.8)$$

$$= \frac{p(\mathbf{t}_n | \mathbf{x}_i, \mathbf{W}_{\text{old}}, \beta_{\text{old}})}{\sum_{i'=1}^{K} p(\mathbf{t}_n | \mathbf{x}_{i'}, \mathbf{W}_{\text{old}}, \beta_{\text{old}})}. \qquad (2.9)$$

We now consider the expectation of the complete-data log likelihood in the form

$$\langle \mathcal{L}_{\text{comp}}(\mathbf{W}, \beta) \rangle = \sum_{n=1}^{N} \sum_{i=1}^{K} R_{in}(\mathbf{W}_{\text{old}}, \beta_{\text{old}}) \ln \{ p(\mathbf{t}_n | \mathbf{x}_i, \mathbf{W}, \beta) \}. \qquad (2.10)$$

Maximizing equation 2.10 with respect to $\mathbf{W}$ and using equations 2.1 and 2.7, we obtain

$$\sum_{n=1}^{N} \sum_{i=1}^{K} R_{in}(\mathbf{W}_{\text{old}}, \beta_{\text{old}}) \{ \mathbf{W}_{\text{new}} \boldsymbol{\phi}(\mathbf{x}_i) - \mathbf{t}_n \} \boldsymbol{\phi}^{\text{T}}(\mathbf{x}_i) = 0. \qquad (2.11)$$

This can conveniently be written in matrix notation in the form

$$\boldsymbol{\Phi}^{\text{T}} \mathbf{G}_{\text{old}} \boldsymbol{\Phi} \mathbf{W}_{\text{new}}^{\text{T}} = \boldsymbol{\Phi}^{\text{T}} \mathbf{R}_{\text{old}} \mathbf{T}, \qquad (2.12)$$

where $\boldsymbol{\Phi}$ is a $K \times M$ matrix with elements $\Phi_{ij} = \phi_j(\mathbf{x}_i)$, $\mathbf{T}$ is a $N \times D$ matrix with elements t_{nk}, $\mathbf{R}$ is a $K \times N$ matrix with elements R_{in}, and $\mathbf{G}$ is a $K \times K$ diagonal matrix with elements

$$G_{ii} = \sum_{n=1}^{N} R_{in}(\mathbf{W}, \beta). \qquad (2.13)$$

We can now solve equation 2.12 for $\mathbf{W}_{\text{new}}$ using standard matrix techniques, based on singular value decomposition to allow for possible ill conditioning. Note that the matrix $\boldsymbol{\Phi}$ is constant throughout the algorithm and so needs only to be evaluated once at the start.

Similarly, maximizing equation 2.10 with respect to β, we obtain the following reestimation formula:

$$\frac{1}{\beta_{\text{new}}} = \frac{1}{ND} \sum_{n=1}^{N} \sum_{i=1}^{K} R_{in}(\mathbf{W}_{\text{old}}, \beta_{\text{old}}) \| \mathbf{W}_{\text{new}} \boldsymbol{\phi}(\mathbf{x}_i) - \mathbf{t}_n \|^2. \qquad (2.14)$$

Generative Topographic Mapping

The EM algorithm alternates between the E-step, corresponding to the evaluation of the posterior probabilities in equation 2.9, and the M-step, given by the solution of equations 2.12 and 2.14. Jensen's inequality can be used to show that at each iteration of the algorithm, the objective function will increase unless it is already at a (local) maximum, as discussed, for example, in Bishop (1995). Typically the EM algorithm gives satisfactory convergence after a few tens of cycles, particularly since we are primarily interested in convergence of the distribution, and this is often achieved much more rapidly than convergence of the parameters themselves.

If desired, a regularization term can be added to the objective function to control the mapping $y(x; W)$. This can be interpreted as a MAP (maximum a posteriori) estimator corresponding to a choice of prior over the weights W. In the case of a radially symmetric gaussian prior of the form

$$p(W|\lambda) = \left(\frac{\lambda}{2\pi}\right)^{MD/2} \exp\left\{-\frac{\lambda}{2}\sum_{j=1}^{M}\sum_{k=1}^{D} w_{jk}^2\right\}, \qquad (2.15)$$

where λ is the regularization coefficient, this leads to a modification of the M-step (equation 2.12) to give

$$(\Phi^T G_{old} \Phi + (\lambda/\beta) I) W_{new}^T = \Phi^T R_{old} T, \qquad (2.16)$$

where I is the identity matrix.

2.2 Data Visualization. One application for GTM is in data visualization, in which Bayes' theorem is used to invert the transformation from latent space to data space. For the particular choice of prior distribution given by equation 2.4, the posterior distribution is again a sum of delta functions centered at the lattice points, with coefficients given by the responsibilities R_{in}. These coefficients can be used to provide a visualization of the posterior responsibility map for individual data points in the two-dimensional latent space. If it is desired to visualize a set of data points, then a complete posterior distribution for each data point may provide too much information, and it is often convenient to summarize the posterior by its mean, given for each data point t_n by

$$\langle x|t_n, W^*, \beta^* \rangle = \int p(x|t_n, W^*, \beta^*) x \, dx \qquad (2.17)$$

$$= \sum_{i=1}^{K} R_{in} x_i. \qquad (2.18)$$

Keep in mind, however, that the posterior distribution can be multimodal, in which case the posterior mean can give a very misleading summary of the true distribution. An alternative approach is therefore to evaluate the mode of the distribution, given by

$$i^{\max} = \arg\max_{\{i\}} R_{in}. \tag{2.19}$$

In practice, it is often convenient to plot both the mean and the mode for each data point, because significant differences between them can be indicative of a multimodal distribution.

2.3 Choice of Model Parameters. The problem of density estimation from a finite data set is fundamentally ill posed, since there exist infinitely many distributions that could have given rise to the observed data. An algorithm for density modeling therefore requires some form of "prior knowledge" in addition to the data set. The assumption that the distribution can be described in terms of a reduced number of latent variables is itself part of this prior. In the GTM algorithm, the prior distribution over mapping functions $y(x; W)$ is governed by the prior over weights W, given, for example, by equation 2.15, as well as by the basis functions. We typically choose the basis functions $\phi_j(x)$ to be radially symmetric gaussians whose centers are distributed on a uniform grid in x-space, with a common width parameter σ, whose value, along with the number and spacing of the basis functions, determines the smoothness of the manifold. Examples of surfaces generated by sampling the prior are shown in Figure 3.

In addition to the basis functions $\phi_i(x)$, it is also necessary to select the latent space sample points $\{x_i\}$. Note that if there are too few sample points in relation to the number of basis functions, then the gaussian mixture centers in data space become relatively independent, and the desired smoothness properties can be lost. Having a large number of sample points, however, causes no difficulty beyond increased computational cost. In particular, there is no overfitting if the number of sample points is increased since the number of degrees of freedom in the model is controlled by the mapping function $y(x; W)$. One way to view the role of the latent space samples $\{x_i\}$ is as a Monte Carlo approximation to the integral over x in equation 2.2 (MacKay, 1995; Bishop, Svensén, & Williams, 1996). The choice of the number K and location of the sample points x_i in latent space is not critical, and we typically choose gaussian basis functions and set K so that, in the case of a two-dimensional latent space, $O(100)$ sample points lie within 2σ of the center of each basis function.

Note that we have considered the basis function parameters (widths and locations) to be fixed, with a gaussian prior on the weight matrix W. In principle, priors over the basis function parameters could also be introduced, and these could again be treated by maximum a posteriori (MAP) estimation or by Bayesian integration.

We initialize the parameters W so that the GTM model initially approximates principal component analysis (PCA). To do this, we first evaluate the

Generative Topographic Mapping

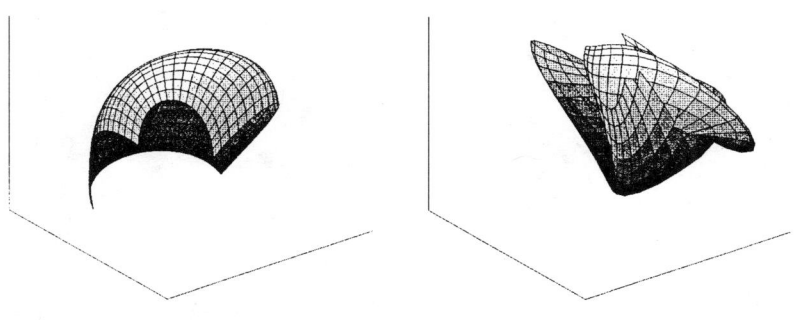

Figure 3: Examples of manifolds generated by sampling from the prior distribution over **W** given by equation 2.15, showing the effect of the choice of basis functions on the smoothness of the manifold. Here the basis functions are gaussian with width $\sigma = 4s$ in the left-hand plot (where s is the spacing of the basis function centers) and $\sigma = 2s$ in the right-hand plot. Different values of λ simply affect the linear scaling of the embedded manifold.

data covariance matrix and obtain the first and second principal eigenvectors, and then we determine **W** by minimizing the error function,

$$E = \frac{1}{2} \sum_i \|\mathbf{W}\phi(\mathbf{x}_i) - \mathbf{U}\mathbf{x}_i\|, \qquad (2.20)$$

where the columns of **U** are given by the eigenvectors. This represents the sum-of-squares error between the projections of the latent points into data space by the GTM model and the corresponding projections obtained from PCA. The value of β^{-1} is initialized to be the larger of either the $L+1$ eigenvalue from PCA (representing the variance of the data away from the PCA plane) or the square of half of the grid spacing of the PCA-projected latent points in data space.

Finally, we note that in a numerical implementation, care must be taken over the evaluation of the responsibilities since this involves computing the exponentials of the distances between the projected latent points and the data points, which may span a significant range of values.

2.4 Summary of the GTM Algorithm. Although the foregoing discussion has been somewhat detailed, the underlying GTM algorithm itself is straightforward and is summarized here for convenience.

GTM consists of a constrained mixture of gaussians in which the model parameters are determined by maximum likelihood using the EM algorithm. It is defined by specifying a set of points $\{\mathbf{x}_i\}$ in latent space, together

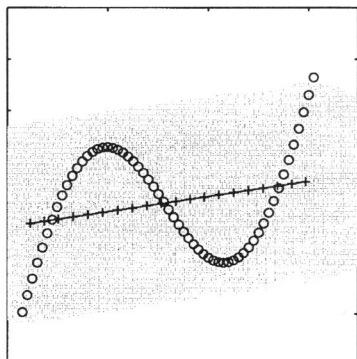 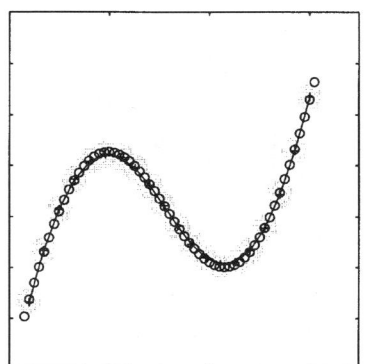

Figure 4: Results from a toy problem involving data (○) generated from a one-dimensional curve embedded in two dimensions, together with the projected latent points (+) and their gaussian noise distributions (filled circles). The initial configuration, determined by principal component analysis, is shown on the left, and the converged configuration, obtained after 15 iterations of EM, is shown on the right.

with a set of basis functions $\{\phi_j(\mathbf{x})\}$. The adaptive parameters $\mathbf{W}$ and β define a constrained mixture of gaussians with centers $\mathbf{W}\phi(\mathbf{x}_i)$ and a common covariance matrix given by $\beta^{-1}\mathbf{I}$. After initializing $\mathbf{W}$ and β, training involves alternating between the E-step in which the posterior probabilities are evaluated using equation 2.9, and the M-step in which $\mathbf{W}$ and β are reestimated using equations 2.12 and 2.14, respectively. Evaluation of the log likelihood using equation 2.6 at the end of each cycle can be used to monitor convergence.

3 Experimental Results

We now present results from the application of this algorithm first to a toy problem involving data in two dimensions and then to a more realistic problem involving 12-dimensional data arising from diagnostic measurements of oil flows along multiphase pipelines. In both examples, we choose the basis functions $\phi_j(\mathbf{x})$ to be radially symmetric gaussians whose centers are distributed on a uniform grid in x-space, with a common width parameter chosen equal to twice the separation of neighboring basis function centers. Results from a toy problem for the case of a two-dimensional data space and a one-dimensional latent space are shown in Figure 4.

Generative Topographic Mapping

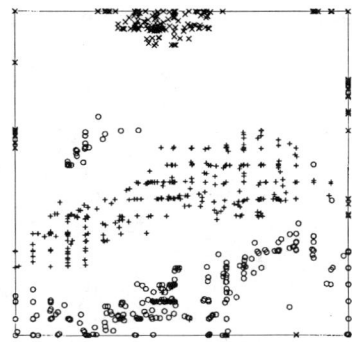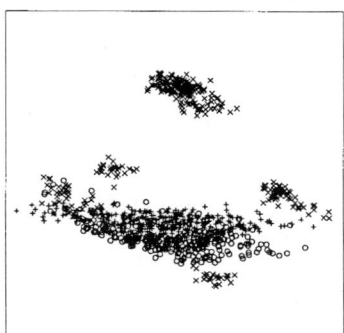

Figure 5: The left plot shows the posterior-mean projection of the oil flow data in the latent space of the GTM model; the plot on the right shows the same data set visualized using principal component analysis. In both plots, crosses, circles, and plus signs represent stratified, annular, and homogeneous multiphase configurations, respectively. Note how the nonlinearity of GTM gives an improved separation of the clusters.

3.1 Oil Flow Data. Our second example arises from the problem of determining the fraction of oil in a multiphase pipeline carrying a mixture of oil, water, and gas (Bishop & James, 1993). Each data point consists of 12 measurements taken from dual-energy gamma densitometers measuring the attenuation of gamma beams passing through the pipe. Synthetically generated data are used that model accurately the attenuation processes in the pipe, as well as the presence of noise (arising from photon statistics). The three phases in the pipe (oil, water, and gas) can belong to one of three different geometrical configurations, corresponding to laminar, homogeneous, and annular flows, and the data set consists of 1000 points drawn with equal probability from the three configurations. We take the latent variable space to be two-dimensional, since our goal is data visualization.

Figure 5 shows the oil data visualized in the latent variable space in which, for each data point, we have plotted the posterior mean vector. Each point has then been labeled according to its multiphase configuration. For comparison, Figure 5 also shows the corresponding results obtained using PCA.

4 Relation to the Self-Organizing Map

Since one motivation for GTM is to provide a principled alternative to the SOM, it is useful to consider the precise relationship between GTM and SOM. Focusing on the batch versions of both algorithms helps to make the relationship particularly clear.

The batch version of the SOM algorithm (Kohonen, 1995) can be described as follows. A set of K reference vectors z_i is defined in the data space, in which each vector is associated with a node on a regular lattice in a (typically) two-dimensional feature map (analogous to the latent space of GTM). The algorithm begins by initializing the reference vectors (for example, by setting them to random values, setting them equal to a random subset of the data points, or using PCA). Each cycle of the algorithm then proceeds as follows. For every data vector t_n, the corresponding "winning node" $j(n)$ is identified, corresponding to the reference vector z_j having the smallest Euclidean distance $\|z_j - t_n\|^2$ to t_n. The reference vectors are then updated by setting them equal to weighted averages of the data points given by

$$z_i = \frac{\sum_n h_{ij(n)} t_n}{\sum_n h_{ij(n)}}, \qquad (4.1)$$

in which h_{ij} is a neighborhood function associated with the ith node. This is generally chosen to be a unimodal function of the feature map coordinates centered on the winning node, for example, a gaussian. The steps of identifying the winning nodes and updating the reference vectors are repeated iteratively. A key ingredient in the algorithm is that the width of the neighborhood function h_{ij} starts with a relatively large value and is gradually reduced after each iteration.

4.1 Kernel versus Linear Regression. As pointed out by Mulier and Cherkassky (1995), the value of the neighborhood function $h_{ij(n)}$ depends only on the identity of the winning node j and not on the value of the corresponding data vector t_n. We can therefore perform partial sums over the groups $\mathcal{G}_j$ of data vectors assigned to each node j, and hence rewrite equation 4.1 in the form

$$z_i = \sum_j K_{ij} m_j, \qquad (4.2)$$

in which m_j is the mean of the vectors in group $\mathcal{G}_j$ and is given by

$$m_j = \frac{1}{N_j} \sum_{n \in \mathcal{G}_j} t_n, \qquad (4.3)$$

where N_j is the number of data vectors in group $\mathcal{G}_j$. The result (equation 4.2) is analogous to the Nadaraya-Watson kernel regression formula (Nadaraya, 1964; Watson, 1964) with the kernel functions given by

$$K_{ij} = \frac{h_{ij} N_j}{\sum_{j'} h_{ij'} N_{j'}}. \tag{4.4}$$

Thus the batch SOM algorithm replaces the reference vectors at each cycle with a convex combination of the node means $\mathbf{m}_j$, with coefficients determined by the neighborhood function. Note that the kernel coefficients satisfy $\sum_j K_{ij} = 1$ for every i.

In the GTM algorithm, the centers $\mathbf{y}(\mathbf{x}_i; \mathbf{W})$ of the gaussian components can be regarded as analogous to the reference vectors $\mathbf{z}_i$ of the SOM. We can evaluate $\mathbf{y}(\mathbf{x}_i; \mathbf{W})$ by solving the M-step equation (2.12) to find $\mathbf{W}$ and then using $\mathbf{y}(\mathbf{x}_i; \mathbf{W}) = \mathbf{W}\boldsymbol{\phi}(\mathbf{x}_i)$. If we define the weighted means of the data vectors by

$$\boldsymbol{\mu}_i = \frac{\sum_n R_{in} \mathbf{t}_n}{\sum_n R_{in}}, \tag{4.5}$$

then we obtain

$$\mathbf{y}(\mathbf{x}_i; \mathbf{W}) = \sum_j F_{ij} \boldsymbol{\mu}_j, \tag{4.6}$$

where we have introduced the effective kernel F_{ij} given by

$$F_{ij} = \boldsymbol{\phi}^T(\mathbf{x}_i) \left(\boldsymbol{\Phi}^T \mathbf{G} \boldsymbol{\Phi}\right)^{-1} \boldsymbol{\phi}(\mathbf{x}_j) G_{jj}. \tag{4.7}$$

Note that the effective kernel satisfies $\sum_j F_{ij} = 1$. To see this, we first use equation 4.7 to show that $\sum_j F_{ij} \phi_l(\mathbf{x}_j) = \phi_l(\mathbf{x}_i)$. Then if one of the basis functions l corresponds to a bias, so that $\phi_l(\mathbf{x}) = \text{const.}$, the result follows.

The solution for $\mathbf{y}(\mathbf{x}_i; \mathbf{W})$ given by equations 4.6 and 4.7 can be interpreted as a weighted least-squares regression (Mardia, Kent, & Bibby, 1979) in which the target vectors are the $\boldsymbol{\mu}_i$, and the weighting coefficients are given by G_{jj}.

Figure 6 shows an example of the effective kernel for GTM corresponding to the oil flow problem discussed in section 3.

From equations 4.2 and 4.6 we see that both GTM and SOM can be regarded as forms of kernel smoothers. However, there are two key differences. The first is that in SOM, the vectors that are smoothed, defined by equation 4.3, correspond to hard assignments of data points to nodes, whereas the corresponding vectors in GTM, given by equation 4.5, involve soft assignments, weighted by the posterior probabilities. This is analogous

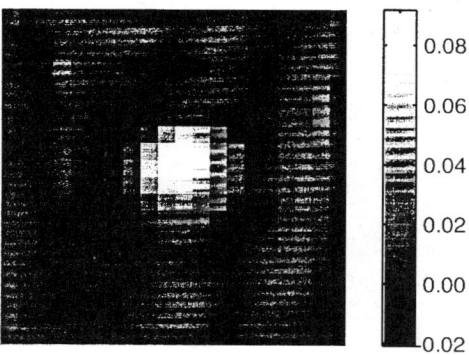

Figure 6: Example of the effective kernel F_{ij} plotted as a function of the node j for a given node i, for the oil flow data set after three iterations of EM. This kernel function is analogous to the (normalized) neighborhood function in the SOM algorithm.

to the distinction between K-means clustering (hard assignments) and fitting a standard gaussian mixture model using EM (soft assignments).

The second key difference is that the kernel function in SOM is made to shrink during the course of the algorithm in an arbitrary, handcrafted manner. In GTM, the posterior probability distribution in latent space, for a given data point, forms a localized bubble and the radius of this bubble shrinks automatically during training, as shown in Figure 7. This responsibility bubble governs the extent to which individual data points contribute toward the vectors μ_i in equation 4.5 and hence toward the updating of the gaussian centers $\mathbf{y}(\mathbf{x}_i; \mathbf{W})$ via equation 4.6.

4.2 Comparison of GTM with SOM. The most significant difference between the GTM and SOM algorithms is that GTM defines an explicit probability density given by the mixture distribution in equation 2.5. As a consequence there is a well-defined objective function given by the log likelihood (see equation 2.6), and convergence to a (local) maximum of the objective function is guaranteed by the use of the EM algorithm (Dempster et al., 1977). This also provides a direct means to compare different choices of model parameters and even to compare a GTM solution with another density model by evaluating the likelihood of a test set under the generative distributions of the respective models. For the SOM algorithm, however, there is no probability density and no well-defined objective function that is being minimized by the training process. Indeed it has been proved (Erwin,

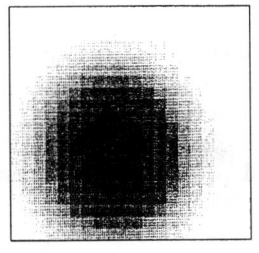 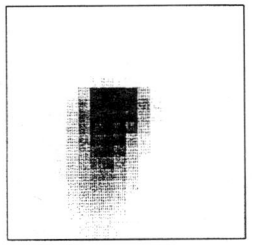 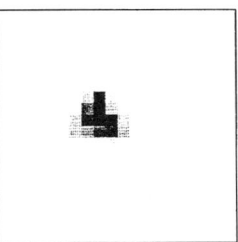

Figure 7: Examples of the posterior probabilities (responsibilities) R_{in} of the latent space points at an early stage (left), intermediate stage (center), and late stage (right) during the convergence of the GTM algorithm. These have been evaluated for a single data point from the training set in the oil flow problem discussed in section 3 and are plotted using a nonlinear scaling of the form $p(\mathbf{x}|\mathbf{t}_n)^{0.1}$ to highlight the variation over the latent space. Notice how the responsibility bubble, which governs the updating of the weight matrix, and hence the updating of the data-space vectors $\mathbf{y}(\mathbf{x}_i; \mathbf{W})$, shrinks automatically during the learning process.

Obermayer, & Schulten 1992) that such an objective function cannot exist for the SOM.

A further limitation of the SOM, highlighted in Kohonen (1995, p. 234), is that the conditions under which so-called self-organization of the SOM occurs have not been quantified, and so in practice it is necessary to confirm empirically that the trained model does indeed have the desired spatial ordering. In contrast, the neighborhood-preserving nature of the GTM mapping is an automatic consequence of the choice of a continuous function $\mathbf{y}(\mathbf{x}; \mathbf{W})$.

Similarly, the smoothness properties of the SOM are determined indirectly by the choice of neighborhood function and by the way in which it is changed during the course of the algorithm and is therefore difficult to control. Thus, prior knowledge about the form of the map cannot easily be specified. The prior distribution for GTM, however, can be controlled directly, and properties such as smoothness are governed explicitly by basis function parameters, as illustrated in Figure 3.

Finally, we consider the relative computational costs of the GTM and SOM algorithms. For problems involving data in high-dimensional spaces, the dominant computational cost of GTM arises from the evaluation of the Euclidean distances from every data point to every gaussian center $\mathbf{y}(\mathbf{x}_i; \mathbf{W})$. Since exactly the same calculations must be done for SOM (involving the distances of data points from the reference vectors $\boldsymbol{\mu}_i$), we expect one iteration of either algorithm to take approximately the same time. An empirical comparison of the computational cost of GTM and SOM was obtained by running each algorithm on the oil flow data until convergence (defined as no discernible change in the appearance of the visualization map). The GTM algorithm took 1058 sec (40 iterations), while the batch SOM took 1011 sec (25 iterations) using a gaussian neighborhood function. With a simple top-hat neighborhood function, in which each reference vector is updated at each iteration using only data points associated with nearby reference vectors, the CPU time for the SOM algorithm is reduced to 305 sec (25 iterations). One potential advantage of GTM in practical applications arises from a reduction in the number of experimental training runs needed since both convergence and topographic ordering are guaranteed.

5 Relation to Other Algorithms

Several algorithms in the published literature have close links with GTM. Here we review briefly the most significant of these.

The elastic net algorithm of Durbin and Willshaw (1987) can be viewed as a gaussian mixture density model, fitted by penalized maximum likelihood. The penalty term encourages the centers of gaussians corresponding to neighboring points along the (typically one-dimensional) chain to be close in data space. It differs from GTM in that it does not define a continuous data space manifold. Also, the training algorithm generally involves a handcrafted annealing of the weight penalty coefficient.

There are also similarities between GTM and principal curves and principal surfaces (Hastie & Stuetzle, 1989; LeBlanc & Tibshirani 1994), which again involve a two-stage algorithm consisting of projection followed by smoothing, although these are not generative models. It is interesting to note that Hastie and Stuetzle (1989) propose reducing the spatial width of the smoothing function during learning, in a manner analogous to the shrinking of the neighborhood function in the SOM. A modified form of the principal curves algorithm (Tibshirani, 1992) introduces a generative distribution based on a mixture of gaussians, with a well-defined likelihood function, and is trained by the EM algorithm. However, the number of gaussian components is equal to the number of data points, and smoothing is imposed by penalizing the likelihood function with the addition of a derivative-based regularization term.

The technique of parameterized self-organizing maps (PSOMs) involves first fitting a standard SOM model to a data set and then finding a manifold in data space that interpolates the reference vectors (Ritter, 1993). Although this defines a continuous manifold, the interpolating surface does not form part of the training algorithm, and the basic problems in using SOM, discussed in section 4.2, remain.

The SOM has also been used for vector quantization. In this context it has been shown how a reformulation of the vector quantization problem

(Luttrell, 1990; Buhmann & Kühnel 1993; Luttrell, 1994; Luttrell, 1995) can avoid many of the problems with the SOM procedure discussed earlier.

Finally, the density network model of MacKay (1995) involves transforming a simple distribution in latent space to a complex distribution in data space by propagation through a nonlinear network. A discrete distribution in latent space is again used, which is interpreted as an approximate Monte Carlo integration over the latent variables needed to define the data space distribution. GTM can be seen as a particular instance of this framework in which the sampling of latent space is regular rather than stochastic, a specific form of nonlinearity is used, and the model parameters are adapted using EM.

6 Discussion

In this article, we have introduced a form of nonlinear latent variable model that can be trained efficiently using the EM algorithm. Viewed as a topographic mapping algorithm, it has the key property that it defines a probability density model.

As an example of the significance of having a probability density, consider the important practical problem of dealing with missing values in the data set (in which some components of the data vectors t_n are unobserved). If the missing values are missing at random (Little & Rubin, 1987) then the likelihood function is obtained by integrating out the unobserved values. For the GTM model, the integrations can be performed analytically, leading to a simple modification of the EM algorithm.

A further consequence of having a probabilistic approach is that it is straightforward to consider a mixture of GTM models. In this case, the overall density can be written as

$$p(\mathbf{t}) = \sum_r P(r) p(\mathbf{t}|r), \qquad (6.1)$$

where $p(\mathbf{t}|r)$ represents the rth model, with its own set of independent parameters, and $P(r)$ are mixing coefficients satisfying $0 \leq P(r) \leq 1$ and $\sum_r P(r) = 1$. Again, it is straightforward to extend the EM algorithm to maximize the corresponding likelihood function.

The GTM algorithm can be extended in other ways, for instance, by allowing independent mixing coefficients π_i (prior probabilities) for each of the gaussian components, which again can be estimated by a straightforward extension of the EM algorithm. Instead of being independent parameters, the π_i can be determined as smooth functions of the latent variables using a normalized exponential applied to a generalized linear regression model, although in this case the M-step of the EM algorithm would involve nonlinear optimization. Similarly, the inverse noise variance β can be generalized to a function of $\mathbf{x}$. An important property of GTM is the existence of a smooth manifold in data space, which allows the local magnification factor between latent and data space to be evaluated as a function of the latent space coordinates using the techniques of differential geometry (Bishop, Svensén, & Williams, in press). Finally, since there is a well-defined likelihood function, it is straightforward in principle to introduce priors over the model parameters (as discussed in section 2.1) and to use Bayesian techniques in place of maximum likelihood.

Throughout this article, we have focused on the batch version of the GTM algorithm in which all of the training data are used together to update the model parameters. In some applications, it will be more convenient to consider sequential adaptation in which data points are presented one at a time. Since we are minimizing a differentiable cost function, given by equation 2.6, a sequential algorithm can be obtained by appealing to the Robbins-Monro procedure (Robbins & Monro, 1951; Bishop, 1995) to find a zero of the objective function gradient. Alternatively, a sequential form of the EM algorithm can be used (Titterington, Smith, & Makov, 1985).

A Web site for GTM is provided at: http://www.ncrg.aston.ac.uk/GTM/, which includes postscript files of relevant papers, a software implementation in Matlab (a C implementation is under development), and example data sets used in the development of the GTM algorithm.

Acknowledgments

This work was supported by EPSRC grant GR/K51808: Neural Networks for Visualization of High-Dimensional Data. We thank Geoffrey Hinton, Iain Strachan, and Michael Tipping for useful discussions. Markus Svensén thanks the staff of the SANS group in Stockholm for their hospitality during part of this project.

References

Bishop, C. M. (1995). *Neural networks for pattern recognition.* New York: Oxford University Press.
Bishop, C. M., & James, G. D. (1993). Analysis of multiphase flows using dual-energy gamma densitometry and neural networks. *Nuclear Instruments and Methods in Physics Research, A327,* 580–593.
Bishop, C. M., Svensén, M., & Williams, C. K. I. (1996). A fast EM algorithm for latent variable density models. In D. S. Touretzky, M. C. Mozer, & M. E. Hasselmo (Eds.), *Advances in neural information processing systems, 8* (pp. 465–471). Cambridge, MA: MIT Press.
Bishop, C. M., Svensén, M., & Williams, C. K. I. (in press). Magnification factors for the GTM algorithm. In *Proceedings of the Fifth IEE International Conference on Artificial Neural Networks.* Cambridge, U.K., IEE, (pp. 64–69).
Buhmann, J., & Kühnel, K. (1993). Vector quantization with complexity costs. *IEEE Transactions on Information Theory, 39*(4), 1133–1145.

Dempster, A. P., Laird, N. M., & Rubin, D. B. (1977). Maximum likelihood from incomplete data via the EM algorithm. *Journal of the Royal Statistical Society, B 39*(1), 1–38.
Durbin, R., & Willshaw, D. (1987). An analogue approach to the travelling salesman problem. *Nature, 326*, 689–691.
Erwin, E., Obermayer, K., & Schulten, K. (1992). Self-organizing maps: Ordering, convergence properties and energy functions. *Biological Cybernetics, 67*, 47–55.
Hastie, T., & Stuetzle, W. (1989). Principal curves. *Journal of the American Statistical Association, 84*(406), 502–516.
Hinton, G. E., Williams, C. K. I., & Revow, M. D. (1992). Adaptive elastic models for hand-printed character recognition. In J. E. Moody, S. J. Hanson, & R. P. Lippmann (Eds.), *Advances in neural information processing systems, 4* (pp. 512–519). San Mateo, CA: Morgan Kauffman.
Kohonen, T. (1982). Self-organized formation of topologically correct feature maps. *Biological Cybernetics, 43*, 59–69.
Kohonen, T. (1995). *Self-organizing maps*. Berlin: Springer-Verlag.
LeBlanc, M., & Tibshirani, R. (1994). Adaptive principal surfaces. *Journal of the American Statistical Association, 89*(425), 53–64.
Little, R. J. A., & Rubin, D. B. (1987). *Statistical analysis with missing data*. New York: John Wiley.
Luttrell, S. P. (1990). Derivation of a class of training algorithms. *IEEE Transactions on Neural Networks, 1*(2), 229–232.
Luttrell, S. P. (1994). A Bayesian analysis of self-organizing maps. *Neural Computation, 6*(5), 767–794.
Luttrell, S. P. (1995). Using self-organizing maps to classify radar range profiles. *Proc. 5th IEE Conf. on Artificial Neural Networks*, 335–340.
MacKay, D. J. C. (1995). Bayesian neural networks and density networks. *Nuclear Instruments and Methods in Physics Research, A 354*(1), 73–80.
Mardia, K., Kent, J., & Bibby, M. (1979). *Multivariate analysis*. New York: Academic Press.
Mulier, F., & Cherkassky, V. (1995). Self-organization as an iterative kernel smoothing process. *Neural Computation, 7*(6), 1165–1177.
Nadaraya, É. A. (1964). On estimating regression. *Theory of Probability and Its Applications, 9*(1), 141–142.
Ritter, H. (1993). Parameterized self-organizing maps. In *Proceedings ICANN'93 International Conference on Artificial Neural Networks, Amsterdam* (pp. 568–575). Berlin: Springer-Verlag.
Robbins, H., & Monro, S. (1951). A stochastic approximation method. *Annals of Mathematical Statistics, 22*, 400–407.
Tibshirani, R. (1992). Principal curves revisited. *Statistics and Computing, 2*, 183–190.
Tipping, M. E., & Bishop, C. M. (1997). Probabilistic Principal Component Analysis. Tech. Rep. NCRG/97/010, *Neural Computing Research Group, Dept. of Computer Science & Applied Mathematics*, Aston Univ., Birmingham B4 7ET, U.K.
Titterington, D. M., Smith, A. F. M., & Makov, U. E. (1985). *Statistical analysis of finite mixture distributions*. New York: Wiley.

Watson, G. S. (1964). Smooth regression analysis. *Sankhyā: The Indian Journal of Statistics, series A, 26,* 359–372.

16

Self-Organization as an Iterative Kernel Smoothing Process

Filip Mulier
Vladimir Cherkassky
Department of Electrical Engineering, University of Minnesota,
Minneapolis, MN 55455 USA

Kohonen's self-organizing map, when described in a batch processing mode, can be interpreted as a statistical kernel smoothing problem. The batch SOM algorithm consists of two steps. First, the training data are partitioned according to the Voronoi regions of the map unit locations. Second, the units are updated by taking weighted centroids of the data falling into the Voronoi regions, with the weighing function given by the neighborhood. Then, the neighborhood width is decreased and steps 1, 2 are repeated. The second step can be interpreted as a statistical kernel smoothing problem where the neighborhood function corresponds to the kernel and neighborhood width corresponds to kernel span. To determine the new unit locations, kernel smoothing is applied to the centroids of the Voronoi regions in the topological space. This interpretation leads to some new insights concerning the role of the neighborhood and dimensionality reduction. It also strengthens the algorithm's connection with the Principal Curve algorithm. A generalized self-organizing algorithm is proposed, where the kernel smoothing step is replaced with an arbitrary nonparametric regression method.

1 Batch Self-Organizing Map Algorithm

The self-organizing map (SOM) (Kohonen 1982) is a neural network model that is capable of projecting high-dimensional data onto a low-dimensional array. The projection is done adaptively and preserves characteristic features of the data. The algorithm has been successfully used for a number of statistical applications: density estimation, vector quantization, and data visualization. However, the relationship between SOM and other statistical tools is not clear. Like many other neural network methods, the SOM algorithm was originally an explanation for biological phenomena, and not motivated by statistical considerations. This makes interpretation of SOM output difficult for statistical applications. Viewing the SOM algorithm in terms of statistical notions gives an understanding of the algorithm's usefulness and limitations as a statistical tool.

Also, improvements can be made based on statistical considerations, so the algorithm can be tailored depending on application.

The SOM algorithm is usually formulated in a flowthrough fashion, where individual training samples are presented one at a time. It is also possible to perform self-organization in the batch mode (Luttrell 1990; Kohonen 1993), using the whole training set in each iteration. Batch SOM has provided faster training time based on empirical tests (Kohonen, 1993). Because of the nature of batch processing, presentation order of the training set has no effect on the final unit positions and there is no learning rate schedule required. This is not the case with the original flowthrough version, where presentation order may have an effect on the final map. The batch algorithm is similar to the LBG (Linde *et al.* 1980) algorithm for vector quantization (Luttrell 1990) except for the use of a neighborhood in Kohonen's algorithm. The LBG algorithm minimizes a simple objective function. However, because of the decreasing neighborhood, the SOM algorithm minimizes (approximately) an objective function which changes over time (Luttrell 1990). Assume vector training data $\mathbf{x}_k \in \Re^N$ ($k = 1, \ldots, K$) where K is the number of samples and k is a sample index rather than the iteration step, since we are performing batch processing. To make the connection between SOM and statistical kernel smoothing clearer, we will change the notation for indexing the units. The unit locations in the sample space are $\mathbf{w}(\theta_j)$ and $\theta_j \in \Re^M$ is the coordinate location of unit j in the M-dimensional topological space. The locations of the units in the topological space are fixed. Usually, the set of locations is taken from points in an M-dimensional integer lattice, $\Theta = \{\theta_j; j = 1, \ldots, J\}$, $\theta_j = (\lambda_1, \ldots, \lambda_M)$ where each λ_i is an integer, $1 \leq \lambda_i \leq S_0$, S_0 is the number of units per dimension, and J is the total number of units. Notice that a unit can be uniquely specified by index $j, j = 1, \ldots, J$ or $\theta_j \in \Theta$. Explicitly indexing the units using their topological coordinates will prove useful when interpreting self-organization as a process involving kernel smoothing in the topological space. The batch SOM algorithm is a two-step process (Luttrell 1990; Kohonen 1993):

1. *Voronoi Partitioning*: Partition the training data according to the Voronoi regions of the units. For each sample, store the index of the nearest (Euclidean distance) unit to that sample:

$$i(k) = \arg\min_j \left\| \mathbf{x}_k - \mathbf{w}(\theta_j) \right\| \quad k = 1, \ldots, K \tag{1.1}$$

2. *Weighted Centroid Update*: Update each unit according to a weighted centroid of the data, where the weights correspond to the neighborhood function of the original flowthrough SOM algorithm. For each unit

$$\mathbf{w}(\theta_j) = \frac{\sum_{k=1}^{K} \mathbf{x}_k C(\theta_{i(k)} - \theta_j)}{\sum_{k=1}^{K} C(\theta_{i(k)} - \theta_j)} \quad j = 1, \ldots, J \tag{1.2}$$

where the neighborhood function $C(\theta)$ is defined in the topological space and decreases monotonically. Neighborhood functions for the flowthrough SOM algorithm, such as the gaussian (Ritter et al. 1992), are used for this algorithm as well.

3. *Neighborhood Decrease*: Decrease the width of the neighborhood and iterate.

The weighted centroid update step of the batch SOM algorithm can be given in a form that simplifies further analysis. This can be done because the value of the neighborhood function is not directly dependent on the value of the input sample itself, but only on the Voronoi region the sample lies in. For all samples in a particular Voronoi region, each will have the same neighborhood weight in the updating of a particular unit. In this case, 1.2 can be rewritten using the sum of the samples in each Voronoi region:

$$\mathbf{w}(\theta_j) = \frac{\sum_{l=1}^{J} \left[C(\theta_l - \theta_j) \sum_{k=1}^{K} \mathbf{x}_k I(k,l) \right]}{\sum_{l=1}^{J} \left[C(\theta_l - \theta_j) \sum_{k=1}^{K} I(k,l) \right]} \quad (1.3)$$

where $I(k,l)$ is an indicator function indicating Voronoi regions, i.e., $I(k,l) = 1$ if sample k is in the Voronoi region corresponding to unit l. Equation 1.3 can be simplified to require only the centroids to determine the location of the units (De Haan and Egecioglu 1991):

$$\mathbf{w}(\theta_j) = \frac{\sum_{l=1}^{J} C(\theta_l - \theta_j) K_l \mathbf{m}_l}{\sum_{l=1}^{J} C(\theta_l - \theta_j) K_l} \quad (1.4)$$

where $\mathbf{m}_l$ is the standard centroid of the Voronoi region of unit l and K_l is the number of samples in the Voronoi region. Assuming that $C(\theta) \geq 0$, unit locations are given by a convex combination of the centroids at each iteration (Fig. 1).

2 Viewing SOM as a Regression Problem

Using the interpretation given by 1.4, it is possible to view the SOM algorithm as a statistical nonparametric regression problem. Specifically, it is possible to write one iteration of the batch SOM algorithm as one iteration of the LBG algorithm followed by a kernel smoothing done on the centroids in the topological space. The form of 1.4 is very similar to the Nadaraya–Watson kernel estimator (Nadaraya 1964; Watson 1964):

$$\hat{y}(x) = \frac{\sum_{k=1}^{K} H(x - x_k) y_k}{\sum_{k=1}^{K} H(x - x_k)} \quad \text{where } x, y \in \Re^1 \quad (2.1)$$

Due to the similarities, 1.4 can be interpreted as a kernel estimate. The neighborhood function C (except for the normalizing factor K_l) plays the role of the kernel H and the neighborhood width parameter defines

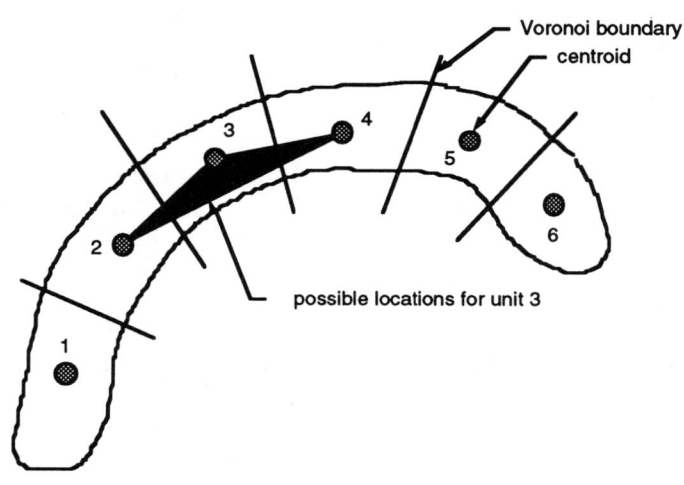

Figure 1: Unit locations are always at the convex combination of neighboring centroids. Based on a neighborhood width of three units, possible unit locations are shown for unit 3.

the span of the kernel. Equation 1.4 defines a vector valued function, which can be viewed as a set of scalar valued functions, one for each coordinate of the sample space. Each coordinate of the sample space can be treated as a "response variable" for a separate kernel smoother. The "predictor variables" for each smoother are the coordinates of θ, which have values indicating the location of a particular unit in the topological space. The problem can be considered a fixed design problem, since the locations of the units are fixed in the topological space and therefore the predictor variables of the smoothers are not random variables. Note that this interpretation of 1.4 does not imply that the results of SOM are similar to the results of kernel smoothing. The SOM algorithm applies kernel smoothing to the centroids iteratively using a kernel span that gradually decreases. The locations of the centroids of the Voronoi regions change with each iteration, depending on the results of past kernel estimates. Also, the kernel smoothing is done in the topological space, not in the sample space. However, interpreting 1.4 as kernel smoothing does help explain some aspects of self-organization.

3 Insights Provided by SOM as a Kernel Smoothing Problem

This connection between Kohonen self-organizing maps, the LBG algorithm, and kernel smoothing leads to some interesting insights into the nature of self-organization. Because the SOM algorithm can be directly interpreted as a kernel smoothing problem, known properties of kernel smoothers can be used to explain some of the strengths and limitations of SOM. The vast literature dealing with kernel smoothing and nonparametric regression in general can also give suggestions on how to improve the SOM algorithm. For example, research on kernel shape, span selection, confidence limit estimates, and even computational shortcuts may be applied to SOM. The interpretation leads to three important insights of the SOM algorithm.

3.1 Continuous Mapping. It has been shown that the SOM is a continuous mapping from sample space to topological space, as long as the distance measure used in the Voronoi partitioning and weighted centroid update step is continuous with respect to the Euclidean distance measure (Grunewald 1992). The units themselves describe this mapping at discrete points in each space, but the kernel smoothing function 1.4 provides a continuous functional mapping between the topological space and the sample space for any point in the topological space. Even though the units fall on an integer grid in the topological space, it is also possible to evaluate the kernel smoothing at arbitrary points in the topological space (between the grid points) to determine the corresponding sample space location. In this way we can construct a continuous mapping between the two spaces. Because of this continuous mapping, the number of units as well as the topology of the map can be changed as self-organization proceeds. For example, new units could be added along one dimension of the map, lengthening it, or the lattice structure of the map could be changed from rectangular regions to hexagonal.

3.2 Process of Dimensionality Reduction. Many studies have shown that the SOM algorithm is capable of performing dimensionality reduction in situations where the sample space may be high-dimensional, but constraints between the variables lead to a small intrinsic dimensionality (Ritter *et al.* 1992). In fact, most applications of SOM use maps with one- or two-dimensional topologies. Higher dimensional topologies are rarely used. Taking into account the previous analysis, the dimensionality of the map corresponds to the dimensionality of θ, the "predictor variables" seen by the kernel smoother. It is well known that the estimation error of kernel smoothers increases for a fixed sample size as the problem dimensionality increases. This indicates that the SOM algorithm may not perform well with high-dimensional maps (assuming the same number of training samples), and may explain a lack of published results.

3.3 Possible Improvements in Computational Speed. From 1.4, the batch SOM algorithm requires $O(K)$ operations to determine the centroid values and $O(J^2)$ operations to perform the kernel smoothing with an *arbitrary* kernel function. However, there are some more restrictive classes of kernel smoothers that require less computation. If the map is one-dimensional and a simple moving average smoother is used, then smoothing can be done with $O(J)$ operations. A local linear smoother could be used in this case as well, also requiring $O(J)$ operations (Friedman and Stuetzle 1982). Computation speed can also be improved by using a small number of units initially and then increasing the number during self-organization (Luttrell 1988; Rodrigues and Almeida 1991). This procedure would provide considerable speedup using the new formulation, since in the most general case, the update is quadratic in J. Using the old formulation, the insertion of units into the map required an interpolation scheme to determine the values of the newly inserted units. Because 1.4 defines a continuous mapping, inserting units can be done by simply using a finer mesh of design points in the kernel smoothing step.

4 Relationship of SOM Algorithm with the LBG Algorithm

The solution provided by the batch SOM algorithm as a substitute for the LBG (Linde *et al.* 1980) algorithm for vector quantization can be clearly understood by the above description of the SOM algorithm. One problem the LBG algorithm has, which is absent in the SOM algorithm, is the problem of unused centers, especially in the initial iterations of each algorithm. The extra step of kernel smoothing in the SOM algorithm effectively updates every center—even those without samples in their Voronoi regions. During the final stages of self-organization, the kernel width is usually decreased to include only one unit, so both the SOM and the LBG algorithm are equivalent at this point. Note that this does not imply that the resulting quantization centers generated by each algorithm are necessarily equivalent.

4.1 Analytical Comparison for the Case of Two Units. It may be possible to find a relationship between the minimal solution of the LBG algorithm and the SOM algorithm, considering that one iteration of the SOM algorithm can be broken down into one iteration of LBG followed by a kernel smoothing. A question that arises is whether the solution provided by the SOM algorithm can be written in terms of the solution of LBG after applying kernel smoothing. Because the LBG and SOM equilibrium conditions involve nonlinear equations, only special cases can be solved analytically. One simple special case where the solutions of SOM and LBG can be related is for a topological map of two units. In this case, the location of the units can be determined analytically for a

Self-Organization as a Kernel Smoothing Process

univariate symmetric density. We will restrict ourselves to the SOM algorithm using a neighborhood that does not decrease over time, since the results of the SOM algorithm with a decreasing neighborhood approach the results of the LBG algorithm as the number of samples approaches infinity. The analysis is based on a generalization of results for principal points (Flury 1990). Suppose the random variable X has a density $f(x)$ and distribution $F(x)$, with $f(x) = f(-x)$, and $E(X^2) = s^2 < \infty$. For a map with two units, the following general neighborhood function can be defined:

$$C(i,j) = \begin{cases} a & i = j \\ 1 - a & i \neq j \end{cases} \quad 1 \leq a \leq 1/2 \tag{4.1}$$

where i is the index of the winning unit, j is the index of the unit being updated, and a is a constant defining the neighborhood. The solution for the two unit values y_1 and y_2 can be found by using the substitution $y_1 = c - h$, $y_2 = c + h$ and minimizing:

$$\begin{aligned} H(c,h) &= \int_{-\infty}^{c} \left[a(x - c + h)^2 + (1-a)(x - c - h)^2 \right] f(x)\, dx \\ &+ \int_{c}^{\infty} \left[(1-a)(x - c + h)^2 + a(x - c - h)^2 \right] f(x)\, dx \end{aligned} \tag{4.2}$$

over $c, h \geq 0$. Setting first derivatives equal to zero gives the local minimal solution and the second derivative matrix gives the positive definite condition:

$$y_1 = -(2a - 1)E(|X|), \qquad y_2 = (2a - 1)E(|X|)$$
$$\text{if and only if } f(0)E(|X|) < \tfrac{1}{2}(2a - 1)^{-2} \tag{4.3}$$

By substituting $a = 1$ we can determine the local minimal solution if no neighborhood is used:

$$m_1 = -E(|X|) \qquad m_2 = E(|X|) \quad \text{if and only if } f(0)E(|X|) < \frac{1}{2} \tag{4.4}$$

One important point shown by these solutions is that 4.3 can be written in terms of a weighted average of solution 4.4, with weights given by the neighborhood function. Although the neighborhood width is held fixed in this example, the results still give insight about why decreasing the neighborhood width during self-organization is useful. Notice that as the width parameter of the neighborhood is increased, the condition for positive definiteness is relaxed, indicating that for some symmetric distributions, solution 4.4 may not be symmetric, but solution 4.3 will be symmetric. This shows that starting self-organization with a wide neighborhood guarantees initial symmetric solutions, but at some point the solution may become asymmetric. It is important to note that a two unit map cannot uniquely specify a topological dimension. All one can say is that the two unit map has a topological dimension $M \geq 1$.

5 Relationship of SOM Algorithm With the Principal Curves Algorithm

In statistics, the notion of principal curves (or manifolds) has been introduced by Hastie and Stuetzle (Hastie 1984; Hastie and Stuetzle 1989) to approximate a scatterplot of points from an unknown probability distribution. They use a smooth nonlinear curve called a principal curve to approximate the joint behavior of the two variables. Obviously, the objectives of the Kohonen method are similar to the goal of finding principal curves, even though Hastie and Stuetzle, evidently, were not familiar with Kohonen's work. It has been noted that Kohonen's method can be viewed as a computational procedure for finding discrete approximation of principal curves (or surfaces) by means of a topological map of units (Ritter et al. 1992). Surprisingly, there is a lot of similarity between Hastie and Stuetzle's algorithm for finding principal curves (PC algorithm), and the batch SOM with a one-dimensional map. For example, the PC algorithm for finding principal curves consists of two steps:

1. The *Projection Step* of finding for each data point in the sample its projection (or the closest point) on the curve. This is similar to the Voronoi partitioning in SOM.
2. The *Conditional-Expectation Step*, implemented via scatterplot smoothing. Scatterplot smoothing is applied to the projected values along the length of the principal curve, which is parameterized according to arc length. Hastie and Stuetzle suggest the following "most successful" empirical strategy for choosing span selection: "initially use a large span, and then decrease it gradually." This is similar to neighborhood reduction in SOM.

There are some differences between the SOM algorithm and the PC algorithm in terms of representation and estimation. The PC algorithm uses line segments to approximate the curve between the data points, while the SOM algorithm uses a piecewise constant approximation between map units. The PC algorithm creates curves that are parameterized according to arc length, while the self-organizing map is parameterized according to topological coordinates of the units. The results of the two algorithms are also different due to the choice of smoothers used for conditional expectation estimation. In the most general form of the PC algorithm, any type of smoother could be used. However, practical implementation of the PC algorithm used locally weighted linear smoothing (Hastie 1984). The SOM algorithm effectively uses a kernel smoother (weighted average). This distinction causes qualitative differences in the structure of the principal curve compared to the SOM, especially in the initial stages of operation for each algorithm. At the start of self-organization, when the neighborhood width is large, the units of the map form a tight cluster around the centroid of the data distribution. This occurs because estimation using a kernel smoothing with a wide span corresponds (approximately) to estimation using the mean. On the other hand, the PC algorithm using local linear smoothing approximates the first principal component line during the initial iterations (when a high degree of smoothing is applied) since smoothing with a wide span approximates global linear regression. In Section 6, we will show a generalized algorithm for self-organization where the kernel smoother in the SOM algorithm is replaced by any estimate for conditional expectation. Empirical examples of self-organizing maps will be shown where a locally weighted linear smoother is used within the SOM algorithm. These maps show a remarkable resemblance to the resulting curves of the PC algorithm, due to the use of a local linear smoother.

6 A Generalized Form of Self-Organization

The choice for regression estimate in the formulation of 1.2 does not have to be limited to kernel smoothing. Any conditional expectation estimate can be applied to estimate the new unit locations using the results of the Voronoi partitioning step. To generalize the regression estimate, the winning unit found for each data sample will be indexed by its topological coordinate θ_j, rather than by scalar index j, as was done in 1.1. It is possible to generalize the SOM algorithm as follows:

1. *Voronoi Partitioning*: Partition the data according to the Voronoi regions of the units. For each sample x_k associate the topological coordinate of the nearest unit (ϕ_k) to that sample:

$$\phi_k = \arg\min_\theta \|x_k - w(\theta)\|, \quad \theta \in \Theta, k = 1, \ldots, K \qquad (6.1)$$

2. *Conditional Expectation Estimate*: Determine the nonparametric regression estimate using the data samples $[\phi_k, x_k]$, $k = 1, \ldots, K$. Treat the winning unit coordinates ϕ_k as predictor variables and x_k as response variables to get the new unit values at the estimation points $\theta_j, j = 1, \ldots, J$:

$$w(\theta_j) = \text{estimate of } E(x \mid \theta = \theta_j), \quad j = 1, \ldots, J \qquad (6.2)$$

3. *Decrease Smoothing*: Gradually decrease the amount of smoothing of the nonparametric regression estimate with each iteration.

The LBG algorithm and Kohonen's SOM algorithm are special cases of this general form. If the conditional expectation is estimated by an average over each Voronoi region, then the steps describe LBG. If the conditional expectation is estimated using kernel smoothing, then we have the SOM algorithm. There is no reason to limit ourselves to kernel smoothing. If locally weighted linear smoothing (Cleveland and Devlin 1988) is used, self-organization approximates the results of the Principal Curve algorithm (Hastie and Stuetzle 1989) (Fig. 2). Spline smoothing may be particularly attractive due to the fixed design nature of the smoothing problem. Also, using specially formulated kernels, one can use kernel smoothing to estimate derivatives of functions (Hardle 1990). Using these kernels with SOM would allow the map to give estimates of the gradient of the training data along the topological dimensions, which can be useful for sensitivity analysis. This may also be useful when the goal of self-organization is to place more units in areas where the map has high curvature (Najafi and Cherkassky 1994). In all these modifications, the neighborhood decrease is equivalent to decreasing the smoothing parameter of the regression method and the regression method is chosen based on the goal of self-organization.

7 Interpretations of Neighborhood Decrease Rate

Interpreting an iteration of the SOM algorithm as a kernel smoothing problem gives some insight on how the neighborhood affects the smoothness of the map in a static sense (that is, assuming a fixed neighborhood width). However, it does not supply many clues about the effects of decreasing the neighborhood as iterations progress. Empirical studies (Kohonen 1989; Ritter *et al.* 1992) all show that starting with a wide neighborhood and decreasing seems to provide the best qualitative results. Not much is known about the optimal rate of decrease, the initial width, or the final width. One can view the problem as an example of deterministic annealing, which is a dynamic process, or as a model parameter selection problem, which assumes the map changes quasistatically.

7.1 As Temperature in Deterministic Annealing. It has been proposed that the self-organization process is similar to deterministic annealing (Martinetz *et al.* 1993). The neighborhood is interpreted as the pdf of the noise process in annealing. Decreasing the neighborhood then corresponds to decreasing the temperature of an annealing process. The study of simulated deterministic annealing for optimization is still in its infancy, so not much is known about optimal temperature schedules.

Luttrell (1990) provides an interesting interpretation of self-organization that can be related to the simulated annealing viewpoint. The SOM can be viewed as a vector quantizer for cases where the encoded symbols are corrupted with noise. In this interpretation, the neighborhood function corresponds to the pdf of the corrupting noise. Decreasing the neighborhood width during self-organization corresponds to starting with a vector quantizer designed for high noise and gradually moving toward a solution for a vector quantizer designed for no noise.

7.2 As an Increasing Model Complexity Parameter. In Section 2 we showed that the neighborhood width controls the amount of smoothing performed at each iteration of the SOM algorithm. If the neighborhood

Self-Organization as a Kernel Smoothing Process

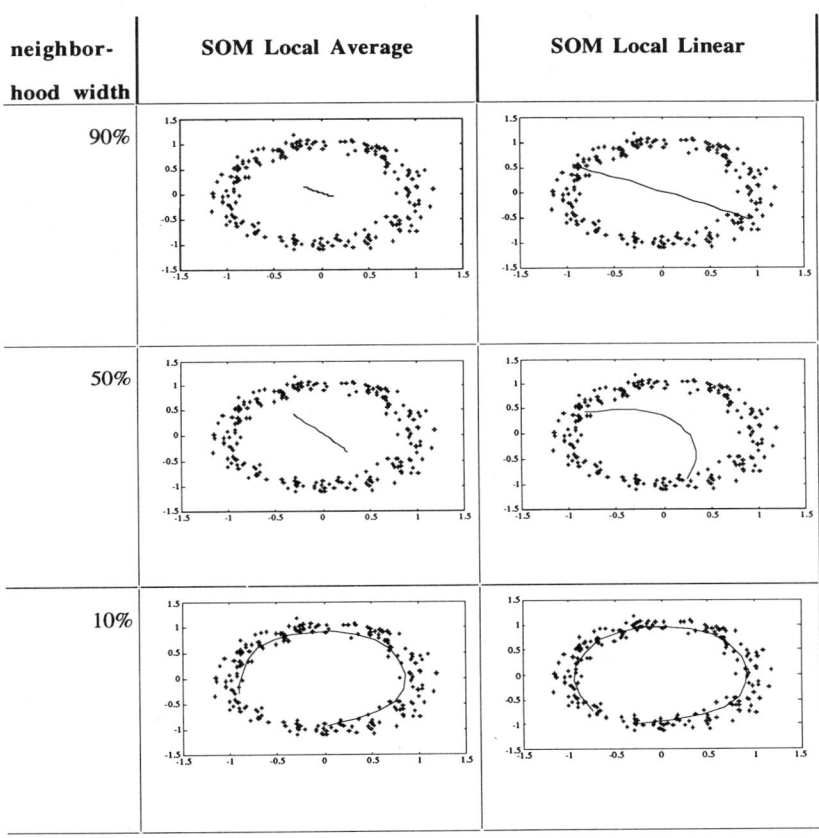

Figure 2: Comparison of SOM maps generated using the standard locally weighted average estimate of conditional expectation versus using a locally weighted linear estimate.

width is decreased at a very slow rate, the SOM algorithm provides a sequence of models in order of increasing complexity. In this case starting with a wide neighborhood and decreasing it is equivalent to assuming a simple regression model for the early iterations and moving towards a more complex one. Asymptotically optimal spans for kernel estimators have been developed, based on number of samples, curvature of underlying function, and variance of noise (Hardle 1990). It is not clear at this point if these bounds can be applied, because of the complex iterative nature of self-organization. Much theoretical work has been done in proving the convergence and consistency of iterative regression estimators (Ahmad and Lin 1976; Rutkowski 1985). These proofs place requirements on the rate of decrease of the kernel span as a function of the number of samples presented to the algorithm. These results may apply to the case of the original flowthrough version of SOM, but it is unclear how they would apply to the batch version. However, interpreting the output of the SOM algorithm as a sequence of models is useful in determining when to stop training. Assuming that the neighborhood width is decreased slowly, determining the final neighborhood width becomes a model selection problem, which has a number of statistical solutions (for example, cross-validation).

Since the output of the SOM algorithm can be interpreted as a sequence of models of increasing complexity, the neighborhood decrease rate controls the range of models created as well as the distribution of models with certain levels of complexity. For example, if the neighborhood width decreases very gradually initially, but then falls off rapidly near the final iterations, the SOM algorithm will produce many models with low complexity and only a few models with high complexity. So qualitatively at least, the neighborhood decrease rate should be used to encode the prior probability that a model with a particular complexity level is the correct model.

8 Summary

This paper focused on the effects of the neighborhood in self-organization. The SOM algorithm can be described in batch mode so that no learning rate is required, isolating the effects of the neighborhood. Each iteration of this algorithm can be seen as a statistical kernel smoothing problem where the neighborhood function is the kernel and smoothing is done in the topological space. This interpretation leads to three new insights of self-organization. First, the kernel smoothing provides a continuous functional mapping from the topological space to the samples space. Second, that the kernel smoothing is performed in the topological space, rather than the samples space, providing dimensionality reduction. Third, that computational speedups are possible because of the efficient implementations of kernel smoothing. The kernel smoothing interpretation also provides a connection between the SOM algorithm, the LBG algorithm, and the Principal Curve algorithm, and makes it possible to generalize self-organization to include these three algorithms as variants.

References

Ahmad, I. A., and Lin, P. 1976. Nonparametric sequential estimation of a multiple regression function, *Bull. Math. Statist.* **17**, 63–75.

Cleveland, W. S., and Delvin, S. J. 1988. Locally weighted regression: An approach to regression analysis by local fitting. *JASA* **83**(403), 596–610.
De Haan, G., and Egecioglu, Ö. 1991. Links between self-organizing feature maps and weighted vector quantization. *Proc. IEEE Int. Joint Conf. Neural Networks*, Singapore, 887–892.
Flury, B. A. 1990. Principal points. *Biometrika* **77**(1), 33–41.
Friedman, J. H., and Stuetzle, W. 1982. *Smoothing of Scatterplots*. Dept. of Statistics. Tech. Rep. Orion 3, Stanford University, Stanford, CA.
Grunewald, A. 1992. Neighborhoods and trajectories in Kohonen maps. *Proc. SPIE Conf. Science Artificial Neural Nets*, **1710**, 670–679.
Hardle, W. 1990. *Applied Nonparametric Regression*. Cambridge University Press, Cambridge.
Hastie, T. 1984. *Principle Curves and Surfaces*. Tech. Rep. no. 11, Department of Statistics, Stanford University, Stanford, CA.
Hastie, T., and Stuetzle, W. 1989. Principal curves. *JASA* **84**(406), 502–516.
Kohonen, T. 1982. Clustering, taxonomy, and topological maps of patterns. *Proc. 6th Int. Conf. on Pattern Recognition* Munich, 114–128.
Kohonen, T. 1989. *Self-Organization and Associative Memory*, 3rd ed. Springer-Verlag, Berlin.
Kohonen, T. 1993. Things you haven't heard about the self-organizing map. *Proc. IEEE Int. Joint Conf. Neural Networks*, San Francisco, 1147–1156.
Linde, Y., Buzo, A., and Gray, R. M. 1980. An algorithm for vector quantizer design. *IEEE Trans. Commun.* **28**, 84–95.
Luttrell, S. P. 1988. Self-organizing multilayer topographic mappings. *Proc. IEEE Int. Joint Conf. Neural Networks*, San Diego, **1**, 93–100.
Luttrell, S. P. 1990. Derivation of a class of training algorithms. *IEEE Trans. Neural Networks* **1**, 229–232.
Martinetz, T., Berkovich, S., and Schulten, K. 1993. "Neural-gas" network for vector quantization and its application to time series prediction. *IEEE Trans. Neural Networks* **4**, 558–569.
Nadaraya, E. A. 1964. On estimating regression. *Theory Prob. Appl. 10* **74**, 743–750.
Najafi, H. L., and Cherkassky, V. 1994. Adaptive knot placement for nonparametric regression. In *Advances in Neural Information Processing Systems 6*, J. D. Cowan *et al.*, eds., pp. 247–254. Morgan Kaufmann, San Mateo, CA.
Ritter, H., Martinetz, T., and Schulten, K. 1992. *Neural Computation and Self-Organizing Maps: An Introduction*. Addison-Wesley, Reading, MA.
Rodrigues, J. S., and Almeida, L. B. 1991. Improving the convergence in Kohonen topological maps. In *Neural Networks: Advances and Applications*, E. Gelenbe, ed., pp. 63–78. North-Holland.
Rutkowski, L. 1985. Nonparametric identification of quasi-stationary systems. *Syst. Control Lett.* **6**, 33–35.
Watson, G. S. 1964. Smooth regression analysis. *Sankhya*, Series A **26**, 359–372.

V

Extensions of Self-Organizing Maps

17

A Stochastic Self-Organizing Map for Proximity Data

Thore Graepel
Klaus Obermayer
Department of Computer Science, Technical University of Berlin, Berlin, Germany

We derive an efficient algorithm for topographic mapping of proximity data (TMP), which can be seen as an extension of Kohonen's self-organizing map to arbitrary distance measures. The TMP cost function is derived in a Baysian framework of folded Markov chains for the description of autoencoders. It incorporates the data by a dissimilarity matrix $\mathcal{D}$ and the topographic neighborhood by a matrix $\mathcal{H}$ of transition probabilities. From the principle of maximum entropy, a nonfactorizing Gibbs distribution is obtained, which is approximated in a mean-field fashion. This allows for maximum likelihood estimation using an expectation-maximization algorithm. In analogy to the transition from topographic vector quantization to the self-organizing map, we suggest an approximation to TMP that is computationally more efficient. In order to prevent convergence to local minima, an annealing scheme in the temperature parameter is introduced, for which the critical temperature of the first phase transition is calculated in terms of $\mathcal{D}$ and $\mathcal{H}$. Numerical results demonstrate the working of the algorithm and confirm the analytical results. Finally, the algorithm is used to generate a connection map of areas of the cat's cerebral cortex.

1 Introduction

Exploratory data analysis and visualization have received a lot of attention, since electronic data processing has made available large amounts of data from different sources all over the world. With respect to unsupervised learning, researchers have focused on analysis methods for data, which are given as vectors in a space that is assumed to be Euclidean. Examples for this kind include principal component analysis (PCA) (Jolliffe 1986; Tipping & Bishop, 1997), independent component analysis (ICA) (Bell & Sejnowski, 1995), vector quantization (VQ) (MacQueen, 1967), latent variable models (Bishop, Svensén, & Williams, 1997), or self-organizing maps (SOM) (Kohonen, 1982; Ritter, Martinetz, & Schulten, 1992). Often, however, data items are not given as points in a Euclidean data space, but one has to restrict oneself to the set of pairwise proximities as measured in particular in empirical sciences like biochemistry, economics, linguistics, or psychology. Here, two strategies for data analysis have been pursued for some time: pairwise clustering, which detects cluster structure in dissimilarity data (Hofmann & Buhmann, 1994; Duda & Hart, 1973), and metric multidimensional scaling (MMDS), which deals with the embedding of pairwise proximity data in a Euclidean space for the purpose of visualization (Borg & Lingoes, 1987). Recently, both approaches were combined by Hofmann and Buhmann (1997), who restrict the mean-fields from the clustering cost function to squared Euclidean distances between data points and cluster centers in the embedding space. The coupling between clusters, however, is maintained only at finite temperatures.

Here we present another approach to combine clustering and the visualization of proximity data, which is based on an extension of Kohonen's (1982) SOM. Data items characterized by mutual dissimilarities are mapped in a many-to-one fashion (clustering) to a set of neurons with predefined neighborhood relations (visualization), according to their similarities. To this extent, we first derive a general cost function for probabilistic autoencoders in the spirit of Luttrell (1994), but with arbitrary distortion measures. This cost function is then minimized by deterministic annealing, which shares the robustness properties of maximum entropy inference. Then the same approximation that leads from Luttrell's (1991) topographic vector quantization (TVQ) to Kohonen's (1982) SOM for the Euclidean case is introduced in order to achieve higher computational efficiency.

The article is structured as follows. In section 2 we derive the cost function for topographic mapping of proximity data (TMP) and discuss its properties. We then derive an optimization algorithm based on deterministic annealing using a mean-field approximation (see Graepel & Obermayer, 1998, for a kernel-based method leading to similar equations in a different context). In section 3 we analytically determine the critical temperature of the first/phase-transition during the annealing as a function of the dissimilarity matrix $\mathcal{D}$ of the data and the coupling matrix $\mathcal{H}$, which determines the neighborhood relations of the set of neurons. In section 4, we apply the algorithm to a toy example and discuss the effects of the approximations made. As an example of how the algorithm works in practice, we finally use the TMP algorithm to group the areas in the cat's cerebral cortex based on their corticocortical connectivity patterns.

2 Derivation of the Topographic Mapping for Proximity Data

2.1 Two-stage Folded Markov Chain. According to Luttrell (1994) the cost functional for a probabilistic autoencoder with two stages as shown in Figure 1 can be expressed as

$$E^{FMC} = \sum_{i,j} \sum_{\mathbf{r},\mathbf{r}'} \sum_{\mathbf{s},\mathbf{s}'} P_0(i) P_1(\mathbf{r}|i) P_2(\mathbf{s}|\mathbf{r}) \delta(\mathbf{s}'|\mathbf{s}) \tilde{P}_2(\mathbf{r}'|\mathbf{s}') \tilde{P}_1(j|\mathbf{r}') d(i,j), \quad (2.1)$$

where i and j are data items, whose dissimilarity is given by $d(i, j)$. $P_0(i)$ is the probability of item i, and $P_1(\mathbf{r}|i)$ and $P_2(\mathbf{s}|\mathbf{r})$ are probabilistic encoders. Their corresponding probabilistic decoders are $\tilde{P}_1(j|\mathbf{r}')$ and $\tilde{P}_2(\mathbf{r}'|\mathbf{s}')$, respectively. A probabilistic encoder is related to its corresponding decoder by Bayes' theorem,

$$\tilde{P}_1(j|\mathbf{r}') = \frac{P_1(\mathbf{r}'|j)P_0(j)}{P_1(\mathbf{r}')}$$
$$\tilde{P}_2(\mathbf{r}'|\mathbf{s}') = \frac{P_2(\mathbf{s}'|\mathbf{r}')P_1(\mathbf{r}')}{P_2(\mathbf{s}')}. \quad (2.2)$$

Inserting equations 2.2 into equation 2.1, cancelling $P_1(\mathbf{r}')$, performing the sum over $\mathbf{s}'$, and assuming $P_2(\mathbf{s}|\mathbf{r})$ to be given yields

$$E^{FMC}(P_1) = \sum_{i,\mathbf{r},\mathbf{s},\mathbf{r}',j} P_0(i)P_1(\mathbf{r}|i)P_2(\mathbf{s}|\mathbf{r})P_1(\mathbf{r}'|j)P_0(j)\frac{P_2(\mathbf{s}|\mathbf{r}')}{P_2(\mathbf{s})}d(i,j). \quad (2.3)$$

This equation does not depend on the decoders anymore, but instead we had to introduce $P_2(\mathbf{s})$,

$$P_2(\mathbf{s}) = \sum_{i,\mathbf{r}} P_2(\mathbf{s}|\mathbf{r})P_1(\mathbf{r}|i)P_0(i), \quad (2.4)$$

as a consequence of Bayes' theorem.

Let us now choose the hitherto probabilistic encoder $P_1(\mathbf{r}|i)$ to be deterministic. In this case, we can express the encoder in terms of a stochastic matrix $\mathcal{M} = (m_{i\mathbf{r}})_{i=1,\ldots,D,\,\mathbf{r}=1,\ldots,N} \in \mathcal{R}^{D \times N}$, whose elements are binary assignment variables $P_1(\mathbf{r}|i) \stackrel{def}{=} m_{i\mathbf{r}}$, $\sum_{\mathbf{r}} m_{i\mathbf{r}} = 1$, $\forall i$, and may take only values from the set $\{0, 1\}$. In order to make contact with the SOM literature (Kohonen, 1982), we denote the second encoder $P_2(\mathbf{s}|\mathbf{r}) \stackrel{def}{=} h_{\mathbf{rs}}$, subject to the constraints $\sum_{\mathbf{s}} h_{\mathbf{rs}} = 1$, $\forall \mathbf{r}$. In the literature on Kohonen's SOM, $h_{\mathbf{rs}}$ is called a neighborhood function in the space of neurons and determines the coupling between neurons $\mathbf{r}$ and $\mathbf{s}$ due to their spatial arrangement in a neural lattice. The data are given by a dissimilarity matrix $\mathcal{D} = (d_{ij})_{i,j=1,\ldots,D} \in \mathcal{R}^{D \times D}$. With these notational conventions, we then arrive at the following cost function for the topographic mapping of D data items onto N neurons,

$$E^{TMP}(\mathcal{M}) = \frac{1}{2}\sum_{i,j=1}^{D}\sum_{\mathbf{r},\mathbf{s},t=1}^{N} \frac{m_{i\mathbf{r}}h_{\mathbf{rs}}m_{j t}h_{t\mathbf{s}}}{\sum_{k=1}^{D}\sum_{\mathbf{u}=1}^{N} m_{k\mathbf{u}}h_{\mathbf{us}}}d_{ij}, \quad (2.5)$$

via their dissimilarity values d_{ij}. The factor 1/2 has been introduced for computational convenience. Let us consider three special cases of the above cost function E^{TMP}:

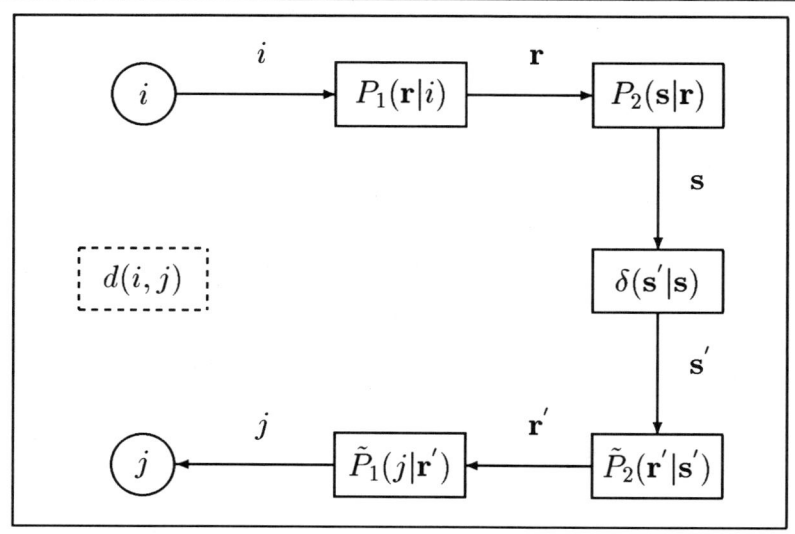

Figure 1: Illustration of a probabilistic autoencoder in the form of a two-stage folded Markov chain. A data item i is encoded by probabilistic encoders $P_1(\mathbf{r}|i)$ and $P_2(\mathbf{s}|\mathbf{r})$ and recovered by corresponding decoders $\tilde{P}_2(\mathbf{r}'|\mathbf{s}')$ and $\tilde{P}_1(j|\mathbf{r}')$ leading to data item j. The resulting distortion is measured as $d(i, j)$.

1. If the dissimilarity values d_{ij} are taken as the squared Euclidean distance $|\vec{x}_i - \vec{x}_j|^2$ of data points $\vec{x}_i$ in a Euclidean space, E^{TMP} is equivalent to the TVQ cost function introduced by Luttrell (1991).

2. If, however, the second encoder or neighborhood matrix is taken to be $h_{\mathbf{rs}} = \delta_{\mathbf{rs}}$, then we recover a cost function that is equivalent to Hofmann and Buhmann's (1997) for pairwise clustering. The normalizing denominator in equation 2.5 then becomes $\sum_{k=1}^{D} m_{ks}$ and was introduced by Hofmann and Buhmann (1997) based on heuristic arguments about cluster coherency. In our derivation, it appears as a natural consequence of Bayes' theorem applied to a probabilistic autoencoder.

3. In the special case of a one-to-one mapping, that is, $N = D$ and $\sum_i m_{ir} = 1, \forall \mathbf{r}$, we recover a form equivalent to the C measure, which was introduced by Goodhill and Sejnowski (1997) as a unifying objective function for topographic one-to-one mappings.

2.2 EM Algorithm and Deterministic Annealing. In order to obtain a robust optimization scheme, we apply the principle of maximum entropy

Stochastic Self-Organizing Map for Proximity Data

(Jaynes, 1957) and obtain a Gibbs distribution,

$$P(\mathcal{M}) = \frac{1}{Z_P} \exp(-\beta E^{TMP}(\mathcal{M})), \qquad (2.6)$$

where β is the inverse temperature and Z_P the partition function, which can be interpreted as the likelihood of the dissimilarity data. The summation in the partition function is over all "legal" assignment matrices $\{\mathcal{M}\}$. Since the cost function $E^{TMP}(\mathcal{M})$ depends on the assignment variables m_{ir} in a nonlinear fashion, this probability distribution does not factorize and, as a consequence, it is difficult to calculate averages with respect to it. Following Saul and Jordan (1996) and Hofmann and Buhmann (1997), we make a parameterized ansatz for a probability distribution $Q(\mathcal{M}, \mathcal{E})$,

$$Q(\mathcal{M}, \mathcal{E}) = \frac{1}{Z_Q} \exp\left(-\beta \sum_{i=1}^{D} \sum_{r=1}^{N} m_{ir} e_{ir}\right), \qquad (2.7)$$

which factorizes, and choose the partial assignment costs $\mathcal{E} = \{e_{ir}\}$ in such a way as to minimize the Kullback-Leibler (KL) divergence $KL(Q|P) = \sum_{\{\mathcal{M}\}} Q \ln(Q/P)$. Note that this approach implicitly assumes that assignments of data items to neurons are independent in the sense that $\langle m_{ir} m_{jr} \rangle = \langle m_{ir} \rangle \langle m_{jr} \rangle$, an assumption that is most likely to be valid in the case $D \gg N$. We obtain

$$\frac{\partial \langle E^{TMP}(\mathcal{M}) \rangle}{\partial e_{kv}} - \sum_{r=1}^{N} \frac{\partial \langle m_{kr} \rangle}{\partial e_{kv}} e_{kr}^* \stackrel{!}{=} 0, \forall k, \mathbf{v}, \qquad (2.8)$$

from which the mean-fields e_{kr}^* can be calculated as detailed in the appendix. We note that the cost function (see equation 2.5) is invariant under the substitution $d_{ij} = d_{ji} \leftarrow (d_{ij} + d_{ji})/2$. We also make the simplifying assumption of zero self-dissimilarity, $d_{ii} = 0$, and we neglect terms of order $\mathcal{O}(1/D)$. The optimal mean-fields e_{kr}^* are then given by

$$e_{kr}^* = \sum_{s=1}^{N} h_{\mathbf{rs}} \sum_{j=1}^{D} \frac{\sum_{t=1}^{N} \langle m_{jt} \rangle h_{\mathbf{ts}}}{\sum_{l=1}^{D} \sum_{u=1}^{N} \langle m_{lu} \rangle h_{\mathbf{us}}}$$
$$\times \left(d_{kj} - \frac{1}{2} \sum_{i=1}^{D} \frac{\sum_{u=1}^{N} \langle m_{iu} \rangle h_{\mathbf{us}}}{\sum_{l=1}^{D} \sum_{u=1}^{N} \langle m_{lu} \rangle h_{\mathbf{us}}} d_{ij} \right), \qquad (2.9)$$

where

$$\langle m_{kr} \rangle = \frac{\exp(-\beta e_{kr}^*)}{\sum_{s=1}^{N} \exp(-\beta e_{ks}^*)}. \qquad (2.10)$$

The self-consistent equations (2.9 and 2.10) can be solved by fixed-point iteration at any given value of the temperature parameter β. This constitutes an EM algorithm (Dempster, Laird, & Rubin, 1977), where the missing variables m_{kr} are estimated in the E step, equation 2.10, and the recalculation of the mean-fields, equation 2.9, corresponds to the M step. Since we are interested in globally optimal solutions, we employ deterministic annealing in β. The annealing scheme starts from high temperature, $\beta < \beta^*$ (see equation 3.7), where the unique maximum of the likelihood is found using the expectation-maximization (EM) algorithm. This maximum is then tracked through higher values of β. At sufficiently high β, the solution is expected to correspond to a good minimum of the original cost function.

2.3 SOM Approximation for TMP. According to Luttrell (1991), Kohonen's (1982) SOM can be considered an approximation to what Luttrell calls TVQ (Luttrell, 1991; Graepel, Burger, & Obermayer, 1997). TVQ corresponds to the optimization of the cost functional (see equation 2.1) for the case that $d(i, j) = |\vec{x}_i - \vec{x}_j|^2$ for data vectors $\vec{x}_i$ and the SOM approximation uses the nearest-neighbor winning rule $r_{win} = argmin_s |\vec{x} - \vec{w}_s|$ instead of the minimum distortion prescription $r_{win} = argmin_s \sum_t h_{st} |\vec{x} - \vec{w}_t|$ for data points $\vec{x}$ and weight vectors $\vec{w}_s$. Let us now introduce an equivalent approximation to TMP. The E-step, equation 2.10, can be seen as a softmax function with respect to the mean-fields e_{kr}^*. Leaving out the convolution with h_{rs} thus leads to a new prescription for the calculation of the mean fields,

$$e_{kr}^* = \sum_{j=1}^{D} \frac{\sum_{t=1}^{N} \langle m_{jt} \rangle h_{tr}}{\sum_{l=1}^{D} \sum_{u=1}^{N} \langle m_{lu} \rangle h_{ur}}$$

$$\times \left(d_{kj} - \frac{1}{2} \sum_{i=1}^{D} \frac{\sum_{u=1}^{N} \langle m_{iu} \rangle h_{ur}}{\sum_{l=1}^{D} \sum_{u=1}^{N} \langle m_{lu} \rangle h_{ur}} d_{ij} \right), \qquad (2.11)$$

the SOM approximation. This approximation is computationally more efficient than the exact update given in equation 2.9. However, it has the drawback that the iteration scheme, equations 2.10 and 2.11, no longer performs an exact maximum likelihood estimate. However, the robustness of the SOM algorithm, being based on the same approximation (Burger, Graepel, & Obermayer, 1998), and our numerical results demonstrate the usefulness of the approximation.

3 Critical Temperature of the First-Phase Transition

For soft clustering it is known that during the annealing process in β, the cluster representation undergoes a series of splittings (Rose, Gurewitz, & Fox, 1990, 1992; Buhmann & Kühnel, 1993). In the topographic case, weight vectors in data space split along the principal axis of the data according to the eigenstructure of the coupling matrix $\mathcal{H}$ (Graepel et al., 1997). Although there exists no Euclidean data space in our dissimilarity approach, we can examine the critical behavior of the neuron assignments with decreasing temperature.

Let us consider the case of infinite temperature, $\beta = 0$. Using $\langle m_{kr}\rangle^0 = 1/N$ in equation 2.10, the mean-fields e^0_{kr} for $\beta = 0$ are given by

$$e^0_{kr} = \frac{1}{D}\sum_{j=1}^{D}\left(d_{kj} - \frac{1}{2D}\sum_{i=1}^{D}d_{ij}\right). \tag{3.1}$$

We now linearize the right-hand side of equation 2.9 around e^0_{kr} by performing a Taylor expansion in $e^*_{mv} - e^0_{mv}$:

$$e^*_{kr} - e^0_{kr} = \sum_{m=1}^{D}\sum_{v=1}^{N}\left[\frac{\partial e^*_{kr}}{\partial e^*_{mv}}\right]_{e^0_{kr}}\left(e^*_{mv} - e^0_{mv}\right) + \cdots. \tag{3.2}$$

Evaluation of this expression yields

$$e^*_{kr} - e^0_{kr} = \beta\sum_{m=1}^{D}\sum_{v=1}^{N}\Delta_{km}\Gamma_{rv}\left(e^*_{mv} - e^0_{mv}\right) \tag{3.3}$$

with

$$\Delta_{km} = \frac{1}{D}\left(\frac{1}{D}\sum_{i=1}^{D}d_{im} + \frac{1}{D}\sum_{j=1}^{D}d_{kj} - d_{km} - \frac{1}{D^2}\sum_{i,j=1}^{D}d_{ij}\right) \tag{3.4}$$

and

$$\Gamma_{rv} = \sum_{s}h_{rs}\left[h_{vs} - \frac{1}{N}\right]. \tag{3.5}$$

Equation 3.3 can be decoupled by transforming the shifted mean-fields $e^*_{kr} - e^0_{kr}$ into the eigenbases of Δ and Γ. Denoting the transformed mean-fields $\tilde{e}_{\kappa\rho}$, we arrive at

$$\tilde{e}_{\kappa\rho} = \beta\Delta\Gamma\tilde{e}_{\kappa\rho}. \tag{3.6}$$

Assuming $h_{rs} = h_{sr}$, this equation has only nonvanishing solutions for $\beta\lambda^{\Delta}\lambda^{\Gamma} = 1$, where λ^{Δ} and λ^{Γ} are eigenvalues of Δ and Γ, respectively. This means that the fixed-point state from equation 3.1 first becomes unstable during the increase of β at

$$\beta^* = \frac{1}{\lambda^{\Delta}_{max}\lambda^{\Gamma}_{max}}, \tag{3.7}$$

where $\lambda_{\max}^{\Delta}$ and $\lambda_{\max}^{\Gamma}$ denote the largest eigenvalues of Δ and Γ, respectively. The instability, which is also referred to as the automatic selection of feature dimensions (Kohonen, 1988), is characterized by the corresponding eigenvectors $v_{\max}^{\Delta}$ and $v_{\max}^{\Gamma}$. While $v_{\max}^{\Gamma}$ determines the mode in neuron space that first becomes unstable (for details, see Graepel et al., 1997), $v_{\max}^{\Delta}$ can be identified as the principal coordinate from classical metric multidimensional scaling (Gower, 1966). It is instructive to consider a special case of Δ to understand its meaning. Assume that the dissimilarity matrix $\mathcal{D}$ represents the squared Euclidean distances $d_{ij} = |\vec{x}_i - \vec{x}_j|^2/2$ of D data vectors $\vec{x}$ with zero mean in an S-dimensional Euclidean space. Then it is easy to show from equation 3.4 that

$$\Delta_{km} = \frac{1}{D}\vec{x}_k \cdot \vec{x}_m. \tag{3.8}$$

In this case the $D \times D$ matrix Δ can at maximum have rank S. From singular value decomposition, it can be seen that the nonzero eigenvalues of Δ are the same as those of the covariance matrix $\mathcal{C}$ of the data. Since the eigenvectors of $\mathcal{C}$ correspond to the principal axes in data space, and its eigenvalues are the associated variances, the maximum variance in data space determines the critical temperature, whereby the instability occurs along the principal axis. In the general case of dissimilarities, we conclude that Δ can be interpreted as determining the width or pseudovariance of the ensemble of dissimilarity items.

The results of this section can be extended to the TMP with SOM approximation. The matrix Γ as given in equation 3.5 is modified by omitting one convolution with h_{rs}, resulting in

$$\Gamma_{rv}^{SOM} = \left[h_{vr} - \frac{1}{N}\right]. \tag{3.9}$$

4 Numerical Simulations

4.1 Toy Example: Noisy Spiral. In this section, we examine the ability of TMP to generate a topographic representation of a one-dimensional noisy spiral (see Figure 2, left) in a three-dimensional Euclidean space using distance data only. One hundred data points $\vec{x}$ were generated via

$$\begin{aligned} x &= \sin(\theta) + n_x \\ y &= \cos(\theta) + n_y \\ z &= \frac{\theta}{\pi} + n_z, \end{aligned} \tag{4.1}$$

where $\theta = [0, 4\pi]$ and $\vec{n}$ is gaussian noise with zero mean and standard deviation $\sigma_{\vec{n}} = 0.3$. The dissimilarity matrix $\mathcal{D}$ was calculated from the

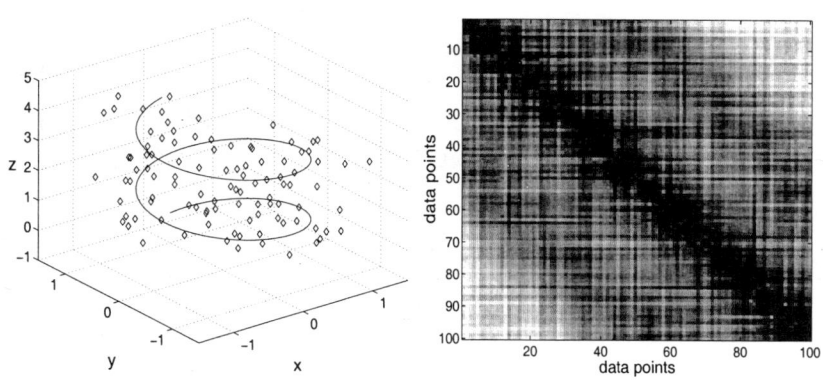

Figure 2: Plots of a noisy spiral (left) and corresponding dissimilarity matrix (right). One hundred data points were generated according to equation 4.1 with $\theta = [0, 4\pi]$ and $\sigma_{\bar{n}} = 0.3$. The dissimilarity matrix was obtained as $d_{ij} = |\vec{x}_i - \vec{x}_j|^2/2$ and was plotted such that the rows from top down and the columns from left to right correspond to the data points in order of their generation along the spiral with increasing θ.

squared Euclidean distances between the data points, $d_{ij} = |\vec{x}_i - \vec{x}_j|^2/2$, and is depicted in Figure 2 (right). The neighborhood matrix $\mathcal{H}$ was chosen such that it reflects the topology of a chain of 10 neurons, with the coupling strength decreasing as a gaussian function of distance,

$$h_{\mathbf{rs}} = \exp(-|\mathbf{r} - \mathbf{s}|^2/2\sigma_h^2)/c. \qquad (4.2)$$

$\sigma_h = 0.5$ and $h_{\mathbf{rs}}$ is normalized to unit probability over all neurons by c. Note that this choice of σ_h corresponds to a very narrow neighborhood. Without annealing, it would lead to topological defects in the representation. We applied TMP both with and without the SOM approximation, choosing an exponential annealing schedule (Graepel et al., 1997) according to $\beta^{t+1} = 1.1\,\beta^t$ with $\beta^0 = 0.1$.

As can be seen from Figure 3, both variants of TMP converge to the same final value of the average cost function at low temperature. The first split occurs close to $\beta^* = 0.71$, the value predicted by equation 3.7, indicated as a vertical line in the plot. Due to the weak coupling, the SOM approximation induces only a slightly earlier transition at $\beta_S^* = 0.70$ in accordance with equation 3.9. TMP detects the reduced dimensionality of the spiral and correctly forms groups along the spiral. Figure 4 shows the assignment matrix of the data points in order of their generation in the spiral to the chain of neurons. At high temperature (see Figure 4, left) the assignments

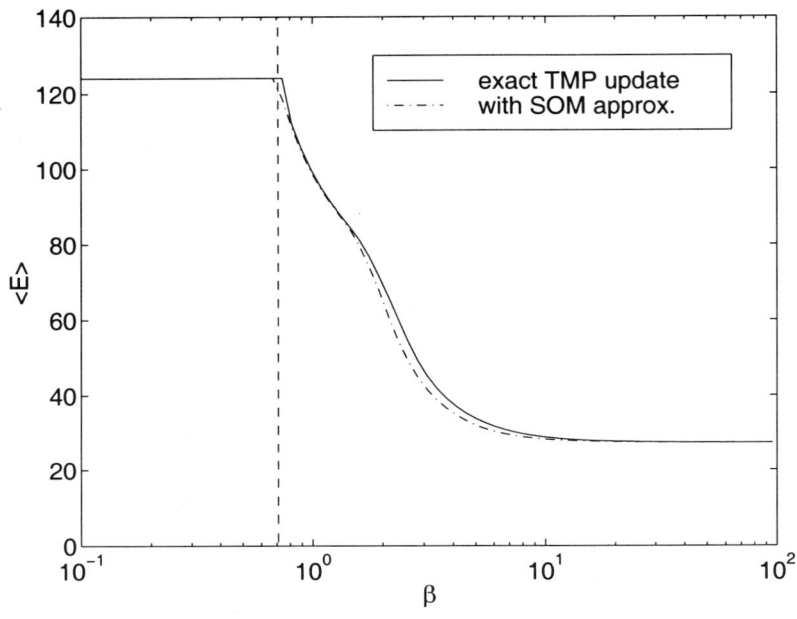

Figure 3: Plot of the average assignment cost $\langle E \rangle$ as a function of the temperature parameter β for TMP with and without SOM approximation applied to the dissimilarity matrix of the noisy spiral from Figure 2. The topology of the neurons was that of a chain given by equation 4.2 with $\sigma_h = 0.5$. β was varied according to $\beta^{t+1} = 1.1\,\beta^t$ with $\beta^0 = 0.1$. The convergence criterion for the EM algorithm was given by $|e_{ir}^{t+1} - e_{ir}^t| < 10^{-7}$, $\forall i, \mathbf{r}$. The average cost $\langle E \rangle$ was calculated using equation 2.5 with the binary assignment variables $m_{i\mathbf{r}}$ replaced by their averages $\langle m_{i\mathbf{r}} \rangle$. The vertical line indicates the value $\beta^* = 0.71$ as calculated from equation 3.7.

are fuzzy, but the emerging topography is visible immediately after the phase transition. The diagonal structure of the assignment matrix at low temperature (see Figure 4, right) indicates the topography of the map, while the small defects stem from the gaussian noise on the data.

4.2 Topographic Map of the Cat's Cerebral Cortex. Let us now consider an example, that cannot in any sense be interpreted as representing a Euclidean space. The input data consist of a matrix of connection strengths between cortical areas of the cat. The data were collected by Scannell, Blake-

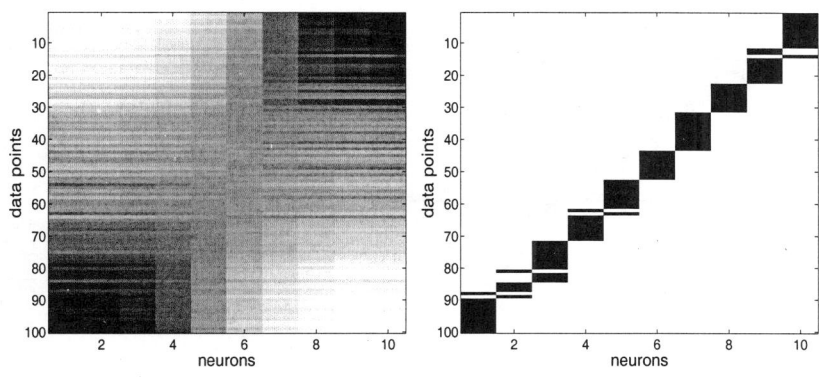

Figure 4: Plot of the average assignments $\langle m_{i\mathbf{r}}\rangle$ at high temperature $\beta = 0.81$ (left) and low temperature $\beta = 186.21$ (right) for TMP without SOM approximation applied to the noisy spiral. Dark corresponds to high probability of assignment. Data and parameters as in Figure 3.

more, and Young (1995) from text and figures of the available anatomical literature, and the connections are assigned dissimilarity values d as follows: self-connection ($d = 0$), strong and dense connection ($d = 1$), intermediate connection ($d = 2$), weak connection ($d = 3$), and absent or unreported connection ($d = 4$). Scannell et al. (1995) analyze these data as ordinal data, but we make the stronger assumption that the dissimilarity values represent a ratio scale. Since the true values of the connection strength are not known, this is a very crude approximation. However, it serves well for demonstration purposes and shows the robustness of the described method. Although the original matrix d'_{ij} was not completely symmetrical due to differences between afferent and efferent connections, the application of TMP is equivalent to the substitution $d_{ij} = (d'_{ij} + d'_{ji})/2$. Since the original matrix was nearly symmetrical, this introduces only a small mean square deviation per dissimilarity from the true matrix, $\sum_{i,j}(d_{ij} - d'_{ij})^2/D^2 \approx 0.1$).

The topology was chosen as a two-dimensional map of 5×5 neurons coupled in accordance with equation 4.2 with two-dimensional index vectors and $\sigma_h = 0.4$. Figure 5 shows the dissimilarity matrix sorted according to the TMP assignment results. The dominant block diagonal structure reflects the fact that areas assigned to the same neuron are very similar. Additionally, it can be seen that areas assigned to neurons far apart in the lattice are less similar to each other than those assigned to neighboring neurons.

Figure 6 displays the areas as assigned to neurons on the map by TMP. Four coherent regions on the map can be seen to represent four cortical

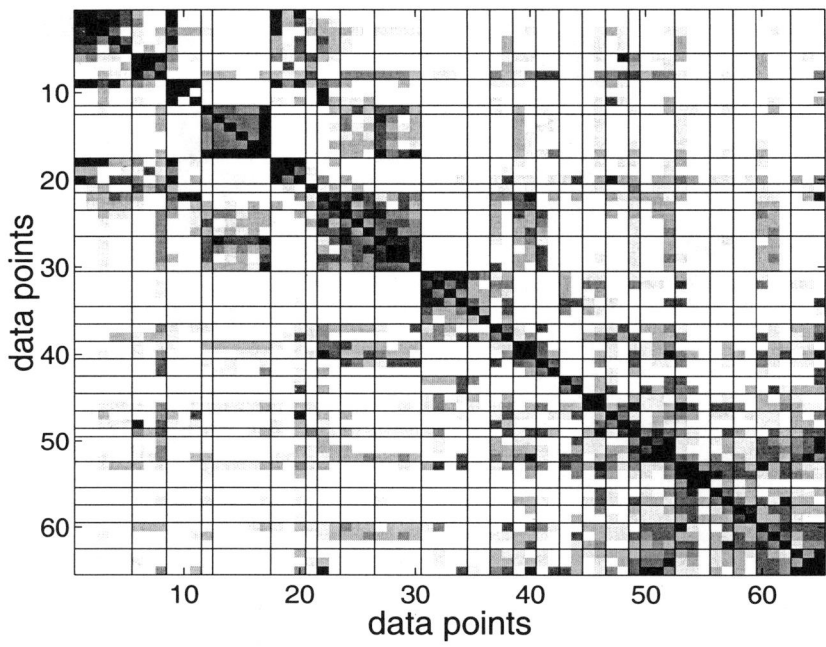

Figure 5: Dissimilarity matrix of areas of the cat's cerebral cortex. The areas are sorted according to their neuron assignments from top down and from left to right. The horizontal and vertical lines show groups of areas as assigned to neurons. Dark means similiar. The topology of the neurons was that of a 5×5 lattice as given by equation 4.2 with $\sigma_h = 0.4$. The annealing scheme was $\beta^{t+1} = 1.05\,\beta^t$ with $\beta^0 = 2.5 < 2.7265 = \beta^*$. The convergence criterion for the EM algorithm was $|e_{i\mathbf{r}}^{t+1} - e_{i\mathbf{r}}^t| < 10^{-10}$, $\forall i, \mathbf{r}$.

systems: visual, auditory, somatosensory, and frontolimbic. The visual areas 20b and PS are an exception and occupy a neuron that is not part of the main visual region. Their position is justified, however, by the fact that these areas have many connections to the frontolimbic system. In general, it is observed that primary areas such as areas 17 and 18 for the visual system, areas 1, 2, 3a, 3b, and SII for the somatosensory system, and areas AI and AII for the auditory system are placed at corners or at an edge of the map. Higher areas with more crosstalk are found more centrally located on the map. An example is EPp, the posterior part of the posterior ectosylvian gyrus, a visual

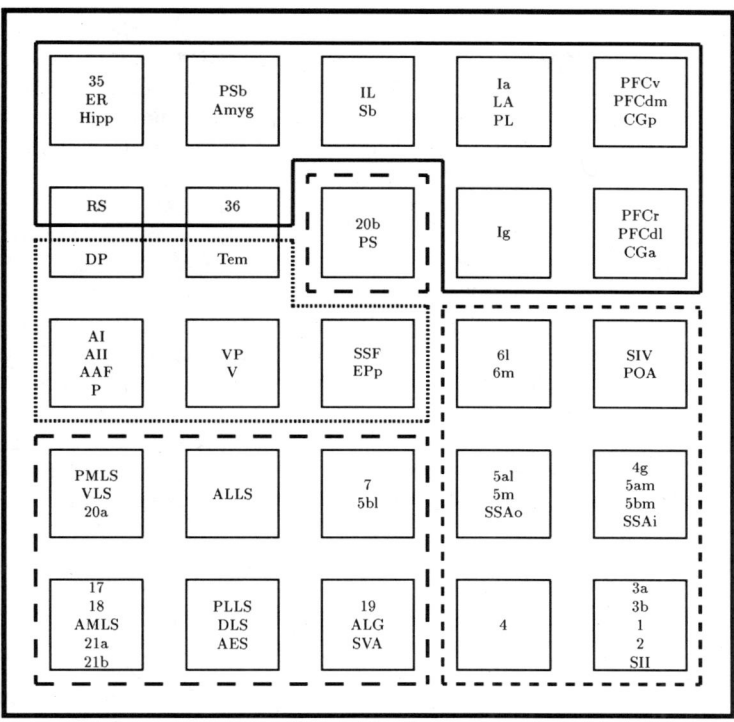

Figure 6: Connection map of the cat's cerebral cortex. The map shows 65 cortical areas mapped to a lattice of 5 × 5 neurons. The four cortical systems—frontolimbic (——), visual (— —), auditory (· · ·), and somatosensory (- -)—have been mapped to coherent regions except for the visual areas 20b and PS, which occupy a neuron apart from the main visual region. Parameters as in Figure 5.

and auditory association area (Scannell et al., 1995) represented at the very center of the map with two direct visual neighbors. In summary, the map in Figure 6 is a plausible visualization of the connection patterns found in the cat's cerebral cortex. It is clear, however, that the rather arbitrary and coarse topography of the 5 × 5 square map cannot fully express the rich cortical structures. Prior knowledge about the connection patterns, if available, could be encoded in the topology of the neurons to improve the representation.

5 Conclusion

We proposed a robust algorithm for TMP, which extends the applicability of topographic mapping algorithms, such as Kohonen's SOM, beyond the standard Euclidean data space used. The deterministic annealing scheme ensures fast convergence and thus leaves the neighborhood matrix $\mathcal{H}$ free to encode the desired spatial relations of the neurons onto which the data items are to be mapped. Besides the potential use of TMP as a more flexible alternative to multidimensional scaling, we envision its application to problems such as the generation of topographic maps of symbol strings, which is useful for large-scale data mining, such as in the World Wide Web (Kohonen, Kaski, Lagus, & Honkela, 1996). However, since the number of dissimilarities scales quadratically with the number of data items, it is computationally expensive to determine the pairwise dissimilarities and to process them. As a consequence, a mechanism for active data selection, for example, based on the expected information gain (MacKay, 1992), would be useful for determining those proximity values most important for the representation of the data. Combined with an estimation procedure for missing data based on the EM algorithm (Tresp, Ahmad, & Neuneier, 1994), this would lead to a system capable of performing data mining and visualization of proximity data on an even larger scale.

Appendix: Derivation of Mean-Field Equations

Using the relations

$$\frac{m_{kr}}{\sum_l \sum_{\mathbf{u}} m_{l\mathbf{u}} h_{\mathbf{us}}} = \frac{m_{kr}}{\sum_{l \neq k} \sum_{\mathbf{u}} m_{l\mathbf{u}} h_{\mathbf{us}} + h_{rs}} \quad \text{(A.1)}$$

and, from $1/(a+b) = 1/a - b/(a(a+b))$,

$$\frac{1}{\sum_l \sum_{\mathbf{u}} m_{l\mathbf{u}} h_{\mathbf{us}}}$$
$$= \frac{1}{\sum_{l \neq k} \sum_{\mathbf{u}} m_{l\mathbf{u}} h_{\mathbf{us}} + \sum_{\mathbf{u}} m_{k\mathbf{u}} h_{\mathbf{us}}}$$
$$= \frac{1}{\sum_{l \neq k} \sum_{\mathbf{u}} m_{l\mathbf{u}} h_{\mathbf{us}}}$$
$$- \sum_{\mathbf{w}} h_{\mathbf{ws}} \frac{m_{kw}}{\sum_{l \neq k} \sum_{\mathbf{u}} m_{l\mathbf{u}} h_{\mathbf{us}} (\sum_{l \neq k} \sum_{\mathbf{u}} m_{l\mathbf{u}} h_{\mathbf{us}} + h_{\mathbf{ws}})}. \quad \text{(A.2)}$$

We obtain for the derivative of the averaged cost function $\langle E^{TMP} \rangle$,

$$\frac{\partial \langle E^{TMP} \rangle}{\partial e_{kv}} = \frac{1}{2} \sum_{r,s,t} h_{rs} h_{ts} \sum_{i,j} \frac{\partial}{\partial e_{kv}} \left\langle \frac{m_{ir} m_{jt}}{\sum_l \sum_{\mathbf{u}} m_{l\mathbf{u}} h_{\mathbf{us}}} \right\rangle d_{ij}$$

$$= \frac{1}{2} \sum_{r,s,t} h_{rs} h_{ts} \left[\sum_{j \neq k} \frac{\partial \langle m_{kr} \rangle}{\partial e_{kv}} \left\langle \frac{m_{jt}}{\sum_{l \neq k} \sum_{u} m_{lu} h_{us} + h_{rs}} \right\rangle d_{kj} \right.$$

$$+ \sum_{i \neq k} \frac{\partial \langle m_{kt} \rangle}{\partial e_{kv}} \left\langle \frac{m_{ir}}{\sum_{l \neq k} \sum_{u} m_{lu} h_{us} + h_{ts}} \right\rangle d_{ik}$$

$$+ \delta_{rt} \frac{\partial \langle m_{kr} \rangle}{\partial e_{kv}} \left\langle \frac{1}{\sum_{l \neq k} \sum_{u} m_{lu} h_{us} + h_{rs}} \right\rangle d_{ii}$$

$$\left. - \sum_{i \neq k} \sum_{j \neq k} \sum_{w} \frac{\partial \langle m_{kw} \rangle}{\partial e_{kv}} h_{ws} \left\langle \frac{m_{jt} m_{ir}}{\sum_{l \neq k} \sum_{u} m_{lu} h_{us} + h_{rs}} \right\rangle d_{ij} \right]. \quad (\text{A}.3)$$

With $d_{ii} = 0$ and $d_{ij} = d_{ji}$ we obtain

$$\frac{\partial \langle E^{TMP} \rangle}{\partial e_{kv}} = \sum_{r} \frac{\partial \langle m_{kr} \rangle}{\partial e_{kv}} \sum_{s,t} h_{rs} h_{ts} \sum_{j \neq k} \left\langle \frac{m_{jt}}{\sum_{l \neq k} \sum_{u} m_{lu} h_{us} + h_{rs}} \right\rangle$$

$$\times \left[d_{kj} - \sum_{i \neq k} \sum_{w} h_{ws} \left\langle \frac{m_{iw}}{\sum_{l \neq k} \sum_{u} m_{lu} h_{us} + h_{ws}} \right\rangle d_{ij} \right] \quad (\text{A}.4)$$

and, comparing equations A.4 and 2.8 optimal mean-fields e_{kr}^*, equation 2.9.

Acknowledgments

This project was funded by the Technical University of Berlin via the Forschungsinitiativprojekt FIP 13/41.

References

Bell, A. J., & Sejnowski, T. J. (1995). An information-maximization approach to blind separation and blind deconvolution. *Neural Computation, 7*, 1129–1159.

Bishop, C. M., Svensén, M., & Williams, C. K. I. (1997). GTM: The generative topographic mapping. *Neural Computation, 10*, 215–234.

Borg, I., & Lingoes, J. (1987). *Multidimensional similarity structure analysis*. Berlin: Springer-Verlag.

Buhmann, J. M., & Kühnel, H. (1993). Vector quantization with complexity costs. *IEEE Transactions on Information Theory, 39*, 1133–1145.

Burger, M., Graepel, T., & Obermayer, K. (1998). An annealed self-organizing map for source channel coding. In *Advances in neural information processing systems, 10* (pp. 430–436). Cambridge, MA: MIT Press.

Dempster, A. P., Laird, N. M., & Rubin, D. B. (1977). Maximum likelihood from incomplete data via the EM algorithm. *Journal of the Royal Statistical Society, 39*, 1–22.

Duda, R. O., & Hart, P. E. (1973). *Pattern classification and scene analysis*. New York: Wiley.

Goodhill, G. J., & Sejnowski, T. J. (1997). A unifying objective function for topographic mappings. *Neural Computation, 9*, 1291–1303.

Gower, J. C. (1966). Some distance properties of latent root and vector methods used in multivariate analysis. *Biometrika, 9*, 325–328.

Graepel, T., Burger, M., & Obermayer, K. (1997). Phase transitions in stochastic self-organizing maps. *Physical Review E, 56*, 3876–3890.

Graepel, T., & Obermayer, K. (1998). Fuzzy topographic kernel clustering. In W. Brauer (Ed.), *Proceedings of the 5th GI Workshop Fuzzy Neuro Systems '98* (pp. 90–97).

Hofmann, T., & Buhmann, J. (1994). Central and pairwise data clustering by competitive neural networks. In J. D. Cowan, G. Tesauro, & J. Alspector (Eds.), *Advances in neural information processing systems, 6* (pp. 104–111). San Mateo, CA: Morgan Kaufmann.

Hofmann, T., & Buhmann, J. (1997). Pairwise data clustering by deterministic annealing. *IEEE Transactions on Pattern Analysis and Machine Intelligence, 19*, 1–14.

Jaynes, E. T. (1957). Information theory and statistical mechanics. *Physical Review, 106*, 620–630.

Jolliffe, I. (1986). Principal component analysis. Berlin: Springer-Verlag.

Kohonen, T. (1982). Self-organized formation of topologically correct feature maps. *Biological Cybernetics, 43*, 59–69.

Kohonen, T. (1988). *Self-organization and associative memory* (3rd ed.). Berlin: Springer-Verlag.

Kohonen, T., Kaski, S., Lagus, K., & Honkela, T. (1996). Very large two-level som for the browsing of newsgroups. In C. v. d. Malsburg, J. C. Vorbrüggen, W. v. Seelen, & B. Sendhoff (Eds.), *Artificial neural networks–ICANN '96* (pp. 833–838). Berlin: Springer-Verlag.

Luttrell, S. P. (1991). Code vector density in topographic mappings: Scalar case. *IEEE Transactions on Neural Networks, 2*, 427–436.

Luttrell, S. P. (1994). A Bayesian analysis of self-organizing maps. *Neural Computation, 6*, 767–794.

MacKay, D. J. C. (1992). Information-based objective functions for active data selection. *Neural Computation, 4*, 586–603.

MacQueen, J. (1967). Some methods for classification and analysis of multivariate observations. In L. M. LeCam & J. Neyman (Eds.), *Proceedings of the Fifth Berkeley Symposium on Mathematical Statistic and Probability* (pp. 281–297). Berkeley: University of California Press.

Ritter, H. J., Martinetz, T., & Schulten, K. J. (1992). *Neural computation and self-organizing maps: An introduction*. Reading, MA: Addison-Wesley.

Rose, K., Gurewitz, E., & Fox, G. C. (1990). Statistical mechanics and phase transitions in clustering. *Physical Review Letters, 65*, 945–948.

Rose, K., Gurewitz, E., & Fox, G. C. (1992). Vector quantization by deterministic annealing. *IEEE Transactions on Information Theory, 38*, 1249–1257.

Saul, L. K., & Jordan, M. I. (1996). Exploiting tractable substructures in intractable networks. In D. S. Touretzky, M. C. Mozer, & M. E. Hasselmo (Eds.), *Advances in neural information processing systems, 8* (pp. 486–492). Cambridge, MA: MIT Press.

Scannell, J. W., Blakemore, C., & Young, M. P. (1995). Analysis of connectivity in the cat cerebral cortex. *Journal of Neuroscience, 15,* 1463–1483.

Tipping, M. E., & Bishop, C. M. (1997). *Mixtures of principal component analysers* (Tech. Rep. NCRG/97/003). Birmingham: Aston University.

Tresp, V., Ahmad, S., & Neuneier, R. (1994). Training neural networks with deficient data. In J. D. Cowan, G. Tessauro, & J. Alspector (Eds.), *Advances in neural information processing systems, 6* (pp. 128–135). San Mateo, CA: Morgan Kaufman.

18

Self-Organized Formation of Various Invariant-Feature Filters in the Adaptive-Subspace SOM

Teuvo Kohonen
Samuel Kaski
Harri Lappalainen
Helsinki University of Technology, Neural Networks Research Centre, Espoo, Finland

The adaptive-subspace self-organizing map (ASSOM) is a modular neural network architecture, the modules of which learn to identify input patterns subject to some simple transformations. The learning process is unsupervised, competitive, and related to that of the traditional SOM (self-organizing map). Each neural module becomes adaptively specific to some restricted class of transformations, and modules close to each other in the network become tuned to similar features in an orderly fashion. If different transformations exist in the input signals, different subsets of ASSOM units become tuned to these transformation classes.

1 Introduction

A long-standing problem in artificial perception has been to recognize patterns subject to simple transformations, such as translation, rotation, or scaling. A frequently held view is that invariances can be achieved by filtering of the pattern features that then become mapped into respective invariance classes. Another problem, equally important and intriguing, then ensues: how to determine a set of effective feature filter functions for arbitrary statistics of dynamic signals. These problems seem to have been solved in biological systems in some effective way. In this article, we devise a corresponding technical solution.

In traditional image analysis and pattern recognition techniques, the primary observations are usually preprocessed in a separate stage that extracts a number of invariant features. On the basis of these features, a statistical decision-making machine is then able to identify or classify the target invariantly. In applications where no prior standardization of the samples is possible—for instance, when the targets are moving or their illumination is varying—the wavelet transforms such as the Gabor transforms (Gabor, 1946; Daubechies, 1990) have become popular as extractors of approximately invariant local features. These transforms, although optimizable by standard techniques, have the limitation that their mathematical forms must be fixed a priori.

The learning scheme discussed in this article differs from all the previous approaches in that the forms of the filter functions are learned directly from short segments or episodes of dynamical signals or pattern samples. If the samples of the episode can be derived from each other by some linear transformation such as translation, they span a special manifold in the input signal space, namely, a linear subspace.

The ASSOM (adaptive-subspace self-organizing map) architecture discussed in this article was introduced by one of the authors in 1995 (Kohonen 1995a, 1995b, 1995c, 1996); this article is a continuing study of it. In this scheme, the various feature filters emerge in learning and become tuned to those manifolds of input patterns that are defined only transiently in short segments of signals but that occur sufficiently often. These filters thus learn not the pattern prototypes as such, but the different low-dimensional manifolds spanned by the consecutive signal pattern vectors.

The discussion here constitutes a viable alternative to the standard principal component analysis (PCA) methods of feature extraction (Hotelling, 1933) for which neural approaches have been presented (Oja, 1983, 1992; Rubner & Tavan, 1989; Cichocki & Unbehauen, 1993). The PCA extracts average features that reflect the global stationary statistical properties of the pattern sequence. The ASSOM, on the contrary, creates a set of statistical representations referring to different temporal events, and by competitive (winner-take-all) selection and learning, each of the representations selectively concentrates on a different class of temporal episodes. Moreover, due to the spatial interactions between the processing units of the ASSOM during learning, characteristic of all the SOM (self-organizing map) methods (Kohonen, 1982, 1995c) in general, the various feature filters emerging in this process will be organized spatially, processing units being ordered along some characteristic feature coordinates.

We should mention a couple of recent works (Földiák, 1991; Wallis, Rolls, & Földiák, 1993) in which neural units learn sequences of simple patterns. In these works, a fixed input layer of a two-layer architecture projects to a competitive second layer, where the winning unit learns a trace of successive inputs. The results obtained with the model do not, however, explain the emergence of the input-layer filters, which are essential for learning arbitrary manifolds. Effective and organized nontrivial invariant-feature filters can ensue only from the cooperation of several kinds of neural components, such as those constituting the ASSOM network architecture discussed here.

2 Auxiliary Concepts

First we set out to discuss the following subproblems in this section: invariant recognition of a pattern as invariant recognition of all its feature components, definition of invariance classes for feature components as linear subspaces, and adaptive learning of the invariance classes from short sequences of input patterns called the episodes.

Formation of Invariant-Feature Filters 347

2.1 Decomposition of a Pattern into Features Mapped into Invariance Classes. Vectors that represent dynamic sensory environments are usually distributed along manifolds, which are continuous subsets or zones in the vector space. Consider tentatively that the input pattern represents some fundamental feature component of a more complex object and is thus very simple, such as the Gabor functions are. Its variations, caused by a particular class of transformations of the basic pattern such as translation, can then be thought to span a low-dimensional manifold. For the simplest transformations, the manifold can even be represented by a linear subspace, in which every vector is linearly dependent on the others. The class of linear transformations of the same fundamental component will be mapped into the same linear subspace, which is then regarded as an invariance class.

If a more complex pattern can then be decomposed into a sum of such simple feature components, approximately at least, then all terms in the sum become mapped into their respective linear subspaces invariantly, whereby the whole pattern will be represented invariantly with respect to this same linear transformation.

2.2 Sample Vectors. The input to a neural network model may be described by a real vector $\mathbf{x} \in \Re^n$. Here we consider sample vectors that consist of scalar samples collected from some time-domain function I at different time lags v_i referred to some instant of time t:

$$\mathbf{x}(t) = [I(t - v_1), I(t - v_2), \ldots, I(t - v_n)]^T. \tag{2.1}$$

Alternatively, the input vector $\mathbf{x}$ may be composed of samples of a two-dimensional input image, collected from points with intensity I around a time-dependent reference point $\mathbf{r} = \mathbf{r}(t) \in \Re^2$. These sampling points are displaced relative to $\mathbf{r}$ by the amounts $\mathbf{s}_i \in \Re^2$:

$$\mathbf{x}(t) = \mathbf{x}[\mathbf{r}(t)] = [I(\mathbf{r}(t) - \mathbf{s}_1), I(\mathbf{r}(t) - \mathbf{s}_2), \ldots, I(\mathbf{r}(t) - \mathbf{s}_n)]^T. \tag{2.2}$$

The v_i and $\mathbf{s}_i$, respectively, form a regular or irregular sampling grid. The time series and the images, as well as patterns eventually representable in higher-dimensional domains, will be discussed below in the framework of the general vector space formalism.

2.3 Episodes, Signal Subspaces, and Orthogonal Projections. One of the basic problems is how the linear subspaces, the invariance classes, can be defined; another is how to test whether an unknown pattern belongs to a subspace. Consider, for instance, time-domain signals. If N sample vectors ($N < n$) are collected from successive reference points t_p, the set of the nearby sample vectors $\{\mathbf{x}(t_p)\}$ spans some linear signal subspace of the total input space. The set of the reference time instants $\mathcal{S} = \{t_p\}$ will be called an episode. The maximum dimensionality of this subspace is equal to the number of sampling instants in $\mathcal{S}$, but the dimensionality can be much smaller if the sample vectors are dependent, as is often the case. The connection between subspaces and invariances lies in realizing that the signal subspace itself is an invariant feature of the input vector **x**.

A linear subspace $\mathcal{L}$ of dimensionality H is in general completely defined by the general linear combination of the linearly independent basis vectors $\mathbf{b}_1, \ldots, \mathbf{b}_H$. However, the choice of the $\mathbf{b}_h$ is not unique; there exist infinitely many equivalent combinations of the $\mathbf{b}_h$ for the same $\mathcal{L}$, in some of which the $\mathbf{b}_h$ can be orthonormal. If a set of basis vectors is known, a set of equivalent orthonormal basis vectors for $\mathcal{L}$ can be computed by the familiar Gram-Schmidt process (for a textbook account, cf. Kohonen 1989, 1995c).

The basic operation to determine whether an unknown vector **x** belongs to $\mathcal{L}$ is the orthogonal projection of **x** on $\mathcal{L}$, denoted $\hat{\mathbf{x}}$. If $\hat{\mathbf{x}} = \mathbf{x}$, then **x** belongs to $\mathcal{L}$. For an arbitrary **x**, one can define its distance from $\mathcal{L}$ as $\|\tilde{\mathbf{x}}\| = \|\mathbf{x} - \hat{\mathbf{x}}\|$, where the norm is Euclidean.

The orthogonal projection $\hat{\mathbf{x}}$ can be computed as either of the following simple expressions, provided that the $\mathbf{b}_h$ are orthonormal:

$$\hat{\mathbf{x}} = \left(\sum_{h=1}^{H} \mathbf{b}_h \mathbf{b}_h^T \right) \mathbf{x} = \sum_{h=1}^{H} (\mathbf{b}_h^T \mathbf{x}) \mathbf{b}_h . \tag{2.3}$$

The latter expression is computationally lighter.

In the case that **x** does not belong to any subspace exactly, it can still be identified with the closest one. The factor in the first parenthesis of equation 2.3 is a projection operator matrix abbreviated P, and there holds $P^2 = P$, $P^T = P$. The pattern space is divided into pattern zones, each of which contains one of the above subspaces. The optimal separating surface between the ith and jth zone is the set of those points **x**, the projections of which on the respective subspaces $\mathcal{L}^{(i)}$ and $\mathcal{L}^{(j)}$ have equal norms. The separating surface is thus defined by the following quadratic equation in **x**:

$$\mathbf{x}^T P^{(i)2} \mathbf{x} - \mathbf{x}^T P^{(j)2} \mathbf{x} = \mathbf{x}^T (P^{(i)} - P^{(j)}) \mathbf{x} = 0, \tag{2.4}$$

where $P^{(i)}$ and $P^{(j)}$ are the projection operators to $\mathcal{L}^{(i)}$ and $\mathcal{L}^{(j)}$, respectively.

2.4 The Network Model. It may be helpful to imagine that the set of subspaces, the invariance classes, corresponds to a two-layered neural architecture, organized into modules that function as processing units (see Figure 1). Each of the modules represents a subspace denoted by $\mathcal{L}^{(i)}$. The neurons in the input layer are linear; if the weight vector of neuron h in the input layer of module i is denoted by $\mathbf{b}_h^{(i)}$ and the input by **x**, respectively, the output of this neuron is $\mathbf{x}^T \mathbf{b}_h^{(i)}$. The weight vectors $\mathbf{b}_h^{(i)}$ form the basis of the subspace $\mathcal{L}^{(i)}$, and they will be referred to as basis vectors. The neurons in the output layer have some quadratic transfer function Q. If in practical

Formation of Invariant-Feature Filters

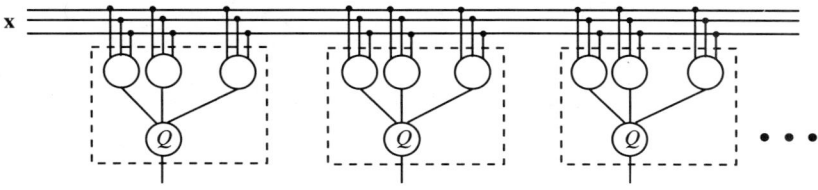

squared lengths of projections of **x** on the due subspaces

Figure 1: Neural network that consists of linear-subspace modules. The modules are separated by dashed lines. Q: quadratic neuron.

simulations the vectors $\mathbf{b}_h^{(i)}$ in each module are kept mutually orthonormal, Q is simply the sum of squares of the inputs of the second-layer neuron.

The sum of squares formed by the output neuron in each module equals the squared norm of the projection $\hat{x}^{(i)}$ of the input on the subspace $\mathcal{L}^{(i)}$, or $\|\hat{x}^{(i)}\|^2$. The output of the module can then be interpreted as the degree of matching between the input and the subspace. Thus, the output of each module is invariant (neglecting eventual changes in the norm of the input) to restricted linear transformations that occur within the subspace represented by the module. In the competitive learning process discussed below, the modules learn to represent different invariance classes.

Competitive learning in this network also involves neighborhood interactions between the modules similar to the neighborhood function in the standard SOM algorithm (Kohonen 1982, 1995c). Due to these interactions, neighboring modules learn to represent similar features, or similarly transformed features, and the array of the modules becomes tuned to the features in an orderly fashion. In the larger scale, different areas in the network may become specialized to different input types, such as transforms, as a result of these interactions.

3 Theory of the ASSOM

In this article, we not only want to create sets of feature filters; we also want these filters to become self-organized into a spatial order that reflects the similarity of the feature values they detect. Such a "map" is easier to inspect, and the artificially produced "maps" can then be better compared with those existing in the neural realms.

3.1 Learning. The ASSOM units learn to become invariant, approximately at least, to the transformations that exist in their environment by modifying their own subspaces to improve matching with the input signal subspaces. The latter are spanned by the successive samples in the episodes $\mathcal{S}$, as discussed in section 2.3.

In order to approximate the input episodes by subspaces of low dimensionality, in the experiments described here, we fixed the ASSOM modules to have two input neurons, the minimum number required to extract invariant features (cf. Gabor filters). It is also quite possible to use more input neurons. When these modules are made to compete on the input signal subspaces, the module that represents a given signal subspace best wins the competition, and it, together with its neighbors in the array, is adapted to represent the input subspace even better. In this way the different modules become gradually specialized to represent different types of input subspaces.

As the modules in the neighborhood of the winner are also adapted to represent the input better, the neighboring modules gradually learn to represent similar inputs; this effect can be regarded as a kind of smoothing of the neighboring representations. Such "neighborhood learning" was also the basis of the SOM algorithm, where the weight vectors of processing units become spatially ordered in the map array.

The ASSOM learning process can be summarized in general terms as follows:

1. Locate the module ("winner") c, the subspace $\mathcal{L}^{(c)}$ of which is closest to the signal subspace of the input episode $\mathcal{S}$.
2. Adjust the subspace $\mathcal{L}^{(c)}$ of the winning module and modules in its neighborhood in the ASSOM array closer to the signal subspace.

Direct comparison of the signal subspace with the subspaces of the neural modules could be rather difficult, for instance, because the dimensionality of the input signal subspace may be defined vaguely due to noise in the samples. A simpler and much more robust definition of match between the input subspace and the neural subspaces is comparison of each input sample of the episode separately with the neural subspaces, and computation of the "energy" (sum of squares) of the projections of the input samples of the episode on each of the subspaces of the ASSOM modules. The module with the largest energy—the sum of the squared projections of the samples collected during an episode—wins the competition. Denote the projections of the samples collected during $\mathcal{S}$ by $\hat{\mathbf{x}}^{(i)}(t_p)$. The representative winner for the whole episode $\mathcal{S}$, again indexed by c, is then defined by the expression

$$c = \arg\max_i \left\{ \sum_{t_p \in \mathcal{S}} \|\hat{\mathbf{x}}^{(i)}(t_p)\|^2 \right\},$$

or equivalently,

$$c = \arg\min_i \left\{ \sum_{t_p \in \mathcal{S}} \|\tilde{\mathbf{x}}^{(i)}(t_p)\|^2 \right\}. \tag{3.1}$$

The final goal in the competitive learning of subspaces is to minimize the

Formation of Invariant-Feature Filters

average expected error when a stochastically selected input subspace is represented by the subspace of the winning module. A somewhat related error principle was also used in the classical vector quantization (Gersho, 1979; Gray, 1984; Makhoul, Roucos, & Gish, 1985). The distance between the subspace spanned by the input samples and the subspace $\mathcal{L}^{(i)}$ will here be measured in terms of the energy of the relative projection errors of the input samples.

Consider tentatively that no neighborhood interactions between the modules are yet taken into account and that the input vectors are normalized. The average expected distance between the input subspace and the subspace of the winning module, computed over the space of all possible Cartesian products X of input samples collected during the episodes $\mathcal{S}$, can be measured in terms of the projection error $\tilde{\mathbf{x}}^{(c)}$ and is expressed by the objective function

$$E = \int \sum_{t_p \in \mathcal{S}} \|\tilde{\mathbf{x}}^{(c)}(t_p)\|^2 p(X) \, dX. \tag{3.2}$$

Here $p(X)$ is the probability density of the X, and dX is a shorthand notation for a volume differential in the integration space, the Cartesian product of all the samples of the episode.

The index of the winning module c depends on the whole episode, as well as on the subspaces $\mathcal{L}^{(i)}$ of all modules i. Thus the exact minimization of equation 3.2 by differentiation may be very complicated (Kohonen, 1991, 1995c; for recent alternative treatments, see Buhmann & Kühnel, 1993; Luttrell, 1994). Therefore we shall resort to the classical Robbins-Monro stochastic approximation (Robbins & Monro, 1951) in minimizing equation 3.2 in the same way as in the derivation of the traditional SOM algorithms (Kohonen, 1991, 1995c). The objective function need not be a Lyapunov or energy function; nonetheless, the convergence of the stochastic approximation has been established generally (Albert & Gardner, 1967; Kushner & Clark, 1978; Wasan, 1969).

The objective function (see equation 3.2) describes the goal of pure unordered competitive learning. In Kohonen (1991, 1995c), to enforce ordering to the old vector quantization problems, the integrand in the error function E was smoothed locally with respect to the processing modules, which leads to the SOM algorithms. The same modification can also be made here by multiplying the integrand with the neighborhood kernel $h_c^{(i)}$, which is a decreasing function of the distance between the modules c and i in the ASSOM array. The new objective function then reads

$$E_1 = \int \sum_i h_c^{(i)} \sum_{t_p \in \mathcal{S}} \|\tilde{\mathbf{x}}^{(i)}(t_p)\|^2 p(X) \, dX. \tag{3.3}$$

Although attempts to optimize cost functions of the type in equation 3.3

have not succeeded in closed form, it has been possible to use the Robbins-Monro stochastic approximation to derive the SOM algorithm (Kohonen, 1991, which also compared the exact and approximate optima). In this approximation, the gradient of E_1 is evaluated on the basis of the last input $\mathbf{x}$ and the last values of $\mathbf{b}_h^{(i)}$ during the sampling sequence. Here the whole set $X = X(t)$ is regarded as constituting a "sample" in the stochastic approximation. Thus, instead of optimizing the original objective function E_1, in this approximation a step in the direction of the negative gradient of the sample function, $E_2(t)$, is taken:

$$E_2(t) = \sum_i h_c^{(i)} \sum_{t_p \in S(t)} \|\tilde{\mathbf{x}}^{(i)}(t_p)\|^2. \tag{3.4}$$

Let us recall that $\tilde{\mathbf{x}}^{(i)} = \mathbf{x} - \hat{\mathbf{x}}^{(i)}$, where $\hat{\mathbf{x}}^{(i)}$, as a function of the $\mathbf{b}_h^{(i)}$, is given by equation 2.3. If the basis vectors are kept orthonormal, the gradient of the sample function with respect to basis vector $\mathbf{b}_h^{(i)}$ is

$$\frac{\partial E_2}{\partial \mathbf{b}_h^{(i)}} = -2h_c^{(i)} \sum_{t_p \in S(t)} \left[\mathbf{x}(t_p) \mathbf{x}(t_p)^T \right] \mathbf{b}_h^{(i)}. \tag{3.5}$$

Comment 1. As index c would be changed abruptly when the signal subspace passes the border between its two closest subspaces $\mathcal{L}^{(i)}$, it will be necessary to stipulate that the signal subspace does not belong to the infinitesimal neighborhood of such a border in equation 3.5. For continuous, stochastic signals, this possibility can be neglected. (See a similar discussion in Kohonen, 1991, 1995c.)

Comment 2. Because the basis vectors that span a subspace are not unique, it might seem that the gradient-descent method cannot be used because the optimum is not unique. Notwithstanding, it may be clear that any of these optima (for which E_2 is minimized) is an equivalent solution, so it will suffice if one optimal basis is found.

With a step length of $\lambda(t)/2$ in the direction of the negative gradient, we obtain the rule

$$\mathbf{b}_h^{(i)}(t+1) = \mathbf{b}_h^{(i)}(t) - \frac{1}{2}\lambda(t) \frac{\partial E_2}{\partial \mathbf{b}_h^{(i)}}$$

$$= \left[I + \lambda(t) h_c^{(i)} \sum_{t_p \in S(t)} \mathbf{x}(t_p) \mathbf{x}(t_p)^T \right] \mathbf{b}_h^{(i)}(t). \tag{3.6}$$

The parameter $\lambda(t)$ is called the learning-rate factor. In stochastic approximation, the $\lambda(t)$ must satisfy the following conditions (Robbins & Monro, 1951; Kushner & Clark, 1978): $\sum_{t=0}^{\infty} \lambda(t) = \infty$, $\sum_{t=0}^{\infty} \lambda^2(t) < \infty$.

Formation of Invariant-Feature Filters 353

In the learning law (see equation 3.6) the operator,

$$R_1(\lambda(t)) = I + \lambda(t) h_c^{(i)} \sum_{t_p \in \mathcal{S}(t)} \mathbf{x}(t_p) \mathbf{x}(t_p)^{\mathrm{T}}, \qquad (3.7)$$

is applied to the basis vector $\mathbf{b}_h^{(i)}$. In the derivation of the learning law, the input vectors were tentatively assumed to be normalized. If they are not, the normalization can be incorporated into the objective function (see equation 3.3) by considering relative projection errors $\|\tilde{\mathbf{x}}^{(i)}(t_p)\|^2 / \|\mathbf{x}(t_p)\|$. Then the rotation operator (see equation 3.7) becomes

$$R_2(\lambda(t)) = I + \lambda(t) h_c^{(i)} \sum_{t_p \in \mathcal{S}(t)} \frac{\mathbf{x}(t_p) \mathbf{x}(t_p)^{\mathrm{T}}}{\|\mathbf{x}(t_p)\|^2}. \qquad (3.8)$$

Earlier (Kohonen, 1995c, 1996) we showed that the following slightly different law, a product of unnormalized rotation operators, can be used for the competing neural units to learn the different input subspaces:

$$R_3(\lambda(t)) = \prod_{t_p \in \mathcal{S}(t)} \left[I + \lambda(t) h_c^{(i)} \frac{\mathbf{x}(t_p) \mathbf{x}(t_p)^{\mathrm{T}}}{\|\mathbf{x}(t_p)\|^2} \right]. \qquad (3.9)$$

When $\lambda(t)$ is small, equations 3.8 and 3.9 can immediately be found equivalent. In fact, equation 3.8 can be seen as a batch version of equation 3.9, where the whole episode is used in one operation. One of the authors earlier proved the so-called adaptive-subspace theorem (Kohonen, 1996), which states that if there is only one subspace $\mathcal{L}^{(i)}$, it will converge to $\mathcal{L}^* \subseteq \mathcal{L}^{(s)}$ almost surely, where $\mathcal{L}^{(s)}$ is the signal subspace from which the samples $\mathbf{x}(t_p)$ are picked at random.

We shall henceforth use the operator $R_3(\lambda(t))$, because it applies the input samples $\mathbf{x}(t_p)$ in succession, and some extra operations explained in section 3.2 shall be made after each operation. The operator $R_3(\lambda(t))$ in fact corresponds to Hebb-type learning: the modification of a synapse (a component of a basis vector) is proportional to the product of its input and the output of the neuron.

Since expressions 3.8 and 3.9 do not preserve the norms of the basis vectors, for good performance the basis vectors should be orthonormalized, at least after some number (e.g., a few dozen) of learning steps.

3.2 Enhancement of the Organizing Power. In order to achieve a sufficient stability in the self-organizing process and to obtain well-distributed filter sets, the advice given in this section is necessary.

First, to ensure effective self-organization, any correction made on a neural unit must be a monotonically increasing function of the error. If this were not the case, the corrections made in neighboring units would strongly depend on their basis vectors before correction, which would lead to unstable self-organization.

The magnitude of the correction made on the subspace $\mathcal{L}^{(i)}$ should be a monotonically increasing function of the true error $\|\tilde{\mathbf{x}}^{(i)}\| = \|\mathbf{x} - \hat{\mathbf{x}}^{(i)}\|$ or a monotonically decreasing function of $\|\hat{\mathbf{x}}^{(i)}\|$. In the projective methods, the correction (see equation 3.6) would be proportional to $\mathbf{x}(t_p)^T \mathbf{b}_h^{(i)}$, which decreases with increasing angle between $\mathbf{x}(t_p)$ and $\mathbf{b}_h^{(i)}$. A simple method for guaranteeing that the correction is an increasing function of error (cf. Kohonen, 1996) is to divide the learning-rate factor $\lambda(t)$ by the scalar value $\|\hat{\mathbf{x}}^{(i)}\|/\|\mathbf{x}\|$, which changes only the effective learning rate. The operator (see equation 3.9) then becomes

$$R^{(i)}(t) = \prod_{t_p \in \mathcal{S}(t)} \left[I + \lambda(t) h_c^{(i)} \frac{\mathbf{x}(t_p)\mathbf{x}(t_p)^T}{\|\hat{\mathbf{x}}^{(i)}(t_p)\| \|\mathbf{x}(t_p)\|} \right]. \tag{3.10}$$

In the course of our simulations, reported in section 4.2, it turned out that the organization of the ASSOM was not always perfect even when the modified rotation operator (see equation 3.10) was used. For instance, when the input consisted of speech signals, some modules were prone to become tuned to two separate frequency bands. An explanation of this phenomenon is that a high-order linear in general can easily learn a rather complicated passband function, even one with many passbands, and it is mainly by the virtue of the competitive-learning process that single passbands at the filters are at all formed, because the process tries to distribute them in an orderly fashion over the frequency domain. When such two-band filters were formed in self-organization, the frequency range between these two bands remained unrepresented by the ASSOM array; that is, a gap in the distribution was formed (see section 4.2).

Without further speculation it may be mentioned that this instability can be eliminated by the following simple method, which has been empirically demonstrated to produce filters that are much better distributed in the frequency domain. If, after each learning step, the magnitude of small components of the basis vectors $\mathbf{b}_h^{(i)}$ is set to zero, then the basis vectors will be forced to approximate the stronger and more fundamental frequency components. If we denote the basis vectors by $\mathbf{b}_h^{(i)} = [b_{h1}^{(i)}, \ldots, b_{hn}^{(i)}]^T \in \Re^n$, then a very simple dissipation effect of this kind can be described by the equation

$$b_{hj}^{\prime(i)} = \text{sgn}(b_{hj}^{(i)}) \max(0, |b_{hj}^{(i)}| - \varepsilon), \tag{3.11}$$

where ε ($0 < \varepsilon < 1$) is a very small term. The amount of dissipation should be a fraction of the magnitude of the correction: $\varepsilon = \varepsilon_h^{(i)}(t) = \delta |\mathbf{b}_h^{(i)}(t) -$

$\mathbf{b}_h^{(i)}(t-1)|$, where δ is a small scalar parameter. The dissipation is applied after each rotation and before normalization.

Other regularizing principles have also increased the stability of self-organization in our experiments. For instance, there exist excessive "parasite" degrees of freedom in the representation of basis vectors because of various symmetries. These parasite degrees of freedom often result in asymmetric filters; for instance, the filters may become centered at any point in the sampling grid. In order to avoid the ASSOM from being organized along irrelevant feature dimensions, there is a simple method for favoring the middle of the sampling grid without significantly affecting the learning process in other respects: weighting the lattice points by a gaussian function centered in the middle. If the function is wide enough, it affects only the components of the basis vectors quite near the edges. Since all input vectors are weighted similarly, this weighting does not alter the transformation group inherent in the input vectors but enhances symmetry.

To speed up the organization process, the gaussian weighting function can also be made time dependent. In the beginning of the organizing process, the function could be selected as rather narrow, in order to fix the middle points first. After that, the width of the gaussian is increased, and the modules learn to represent their inputs more and more accurately using more and more peripheral points of the sampling grid.

Still another method for enhancing the organizing power, a standard method for warranting good organization in ordinary SOMs, is to make the neighborhood kernel dependent on time, $h_c^{(i)} = h_c^{(i)}(t)$. In the beginning of learning, the kernel should be very wide, effectively comprising half or even more of the map. When the width then gradually decreases to its final value, the map approximates its inputs more closely, while at the same time preserving the global ordering achieved in the beginning. In our simulations, we used a simple box-shaped kernel. The modules up to a certain radius from the winner were thereby updated equally $(h_c^{(i)}(t) = 1)$, whereas the other modules were not updated at all during this learning step $(h_c^{(i)}(t) = 0)$.

3.3 Summary: The ASSOM Learning Algorithm. For each learning episode $\mathcal{S}(t)$ consisting of successive time instants $t_p \in \mathcal{S}(t)$ do the following:

- Find the winner, indexed by c:

$$c = \arg\max_i \left\{ \sum_{t_p \in \mathcal{S}(t)} ||\hat{\mathbf{x}}^{(i)}(t_p)||^2 \right\}.$$

- For each sample $\mathbf{x}(t_p)$, $t_p \in \mathcal{S}(t)$:

  1. Rotate the basis vectors of the modules:

  $$\mathbf{b}_h^{(i)}(t+1) = \left[I + \lambda(t) h_c^{(i)}(t) \frac{\mathbf{x}(t_p)\mathbf{x}(t_p)^T}{\|\hat{\mathbf{x}}^{(i)}(t_p)\| \|\mathbf{x}(t_p)\|} \right] \mathbf{b}_h^{(i)}(t).$$

  2. Dissipate the components $b_{hj}^{(i)}$ of the basis vectors $\mathbf{b}_h^{(i)}$:

  $$b'^{(i)}_{hj} = \operatorname{sgn}(b_{hj}^{(i)}) \max(0, |b_{hj}^{(i)}| - \varepsilon),$$

  where

  $$\varepsilon = \varepsilon_h^{(i)}(t) = \delta |\mathbf{b}_h^{(i)}(t) - \mathbf{b}_h^{(i)}(t-1)|.$$

  3. Orthonormalize the basis vectors of each module.

The orthonormalization can also be made more seldom, say, after every hundred steps. Above, $\lambda(t)$ and δ are suitable small scalar parameters.

4 Experiments

We next show what kinds of invariant-feature filters will emerge in the AS-SOM learning process in different sensory environments, that is, when the input to the ASSOM is subjected to various transformations. The emerging filters reflect statistical characteristics of short sequences of input patterns but not waveforms as such. The filters will only learn such pattern components present in short input sequences that satisfy certain linear constraints, such as lying on a linear subspace. Patterns that do not satisfy these constraints will be averaged out in the long run. The resulting basis vectors in fact represent kernels of transforms that produce the invariant outputs.

Before reporting the final results, we first define some details of simulations. Then we demonstrate the enhancement of the organizing power due to the nonlinear dissipation effect introduced in section 3.2.

4.1 Details of the Simulations. In this section we summarize the kinds of input patterns used and how they were transformed.

4.1.1 Translated Speech Signal. In the first experiments, the input signal consisted of digitized time-domain speech waveforms from the TIMIT (1988) speech data set, which contains phrases spoken by a large number of U.S. speakers, sampled at 12.8 kHz. Before picking up the input vectors, high frequencies in the signal were enhanced by taking differences of successive samples (high-pass filtering).

The input vectors consisted of 64 successive samples of the speech waveform. Each learning episode began at a randomly chosen time instant and consisted of eight vectors, each displaced by a random amount (eight sam-

Formation of Invariant-Feature Filters

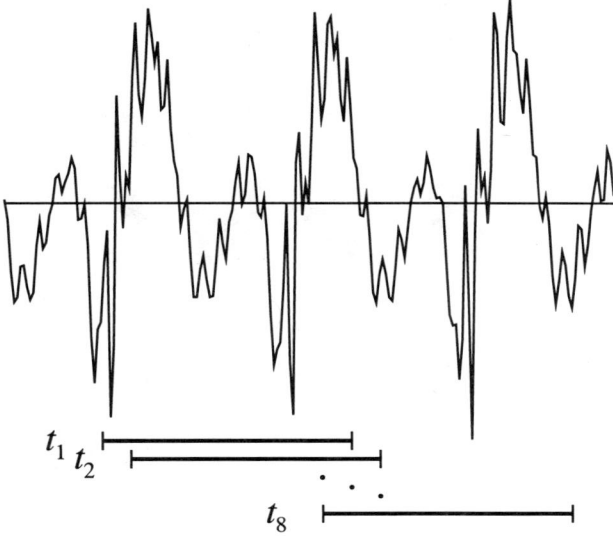

Figure 2: A sample speech waveform. The locations of the eight input vectors (with starting times $t_1, \ldots, t_8$) belonging to an episode are identified with the line segments under the speech waveform.

ples on the average) from the previous one. Thus, the transformation group inherent in the data consisted of translations in time. A segment of the original signal and the eight input vectors forming an episode are shown in Figure 2.

4.1.2 *Two-Dimensional Colored Noise.* Earlier (Kohonen, 1995c) we demonstrated that two-dimensional filters can be formed in response to photographic images. Here we wanted to specify the images statistically. Thus, in the rest of the experiments reported here, two-dimensional patterns consisting of colored noise were used. The patterns were formed by low-pass filtering of white noise with a second-order Butterworth filter that had the cutoff frequency at 60 percent of the Nyquist frequency. The image was sampled with a circular, uniformly spaced sampling grid consisting of 316 pixels.

In the experiments, the inputs were translated horizontally, rotated, or scaled. The center of both the rotation and the scaling operations was fixed to be the center of the sampling grid. The signal subspaces spanned by the samples of the episode can be regarded as low dimensional only if the transformations between the samples are modest. The amount of translation was varied from 0 to 10 pixels, using equal steps and a 10 percent random

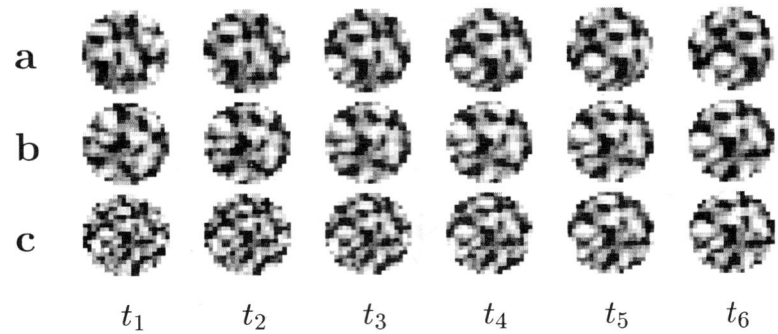

Figure 3: Samples of transformed colored noise patterns. (a) Translated inputs. (b) Rotated inputs. (c) Scaled inputs. Each horizontal row forms an episode.

displacement at each. The amount of rotation ranged from 0 to 1 radian, divided into equal steps and having 10 percent random rotation at each step. The amount of scaling used in the episode increased with equal steps from 1.0 to 1.5, with a 10 percent random variation applied at each step. The translated images were weighted by a vertical gaussian kernel, to force all templates to become vertically centered at the same location (see section 3.2). The other kinds of inputs, scaled and rotated, were not weighted.

The inputs were high-pass-filtered in time by taking differences of successive input vectors to enhance the changing parts of the input. High-pass filtering is necessary, for example, for scaled images where the center of the scaling remains approximately constant. A well-functioning invariance filter would then model predominantly this invariant area instead of the changes in the stimuli produced by scaling. Before filtering, the number of samples in each episode was six, and the number decreased to five after taking the differences.

Exemplary episodes of translated, rotated, and scaled colored noise are shown in Figure 3.

4.1.3 Methods.

The ASSOM lattice consisted, unless otherwise stated, of 24 units organized as a one-dimensional array. Each ASSOM unit contained two basis vectors $\mathbf{b}_1^{(i)}$ and $\mathbf{b}_2^{(i)}$, which were initialized with random values before learning. All inputs were normalized to unit length. The learning process was summarized in section 3.3. The neighborhood kernel $h_c^{(i)}$ was box shaped with $h_c^{(i)} = 1$ in the neighborhood of the winner and $h_c^{(i)} = 0$ for the other units. The basis vectors were orthonormalized after each adaptation step. In case the computing time is critical, orthonormalization

Formation of Invariant-Feature Filters

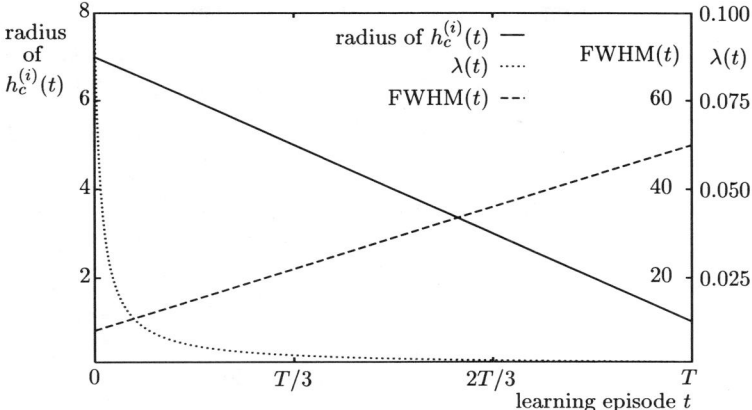

Figure 4: The learning parameters versus number of learning episodes. The learning-rate factor $\lambda(t)$ was of the form $0.1 \cdot T/(T + 99t)$, where T is the total number of episodes during learning. In T steps the radius of the box-shaped neighborhood decreased linearly from seven lattice spacings to one spacing. The gaussian function used for weighting the sampled input pattern changed according to the curve marked by FWHM(t), full width at half maximum, expressed in terms of sampling points. The FWHM increased linearly from 8 to 50 sampling points.

can be made more seldom. During the learning process, the parameters changed according to Figure 4.

4.2 Demonstration of the Enhancement of the Organizing Power.

4.2.1 Preliminary Experiment Without Dissipation. In the first experiment with the ASSOM algorithm, the input consisted of translated speech signals. After 2000 learning episodes, the ASSOM units represented different frequency components in an orderly fashion (see Figure 5). The two basis vectors in each unit, $\mathbf{b}_1^{(i)}$ and $\mathbf{b}_2^{(i)}$, became tuned to an approximately similar frequency band and had a 90-degree phase shift with respect to each other. Each output (squared projection of the input on the subspace of a unit) of the units became selective to a certain frequency band and was invariant to translations in time, as long as the frequency content of the input did not change.

If the learning period was extended, it turned out that the organizing result was not stable. In continued learning, a gap appeared in the representation. Some units had the tendency of representing several, usually two, distinct frequency components instead of one compact frequency band, and

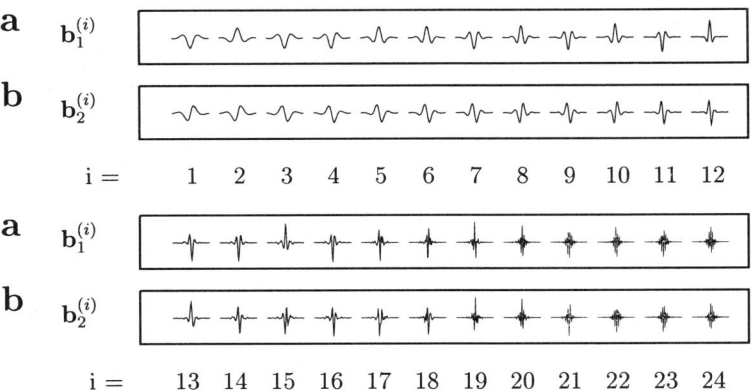

Figure 5: Tentative results with translated speech waveforms as inputs. Notice that the diagrams are in two parts. (a) The first basis vectors of the ASSOM units ($\mathbf{b}_1^{(i)}$). (b) The second basis vectors ($\mathbf{b}_2^{(i)}$).

some range of the input frequencies was left unrepresented. This occurred especially at the minima of the frequency spectrum. Figure 6 shows the filters after a learning process consisting of 100,000 episodes. There is a clear defect in the organization: a wide gap at frequencies 2000 through 3500 Hz in the distribution of the dominant frequencies of the units (see Figure 6e). It is notable that the frequency response, defined as the output of a unit as a function of the input frequency, of unit number 18 (closest to the gap) consists of two separate peaks corresponding to the borders of the frequency gap (see Figure 6d). The ability of the ASSOM filters to represent several frequencies at the same time was discussed in section 3.2.

4.2.2 *Reducing Excessive Degrees of Freedom Using Dissipation.* After the dissipation term discussed in section 3.2 was introduced, the frequency responses of all units obtained a single, relatively narrow passband (see Figure 7d). The value 0.02 was used for the dissipation constant δ. The gap in the distribution of the dominant frequencies of the ASSOM units was thereby closed (see Figure 7e). The steepest slope in the distribution of filters corresponds to a local minimum in the frequency spectrum.

If Figures 7a–b are inspected carefully, the effect of nonlinearity due to dissipation can be seen as small shoulders in the basis vectors at small values.

It may be interesting to note that an effective gaussian-shaped time window was determined by the wavelet shapes (see Figure 7c), and its width seemed to be optimized for each filter separately.

Formation of Invariant-Feature Filters

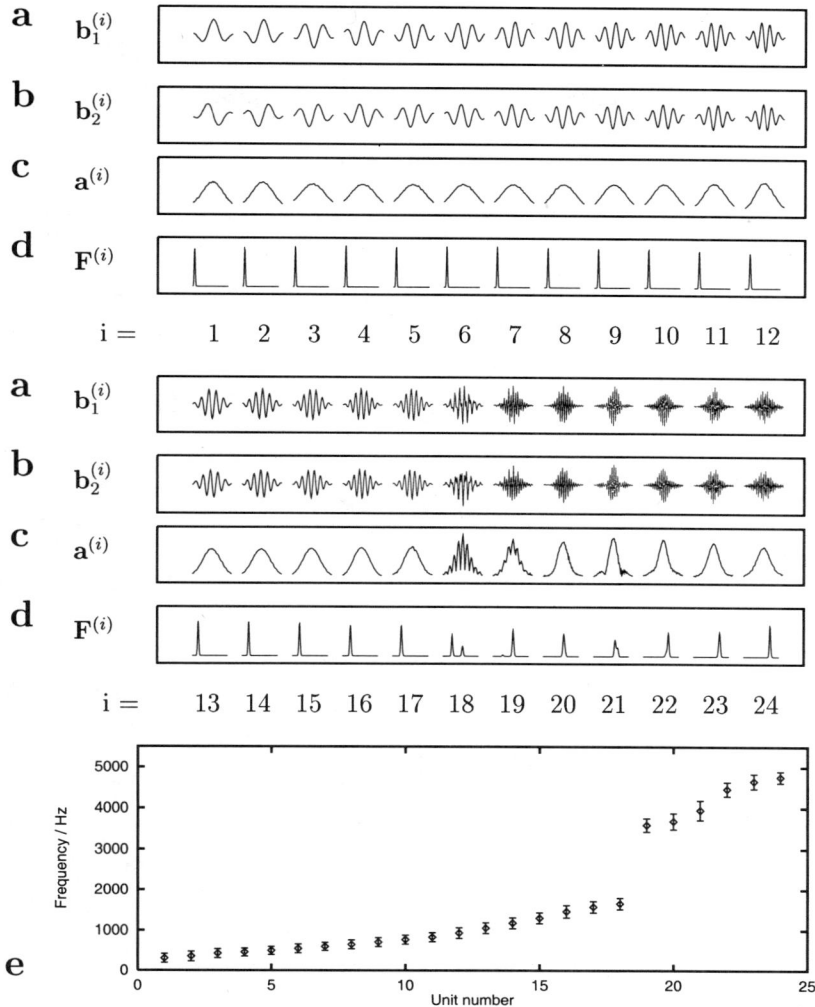

Figure 6: Results after a longer learning process: The tentative results turned out to be unstable in the long run. Notice that the diagrams a–d are in two parts. (a) The first basis vectors of the ASSOM units ($\mathbf{b}_1^{(i)}$). (b) The second basis vectors ($\mathbf{b}_2^{(i)}$). (c) $a_j^{(i)} = (b_{1j}^{(i)})^2 + (b_{2j}^{(i)})^2$, where $\mathbf{b}_1^{(i)} = [b_{1,1}^{(i)}, \ldots, b_{1,64}^{(i)}]^T$, etc. (d) The response of the units to different frequencies, $F_j^{(i)} = (f_{1j}^{(i)})^2 + (f_{2j}^{(i)})^2$, where $\mathbf{f}_1^{(i)}$ and $\mathbf{f}_2^{(i)}$ are the Fourier transforms of the $\mathbf{b}_1^{(i)}$ and $\mathbf{b}_2^{(i)}$, respectively. (e) The dominant frequencies of the units. The bars indicate the FWHM of the frequency responses $\mathbf{F}^{(i)}$.

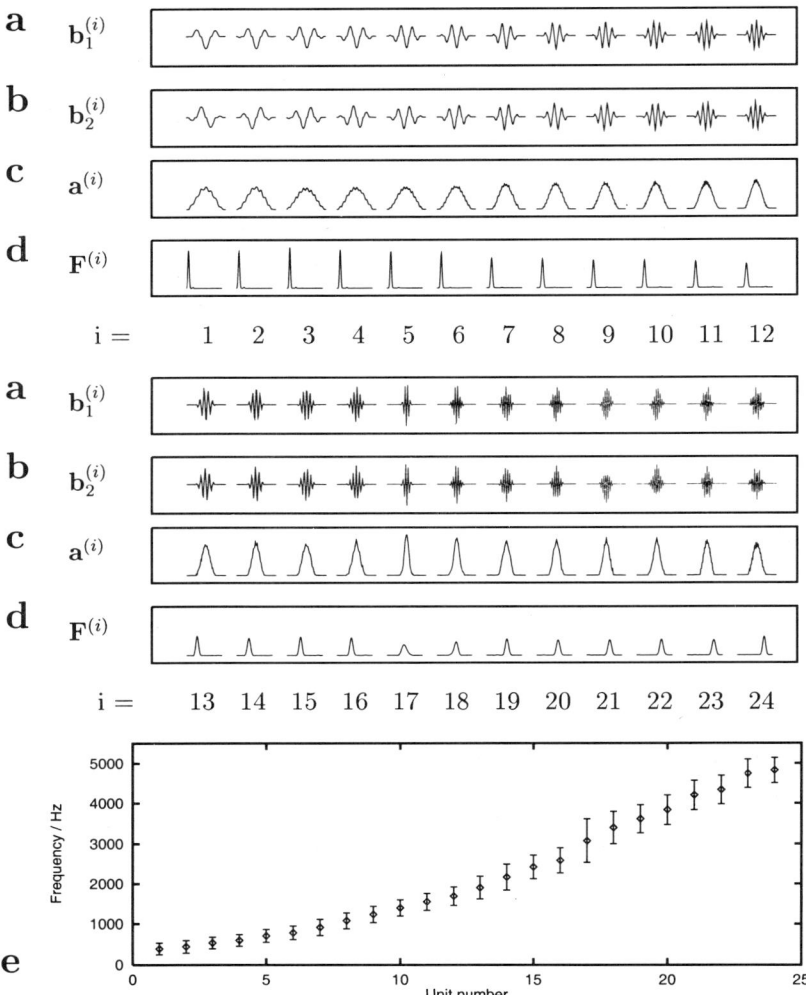

Figure 7: The final results with speech waveforms, when the nonlinear dissipation effect was included. Notice that the diagrams a–d are in two parts. (a) The first basis vectors of the ASSOM units ($\mathbf{b}_1^{(i)}$). (b) The second basis vectors ($\mathbf{b}_2^{(i)}$). (c) $a_j^{(i)} = (b_{1j}^{(i)})^2 + (b_{2j}^{(i)})^2$. (d) The response of the units to different frequencies, $F_j^{(i)} = (f_{1j}^{(i)})^2 + (f_{2j}^{(i)})^2$, where $\mathbf{f}_1^{(i)}$ and $\mathbf{f}_2^{(i)}$ are the Fourier transforms of the $\mathbf{b}_1^{(i)}$ and $\mathbf{b}_2^{(i)}$, respectively. (e) The dominant frequencies of the units. The bars indicate the FWHM of the frequency responses $\mathbf{F}^{(i)}$.

Formation of Invariant-Feature Filters

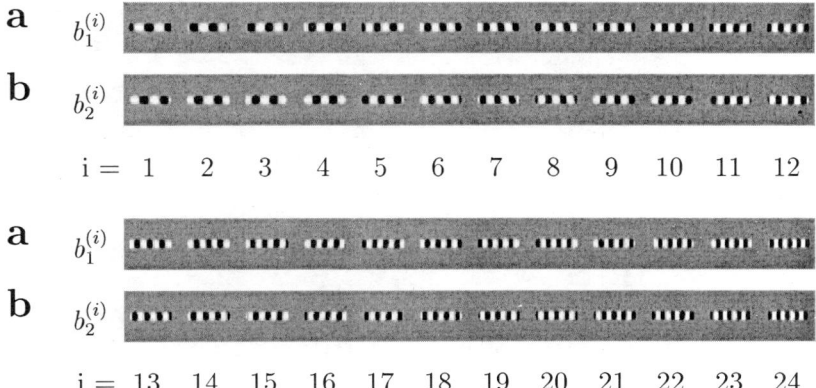

Figure 8: (a) Basis vectors $\mathbf{b}_1^{(i)}$ and (b) basis vectors $\mathbf{b}_2^{(i)}$ of an ASSOM that is invariant to horizontal translations. Notice that the diagrams are in two parts. During learning the FWHM of the vertical gaussian used for weighting the inputs changed from 0.2 to 1.0.

4.3 Formation of Various Invariant Visual-Feature Filters.

The environment—the transforms that modify the inputs—determines what kinds of filters emerge in the learning process. In the previous section, where the input consisted of translated speech signals, the basis vectors developed into wavelet-like templates. In the following experiments, we show that different types of invariant visual-feature filters are learned when the input is translated horizontally, rotated, or scaled. Since the system model was the same all the time and the input samples in all of these experiments consisted of the same type of colored noise, the differences in the resulting filters are totally determined by the characteristics of the transformation type.

A total of $T = 30,000$ episodes, consisting of five transformed sample patterns each, were presented. The value of the dissipation constant δ was 0.0001.

If the inputs are translated randomly in the image plane, in both the horizontal and the vertical directions, basis vectors resembling two dimensional Gabor functions will emerge (Kohonen, 1996). Here we show for comparison that if the translation is mainly restricted to one direction, say horizontal, then the filters will become invariant to movements in that direction. Filters that have emerged when the input was translated horizontally and thereby weighted with a vertical gaussian to eliminate the asymmetries (see section 3.2) are shown in Figure 8. The basis vectors are sinusoidally modulated in the horizontal direction, and the two basis vectors in each unit have a 90-degree phase shift with each other.

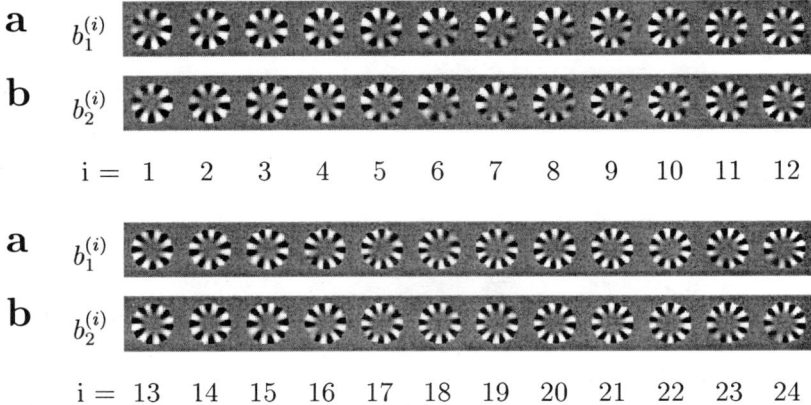

Figure 9: (a) Basis vectors $\mathbf{b}_1^{(i)}$ and (b) basis vectors $\mathbf{b}_2^{(i)}$ of the rotation-invariant ASSOM. Notice that the diagrams are in two parts.

In an environment where differently rotated input patterns are present, sinusoidally modulated basis vectors again emerge. This time the modulation occurs in the azimuthal direction (see Figure 9). The phases of the two basis vectors $\mathbf{b}_1^{(i)}$ and $\mathbf{b}_2^{(i)}$ have a 90-degree phase shift with respect to each other, whereby the responses of the units are invariant to rotation of the inputs.

The ASSOM subspaces can readily represent invariance classes of linear transformations, like rotation and translation. Also, nonlinear transformations can be approximately represented linearly, the better the smaller the amount of transformation. Such linear approximations to a nonlinear operation emerge in the ASSOM when the inputs are scaled with respect to the center of the sampling grid. The basis vectors acquire a sinusoidal modulation in the radial direction outward from the scaling center (see Figure 10). The phases of the two basis vectors in each unit again have a 90-degree phase shift with each other, whereby the responses of the units are invariant to the changing scale of the inputs.

4.4 Competition on Different Transformations. If the input patterns are subjected to several transformation types, each of them active during different episodes, the ASSOM units will also compete on these different transformations. Due to the neighborhood interactions during learning, neighboring units will become invariant to similar transformations, but also areas that are devoted to different transformations will emerge.

To demonstrate the formation of areas specializing to different transformation types, we transformed the input patterns using three different transformation types—horizontal translation, rotation, and scaling—during dif-

Formation of Invariant-Feature Filters

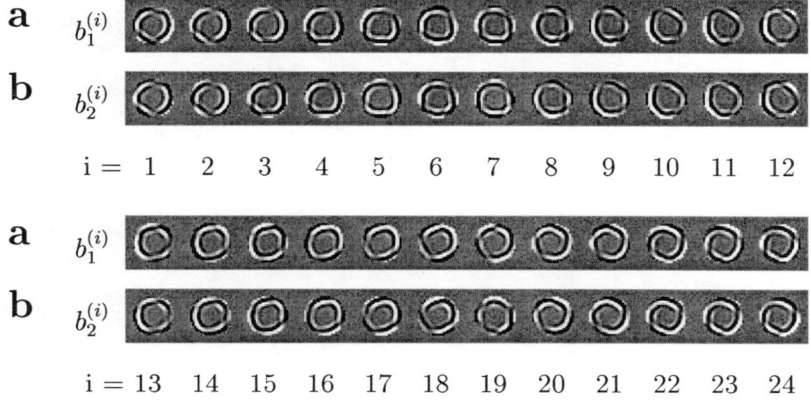

Figure 10: (a) Basis vectors $\mathbf{b}_1^{(i)}$ and (b) basis vectors $\mathbf{b}_2^{(i)}$ of the scale-invariant ASSOM. Notice that the diagrams are in two parts.

ferent episodes. The transformations were defined precisely as in the previous section, except that no gaussian weighting was applied to the inputs. Vertical centering of the templates during horizontal translation was favored by varying the tilt of the pattern with respect to the sampling grid after each translation by a random amount (uniformly distributed between −0.5 and 0.5 radians). The ASSOM lattice consisted of 48 units, and the radius of the neighborhood kernel decreased from 14 units to 1 during learning. Otherwise the learning proceeded exactly as before.

After the learning process, three distinct areas can be discerned in the ASSOM (see Figure 11). The units in the first row have mainly become invariant to scaling, and the units in the last row mainly to rotation. The units in the middle of the ASSOM, especially units 25 to 30, are best described as being invariant to horizontal translations.

5 Discussion

In this article we demonstrated that invariant-feature filters and areas specializing in different transformations can emerge in the ASSOM as a result of Hebbian-type competitive learning. The learning rule was derived by minimizing an error function with the Robbins-Monro stochastic approximation. The objective function describes the average expected error of a random sequence of input samples compared with the corresponding best "neural" representation (subspace of the best-matching processing module).

With the simple nonlinear modifications of the learning rule described in section 3.2, the invariant-feature filters were ordered robustly and reliably

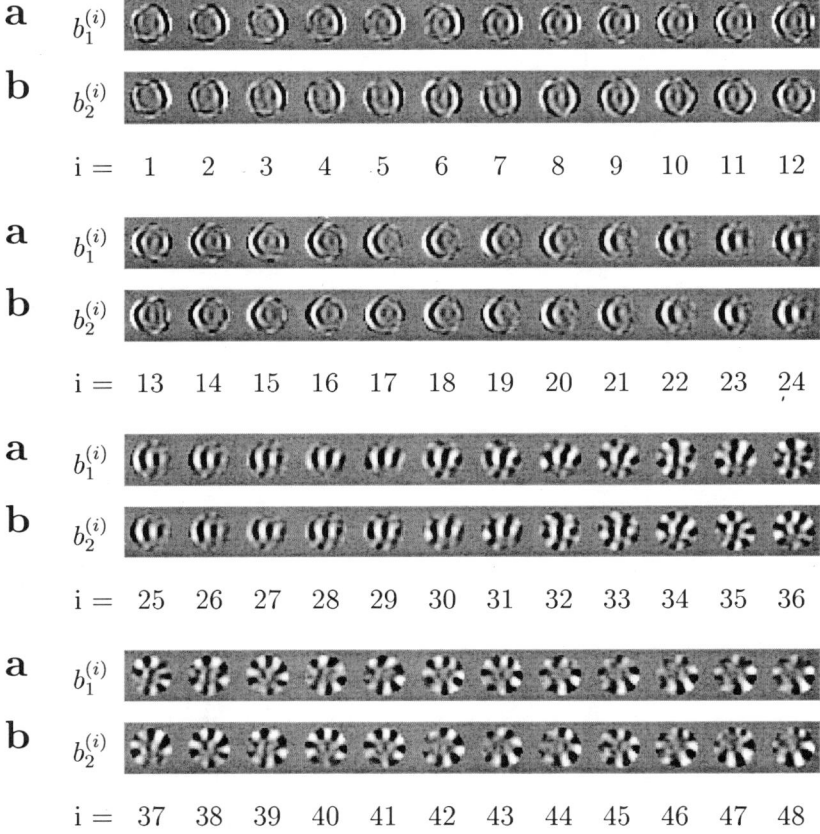

Figure 11: Different areas on an ASSOM have become invariant to different transformations, when the input consisted of horizontally translated, rotated, and scaled patterns. (a) The first basis vectors of the ASSOM units ($\mathbf{b}_1^{(i)}$). (b) The second basis vectors ($\mathbf{b}_2^{(i)}$). Notice that the diagrams are in four parts.

according to the similarity of the transformations. The capability of the network to learn invariant features was demonstrated for both natural speech signals and broadband random images.

Each processing module in the network can be made to become invariant to one transformation type and decode a certain range of features invariantly of this transformation. Different competing modules specialize in representing different kinds of invariant features. The network can thus function as a learning preprocessing stage for invariant-feature extraction.

There were two basis vectors in the neural modules in our experiments.

The resulting two-dimensional subspaces then corresponded to those of the basic wavelet filters. However, there is no restriction on the number of basis vectors in the algorithm, and subspaces of larger dimensions can readily be used to represent more complex features.

An intriguing possibility that the neurons in the ASSOM architecture might have biological counterparts ensues from the forms and operation of the filters in the input and output layers. The receptive fields of the simple cells in the mammalian primary visual cortex have been hypothesized to be describable by Gabor-type functions (Daugman, 1980, 1985; Marcelja, 1980; Jones & Palmer, 1987), and the ASSOM process also produces Gabor-type filters in the first-layer neurons. The output-layer neurons respond invariantly to moving and transforming targets and in this sense resemble the complex cells.

Acknowledgments

We thank Professor Erkki Oja for useful discussions.

References

Albert, A. E., & Gardner, L. A., Jr. (1967). *Stochastic approximation and nonlinear regression*. Cambridge, MA: MIT Press.

Buhmann, J., & Kühnel, H. (1993). Vector quantization with complexity costs. *IEEE Trans. Information Theory* 39:1133–1145.

Cichocki, A., & Unbehauen, R. (1993). *Neural networks for optimization and signal processing*. New York: Wiley.

Daubechies, I. (1990). The wavelet transform, time-frequency localization and signal analysis. *IEEE Trans. Information Theory* 36:961–1005.

Daugman, J. (1980). Two-dimensional spectral analysis of cortical receptive field profiles. *Vision Res.* 20:847–856.

Daugman, J. (1985). Uncertainty relation for resolution in space, spatial frequency, and orientation optimized by two-dimensional visual cortical filters. *J. Opt. Soc. Am. A* 2:1160–1169.

Földiák, P. (1991). Learning invariance from transformation sequences. *Neural Comp.* 3:194–200.

Gabor, D. (1946). Theory of communication. *J. IEE* 93:429–457.

Gersho, A. (1979). Asymptotically optimal block quantization. *IEEE Trans. Information Theory* 25:373–380.

Gray, R. M. (April, 1984). Vector quantization. *IEEE ASSP Magazine*, pp. 4–29.

Hotelling, H. (1933). Analysis of a complex of statistical variables into principal components. *J. Educat. Psych.* 24:498–520.

Jones, J., & Palmer, L. (1987). An evaluation of the two-dimensional Gabor filter model of simple receptive fields in cat striate cortex. *J. Neurophysiol.* 58:1233–1258.

Kohonen, T. (1982). Self-organized formation of topologically correct feature maps. *Biol. Cybern.* 43:59–69.

Kohonen, T. (1989). *Self-organization and associative memory* (3rd ed.). Berlin: Springer-Verlag.

Kohonen, T. (1991). Self-organizing maps: Optimization approaches. In T. Kohonen, K. Mäkisara, O. Simula, & J. Kangas (Eds.), *Artificial Neural Networks* (Vol. 2, pp. 981–990). Amsterdam: North-Holland.

Kohonen, T. (1995a). The adaptive-subspace SOM (ASSOM) and its use for the implementation of invariant feature detection. In F. Fogelman-Soulié & P. Gallinari (Eds.), *Proc. ICANN'95, Int. Conf. on Artificial Neural Networks* (Vol. 1, pp. 3–10). Paris: EC2 et Cie.

Kohonen, T. (1995b). Emergence of invariant-feature detectors in self-organization. In M. Palaniswami, Y. Attikiouzel, R. J. Marks II, D. Fogel, and T. Fukuda (Eds.), *Computational Intelligence. A Dynamic System Perspective* (pp. 17–31). New York: IEEE Press.

Kohonen, T. (1995c). *Self-organizing maps.* Berlin: Springer-Verlag.

Kohonen, T. (1996). Emergence of invariant-feature detectors in the adaptive-subspace SOM. *Biol. Cybern.* 75:281–291.

Kushner, H. J., & Clark, D. S. (1978). *Stochastic approximation methods for constrained and unconstrained systems.* New York: Springer-Verlag.

Luttrell, S. P. (1994). A Bayesian analysis of self-organizing maps. *Neural Comp.* 6:767–794.

Makhoul, J., Roucos, S., & Gish, H. (1985). Vector quantization in speech coding. *Proc. IEEE* 73:1551–1588.

Marcelja, S. (1980). Mathematical description of the responses of simple cortical cells. *J. Opt. Soc. Am.* 70:1297–1300.

Oja, E. (1983). *Subspace methods of pattern recognition.* Letchworth, England: Research Studies Press.

Oja, E. (1992). Principal components, minor components, and linear neural networks. *Neural Networks* 5:927–935.

Robbins, H., & Monro, S. (1951). A stochastic approximation method. *Ann. Math. Statist.* 22:400–407.

Rubner, J., & Tavan, P. (1989). A self-organizing network for principal-component analysis. *Europhys. Lett.* 10:693–698.

TIMIT. (1988). CD-ROM prototype version of the DARPA TIMIT acoustic-phonetic speech database.

Wallis, G., Rolls, E., & Földiák, P. (1993). Learning invariant responses to the natural transformations of objects. In *Proc. IJCNN'93, Int. Joint Conf. on Neural Networks, Nagoya* (pp. 1087–1090). Piscataway, NJ: IEEE Service Center.

Wasan, M. T. (1969). *Stochastic approximation.* Cambridge: Cambridge University Press.

Received April 19, 1996; accepted November 1, 1996.

19

Faithful Representation of Separable Distributions

Juan K. Lin
David G. Grier
Department of Physics, University of Chicago, Chicago, IL 60637, U.S.A.

Jack D. Cowan
Department of Mathematics, University of Chicago, Chicago, IL 60637, U.S.A.

A geometric approach to data representation incorporating information-theoretic ideas is presented. The task of finding a faithful representation, where the input distribution is evenly partitioned into regions of equal mass, is addressed. For input consisting of mixtures of statistically independent sources, we treat independent component analysis (ICA) as a computational geometry problem. First, we consider the separation of sources with sharply peaked distribution functions, where the ICA problem becomes that of finding high-density directions in the input distribution. Second, we consider the more general problem for arbitrary input distributions, where ICA is transformed into the task of finding an aligned equipartition. By modifying the Kohonen self-organized feature maps, we arrive at neural networks with local interactions that optimize coding while simultaneously performing source separation. The local nature of our approach results in networks with nonlinear ICA capabilities.

1 Introduction

Barlow, Linsker, Atick, Redlich, and Field have all noted the primary importance of information theory in modeling sensory coding (Barlow, 1989; Linsker, 1989; Atick & Redlich, 1990; Field, 1994). Recently, Bell and Sejnowski (1995a, 1995b) developed an information theory-based algorithm for blind source separation. In this article, a simple synthesis of current research on coding and processing is presented by geometrically incorporating information-theoretic ideas into self-organized feature maps.

Ritter and Schulten (1986) demonstrated that, contrary to intuition, the steady state of Kohonen's self-organized feature maps (SOFM) (Kohonen, 1995) is not one in which the density of neural units is proportional to the input density. In one dimension, they showed that the Kohonen net underrepresents high-density and overrepresents low-density regions. Intuitively, an ideally formed input representation should have the density of the neural (output) units be strictly proportional to the input density. Loosely speaking, this is what is meant by a "faithful representation." Past faithful representation SOFMs of Linsker (1989) and DeSieno (1988) have relied on a form of memory to track the cumulative activity of individual units, which the authors termed "historical information" and "conscience," respectively. Recently, Bauer, Der, and Herrmann (1996) used an adaptive step size to accomplish the task. This article continues along the same path and presents modifications to both the update rule and the partition to allow the SOFM to perform blind signal processing.

Section 2 provides preliminary definitions. Two modifications of the one-dimensional Kohonen SOFM are presented in section 3, which allow for an arbitrary power law relationship between input (data) and output (representation) densities. Section 4 generalizes the faithful representation SOFMs to higher dimensions for independent component analysis. The implications for source separation and optimal coding via the representations are made clear with examples.

2 Preliminaries

We begin with some preliminary definitions and background results. Given an input set $\{\vec{\xi}\}$ with $\vec{\xi}_j$ in the input vector space V, we say that $\{\vec{\xi}\}$ is a separable (input) distribution if it is constructed from nonsingular mixtures of statistically independent scalar sources. So $\{\vec{\xi}\} = \{A\vec{s}\}$, where A is a nonsingular matrix, and the components of $\vec{s}$ are all statistically independent. Thus the joint probability factorizes: $P(\vec{s}) = \prod P_k(s_k)$. By a representation of $\{\vec{\xi}\}$, we mean a collection $\{\Omega(\vec{w})\}$ of regions in V, $\Omega(\vec{w}_i) \subset V$. The unit $\vec{w}_i$ is said to represent ξ_j if $\xi_j \in \Omega(\vec{w}_i)$. A nonoverlapping representation is defined to be one in which the regions are pairwise disjoint: $\Omega(\vec{w}_i) \cap \Omega(\vec{w}_{i'}) = \emptyset$, for all pairs $i \neq i'$ of regions in the representation. A covering is a representation where $V = \cup_i \Omega(\vec{w}_i)$. So the entire input vector space V is represented in a covering, and any element in V is represented by exactly one unit in a nonoverlapping covering (partition). Focusing on nonoverlapping coverings simplifies things because probability is already normalized, $\sum_i P(\vec{w}_i) = 1$. The assignment of probability in overlapping regions does not have to be considered. For a nonoverlapping covering $\{\Omega(w)\}$ of $\{\xi\}$, $P(w|\xi) = P(w, \xi) = 1$ if w represents ξ, and 0 otherwise. The mutual information $H(\xi; W) = H(W) + \sum P(\xi, w) \log P(w|\xi) = H(W)$. This article deals exclusively with nonoverlapping coverings,

Although equipartition is a better mathematical term, to incorporate some intuition into our terminology, we use the term faithful representation for a nonoverlapping covering in which the probability measures of all the regions are equal. Thus, faithful representations evenly partition the input distribution and maximize the mutual information between the input data and the representation. With M units in the faithful representation, the mutual information of the system is $H(\xi; W) = H(W) = \log M$, the capacity of a noiseless channel (Shannon & Weaver, 1949). In the continuum limit, a faithful input representation's local density of units is proportional to the

Separable Distributions

local input density. We now describe two local algorithms for obtaining faithful representations.

3 Modifications of the One-Dimensional SOFM

For simplicity, we start with the one-dimensional case, $V = \Re$. In a locally translationally invariant network with unit positions $\{w\}$ receiving scalar input ξ, the Kohonen update rule is given by

$$\Delta w_i = \kappa \Lambda(i^* - i)(\xi - w_i), \tag{3.1}$$

where the "winning" unit i^* associated with input ξ is

$$i^* = \{i : |w_i - \xi| \leq |w_j - \xi| \; \forall j\}, \tag{3.2}$$

κ is the learning rate, and the local neighborhood function $\Lambda(i^* - i)$ incorporates the network topology. With care taken with respect to the midpoints between adjacent units, the Kohonen net is a dynamical nonoverlapping covering in our terminology. Here w_i gives the position of the "neural" unit and $\Omega(w_i)$ its "receptive field"—defined to be the region in V that it represents. From a set of points $\{w\}$, equation 3.2 partitions V according to the nearest-neighbor Voronoi tessellation (see, e.g., Preparata & Shamos, 1988).

In this learning rule, the change in position of a unit is proportional to its distance to the data point. Units close to the winning unit are dragged along according to the predefined neighborhood function $\Lambda(i^* - i)$, which is taken to be a gaussian with width σ. For a more general update rule, with $\epsilon = i^* - i$, we scale the learning rule as follows:

$$\Delta w_i = \kappa \Lambda(\epsilon)(\xi - w_i)|\xi - w_i|^{n-1}. \tag{3.3}$$

The extra weighting term allows for a variable relation between the input data and output representation densities. Notice the $n = 0$ form discards the distance to the input data and relies only on a sign term. Consequently it is a purely digital update rule, where w_i can only change by discrete values. Pursuing this idea further, we propose a second modification as follows:[1]

$$\Delta w_i = \kappa \Lambda(\epsilon) \cdot sgn(\epsilon) \cdot |w_{i^*} - w_i|^n. \tag{3.4}$$

In order to extend our results to the boundaries, we also complement equation 3.4 with a movement,

$$\Delta w_{i^*} = \sum_i \Delta w_i, \tag{3.5}$$

---

[1] The sign function $sgn(i)$ takes on a value of 1 for $i > 0$, 0 for $i = 0$ and -1 for $i < 0$.

of the winning unit. The position of the input ξ does not directly enter in the $n = 0$ form of this variant. The network responds only according to its partition of the input space.

Following the continuum limit analysis of Ritter and Schulten (1986), to order $O(\epsilon^2)$, the steady-state configuration of both of the above modified SOFMs is (see appendix A)

$$(w(x)')^{-1} \propto [P(w)]^{(\frac{2}{n+2})}, \tag{3.6}$$

where $(w(x)')^{-1} \equiv D(w)$ is the density of the output units. The Kohonen algorithm is comparable to the $n = 1$ case, with the well-known Ritter and Schulten $D(w) \propto P(w)^{2/3}$ result for the steady state in which the network undersamples high-density and oversamples low-density regions. If $-2 < n < 0$, the network oversamples high-density regions, but the most interesting case occurs for $n = 0$ when $D(w) \propto P(w)$. In this case, the network forms a faithful representation of the input distribution.

We performed simple Monte-Carlo simulations demonstrating the power law behavior for both update rules. The results are shown in Figure 1. For the $n = 0$ digital learning rules, the second variant (see equations 3.4 and 3.5) is not very good at untangling folds in the network because the position of the input has been discarded. Numerically, instead of algorithmically imposing a no-folding constraint, we took a shortcut by sorting and relabeling the units periodically. The second learning rule is purely a counting algorithm for achieving the equipartition steady state, so it must rely on the fact that the proper topology has already been formed. The first variant has the advantage of retaining the direction of ξ relative to the network units, necessary for the formation of the proper topology. However, this advantage comes at the cost of losing the pure counting aspect, which is essential for exact equipartition.

Both $n = 0$ faithful representation learning rules are digital. This is interesting from both biological and computational perspectives; with the addition of an inhibitory population, the update rule can be implemented in a network with only binary communication between its elements!

4 Faithful Representation Networks for Independent Component Analysis

4.1 Branch Net for Finding High-Density Regions. Mixtures of sources with sharply peaked distribution functions will contain high-density directions corresponding to the independent component axes. Blind separation can be performed rapidly for this case in a net with one-dimensional branch topology, the conventional Voronoi partition, and the generalization of the

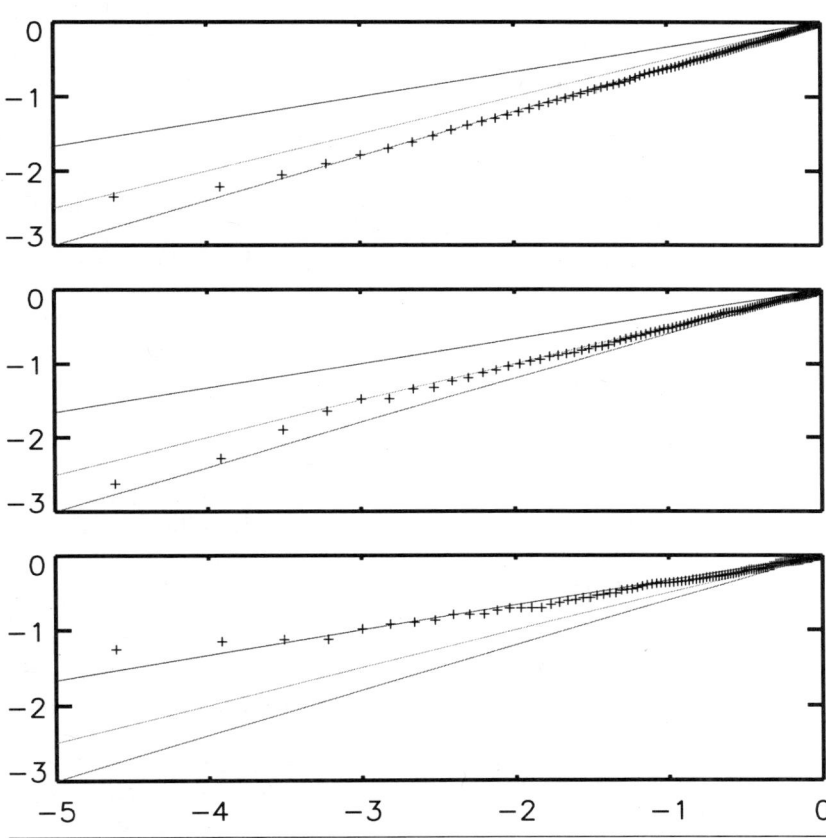

Figure 1: Plot of $\log w(x)$ versus $\log(x)$ for $P(w) \propto w$, showing power law behavior in a network with 100 units. The networks in the top, middle, and bottom plots were trained with $n = 1$, $n = 0$, and $n = -1$ learning rules, respectively. Equations 3.4 and 3.5 were used for $n = 1$ and $n = 0$ simulations; equation 3.3 was used for the $n = -1$ net. The three lines plotted are for $\log(w) \propto (3/5) \log(x)$, $(1/2) \log(x)$, and $(1/3) \log(x)$, corresponding to $D(w) \propto P(w)^{2/3}$, $P(w)$, and $P(w)^2$, respectively. Forty thousand data points were used in the $n = 1$ and $n = 0$ simulations; the units were sorted and relabeled every 5000 data points. For $n = 1$, $\kappa = .005$, $\sigma = 10$ for the first 20,000 points, and $\kappa = .1$, $\sigma = 2$ for the remaining 20,000 points. For $n = 0$, $\kappa = .001$; $\sigma = 10$ for the first 20,000 points, and $\sigma = 5$ for the remaining 20,000 points. For $n = -1$, to reduce the destabilizing effect of the singularity, the $|\xi - w_i|^{-1}$ term was capped at 1000, and the units were sorted every 1000 data points. The learning rate $\kappa = .00002$. For the first 30,000 points, $\sigma = 20$; then it was reduced to $\sigma = 5$ for 10,000 points.

$n = 0$ update rule given in equation 3.3:[2]

$$\Delta \vec{w}_i = \kappa \Lambda(\epsilon) \cdot sgn(\vec{\xi} - \vec{w}_i). \tag{4.1}$$

Numerically, we performed source separation and coding of two mixed signals in a net with the topology of two cross-linked branches (see Figure 2). The elements of the mixing matrix A were chosen randomly with uniform distribution between 1 and -1. The input was first prewhitened following Bell and Sejnowski (1995b) to reduce the amount of dilation and shearing required of the branch net. A typical simulation is shown in Figure 2. As seen in the figure, the branch net rotates very well, and since prewhitening tends to orthogonalize the independent component axes, much of the processing that remains after whitening is rotation to find the independence axes. The net quickly zeroes in on the independent component axes with little annealing. The neighborhood function is taken to be gaussian where ϵ is the distance to the winning unit along the branch structure.

To demonstrate the generality of our approach, we show a faithful representation of a nonlinear mixture. Because our network has local dynamics, with enough units, the network can follow the curved independent component contours of the input distribution. The result is shown in Figure 3. With nonlinear mixtures, however, the transformation must be one-to-one in the region of interest.

To unmix the input, the independent component contours can be found by using parametric least-squares fit to the branch contours. For the source separation in Figure 2, inserting the axes directions into an unmixing matrix W, we find a reduction of the amplitudes of the mixtures to less than 1 percent of the signal.[3] This is typical of the quality of separation obtained in our simulations. Alternatively, taking full advantage of the input representation formed by the net, an approximation of the independent sources can be constructed from the positions in V of the winning unit ($\vec{w}_{i^*}$). Or, as we show in Figure 4 for the nonlinear separation, the cell labels i^* can be used to give a pseudowhitened signal approximation. Since there is only one winning unit along one branch, only one output channel is active at any given time. For sharply peaked source distributions such as speech, this does not hinder the fidelity of the signal approximation much since the input sources hover around zero most of the time. This property also has the potential for utilization in compression. However, for a full, rigorous whitened source representation, we must turn to a network with a topology that matches the dimensionality of the input data.

---

[2] Here the sign function acts componentwise on the vector.

[3] For the separation shown in Figure 2, $WA = \begin{bmatrix} 1 & 0.0068 \\ .0054 & 1 \end{bmatrix}$, where the largest elements of each row have been normalized to one.

Separable Distributions

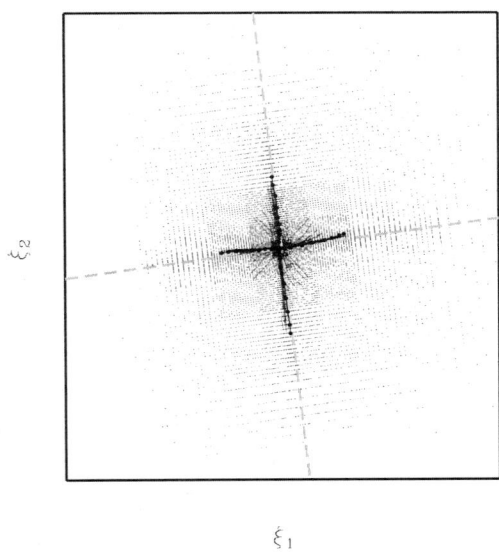

Figure 2: Independent component analysis by a branch architecture network. The two sources are audio files containing spoken Japanese phrases. The input distribution was prewhitened first. The branches initially lie along the $\xi_1 = \xi_2$ and $\xi_1 = -\xi_2$ directions and quickly spiral around to align with the independent component axes (dashed lines). The net is trained on 4000 randomly selected data points. For the annealing, $\kappa = .0007$; $\sigma = 5$ for the first 2000 points and $\sigma = 2$ for the remaining 2000 points. The configuration of the net is shown after every 200 data points, with the final unit positions marked with dots.

4.2 Aligned (M, N) Equipartition Net. The simplest equipartition of a separable distribution is the trivial partition generated from the independent component axes, which decouples the N-dimensional problem into N one-dimensional ones. This partition consists of N distinct hyperplane orientations, with cuts by, say, M parallel hyperplanes along each of the N orientations. We define this to be an (M, N) partition. Thus, the MN hyperplanes partition the input vector space into $(M + 1)^N$ regions. Our goal is to achieve the trivial equipartition using an SOFM with hypercube architecture. Here $M + 1$ is the number of units per dimension in the hypercube. For an (M, N) equipartition, since the number of constraints grows exponentially in N, while the number of degrees of freedom to define the MN hyperplanes grows only quadratically in N, with enough units per dimension

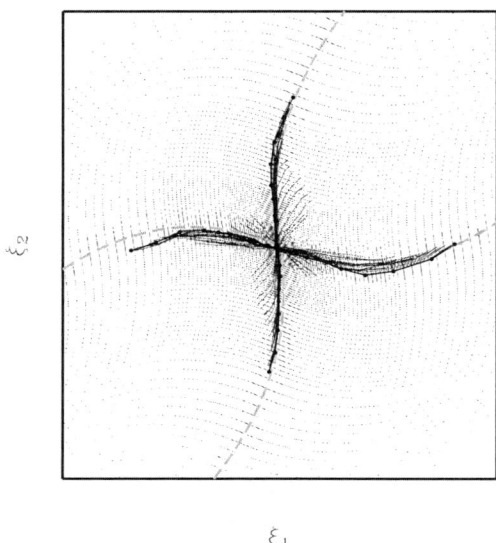

Figure 3: Input representation of a nonlinear mixture. The mixture is given by $\xi_1 = sgn(s_2) \cdot s_2^2 + s_1 - .2s_2$, $\xi_2 = sgn(s_1) \cdot s_1^2 - .4s_1 + s_2$. The network is trained on 6000 data points, with the position of the units shown every 200 data points in the figure. The learning rate $\kappa = .0008$; $\sigma = 5$ for the first 2000 points, $\sigma = 2$ for the next 2000 points, and $\sigma = 1$ for the remaining 2000 points. The independent component contours are drawn in the dashed lines. The units along the branches conform nicely to the statistically independent contours.

in the hypercube, the desired trivial equipartition will be the only (M, N) equipartition. Currently we believe as few as three units per dimension ($M = 2$) suffices for uniqueness. In order to achieve this independent component analysis (ICA) equipartition, the learning rule must be extended to many dimensions, and the definition of the partition needs to be modified.

The second faithful representation learning rule is generalized to multidimensions as follows. With $V = \Re^N$ and $\vec{\epsilon} = \vec{i}^* - \vec{i}$, the learning rule is given by:[4]

$$\Delta \vec{w}_{\vec{i}} = \kappa \Lambda(\vec{\epsilon}) \cdot sgn(\vec{\epsilon}) \qquad (4.2)$$

---

[4] More generally, $\Delta \vec{w}_{\vec{i}} = \kappa \vec{\Gamma}(\vec{\epsilon})$, $\Delta \vec{w}_{\vec{i}^*} = \sum_{\vec{i}} \Delta \vec{w}_{\vec{i}}$, where $\vec{\Gamma}(\vec{\epsilon}) = -\vec{\Gamma}(-\vec{\epsilon})$.

Separable Distributions

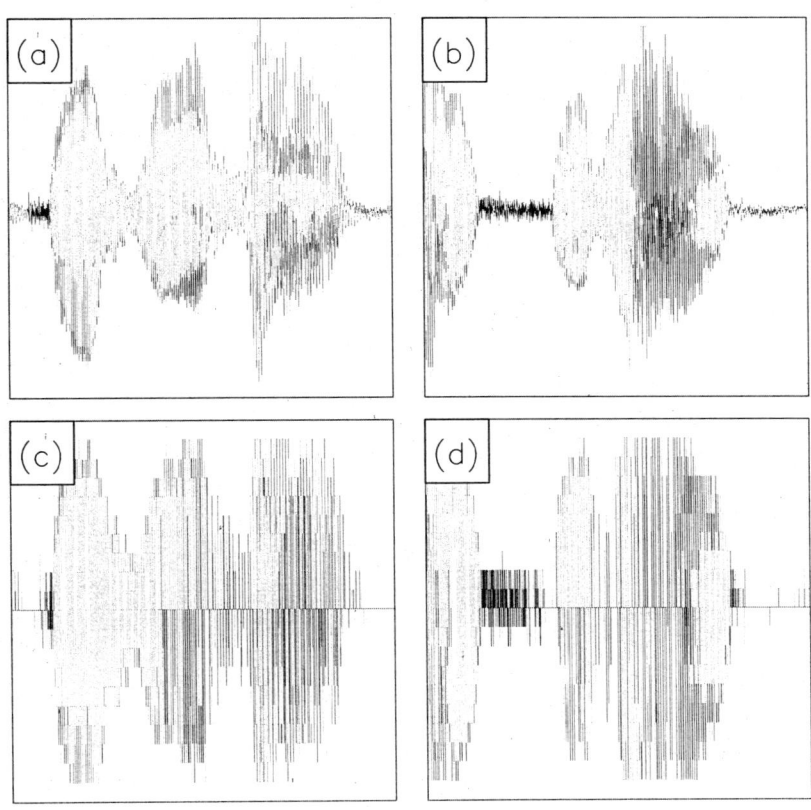

Figure 4: Input representation achieved by the branch net in Figure 3. (a, b) Intensity versus time plots of sections of the two independent input sources (Japanese phrases). (c, d) Winning unit i^* versus time along the corresponding branches of the net.

$$\Delta \vec{w}_{\vec{i}^*} = \sum_{\vec{i}} \Delta \vec{w}_{\vec{i}}, \tag{4.3}$$

where

$$\Lambda(\vec{\epsilon}) = \Lambda(-\vec{\epsilon}). \tag{4.4}$$

Instead of extending the continuum limit analysis for distributions that factorize, we show that a finite discrete network with the dynamics given above has equipartition as a steady state. Let $q_{\vec{i}}$ be the probability measure of unit $\vec{i}$. For the steady state, we require:

$$\begin{aligned}\langle \Delta \vec{w}_{\vec{k}}\rangle &= 0 \\ &= \sum_{\vec{i}} q_{\vec{i}} \cdot \Lambda(\vec{i}-\vec{k}) \cdot sgn(\vec{i}-\vec{k}) + q_{\vec{k}} \sum_{\vec{i}} \Lambda(\vec{k}-\vec{i}) \cdot sgn(\vec{k}-\vec{i}) \\ &= \sum_{\vec{i}} (q_{\vec{i}} - q_{\vec{k}}) \cdot \Lambda(\vec{i}-\vec{k}) \cdot sgn(\vec{i}-\vec{k}),\end{aligned}$$

for all units $\vec{k}$. By inspection, equipartition, where $q_{\vec{i}} = q_{\vec{k}_0}$ for all units $\vec{i}$, is a solution to the equation above. In a two-dimensional rectangular grid network with a range of one for $\Lambda(\vec{e})$ as measured with the city block metric, it can be shown that equipartition is the only steady state of the dynamics (see appendix B). However, it remains to be analyzed more generally the conditions under which this uniqueness property holds.

Although we have shown that the network has a very desirable steady state, our desired ICA equipartition is not a proper Voronoi partition except when the independent component axes are orthogonal. To obtain the ICA aligned equipartition, it is necessary to modify the definition of the winning unit $\vec{i}^*$. Let the input data be given by $\{\vec{\xi}\} = \{A\vec{s}\}$, where $\vec{s}$ is the source vector and A the nonsingular mixing matrix. Let

$$\Omega(\vec{w}_{\vec{i}}) = \{\vec{\xi} \in \Re^N : \vec{i}^* = \vec{i}\} \qquad (4.5)$$

be the winning region of the unit at $\vec{w}_{\vec{i}}$. Since an equipartition invariant to simultaneous linear transformations of the input and representation is desired, we require that

$$\{A\Omega(\vec{w})\} = \{\Omega(A\vec{w})\}, \qquad (4.6)$$

that is, Ω is equivariant under the action of A (see, e.g., Golubitsky, Stewart, & Schaeffer, 1988). This implies that if $\vec{w}$ represents $\vec{\xi}$, then $A\vec{w}$ represents $A\vec{\xi}$.

The Voronoi tessellation resulting from the nearest–neighbor definition of the winning unit (see equation 3.2) satisfies this condition only for rotations and reflections, not nonsingular transformations in general. In two dimensions, we modify the tessellation by dividing up a primitive cell among its constituent units along lines joining the midpoints of the sides. For a primitive cell composed of units at $\vec{a}, \vec{b}, \vec{c}$, and $\vec{d}$, the region of the primitive cell represented by $\vec{a}$ is the simply connected polygon defined by vertices at $\vec{a}$, $(\vec{a}+\vec{b})/2$, $(\vec{a}+\vec{d})/2$, and $(\vec{a}+\vec{b}+\vec{c}+\vec{d})/4$. More generally in N dimensions, the 2^N vertices of the winning polytope region are made up of

$$\binom{N}{j}$$

Separable Distributions

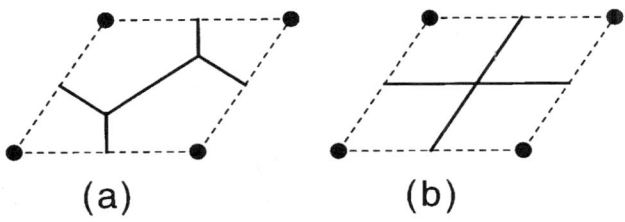

Figure 5: Partition of the primitive cell by the four constituent units. (a) Voronoi partition. (b) Modified equivariant partition.

averages of 2^j unit positions, for all j from 0 to N.[5] The two partitions are contrasted in Figure 5. Our modified partition satisfies equation 4.6 for all nonsingular linear transformations since they are continuous and map polygons to polygons. Note, however, that this partition is valid only for networks with hypercube architecture and defined in the interior of the hypercube. The region outside the hypercube is partitioned by careful extrapolation of the boundary unit partitions.

The learning rule given above was shown to have an equipartition steady state. It remains, however, to align the partitions so that it becomes a valid (M, N) partition. The addition of a local anisotropic coupling that physically, in analogy to elastic nets, might correspond to a bending modulus along the network's axes will tend to align the partitions and enhance convergence to the desired steady state. The algorithmic details are given in appendix C. Numerically, we trained a two-dimensional 9×9 network to represent linear mixtures of two sources faithfully. The result is shown in Figure 6. Using least-squares linear fit to find the independent component axes, the mixture amplitudes are found to be approximately 1 percent of the signal.[6]

Geometrically, the units arrange themselves so that each unit has an equal probability of winning, with the axes of the net aligned with the independent component axes. From a coding perspective, an optimal quantization grid is formed by the network. With the ICA equipartition in place, the components of the winning unit $\vec{i}^*$ give whitened approximations of the independent sources. For compression, given a network with α units, if the elements in

---

[5] Recall $2^N = \sum_{j=0}^{N} \binom{N}{j}$.

[6] The mixing matrix used in Figure 6 is $A = \begin{bmatrix} 0.06 & 0.76 \\ 0.43 & 0.13 \end{bmatrix}$. Using least-squares linear fit for W, we find $WA = \begin{bmatrix} 1 & 0.0041 \\ -0.016 & 1 \end{bmatrix}$.

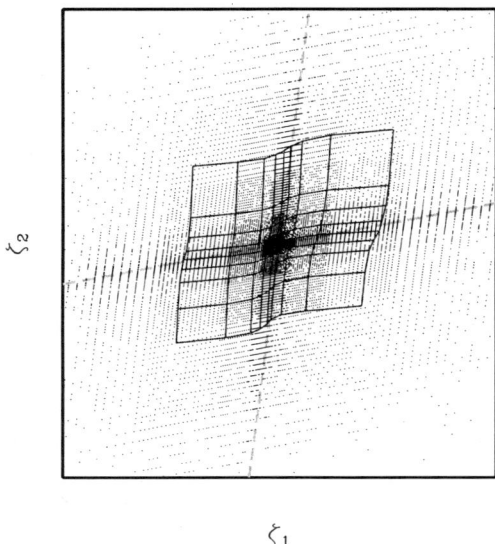

Figure 6: Plot in the $\vec{\xi}$ coordinate frame of the input distribution, independent component axes (dashed lines), and representation formed by the network. The units of the network are located at the grid points of the wire mesh. Initially the units were equally spaced and aligned with the $\hat{\xi}_1$ and $\hat{\xi}_2$ directions. A gaussian with $\sigma = 8$ was used for the neighborhood function $\Lambda(\vec{\epsilon})$, and the learning rate was $\kappa = .00015$. The network is shown after presentation of 4000 randomly chosen points in the input data set. Faithful sampling and alignment of the network along the independent component axes can be seen.

$\{\xi\}$ can be in any one of β states, the compression factor achieved by the net's input representation is $\log \alpha / \log \beta$. This is just the log ratio of the input and representation state-space sizes. If further data compression is desired, the activity of units closer than a threshold need not be differentiated.[7] Often the threshold is set at a characteristic noise or sensitivity level. This practice, standard in the field of wavelet decomposition, can lead to highly compact information coding, especially for sharply peaked input source distributions (see, e.g., Daubechies, 1992; Koornwinder, 1993).

---

[7] Distance as measured in the input vector space V.

5 Discussion

There are a few important differences between the (M, N) equipartition network and past SOFMs. First, the Voronoi partition has been replaced with an equivariant partition specially designed for separable input distributions. Second, in contrast to previous SOFMs, direct dependence on $\vec{\xi}$ and $\vec{w}_i$ has been extracted out. Because the equipartition learning rule (see equations 4.3 and 4.4) is purely in terms of the network's internal architecture ($\vec{e}$), it learns from its own coarse response to stimuli. This is an important aspect of our algorithm, though much work remains to be done on the analysis of these digital learning rules. Also, the question of stability of the steady state, which involves both the digital learning rules and the analog alignment algorithms, needs to be addressed.

The folding problem alluded to earlier is closely tied to this digital counting aspect of our algorithm. For the square blind separation problem where the number of sources is equal to the number of sensors, by starting with a network with no folds and the right topology, the problem can be remedied by the addition of an algorithm that prevents folding. However, a potentially more serious problem arises from the indirectness of defining a partition from the SOFM units. Folds in a network are actually required to define certain partitions by the SOFM units. In practice, this should not pose a serious problem since only a few units per dimension are required for ICA.

For separable input distributions, the (M, N) faithful representation network performs a nonparametric histogram density estimation while separating out statistically independent sources. In contrast to the nonlocal parametric blind separation work of Bell and Sejnowski (1995a, 1995b), this source separation approach is very general in the sense that no a priori assumptions about the individual source probability density distributions are made. They need not be symmetric, sharply peaked, unimodal, or even continuous. Furthermore, because of the local nature of the network, aside from being more robust, nonlinear mixtures of the sources can also be properly represented.

From a coding perspective, intuitively, the most efficient encoding must require an understanding of the input. Arguably, conventional wavelet decompositions encode without processing, since a fixed scaling function ϕ and a derivative mother wavelet ψ are used to encode local mean and detail information, respectively (see, e.g., Daubechies, 1992; Koornwinder, 1993). In neural network terminology, wavelet decomposition is strictly feedforward, while the lateral coupling in our network allows for higher-order processing. Because of the uniqueness of the (M, N) equipartition for separable distributions, faithful representation coding is coupled with blind source separation. In our approach, local coding and processing combine to generate globally optimal coding and processing. In a sense, the units in our network are local independence and activity detectors.

6 Conclusion

The organization principle of maximizing the entropy of a system's response to stimuli ensures that on average there are no overactive or idle units in the network. This demand-based resource allocation principle underlies many of the organizational decisions we make but also provides an organizational basis for coding and processing on a microscopic level. By mixing in elements from statistics, information theory, and self-organized feature maps, we find networks with local dynamics that possess quite general coding and processing capabilities. This approach unifies processing and coding in the sense that the encoding formed is optimized to process previously encountered stimuli. In a network in which the representations are dynamically formed, no distinction is necessary between an early developmental and a late processing stage.

Appendix A: One-Dimensional Continuum Limit Analysis

For the update rule given in equations 3.4 and 3.5, we set the ensemble average $\langle \Delta w \rangle$ to zero and go to the continuum limit with the net parameterized by the continuous variable x. Let $P(\xi)$ be the probability density function of the input, which we take to be differentiable. Taylor expanding about $\epsilon = x^* - x$, and keeping terms of order $O(\epsilon^2)$, we need to solve

$$\langle \Delta w \rangle = 0$$
$$= \int \Lambda(\epsilon) \epsilon |w(x^*) - w(x)|^n P(\xi) d\xi$$
$$\approx \int \Lambda(\epsilon) \epsilon |\epsilon w'|^n \left(1 + \frac{n\epsilon w''}{2w'}\right) (P + \epsilon w' D_w P)(w' + \epsilon w'') d\epsilon,$$

where

$$w' = \left. \frac{dw(x)}{dx} \right|_x,$$

and

$$D_w P = \left. \frac{dP(w(x))}{dw} \right|_{w(x)}.$$

Taking $\Lambda(\epsilon)$ to be an even function, all odd powers of ϵ vanish. The differential equation that remains is:

$$\frac{D_w P \, w'}{P} = -\left(\frac{n+2}{2}\right) \frac{w''}{w'}. \tag{A.1}$$

Its solution is given by

$$(w(x)')^{-1} \propto [P(w)]^{(\frac{2}{n+2})}. \tag{A.2}$$

The calculation for the other learning rule is almost identical and leads to the same result.

Appendix B: Uniqueness of Equipartition Steady State

Here a sketch of the proof is provided for the uniqueness of the equipartition steady state in a two-dimensional rectangular grid network. The range of $\Lambda(\vec{e})$ as measured with the city block metric is one.

The labels for the probability measure of the top two rows of the network are taken to be $q_{(1,1)}, q_{(2,1)}, \ldots, q_{(L,1)}$, and $q_{(1,2)}, q_{(2,2)}, \ldots, q_{(L,2)}$. The steady-state equation for the corner unit at $(1, 1)$ imposes the constraints $q_{(1,2)} - q_{(1,1)} = q_{(2,1)} - q_{(1,1)}$ and $q_{(1,1)} - q_{(2,2)} = q_{(2,1)} - q_{(1,1)}$. Continuing down the row of border units to the other corner unit at $(L, 1)$, the steady-state equations constrain the probability measures of all the units in these two rows to be equal. The equations for the second row units extend the equipartition to the third row. This proceeds until the probability measures of all the units are shown to be equal. Thus, the equipartition steady state is the only steady state of the dynamics.

Appendix C: Alignment Algorithms

Although the exact form of the alignment algorithms is not essential, we describe here some of the simple local algorithms used in our simulations.

First, after each update, the units in the network were moved toward a boxcar convolution of the unit positions. The kernel used was $(1/3, 1/3, 1/3)$ in one dimension and $(1/3, 1/3, 1/3)^t$ in the other dimension. The units were moved a fraction of the distance toward the smoothed positions. For Figure 6, the fraction was set to 0.02. This tends to straighten out the individual rods in the network.

Second, we implemented an algorithm that attempts to make each primitive cell a parallelogram. Unit positions were adjusted to try to equalize the opposing lengths in each primitive cell as follows. In a primitive cell composed of units at $\vec{a}, \vec{b}, \vec{c}$, and $\vec{d}$,

$$\vec{a} \to \vec{a} + \frac{\eta}{2}[(\vec{a} - \vec{d})(-1 + l2/l4) + (\vec{a} - \vec{b})(-1 + l3/l1)],$$

where η is a gain term and $l1, l2, l3, l4$ are the lengths $|\vec{a} - \vec{b}|, |\vec{b} - \vec{c}|, |\vec{c} - \vec{d}|$ and $|\vec{d} - \vec{a}|$. The other three units are also updated accordingly. For Figure 6, η was set to 0.05. This algorithm has the effect of making the individual rods parallel.

Acknowledgments

We thank Trevor Mundel, Alexander Dimitrov, and the anonymous referees for many helpful comments.

References

Atick, J. J., & Redlich, A. N. (1990). Towards a theory of early visual processing. *Neural Comp., 4*, 196–210.

Barlow, H. B. (1989). Unsupervised learning. *Neural Comp., 1*, 295–311.

Bauer, H.-U., Der, R., & Herrmann, M. (1996). Controlling the magnification factor of self-organizing feature maps. *Neural Comp., 8*, 757–771.

Bell, A. J., & Sejnowski, T. J. (1995a). An information-maximization approach to blind separation and blind deconvolution. *Neural Comp., 7*, 1129–1159.

Bell, A. J., & Sejnowski, T. J. (1995b). Fast blind separation based on information theory. In *Proc. 1995 International Symposium on Nonlinear Theory and Applications* (Vol. 1, pp. 43–47). Tokyo: NTA Research Society of IEICE.

Daubechies, I. (1992). *Ten lectures on wavelets*. Philadelphia: SIAM.

DeSieno, D. (1988). Adding a conscience to competitive learning. *IEEE Int. Conf. on Neural Computing, 1*, I117–I124.

Field, D. J. (1994). What is the goal of sensory coding? *Neural Comp., 6*, 559–601.

Golubitsky, M., Stewart, I., & Schaeffer, D. G. (1988). *Singularities and groups in bifurcation theory*. Berlin: Springer-Verlag.

Kohonen, T. (1995). *Self-organizing maps*. Berlin: Springer-Verlag.

Koornwinder, T. (Ed.) (1993). *Wavelets: An elementary treatment of theory and applications*. Singapore: World Scientific.

Linsker, R. (1989). How to generate ordered maps by maximizing the mutual information between input and output signals. *Neural Comp., 1*, 402–411.

Preparata, F. P., & Shamos, M. I. (1988). *Computational geometry: An introduction*. New York: Springer-Verlag.

Ritter, H., & Schulten, K. (1986). On the stationary state of Kohonen's self-organizing sensory mapping. *Biol. Cybern., 54*, 99–106.

Shannon, C. E., & Weaver, W. (1949). *The mathematical theory of communication*. Urbana: University of Illinois Press.

Dynamic Cell Structure Learns Perfectly Topology Preserving Map

Jörg Bruske
Gerald Sommer
*Institut für Informatik und Praktische Mathematik,
Christian-Albrechts-Universität Kiel, Preusserstraße 1-9,
D-24105 Kiel, Germany*

Dynamic cell structures (DCS) represent a family of artificial neural architectures suited both for *unsupervised* and *supervised* learning. They belong to the recently (Martinetz 1994) introduced class of *topology representing networks* (TRN) that build *perfectly topology preserving feature maps*. DCS employ a modified *Kohonen learning rule* in conjunction with *competitive Hebbian learning*. The Kohonen type learning rule serves to adjust the synaptic weight vectors while Hebbian learning establishes a dynamic *lateral connection structure* between the units reflecting the topology of the feature manifold. In case of supervised learning, i.e., function approximation, each neural unit implements a *radial basis function*, and an additional layer of linear output units adjusts according to a *delta-rule*. DCS is the first RBF-based approximation scheme attempting to concurrently learn and utilize a perfectly topology preserving map for improved performance. Simulations on a selection of CMU-Benchmarks indicate that the DCS idea applied to the *growing cell structure* algorithm (Fritzke 1993c) leads to an efficient and elegant algorithm that can beat conventional models on similar tasks.

1 Introduction

Kohonen's self-organizing feature maps (SOM) (Kohonen 1987), besides backpropagation networks, are now the most popular and successful types of artificial neural networks (ANN). This is impressively demonstrated by a constantly growing list of references to SOM-related research and applications available from Helsinki University of Technology containing about 500 entries.[1]

SOMs are used for adaptive vector quantization, clustering, and dimensionality reduction, and can be extended to associative memories

---
[1] Via anonymous FTP from cochlea.hut.fi (130.233.168.48).

like sensorimotor maps simply by adding an output to each neural unit (Ritter *et al.* 1991). Their main features are

- formation of "topology preserving" feature maps, i.e., mapping similar input signals to neighbored neural units (and vice versa) and
- approximation of the input probability distribution, i.e., the number of neural units responding to a certain subset of the input space is proportional to the probability of a stimulus to come from this subspace.

However, it has long been noticed that Kohonen maps have several drawbacks when used for tasks different from visualization of high dimensional data. Mainly these are

1. a fixed number of neural units, making them impractical for applications where the optimal number of units is not known in advance (but only, say, some accuracy parameters),
2. a topology of fixed dimensionality, resulting in problems if this dimensionality does not match the dimensionality of the feature manifold (in this case one cannot claim topology preservation),
3. that classes/clusters have to be separated by hand, whereas an automatic separation is clearly desirable, and
4. unoptimal behavior if, as in the case of sensorimotor maps, one is interested in optimizing the output and not so much in approximating the input density (there may be less interesting regions of high input density but important regions of low input density).

All these problems are topics of ongoing vivid research. In particular, Fritzke's growing cell structures (GCS) (Fritzke 1992, 1993), represent a computationally inexpensive neural algorithm with a variable number of neural units that elegantly combines the merits of RBF networks with an SOM-like topology preserving neighborhood relation between units. A local error measure serves to allocate new units that, since the neighborhood relation between units is known, can be placed in between neighbored units. However, although the topology of GCS is much more flexible than that of the Kohonen map, the problem of fixed topology dimension remains. Further, GCS cause problems when cells are to be deleted.[2]

There have been numerous attempts (e.g., Sebestyen 1962; Hart 1968; Reilly *et al.* 1982; Specht 1990) to realize variable sized clustering and RBF networks (Platt 1991a; Hakala and Eckmiller 1993). In the latter two, units are inserted depending on the overall performance of the net, the center of their receptive field and output being set to the current training input and output. Unlike Kohonen's feature maps these typical RBF networks do not utilize a neighborhood relation between units, nor do

---

[2]This is due to the lateral connection structure between cells, which has to form k-dimensional simplices.

they learn one. We also point out the close relation of all these algorithms to techniques of case based reasoning in symbolic AI and techniques for fuzzy rule generation.

The missing attention to problem (2) turned out to be a problem of missing definition: There has been no rigorous definition of "topology preserving feature mapping" up to the article of Martinetz (1993). A rather intuitive and imprecise notion of "topology preservation" prevailed. Having established this definition Martinetz was able to show that a very simple competitive Hebbian learning rule can learn perfectly topology preserving feature maps if the neural units are "dense." Martinetz (1992) demonstrates that his *neural gas* algorithm enriched by his competitive Hebbian learning rule has the potential to learn perfectly topology preserving mappings. However, the neural gas does not further exploit this information and continues to recompute the k nearest-neighbors of the best matching unit on every presentation of a new stimulus. The very recommendable contribution (Martinetz and Schulten 1994) summarizes these ideas and outlines the relevance of perfect topology preservation for practical applications.

The authors' DCS appear as a natural consequence: Combining the merits of locally tuned processing units with Martinetz's idea of perfectly topology learning we obtain SOM like ANNs that concurrently attempt to learn and utilize a perfectly topology preserving map for an improved training and approximation performance of RBF networks. DCS promise to solve the problem of perfect topology preservation and support automatic cluster separation. Compared to Martinetz's neural gas algorithm, DCS avoid computational burdens by utilizing the lateral connection structure (topology) learned so far.

The particular instance of a DCS algorithm presented in this paper is the *DCS-GCS* algorithm, which rests on Fritzke's GCS. We have chosen GCS because of its increasing popularity and because of encouraging results on a selection of CMU Benchmarks (Fritzke 1993c) to which DCS-GCS can be readily compared. This comparison indicates that DCS-GCS compares well to GCS while beating most conventional algorithms on similar tasks. Unlike GCS, however, DCS-GCS does not use a priori information about the topology of the feature manifold but learns a perfectly topology preserving map and is easier to implement. Similar simulations by Fritzke have confirmed our results (Fritzke, personal communications on ICANN'94).

2 Foundations

In this section we want to recapitulate the definitions and theorems of Martinetz concerning the formation of perfectly topology preserving maps and outline the most important features of Fritzke's GCS. We also indicate how their work is extended and synthesized to GCS-DCS.

2.1 Perfectly Topology Preserving Maps.
In the following, let

- G be a graph (network) with vertices (neural units) i, $1 \leq i \leq N$ and edges (lateral connections) between them weighted by C_{ij}, its adjacency matrix[3] (weight matrix).
- $M \subseteq \Re^D$ be a given manifold of features $v \in M$,
- $S = \{w_1, \ldots, w_N\}$ be a set of pointers (synaptic weight vectors) $w_i \in M$, each of which is attached to a vertex i of G,
- $V_i = \{v \in \Re^D \mid (\|v - w_i\| \leq \|v - w_j\|, 1 \leq j \leq N)\}$ the Voronoi polyhedron belonging to $w_i \in M$, and
- $V_i^{(m)} = V_i \cap M$ the masked Voronoi polyhedron of V_i, $1 \leq i \leq N$.

Definition 1. Two points $w_i, w_j \in S$ are adjacent on M if their masked Voronoi polyhedra $V_i^{(M)}, V_j^{(M)}$ are adjacent (have some boundary points in common), i.e., $V_i^{(M)} \cap V_j^{(M)} \neq \emptyset$.

Definition 2. The graph G forms a perfectly topology preserving map of M, if pointers w_i, w_j, which are adjacent on M, belong to vertices i, j which are adjacent in G ($C_{ij} \neq 0$), and vice versa.

Definition 3. The induced Delaunay triangulation $D_S^{(M)}$ of S, given M, is defined by the graph, which connects two points w_i, w_j iff their masked Voronoi polyhedra $V_i^{(M)}, V_j^{(M)}$ are adjacent, i.e., $(C_{ij} \neq 0) \Leftrightarrow (V_i^{(M)} \cap V_j^{(M)} \neq \emptyset)$.

Definition 4. The set $S = \{w_1, \ldots, w_N\}$ is dense on M if for each $v \in M$ the triangle $\Delta(v, w_{i_0}, w_{i_1})$ formed by the point w_{i_0}, which is closest to v, the point w_{i_1}, which is second closest to v, and v itself lie completely on M, i.e., $\Delta(v, w_{i_0}, w_{i_1}) \subseteq M$ is valid.

We are now able to quote Martinetz's central theorem

Theorem 1 (Martinetz 1993). *If the distribution of pointers $w_i \in S$ is dense on M then the edges (lateral connections) i–j formed by the competitive Hebb rule*

$$\Delta C_{ij} = \begin{cases} y_i \cdot y_j; & y_i \cdot y_j \geq y_k \cdot y_l \, \forall (1 \leq k, l \leq N) \\ 0; & \text{otherwise} \end{cases} \quad (2.1)$$

define a graph (network) G that corresponds to the induced Delaunay triangulation $D_S^{(M)}$ of S and, hence, forms a perfectly topology preserving map of M.

Here, $y_i = R(\|v - w_i\|)$ is the activation of the ith unit with w_i as the center of its receptive field on presentation of stimulus v. The mapping $R(\cdot) : \Re \to [0, 1]$ must be a continuously monotonically decreasing function. Martinetz (1994) coins the term topology representing network (TRN) for networks that use equation 2.1 for topology learning.

---
[3]The adjacency matrix A of a graph G normally is defined by $a_{ij} = 1$ if node i is connected with node j, and $a_{ij} = 0$ otherwise. However, our adjacency matrix C is defined by $0 < c_{ij} \leq 1$ if node i is connected with node j, and $c_{ij} = 0$ otherwise. The c_{ij} may be interpreted as the certainty that i is connected with j.

Of course, when dealing with realistic data from an unknown feature manifold M, we cannot decide whether a given (learned) set $S \subseteq M$ is dense. Instead, only a (possibly small) set of training data $T \subseteq M$ is available, from which a set of points $S(T)$ has to be constructed such that $D_S^{(M)} = D_{S(T)}^{(M)}$ for some dense set $S \subseteq M$. Moreover, we are often interested in smallest dense sets $S \subseteq M$ because these result in the highest data reduction. A third problem arises if the pattern distribution $P(v)$ is not stationary. In this case the neighborhood relation may change with time and thus lateral connections may have to be removed (forgotten): The same problem appears with dynamic data sets S and T.

A straightforward solution to the last problem is to introduce a forgetting constant α, $0 < \alpha < 1$, such that $C_{ij}(t+1) = \alpha C_{ij}(t)$. In DCS we started experiments with the competitive Hebbian learning rule

$$C_{ij}(t+1) = \begin{cases} 1; & y_i \cdot y_j \geq y_k \cdot y_l \; \forall (1 \leq k, l \leq N) \\ 0; & C_{ij}(t) < \theta \\ \alpha C_{ij}(t); & \text{otherwise} \end{cases} \quad (2.2)$$

where θ, $0 < \theta < 1$, serves as a threshold for deleting lateral connections.

For off-line learning with a training set T of fixed size $|T|$,

$$\alpha = \sqrt[|T|]{\theta} \quad (2.3)$$

is likely to be a good choice because once $S(T)$ is dense on M one further epoch of training will yield the induced Delaunay triangulation $D_{S(T)}^{(M)}$. For on-line learning the optimal choice of α will depend on $P(v)$ and the error distribution $P(\Delta v)$ (which most often are unknown). We also conducted experiments with an alternative to equation 2.2, where

$$C_{ij}(t+1) = \begin{cases} \max\{y_i \cdot y_j, C_{ij}(t)\}; & y_i \cdot y_j \geq y_k \cdot y_l \; \forall (1 \leq k, l \leq N) \end{cases} \quad (2.4)$$

Equation 2.4 offers the advantage that the induced connection strength between two units peaks for stimuli lying exactly in between these units. It can be expected to be less sensitive to noise and to perform better if S is not dense. Indeed, best results on the tested Benchmarks have been obtained using equation 2.4.

Martinetz (1992) points out that for reasons of efficiency instead of decreasing all connections one can decrease the connections to the best matching unit only, and that these methods are equivalent if each unit has equal probability of being the best match. Moreover, this method offers an additional advantage for on-line learning situations where equation 2.2 or 2.4 may lead to a total decay of the connection structure in regions of the input space which have not been visited for a longer time.

2.2 Growing Cell Structures and Resources.

In Fritzke's GCS, the network is initialized with a k-dimensional simplex of $N = k + 1$ neural units and $(k+1) \cdot k / 2$ lateral connections (edges). Growing of the network is performed such that after insertion of a new unit the network consists solely of k-dimensional simplices again. Thus, like Kohonen's SOM, GCS can learn a perfectly topology preserving map only if k meets the actual dimension of the feature manifold. Assuming that the lateral connections do reflect the adjacency of units the connections serve to define a neighborhood for a Kohonen-like adaptation of the synaptic vectors w_i and guide the insertion of new units. Insertion happens incrementally and does not necessitate a retraining of the network. The principle is to insert new neurons in such a way that the expected value of a certain local error measure, which Fritzke calls the resource, becomes equal for all neurons. For instance, the number of times a neuron wins the competition, the sum of distances to stimuli for which the neuron wins or the sum of errors in the neuron's output can all serve as a resource and dramatically change the behavior of GCS. Using different error measures and guiding insertion by the lateral connections contributes much to the success of GCS. For more details about GCS the reader is referred to Fritzke (1993c).

DCS-GCS works much like GCS with one essential difference: The topology of the graph G (lateral connection scheme between the neural units) is not of a predefined and fixed dimensionality k but rather is learned on-line (during training) according to 2.4. This not only decreases overhead (Fritzke has to handle sophisticated data structures to maintain the k-dimensional simplex structure after insertion/deletion of units) but offers the possibility of learning real (perfectly) topology preserving feature mappings. Since the isomorphic representation of the topology of the feature manifold M in the lateral connection structure is central to performance, DCS-GCS can be expected to outperform GCS (if k is not constant over M or is not known in advance).

Note that if a DCS algorithm has actually learned a perfectly topology preserving mapping, cluster analysis becomes extremely simple: Clusters that are bounded by regions of $P(v) = 0$ can be identified simply by a connected component analysis. However, without prior knowledge about the feature manifold M it is, in principle, impossible to check for perfect topology preservation or the density of S. Noise in the input data may render perfect topology learning even more difficult. So what can perfect topology learning be used for? The answer is that for every set S of reference vectors perfect topology learning yields maximum topology preservation[4] with respect to this set. So in this sense the learned connection structure C is the best estimate for a topology preserving neighborhood relation if no a priori knowledge of the dimensionality k of M is available. Consequently, this is the case where it should be used for Kohonen-like adaptations of the reference vectors and interpolations between the outputs of neighbored units—the principle of DCS. Con-

---

[4]If topology preservation is measured by the topographic function as defined in Villmann *et al.* (1994).

nected components with respect to C may well serve as an initialization for postprocessing by hierarchical cluster algorithms.

Admittedly, if k is known in advance (a priori knowledge) then SOM-like algorithms that utilize k can be advantageous, especially if training data are sparse.

3 Unsupervised DCS-GCS

In this section we present our algorithm for unsupervised learning DCS-GCS. Simulations serve to illustrate the dynamics.

The unsupervised DCS-GCS algorithm can be obtained from Figure 3, the supervised version, by dropping procedures *calcOutput*(y, v, bmu, σ) and *deltaRule*(y, bmu, u, η) and neglecting the training outputs u. It starts with initializing the network (graph) to two neural units (vertices) $n1$ and $n2$. Their weight vectors w_1, w_1 (centers of receptive fields) are set to points $v_1, v_2 \in M$, which are drawn from M according to $P(v)$ in procedure *getNextExample*(&v, TRAIN). In procedure *enforceConnection*$(n1, n2, 1.0)$ they are connected by a lateral connection of weight $C_{12} = C_{21} = 1$. Note that lateral connections in DCS are always bidirectional and have symmetric weights.

Now the algorithm enters its outer loop, which is repeated until *stoppingCriterion*( ) is fulfilled. This stopping criterion could, for instance, be a test whether the quantization error has already dropped below a predefined accuracy.

The inner loop is repeated λ times. In off-line learning λ can be set to the number of examples in the training set T. In this case, the inner loop just represents an epoch of training.

Within the inner loop, the algorithm first draws an input stimulus $v \in M$ from M according to $P(v)$ by calling *getNextExample*(&v, TRAIN) and then proceeds to calculate the two neural units, which weight vectors are first and second closest to v (by *calcTwoClosest*(&bmu, &$second, v$)].

$$\begin{aligned} \|w_{bmu} - v\| &\leq \|w_i - v\|, \ (1 \leq i \leq N), \\ \|w_{second} - v\| &\leq \|w_i - v\|, \ (1 \leq i \neq bmu \leq N) \end{aligned} \quad (3.1)$$

In the next step, the lateral connections between the neural units are modified according to equation 2.4, a competitive Hebbian learning rule. It is implemented by the procedure *competitiveHebb*$(bmu, second, \alpha, \theta)$. As already mentioned, it is a good idea to set $\alpha = \sqrt[\lambda]{\theta}$ in off-line learning.

Procedure *restrictedKohonen*$(bmu, v, \varepsilon_B, \varepsilon_N)$ adjusts the weight vectors w_i of the best matching unit and its neighbors in a Kohonen-like fashion:

$$\begin{aligned} \Delta w_{bmu} &= \varepsilon_B(v - w_{bmu}) \quad \text{and} \\ \Delta w_j &= \varepsilon_{Nh}(v - w_j), (k = bmu) \land [j \in Nh(bmu)] \end{aligned} \quad (3.2)$$

where the neighborhood $Nh(j)$ of a unit j is defined by

$$Nh(j) = \{i \mid (C_{ji} \neq 0, 1 \leq i \leq N)\} \tag{3.3}$$

The inner loop ends with updating the resource value of the best matching unit. The resource of a neuron is a local error measure attached to each neural unit. As pointed out in Section 2.2, one can choose alternative update functions corresponding to different error measures. For our experiments (Section 3.1) we used the accumulated squared distance to the stimulus, i.e., $\Delta \tau_{bmu} = \|v - w_{bmu}\|^2$.

The outer loop now proceeds by adding a new neural unit r to the network (*addNewNeuron*( )). This unit is located in between the unit l with largest resource value and its neighbor n with second largest resource value.[5]

$$\begin{aligned} \tau_l &\geq \tau_i, & (1 \leq i \leq N) \quad \text{and} \\ \tau_n &\geq \tau_i, & [1 \leq i \neq l \leq N, n \in Nh(l)] \end{aligned} \tag{3.4}$$

The exact location of its center of receptive field w_r is calculated according to the ratio of the resource values τ_l, τ_n, and the resource values of units n and l are redistributed among $r, n,$ and l:

$$\begin{aligned} \gamma &= \tau_n/(\tau_n + \tau_l), & \Delta \tau_l &= \frac{1}{2}(1 - \gamma)\tau_l \quad \text{and} \quad \Delta \tau_n = \frac{1}{2}\gamma \tau_n \tag{3.5} \\ w_r &= w_l + \gamma(w_n - w_l), & \tau_r &= \Delta \tau_n + \Delta \tau_l, \tau_l = \tau_l - \Delta \tau_l, \text{ and} \\ \tau_n &= \tau_n - \Delta \tau_n \end{aligned} \tag{3.6}$$

This gives an estimate of the resource values if the new unit had been in the network from the start. Finally the lateral connections are changed:

$$C_{rl} = C_{lr} = 1, \qquad C_{nr} = C_{rn} = 1 \text{ and } C_{nl} = C_{ln} = 0 \tag{3.7}$$

connecting unit r to unit l and disconnecting n and l.

This heuristic guided by the emerging lateral connection structure and the resource values promises insertion of new units at good initial positions. It is responsible for the better performance of DCS-GCS compared to algorithms that do not exploit the neighborhood relation between existing units.

---

[5]Fritzke inserts new units at a slightly different location, using not the neighbor with second largest resource but the most distant neighbor.

The outer loop closes by decrementing the resource values of all units [in procedure *decrement-ResourceValues(β)*]:

$$\tau_i(t+1) = \beta \tau_i(t), \quad 1 \leq i \leq N \tag{3.8}$$

where $0 < \beta < 1$ is a constant. This last step just avoids overflow of the resource variables. For off-line simulations, $\beta = 0$ is the natural choice.

3.1 Unsupervised Simulation Results. Before turning to the results of two simulations of unsupervised DCS-GCS on artificial data, we want to draw the reader's attention to the kind of data preprocessing necessary to obtain satisfying results with GCS and DCS-GCS. First, due to the insertion strategy, GCS like networks have difficulties unfolding if the starting units are very close to each other. Maximally distant data points are best suited for initialization. Second, because learning constants are usually high and will not be "frozen," the algorithms are very sensitive to the order of data presentation. Therefore, we strongly recommend choosing a random order presentation to prevent erratic oscillations.

In our first example, the training set T consists of 2000 examples drawn from $[0, 100] \times [0, 100] \subset \Re^2$ according to

$$P(v) = \begin{cases} 1/4; & v \in [10, 40] \times [10, 40] \\ 1/4; & v \in [60, 90] \times [10, 40] \\ 1/4; & v \in [60, 90] \times [60, 90] \\ 1/4; & v \in \{p \mid (40 \leq p_x = p_y \leq 60)\} \end{cases} \tag{3.9}$$

Thus our feature manifold M consists of three squares, two of them connected by a line. The development of our unsupervised DCS-GCS network is depicted in Figure 1, with the initial situation of only two units shown in the upper left. Examples are represented by small dots, the centers of receptive fields by small circles, and the lateral connections by lines connecting the circles. From left to right the network is examined after 0, 9, and 31 epochs of training (i.e., after insertion of 2, 11, and 33 neural units).

After 31 epochs the network has built a perfectly topology preserving map of M, the lateral connection structure nicely reflecting the shape of M: Where M is two-dimensional the lateral connection structure is two-dimensional, and it is one-dimensional where M is one-dimensional. Note that a connected component analysis could recognize that the upper right square is separated from the rest of M. The parameters for this simulation were $\varepsilon_B = 0.1$, $\varepsilon_N = 0.006$, $\beta = 0$, and $\alpha = \sqrt[|T|]{\theta}$. The accumulated squared distance to stimuli served as the resource.

The quantization error $E_q = \sum_{v \in T} \|v - w_{bmu(v)}\|^2$ dropped from 100% (3 units) to 3% (33 units).

The second simulation deals with the two-spirals benchmark. Data were obtained by running the program "two-spirals" (provided by CMU) with parameters 5 (density) and 6.5 (spiral radius) resulting in a training

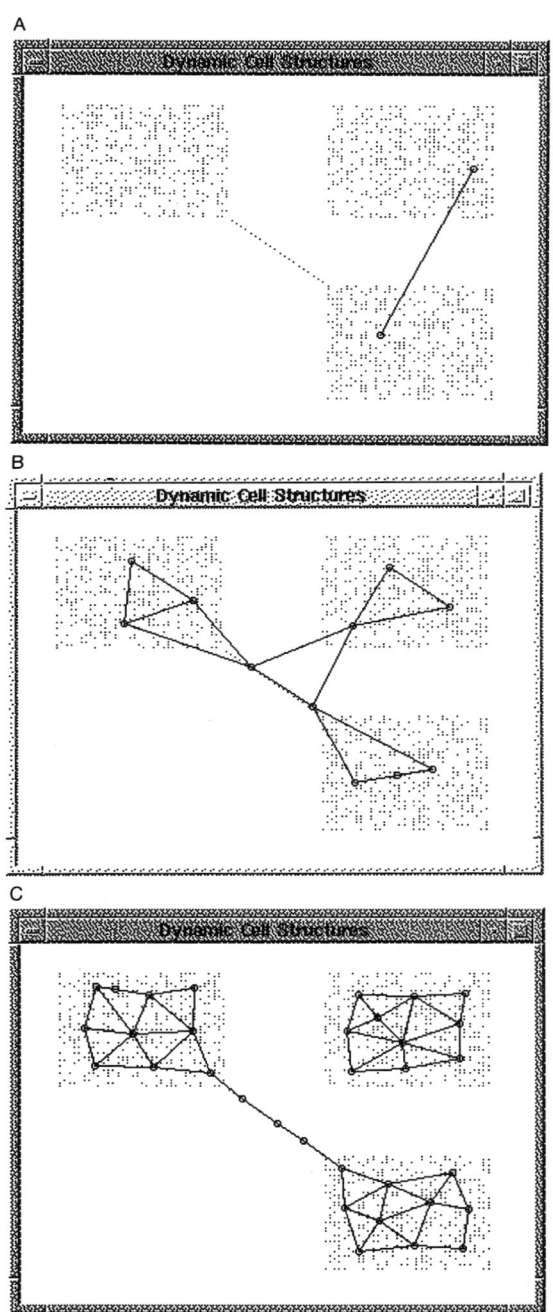

Figure 1: Unsupervised DCS-GCS on artificial data.

DCS Learns Topology Preserving Map

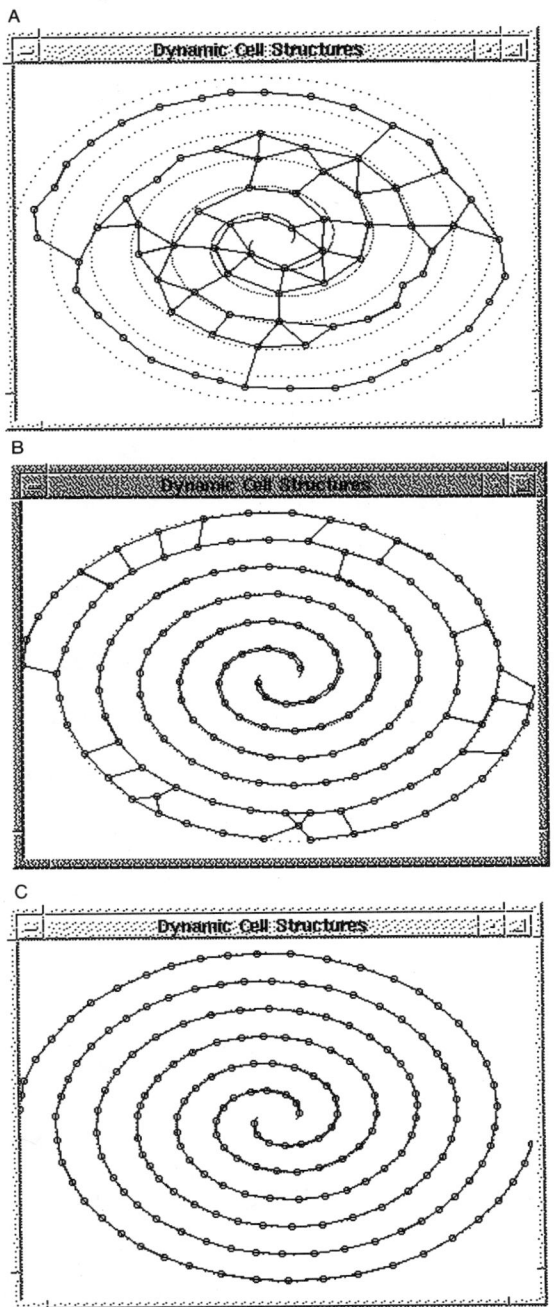

Figure 2: Unsupervised learning of two spirals.

```
void DCS-GCSalgorithm()
{ float $\varepsilon_B$, $\varepsilon_N$, $\eta$, $\alpha$, $\beta$, $\sigma$, $\theta$;
  InputVector v;
  OutputVector u, y;
  neuronP n1, n2, bmu, second;

  getNextExample(&v,&u,TRAIN);
  n1 = insertNewNeuron(v, u);
  getNextExample(&v,&u,TRAIN);
  n2 = insertNewNeuron(v, u);
  enforceConnection(n1, n2, 1.0);
  do{
    for ( $\lambda$ times){
      getNextExample(&v, &u, TRAIN,);
      calculateTwoClosest(&bmu, &second, v);
      competitiveHebb(bmu, second, $\alpha$, $\theta$);
      restrictedKohonen(bmu, v, $\varepsilon_B$, $\varepsilon_N$);
      calculateOutput(y, v, bmu, $\sigma$);
      deltaRule(y, bmu, u, $\eta$);
      updateResource(bmu, v, y, u);
    }
    if (stoppingCriterion())break;
    addNewNeuron();
    decrementResourceValues($\beta$);
  }loop;
}
```

Figure 3: The supervised DCS-GCS algorithm.

set T of 962 examples. The data represent two distinct spirals in the x-y plane. Unsupervised DCS-GCS at work is shown in Figure 2, after insertion of 80, 154, and, finally, 196 units. With 196 units a perfectly topology preserving map of M has emerged, and the two spirals are clearly separated. Note that the algorithm has learned the separation in a totally unsupervised manner, i.e., not using the labels of the data points (which are provided by CMU for supervised learning). Parameters and the type of resource are the same as in the previous simulation.

4 Supervised DCS-GCS

The algorithm for supervised DCS-GCS (see Fig. 3) differs from the unsupervised version in just two lines of code: the calls to procedure *calcOutput*(y, v, bmu, σ) for calculating the output vector y of the network and procedure *deltaRule*(y, bmu, u, η) for adjusting the output vectors o_i, $(1 \leq i \leq N)$ according to the teaching output vector u.

It works very similarly to its unsupervised version except

- when a neuron n_i is inserted by *insertNewNeuron*(v, u) an output vector o_i will be attached to it with $o_i = u$. If it is added by *addNewNeuron*( ) its output vector is initialized by $o_i = o_l + \gamma(o_n - o_l)$

DCS Learns Topology Preserving Map

- the output y of the network is calculated as a weighted sum of the best matching unit's output vector o_{bmu} and the output vectors of its neighbors o_i, $i \in Nh(bmu)$,

$$y = \sum_{i \in \{bmu \cup Nh(bmu)\}} a_i o_i \qquad (3.10)$$

where a_i is the activation of neuron i on stimulus v. We used activation functions

$$a_i = \frac{1}{\sigma \|v - w_i\|^2 + 1} \qquad (3.11)$$

with σ, $\sigma > 0$ representing the size of the receptive fields. In our simulations, the sizes of receptive fields have been equal for all units.

- adaptation of output vectors by $deltaRule(y, bmu, u, \eta)$: A simple delta-rule is employed to adjust the output vectors of the best matching unit and its neighbors:

$$\Delta o_j = \eta a_j (u - y), \qquad j \in bmu \cup Nh(bmu) \qquad (3.12)$$

Most important, the approximation (classification) error can be used for resource updating. This idea of Fritzke leads to insertion of new units in regions where the approximation error is worst, thus promising to outperform algorithms that do not employ such a criterion for insertion. In our simulations we used the accumulated squared distance of calculated and teaching output

$$\Delta \tau_{bmu} = \|y - u\|^2 \qquad (3.13)$$

4.1 Variations on DCS-GCS. In this section we want to discuss some variations on DCS-GCS. While having been tested in our Benchmark simulations but not significantly affecting performance, it may be useful to reconsider them in other applications.

4.1.1 Normalized Radial Basis Functions. Normalized radial basis functions have often been reported to result in better interpolation characteristics. Simply change equations 3.10 and 3.12 accordingly.

4.1.2 Variable Sized and Formed Receptive Fields. In general, one might benefit from variable sized and formed receptive fields instead of fixed σ. Using local covariance matrix estimation, not only the topology of the network but also the form of receptive fields can adapt to the topology of the feature manifold M. However, these modified activation functions can no longer be used for perfect topology learning that has to be done separately.

4.1.3 Error Based Adaptation of Reference Vectors. As stressed by Fritzke, one of the key ideas of GCS is that the distribution of units generally should not depend on the input probability distribution $P(v)$ but should reflect an even distribution of resource values among the units. In GCS, this idea is supported only by the insertion strategy, whereas the Kohonen type adaptation still depends on $P(v)$ only. Thus the larger λ the more the distribution of units will be determined by $P(v)$. A first improvement could be to use the usual stochastic gradient with respect to the output error for updating the weights of the bmu and its topological neighbors. This gradient based adaptation (which is also consistent with the delta rule) would then be responsible for output error minimization, while the insertion process tries to evenly distribute resource values. Alternative ideas for error-weighted adaptation aiming at an even distribution of errors in K-means type algorithms can be found in Chinrungrueng and Sequin (1993).

4.2 Supervised Simulation Results.

We applied our supervised DCS-GCS algorithm to three CMU benchmarks, the supervised two-spiral problem, the speaker independent vowel recognition problem, and the sonar mine/rock separation problem. The first two problems have also been used by Fritzke to test his GCS, so that we have some indication of the performance of DCS-GCS relative to GCS on these problems.

4.2.1 General Method of Simulation. DCS-GCS like any other algorithm using a stochastic gradient (sample by sample) following update rule is sensitive to the order of sample presentation. Moreover, in our simulations the order of sample presentation also determined the two starting units. We therefore repeated our simulations with 20 different random orders of sample presentations[6] and will subsequently report the statistics of these runs. These are e_{min} and n_{min}, the minimal classification error and number of neural units for this error, e_{mean} and n_{mean}, the mean classification error and number of units, and σ_e and σ_n, the standard deviation in classification error and number of units.

The second point that needs to be discussed is the choice of an adequate stopping criterion. Only the two spirals provide a concrete objective: The training error has to be zero. Consequently, this objective together with the (self-imposed) constraint, that the number of units should not exceed the number of training samples, defines the stopping criterion.

Things are different with the vowel recognition and the sonar classification benchmark. Here, one has to be as good as possible but the regulations neither bound classification performance nor number of units. Furthermore, it is well known (Robinson 1989) that the minimum for the training set does not coincide with the minimum for the test set. We

---

[6]Using just 20 successive "seeds" for the random generator used to mix the training sets.

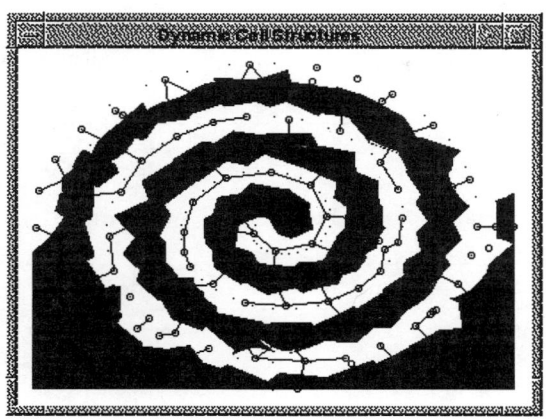

Figure 4: Supervised learning of two spirals.

therefore did not define an explicit stopping criterion but by cross-validation recorded the performance of the network (classification error and number of units) on the test set after each epoch of training. The result of each simulation was then set to the best result thus obtained. A run was terminated if the number of units exceeded the number of training samples.

4.2.2 *The Two Spirals Problem.* Let us first turn to the supervised version of the two-spiral problem already introduced in the previous section. The training set for benchmarking had to be produced by running the "two spirals" program with parameters 1 (density) and 6.5 (radius), producing 194 examples, each consisting of an input vector $v \in \Re^2$ and a binary label indicating to which spiral the point belongs. Obviously the spirals cannot be linearly separated. The task is to train the examples until the learning system can produce the correct output for all of them and to record the time. No test set is provided. While this task is trivial for algorithms doing essentially table-lookup, it is a very hard task for MLPs with sigmoidal activation functions. GCS and DCS-GCS are somewhere in between, using locally tuned units but not directly placing them on data points.

The decision regions learned after 135 epochs of supervised DCS-GCS training are depicted in Figure 4. Black indicates assignment to the first and white assignment to the second spiral. The network and the examples are overlaid. The classification error on the training set (measured in accordance with the CMU regulations) dropped to 0%. Parameters are

Table 1: DCS-GCS Classification Results on Two Spirals Problem.

	Training set performance					Test set performance		
e_{min}	n_{min}	e_{mean}	n_{mean}	σ_e	σ_n	e_{min}	e_{mean}	σ_e
0.0%	135	0.36%	163	0.43%	14	0.7%	1.5%	0.7%

Table 2: Epochs for Supervised Learning of Two Spirals.

Network model	Number of epochs	Reported in
Backpropagation	20000	Lang and Witbrock (1989)
Cross entropy BP	10000	Fahlman and Lebiere (1990)
Cascade-correlation	1700	Fahlman and Lebiere (1990)
GCS	180	Fritzke 1993
DCS-GCS	135	This article

$\varepsilon_B = 0.2$, $\varepsilon_N = 0.012$, $\beta = 0$, $\alpha = \sqrt[|T|]{\theta}$, $\eta = 0.3$, $\sigma = 2.0$, and the accumulated squared output error served for resource updating, $\Delta\tau_{bmu} = \|y-u\|^2$, $y, u \in \{-1, 1\}$. The statistics for this parameter set are presented in Table 1. In 10 of 20 runs the training set performance dropped to zero before utilizing the maximum number of 194 units. Among the other runs, maximally three training samples have been misclassified. The difference in classification reflects the dependency on the order of sample presentation. The performance on the test set is given for reasons of completeness; it is not required by the benchmark.

Supervised spiral learning nicely demonstrates properties of GCS and DCS-GCS: The distribution of units does not reflect the input probability density (which is highest in the center and continuously decreasing toward the periphery) but by trying to equalize resource values is relatively dense at the periphery. This is not surprising, since due to the decreasing probability density classification is most difficult at the periphery. The "unfolding problem" already mentioned in Section 3.1 further contributes to spatially decreasing classification performance (reference vectors at the center have experienced more adaptation steps than those at the periphery). On the other hand, topology preservation is rather bad due to the sparse data.

For comparison we list results obtained by Lang and Witbrok (1989), Fahlman and Lebiere (1990), and Fritzke (1993c) in Table 2.

4.2.3 The Speaker Independent Vowel Recognition Problem. The data for the speaker independent vowel recognition problem comprises a training set of 582 examples and a test set of 462 examples. The input vector is 10-dimensional, $v \in [0, 1]^{10}$, and we used an 11-dimensional output vector

Table 3: DCS-GCS Classification Results on Speaker Independent Vowel Recognition.

	Test set performance					Training set performance		
e_{min}	n_{min}	e_{mean}	n_{mean}	σ_e	σ_n	e_{min}	e_{mean}	σ_e
35%	108	40%	97	2%	32	0.5%	7%	5%

Table 4: Speaker Independent Vowel Recognition.

Classifier	Hidden units	Percent correct
Single layer perceptron		33
Multilayer perceptron	88	51
Modified Kanerva model	528	50
Radial basis function	528	53
Gaussian node network	528	55
Square node network	88	55
Nearest-neighbor		56
3D GCS	158, 165, 154	61, 62, 67
5D GCS	135, 196	66, 66
DCS-GCS	108	65

u with a 1 in the jth position indicating the presence of the jth vowel and -1 in all the other positions. For details about the preprocessing steps yielding these input vectors the interested reader is referred to the thesis of Robinson (1989). With $\varepsilon_B = 0.05$, $\varepsilon_N = 0.006$, $\beta = 0$, $\alpha = \sqrt[|T|]{\theta}$, $\eta = 0.075$, $\sigma = 2.0$ and the same resource as in the previous simulation we obtained a peak performance of 65% correctly classified test samples with 108 neural units. The statistics for this parameter set are presented in Table 3. For comparison, Table 4 shows results obtained by others. The upper part of the table was published by Robinson, reporting final performance figures after about 3000 trials,[7] the lower in Fritzke (1992a), reporting peak performances of some 3D and 5D GCS for particular (unpublished) parameter sets and orders of presentation.

The figures indicate that DCS-GCS beats the conventional methods on this problem with respect to average peak classification performance and qualitatively compares to GCS (peaks above the 60% margin). Since for single simulation runs the fluctuations can easily wipe out any difference between methods, and reporting best results may be considered a questionable method, we do not regard the gap in peak performance between DCS-GCS and GCS as statistically significant. Note that DCS-GCS does

---

[7]Robinson reports a peak performance of about 54% for most models.

Table 5: DCS-GCS Classification Results on Sonar Target Recognition.

Test set performance						Training set performance		
e_{min}	n_{min}	e_{mean}	n_{mean}	σ_e	σ_n	e_{min}	e_{mean}	σ_e
5%	88	8%	85	2%	12	0%	2%	3%

not rely on a prespecified connection structure (but learns it by means of its easy-to-implement competitive Hebb rule).

4.2.4 The Sonar Target Classification Problem. Our last simulation concerns a data set used by Gorman and Sejnowski (1988) in their study on classification of sonar data. The task is to discriminate between sonar signals bounced off a metal cylinder and those bounced off a roughly cylindrical rock. Our input vector is 60-dimensional, $v \in [0,1]^{60}$, and we employ a 2D output vector $u \in \{-1,1\}^2$. The training and the test set contain 104 examples each.

Gorman and Sejnowski (1988) report best results of 90.4% correctly classified test examples for a standard BP network with 12 hidden units and 82.7% for a nearest-neighbor classifier. Supervised DCS-GCS reaches a peak performance of 95% correctly classified test examples after only 88 epochs of training. Parameters were $\varepsilon_B = 0.2$, $\varepsilon_N = 0.006$, $\beta = 0$, $\alpha = |T|/\theta$, $\eta = 0.3$, $\sigma = 0.5$, and the squared output error served as the resource. The statistics for this parameter set are presented in Table 5.

4.3 Complexity of DCS. We restrict our complexity analysis to the time a DCS algorithm needs to process a single stimulus (including response calculation and adaptation).

Here, the main argument in favor of DCS is that the topologically nearest neighbors of the best matching unit can be found in linear time by exploiting the induced Delaunay triangulation. Searching for the best matching unit can obviously be accomplished in linear time,[8] too. Hence, if connection updates (equations 2.2 or 2.4) are restricted to the best matching unit and its neighbors, the serial time complexity for processing a single stimulus is $O(N)$. Yet for planar manifolds it is well known (Preparata and Shamos 1985) that the number of edges of the Delaunay triangulation is $O(N)$, implying linear time complexity even if all connections are updated on each stimulus. The number of edges of the induced Delaunay triangulation also determines the space complexity of DCS. Clearly, $O(N^2)$ is an upper bound (and we are not aware of lower upper bounds except for the planar case).

---

[8]In parallel implementations the best matching unit can be found in constant time, as has been pointed out in Martinetz (1992).

Note that the serial time complexity of the neural gas with k nearest-neighbors is $\Omega(N)$, approaching $O(N \log N)$ for $k \to N$.

5 Conclusion

We introduced the idea of RBF networks that concurrently learn and utilize perfectly topology preserving feature maps for adaptation and interpolation. This family of ANNs, which we termed dynamic cell structures, offers conceptual advantage compared to classical Kohonen-type SOMs since the emerging lateral connection structure maximally preserves topology. We discussed the DCS-GCS algorithm as an instance of DCS. Compared to its ancestor GCS of Fritzke, this algorithm elegantly avoids computational overhead for handling sophisticated data structures. Having linear (serial) worst time complexity, DCS may also be considered as an improvement of Martinetz's neural gas idea. The simulations on CMU-Benchmarks indicate that DCS indeed has practical relevance for classification and approximation.

Thus encouraged, we look forward to applying DCS at various sites in our active computer vision project, including image compression by dynamic vector quantization, sensorimotor maps for the oculomotor system, and hand–eye coordination, cartography, and associative memories.

Acknowledgments

The authors would like to thank their reviewers for numerous hints and for pointing out some earlier works on growing clustering and RBF networks. We also feel indebted to our colleagues, in particular Konstantinos Daniilidis and Josef Pauli, for fruitful discussions and stylistic improvements on this article.

References

Chinrungrueng, Ch., and Sequin, C. H. 1993. Adaptive K-means algorithm with error-weighted deviation measure, *Proc. IJCNN 93* 626–631.

Fahlman, S. E. 1993. *CMU Benchmark Collection for Neural Net Learning Algorithms*. Carnegie Mellon Univ., School of Computer Science, machine-readable data repository, Pittsburgh.

Fahlman, S. E., and Lebiere, C. 1990. The cascade-correlation learning architecture. In *Advances in Neural Information Processing Systems 2*, pp. 524–534. Morgan Kaufmann, San Mateo, CA.

Fritzke, B. 1991. Unsupervised clustering with growing cell structures. *Proc. IJCNN 91* 531–536.

Fritzke, B. 1992. Growing cell structures—a self organizing network in k dimensions. In *Artificial Neural Networks 2*, pp. 1051–1056. North-Holland, Amsterdam.

Fritzke, B. 1993a. Kohonen feature maps and growing cell structures—a performance comparison. In *Advances in NIPS*, Vol. 5, pp. 123–130. Morgan Kaufmann, San Mateo, CA.

Fritzke, B. 1993b. Vector quantization with a growing and splitting elastic net. *Proc. ICANN 93* 580–585.

Fritzke, B. 1993c. *Growing cell structures—a self organizing network for unsupervised and supervised training*. Tech. Rep., tr-93-026, ICSI Berkeley.

Fritzke, B. 1995. Growing cell structures—a self-organizing network for unsupervised and supervised training. *Neural Networks* 7(9), 1441–1460.

Gorman, R. B., and Sejnowski, T. J. 1988. Analysis of hidden units in a layered network trained to classify sonar targets. *Neural Networks* 1, 75–89.

Hakala, J., and Wernteg, H. W. 1992. Node allocation and topographical encoding (NATE) for inverse kinematics of a redundant robot arm. *ICANN'92*, 615–618.

Hakala, J., and Eckmiller, R. 1993. Node allocation and topographical encoding (NATE) for inverse kinematics of a 6-DOF robot arm. *ICANN'93*, 309–312.

Hart, P. E. 1968. The condensed nearest neighbor rule. *IEEE Transact. Inform. Theory* **IT-4**, 515–516.

Kohonen, T. 1987. Adaptive, associative, and self-organizing functions in neural computing. *Appl. Optics* **26**, 4910–4918.

Lang, K. J., and Witbrock, M. J. 1989. Learning to tell two spirals apart. In *Proceedings of the 1988 Connectionist Models Summer School*, pp. 52–59. Morgan Kaufmann, San Mateo, CA.

Martinetz, T. 1992. *Selbstorganisierende neuronale Netzwerke zur Bewegungssteuerung*. Dissertation, DIFKI-Verlag.

Martinetz, T. 1993. Competitive Hebbian learning rule forms perfectly topology preserving maps. *Proc. ICANN 93*, 426–438.

Martinetz, T., and Schulten, K. 1994. Topology representing networks. *Neural Networks* **7**(3), 505–522.

Moody, J., and Darken, C. J. 1989. Fast learning in networks of locally-tuned processing units. *Neural Comp.* **1**(2), 281–294.

Platt, J. 1991a. A resource-allocating network for function interpolation. *Neural Comp.* **2**, 213–225.

Platt, J. 1991b. Learning by combining memorization and gradient descent. *NIPS'91* 714–721.

Preparata, F. P., and Shamos, M. I. 1985. *Computational Geometry—An Introduction*. Springer-Verlag, Berlin.

Reilly, D., Cooper, L., and Elbaum, C. 1982. A neural model for category learning. *Biol. Cybern.* **45**, 35–41.

Ritter, H., Martinetz, T., and Schulten, K. 1991. *Neuronale Netze*. Addison-Wesley, Reading, MA.

Robinson, A. J. 1989. *Dynamic error propagation networks*. Cambridge Univ., Ph.D. thesis.

Sebestyen, G. S. 1962. Pattern recognition by an adaptive process of sample set construction. *IRE Transact. Inform. Theory* **IT-8**, 82–91.

Specht, D. F. 1990. Probabilistic neural networks. *Neural Networks* **3**, 109–118.

Villmann, T., Der, R., and Martinetz, T. 1994. A novel approach to measure the topology preservation of feature maps. *Proc. ICANN 94* 298–301.

21

An Analysis of the Elastic Net Approach to the Traveling Salesman Problem

Richard Durbin*
King's College Research Centre, Cambridge CB2 1ST, England

Richard Szeliski
Artificial Intelligence Center, SRI International, Menlo Park, CA 94025 USA

Alan Yuille
Division of Applied Sciences, Harvard University, Cambridge, MA 02138 USA

This paper analyzes the elastic net approach (Durbin and Willshaw 1987) to the traveling salesman problem of finding the shortest path through a set of cities. The elastic net approach jointly minimizes the length of an arbitrary path in the plane and the distance between the path points and the cities. The tradeoff between these two requirements is controlled by a scale parameter K. A global minimum is found for large K, and is then tracked to a small value. In this paper, we show that (1) in the small K limit the elastic path passes arbitrarily close to all the cities, but that only one path point is attracted to each city, (2) in the large K limit the net lies at the center of the set of cities, and (3) at a critical value of K the energy function bifurcates. We also show that this method can be interpreted in terms of extremizing a probability distribution controlled by K. The minimum at a given K corresponds to the *maximum a posteriori* (**MAP**) Bayesian estimate of the tour under a natural statistical interpretation. The analysis presented in this paper gives us a better understanding of the behavior of the elastic net, allows us to better choose the parameters for the optimization, and suggests how to extend the underlying ideas to other domains.

1 Introduction

The traveling salesman problem (Lawler *et al.* 1985) is a classical problem in combinatorial optimization. The task is to find the shortest possible tour through a set of N cities that passes through each city exactly once. This problem is known to be NP-complete, and it is generally believed

---

*Current address: Department of Psychology, Stanford University, Stanford, CA 94305 USA.

that the computational power needed to solve it grows exponentially with the number of cities. In this paper we analyze a recent parallel analog algorithm based on an elastic net approach (Durbin and Willshaw 1987) that generates good solutions in much less time.

This approach uses a fast heuristic method with a strong geometrical flavor that is based on the tea trader model of neural development (Willshaw and Von der Malsburg 1979). It will work in a space of any dimension, but for simplicity we will assume the two-dimensional plane in this paper. Below we briefly review the algorithm.

Let $\{\mathbf{X}_i\}$, $i = 1$ to N, represent the positions of the N cities. The algorithm manipulates a path of points in the plane, specified by $\{\mathbf{Y}_j\}$, $j = 1$ to M (M larger than N), so that they eventually define a tour (that is, eventually each city $\mathbf{X}_i$ has some path point $\mathbf{Y}_j$ converge to it). The path is updated each time step according to

$$\Delta \mathbf{Y}_j = \alpha \sum_i w_{ij}(\mathbf{X}_i - \mathbf{Y}_j) + \beta K(\mathbf{Y}_{j+1} + \mathbf{Y}_{j-1} - 2\mathbf{Y}_j)$$

where

$$w_{ij} = \frac{e^{-|\mathbf{X}_i - \mathbf{Y}_j|^2/2K^2}}{\sum_k e^{-|\mathbf{X}_i - \mathbf{Y}_k|^2/2K^2}},$$

α and β are constants, and K is the scale parameter. Informally, the α term pulls the path toward the cities, so that for each $\mathbf{X}_i$ there is at least one $\mathbf{Y}_j$ within distance approximately K. The β term pulls neighboring path points toward each other, and hence tries to make the path short. The update equations are integrable, so that $\Delta \mathbf{Y}_j = -K \partial E / \partial \mathbf{Y}_j$ for an "energy" function, E, given by

$$E(\{\mathbf{Y}_j\}, K) = -\alpha K \sum_i \log \sum_j e^{-|\mathbf{X}_i - \mathbf{Y}_j|^2/2K^2} + \beta \sum_j \{\mathbf{Y}_j - \mathbf{Y}_{j+1}\}^2 \quad (1.1)$$

For fixed K the path will converge to a (possibly local) minimum of E. At large values of K the energy function is smoothed and there is only one minimum. At small values of K, the energy function contains many local minima, all of which correspond to possible tours of the cities (we prove this later in the paper), and the deepest minimum is the shortest possible tour. The algorithm proceeds by starting at large K, and gradually reducing K, keeping to a local minimum of E (see Fig. 1). We would like this minimum that is tracked to remain the global minimum as K becomes small. Unfortunately, this can not be guaranteed (see section 3).

The elastic net approach is similar to a number of previously developed algorithms that use elastic matching (Burr 1981), energy-based matching (Terzopoulos et al. 1987), or topographic mapping (Kohonen 1988) to solve vision, speech, and neural development problems. Alternative parallel analog algorithms have also recently been proposed for solving the traveling salesman problem (Hopfield and Tank 1985; Angéniol et al. 1988). The method of Angéniol et al. is closely related

The Elastic Net Approach to the Traveling Salesman Problem

to that discussed here, but is based on Kohonen's self-organization algorithm (Kohonen 1988). It is faster, but for large problems it is marginally less accurate than the elastic method.

An important contribution of this paper is to analyze the behavior of the energy function as the constant K changes and to describe the energy landscape. In particular, we prove results about the behavior of the function for large and small K, confirming the assertions made above about how the algorithm works. First, however, we show that

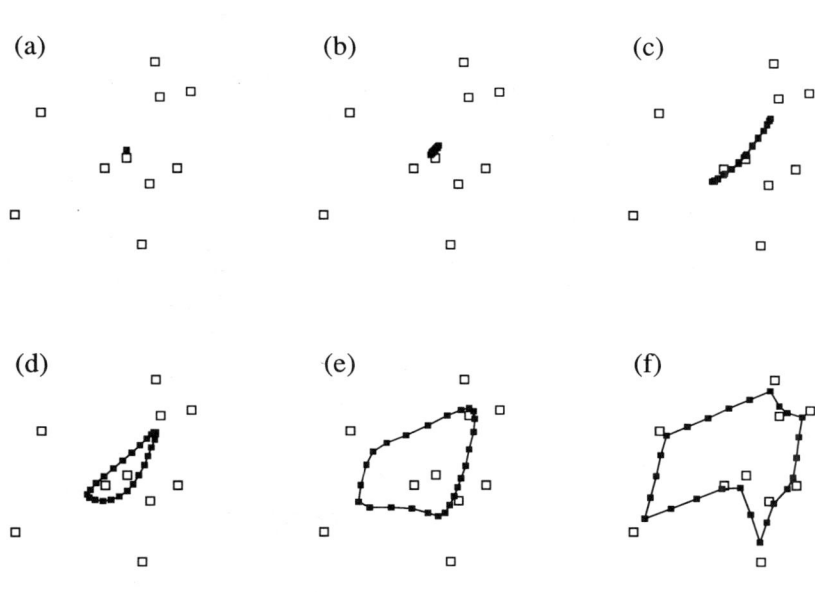

Figure 1: The convergence of the network as a function of K. The white and black squares represent the data (10 cities) and the network (25 path points), respectively. The six figures (a–f) show the configuration found by the network at values $K = 0.261, 0.26, 0.21, 0.20, 0.12, 0.04$. The data set is centered on (0.49, 0.46) and has second-order moments $(K_{xx}, K_{xy}, K_{yy}) = (0.75, -0.23, 0.70)$. We use $\alpha = 0.2$ and $\beta = 1.0$. The first bifurcation, when the origin becomes unstable, can be calculated to occur at $K = 0.2606$ (see Section 5), in agreement with the simulation. The second break temperature is between $K = 0.21$ and $K = 0.20$ for the simulation when the line spreads into a loop. This corresponds well to the point at which the second eigenvalue becomes negative ($K = 0.196$). The correspondence is not exact because nonlinear terms become significant after the first break.

minimizing this cost function can be interpreted in terms of maximizing a probability distribution.

2 The Probabilistic Interpretation

The energy function (1.1) can be related to a probability distribution by exponentiation. This is analogous to use of the Gibbs distribution in statistical mechanics.

$$L(\{\mathbf{Y}_j\}, K) = \frac{1}{(2\pi)^N K^{2N} M^N} e^{-E/\alpha K}$$

$$= \prod_{i=1}^{N} \frac{1}{M} \{\sum_{j=1}^{M} \frac{1}{2\pi K^2} e^{-|\mathbf{X}_i - \mathbf{Y}_j|^2/2K^2}\} \prod_{j=1}^{M} e^{-\frac{\beta}{\alpha K}\{\mathbf{Y}_j - \mathbf{Y}_{j+1}\}^2}$$

Observe that minimizing E with respect to $\{\mathbf{Y}_j\}$ corresponds to maximizing L with respect to $\{\mathbf{Y}_j\}$.

We can interpret L in terms of Bayes' theorem, which states that

$$P(\mathbf{Y}|\mathbf{X}) = \frac{P(\mathbf{X}|\mathbf{Y}) P(\mathbf{Y})}{P(\mathbf{X})} \qquad (2.1)$$

where $P(\mathbf{Y}|\mathbf{X})$ is the probability of a tour ($\mathbf{Y}$) given a set of cities ($\mathbf{X}$). Our algorithm maximizes $P(\mathbf{Y}|\mathbf{X})$ over all possible tours ($\mathbf{Y}$), so the value of $P(\mathbf{X})$ is irrelevant.

The distribution

$$P(\mathbf{Y}) = \prod_{j=1}^{M} e^{-\beta/\alpha K \{\mathbf{Y}_j - \mathbf{Y}_{j+1}\}^2} \qquad (2.2)$$

is the a priori probability of a given tour. This distribution is a correlated gaussian that assigns greater prior probability to shorter tours. The distribution

$$P(\mathbf{X}|\mathbf{Y}) = \prod_{i=1}^{N} \frac{1}{M} \{\sum_{j=1}^{M} \frac{1}{2\pi K^2} e^{-|\mathbf{X}_i - \mathbf{Y}_j|^2/2K^2}\} \qquad (2.3)$$

is the probability of the cities being at ($\mathbf{X}$) given that the tour points are at ($\mathbf{Y}$).

$P(\mathbf{X}|\mathbf{Y})$ is the product of N independent probability distributions

$$P(\mathbf{X}_i|\mathbf{Y}) = \frac{1}{M} \sum_{j=1}^{M} \frac{1}{2\pi K^2} e^{-|\mathbf{X}_i - \mathbf{Y}_j|^2/2K^2}$$

This equation is equivalent to assuming that the measured position of city $\mathbf{X}_i$ was actually derived from one of the tour points in $\{\mathbf{Y}_j\}$ with a two-dimensional gaussian error of variance K^2, but without knowing which tour point $\mathbf{X}_i$ corresponds to. Thus equation 2.1 shows that the elastic net algorithm is computing the most probable tour (finding the

The Elastic Net Approach to the Traveling Salesman Problem

Bayesian MAP estimate) given a prior model (2.2) that favors short tours and a sensor model (2.3) with two-dimensional position uncertainty. Our method thus has an obvious extension to surface interpolation and three-dimensional surface modeling where the correspondence between surface points and measured data points is unknown.

3 Tracking a Minimum

The algorithm devised by Durbin and Willshaw minimizes E at large K and then tracks the minimum energy solution down to small K. At a local minimum (or any extremum), we have

$$\frac{\partial E}{\partial Y_i^\mu} = 0$$

where μ is 1 or 2 and Y_i^1 and Y_i^2 are the x and y components of the position vector $\mathbf{Y}_i$. As we follow the extrema as K changes we get the equation

$$\frac{d}{dK}\left(\frac{\partial E}{\partial Y_i^\mu}\right) = 0$$

which becomes

$$\frac{\partial^2 E}{\partial K \partial Y_i^\mu} + \frac{\partial^2 E}{\partial Y_i^\mu \partial Y_j^\nu}\frac{dY_j^\nu}{dK} = 0$$

To obtain the trajectory we must solve this equation for dY_j^ν/dK. When we are at a true minimum, the Hessian $\partial^2 E/\partial Y_i^\mu \partial Y_j^\nu$ is a positive definite matrix and can be inverted, enabling us to compute dY_j^ν/dK. Bifurcations occur when the Hessian has zero eigenvalues. In this case dY_j^ν/dK is underdetermined and there are several possible solutions.

Computer simulations and our calculations in the large K limit (see below) show that such a bifurcation occurs as the tour initially spreads out from a point. After this, our simulations suggest that the minimum tracks smoothly with K. Other minima of the energy function also appear as K is reduced. For the configuration shown in Figure 1, the number of minima increases rapidly from 1 at $K = 0.12$ to 3 at $K = 0.10$, 9 at $K = 0.08$ (shown in Fig. 2), and very many at $K < 0.05$. The minimum found by tracking K from large to small values is *not* necessarily the optimal (global) minimum (Fig. 2). Nevertheless, empirically the minima found are within a few percent of optimal (Durbin and Willshaw 1987). One possible improvement would be to pick up and track nearby minima by local random perturbation as in simulated annealing (Kirkpatrick et al. 1983).

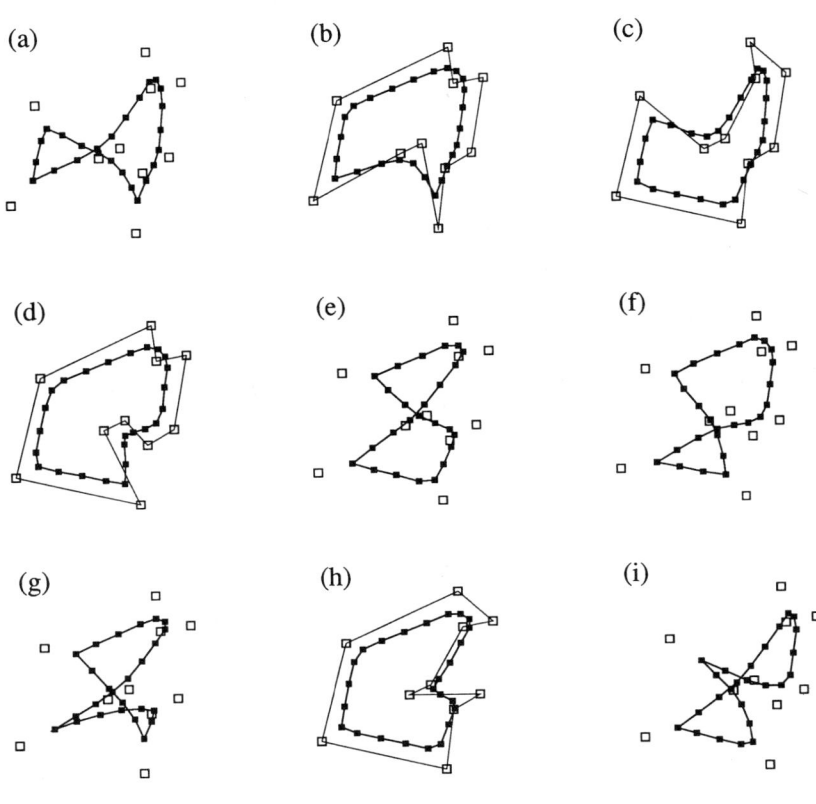

Figure 2: Possible minima of the energy function for the data in Figure 1. To investigate the energy minima we started 1000 simulations at $K = 0.08$ with random initial configurations, hence *without* using the solutions for larger K as initial conditions. In cases that lead to a sensible tour on subsequent slow reduction of K, the lines joining the white boxes (data points) show the tour found by the network. We found nine distinct groups of minima with the following frequencies: (a) 260, (b) 183 (tour length 3.356), (c) 140 (tour length 3.288), (d) 130 (tour length 3.350), (e) 95, (f) 72, (g) 48, (h) 36 (tour length 3.420), and (i) 36. We have probably found all the major forms of minima, since the least frequent happened 36 times. Note that the most frequent pattern (a) is neither the one obtained from tracking K (b) nor the optimal one (c).

4 The Small K Limit

We now consider the behavior of the extrema and the Hessian at these extrema as $K \to 0$. We will show that the only stable extrema occur

The Elastic Net Approach to the Traveling Salesman Problem

when each $\{X_i\}$ has at least one $\{Y_j\}$ arbitrarily close to it. Thus, the extrema all correspond to possible tours.

For any given i let

$$B(K) = \min_j |X_i - Y_j|$$

Then

$$\sum_j e^{-|X_i - Y_j|^2 / 2K^2} \leq M e^{-B^2(K)/2K^2}$$

and

$$-\alpha K \log \sum_j e^{-|X_i - Y_j|^2 / 2K^2} \geq -\alpha K \log M + \frac{B^2(K)\alpha}{2K}$$

Thus, for the energy to be bounded we must have

$$\lim_{K \to 0} \frac{\{B^2(K) - 2K^2 \log M\}\alpha}{2K} = C$$

where C is a constant and hence $B(K) = O(K^{1/2})$.

Thus, in the limit as $K \to 0$, configurations with unmatched Xs will have arbitrarily high energy, and so will not be found by the algorithm. This means that the minima will all correspond to possible tours. Although all the Xs are matched there is no requirement that all the Ys are matched. Indeed, with correct choice of parameters α and β it can be shown that there will be only one tour point at each city. The remaining tour points space themselves evenly in the intercity intervals. A sufficient requirement on the parameters for this to happen is that

$$\frac{\alpha}{\beta} < A$$

where A is the shortest distance from a tour point being attracted to some city to any tour point not being attracted to that city.

To derive this condition on the parameters consider a single city situated at the origin. Define w_j by

$$w_j = \frac{e^{-|Y_j|^2 / 2K^2}}{\sum_k e^{-|Y_k|^2 / 2K^2}}$$

Assume the Y_j are at equilibrium. We wish to consider the stability of an equilibrium in which there are two w_j that stay significantly nonzero as $K \to 0$ (to have a single tour point converge to each city we require instability). We can choose K sufficiently small that there is no significant interaction between these two tour points and any other cities. Consider perturbations $\mathbf{Y}'_j = \mathbf{Y}_j + \varepsilon_j$. We want to find eigenvectors such that

$$\begin{aligned}
\lambda \varepsilon_j &= -K \frac{\partial E}{\partial \mathbf{Y}'_j} \\
&= -\alpha w'_j \mathbf{Y}'_j + \beta K(\mathbf{Y}'_{j+1} + \mathbf{Y}'_{j-1} - 2\mathbf{Y}'_j) \\
&= -\alpha \{w_j \varepsilon_j + \mathbf{Y}_j \sum_k (\frac{\partial w_j}{\partial \mathbf{Y}_k} \cdot \varepsilon_k)\} + \beta K O(\epsilon) + O(\epsilon^2) \\
&= -\alpha \{w_j \varepsilon_j + \sum_k \mathbf{Y}_j \frac{1}{K^2}(w_j w_k \mathbf{Y}_k - \delta_{jk} w_j \mathbf{Y}_j) \cdot \varepsilon_k\} + \beta K O(\epsilon) + O(\epsilon^2) \\
&= -\frac{\alpha w_j}{K^2} \{K^2 \varepsilon_j + \mathbf{Y}_j \sum_k w_k(\mathbf{Y}_k \cdot \varepsilon_k) - \mathbf{Y}_j(\mathbf{Y}_j \cdot \varepsilon_j)\} + \beta K O(\epsilon) + O(\epsilon^2)
\end{aligned}$$

where $\epsilon = \max_j(|\varepsilon_j|)$. In the limit of small K we can ignore the β term as well as the higher order ϵ term. Clearly then for each j $\bar{\varepsilon}_j = \epsilon_j \mathbf{Y}_j$ for some scalar ϵ_j. Let $\mu = -\lambda K^2 / \alpha$, and consider the case where only w_1, w_2 are significant. This leads to the eigenvalue equation

$$\begin{pmatrix} w_1 \left[K^2 - (1 - w_1)Y_1^2\right] - \mu & w_1 w_2 Y_2^2 \\ w_1 w_2 Y_1^2 & w_2 \left[K^2 - (1 - w_2)Y_2^2\right] - \mu \end{pmatrix} \begin{pmatrix} \epsilon_1 \\ \epsilon_2 \end{pmatrix} = 0$$

The criterion for instability is that at least one λ is positive, and hence that the corresponding μ is negative. For large K both eigenvalues μ_1 and μ_2 are clearly positive. Hence for instability we require that K should be below the value at which one eigenvalue (and hence their product) goes negative. The product is

$$\begin{aligned}
\mu_1 \mu_2 &= w_1 w_2 \left[(K^2 - w_2 Y_1^2)(K^2 - w_1 Y_2^2) - w_1 w_2 Y_1 Y_2\right] \\
&= w_1 w_2 K^2 \left[K^2 - (w_2 Y_1^2 + w_1 Y_2^2)\right]
\end{aligned}$$

Therefore we require that

$$K^2 < w_2 Y_1^2 + w_1 Y_2^2$$

Since $w_1 + w_2 = 1$ we will be safe if $\min |\mathbf{Y}_j| > K$. At equilibrium at small K we have $\mathbf{Y}_j = (\beta K / \alpha w_j) \mathbf{A}_j$ where $\mathbf{A}_j = \mathbf{Y}_{j+1} + \mathbf{Y}_{j-1}$. When, as will be usual, $\mathbf{Y}_1$ and $\mathbf{Y}_2$ are neighbors, then $|\mathbf{A}_j|$ is just the distance to the next path point not converging on the city, and a sufficient requirement is that this distance must be greater than α / β.

Since an average tour on N cities has length $(N/2)^{1/2}$ a safe estimate for $A_{\min}$ would be $0.2(N/2)^{1/2}/M$. Alternatively one could choose α to be a decreasing function of K, such as K^p where p is a fixed exponent between zero and one.

5 At Large K

For large K, the energy function (1.1) has a minimum corresponding to the net lying at the center of the cities. At a critical value of K this minimum becomes unstable and the system bifurcates. The initial movement of the net depends only on the second-order moments of the cities.

To show this, we first calculate the first and second derivatives of E with respect to $\mathbf{Y}$.

$$\frac{\partial E}{\partial Y_k^\mu} = \frac{\alpha}{K} \sum_{i=1}^{N} \frac{(Y_k^\mu - X_i^\mu)e^{-|\mathbf{X}_i - \mathbf{Y}_k|^2/2K^2}}{(\sum_{j=1}^{M} e^{-|\mathbf{X}_i - \mathbf{Y}_j|^2/2K^2})}$$
$$+ 2\beta\{2Y_k^\mu - Y_{k+1}^\mu - Y_{k-1}^\mu\} \tag{5.1}$$

$$\frac{\partial^2 E}{\partial Y_k^\mu \partial Y_l^\nu} = \frac{\alpha}{K} \sum_{i=1}^{N} \frac{\delta^{\mu\nu}\delta_{kl}e^{-|\mathbf{X}_i - \mathbf{Y}_k|^2/2K^2}}{(\sum_{j=1}^{M} e^{-|\mathbf{X}_i - \mathbf{Y}_j|^2/2K^2})}$$
$$+ \frac{\alpha}{K^3} \sum_{i=1}^{N} \frac{(Y_k^\mu - X_i^\mu)(Y_l^\nu - X_i^\nu)e^{-|\mathbf{X}_i - \mathbf{Y}_k|^2/2K^2}e^{-|\mathbf{X}_i - \mathbf{Y}_l|^2/2K^2}}{(\sum_{j=1}^{M} e^{-|\mathbf{X}_i - \mathbf{Y}_j|^2/2K^2})^2}$$
$$- \frac{\alpha}{K^3} \sum_{i=1}^{N} \frac{(Y_k^\mu - X_i^\mu)(Y_k^\nu - X_i^\nu)e^{-|\mathbf{X}_i - \mathbf{Y}_k|^2/2K^2}\delta_{kl}}{(\sum_{j=1}^{M} e^{-|\mathbf{X}_i - \mathbf{Y}_j|^2/2K^2})}$$
$$+ 2\beta\delta^{\mu\nu}\{2\delta_{kl} - \delta_{k+1\,l} - \delta_{k-1\,l}\} \tag{5.2}$$

By substituting $\mathbf{Y}_j = 0$ into (5.1) we find that

$$\frac{\partial E}{\partial Y_k^\mu} = \frac{\alpha}{K} \sum_{i=1}^{N} \frac{(-X_i^\mu)e^{-|\mathbf{X}_i|^2/2K^2}}{(\sum_{j=1}^{M} e^{-|\mathbf{X}_i|^2/2K^2})} = -\frac{\alpha}{KM} \sum_{i=1}^{N} X_i^\mu$$

The origin is thus always an extremum, provided that it is chosen at the center of the $\mathbf{X}$s (i.e., $\sum_{i=1}^{N} \mathbf{X}_i = 0$).

To show that the center is a minimum for very large K, we must calculate the eigenvalues of the Hessian. As K decreases, this minimum becomes unstable and a bifurcation occurs. Knowing the value of K at which this occurs will give us a useful starting value for K when we are running the elastic net algorithm. At the origin the Hessian can be written as

$$\frac{\partial^2 E}{\partial Y_k^\mu \partial Y_l^\nu} = \frac{\alpha N}{MK} \delta^{\mu\nu}\delta_{kl} + \frac{\alpha}{K^3 M^2} \sum_{i=1}^{N} X_i^\mu X_i^\nu$$
$$- \frac{\alpha}{K^3 M} \delta_{kl} \sum_{i=1}^{N} X_i^\mu X_i^\nu + 2\beta\delta^{\mu\nu}\{2\delta_{kl} - \delta_{k+1\,l} - \delta_{k-1\,l}\} \tag{5.3}$$

For large K, the eigenvalues of the Hessian are clearly all positive. By inspection of equation 2, we see that throughout the region $|\mathbf{Y}_j| \ll K$ the Hessian is positive definite and so the origin is a unique minimum. For small K, the dominant terms (the second and third terms on the right-hand side of 5.2) have negative trace, so there are some negative eigenvalues. Thus, the origin is a stable state for large K but then becomes unstable as K decreases. To see how this occurs we must explicitly calculate the eigenvectors.

If we compute the eigenvalues of the Hessian (Durbin *et al.* 1989), we find that smallest eigenvalue is

$$\lambda_{\min} = \frac{\alpha N}{KM} - \frac{\alpha \lambda}{K^4 M} + 8\beta \sin^2 \frac{\pi}{M} \tag{5.4}$$

where λ is the principal eigenvalue of the city covariance matrix. The center then becomes unstable and breaks at K s.t. $\lambda_{\min} = 0$. This can be calculated from equation 5.4. Since the eigenvectors depend only on the second-order moments of the distribution of the cities the global minimum for K just below the critical value will also depend chiefly on the second-order moments. As K decreases further the higher order moments will become important. These theoretical results are confirmed by computer simulations (see Fig. 1). The net stays at the origin until the critical value of K and then forms a line along the principal axis of the city distribution. Near the second critical value of K (when the eigenvalue determined by substituting the minor eigenvalue of the city covariance matrix into equation 5.4 becomes negative) the line spreads into a loop.

6 Conclusion

In summary, we have obtained several theoretical results concerning the elastic net method. First, we have shown how the elastic net solution can be interpreted as a *maximum a posteriori* estimate of an unknown tour (circular curve), where some points along the tour have been measured with gaussian uncertainty in position. Second, we have proved that for small K every point $\mathbf{X}_i$ is matched, and that each point must be within $O(K^{1/2})$ of a tour point. Third, we have found a condition on the parameters α, β under which each city becomes matched by only one tour point. Fourth, we have shown that at large K, a single minimum exists for the energy function, with all of the tour points lying at the center of gravity of the cities. Fifth, we have shown how to calculate the bifurcation points for the elastic net as K is reduced.

The first result is particularly interesting since it suggests that this approach can be applied to other interpolation, approximation, and matching problems (such as surface interpolation in computer vision). The important feature here is that we do not need to prespecify which model point matches a data point, allowing "slippery" matching. The second result proves the "correctness" of the elastic net method, in that any final solution must be a valid tour. The third, fourth, and fifth results can be used in selecting parameter values, a starting configuration for the net, and a starting value for K. The elastic net method that we have analyzed provides a simple, effective, and intuitively satisfying algorithm for generating good traveling salesman tours. We believe that similar continuation-based algorithms can be applied to a wide range of optimization and approximation problems.

References

Angéniol, B., de La Croix Vaubois, G., and Le Texier, J.-Y. 1988. Selforganizing feature maps and the travelling salesman problem. *Neural Networks* **1**, 289–293.

Burr, D.J. 1981. Elastic matching of line drawings. *IEEE Trans. Pattern Anal. Machine Intelligence* PAMI-3 **6**, 708–713.

Durbin, R., Szeliski, R., and Yuille, A. 1989. *An Analysis of the Elastic Net Approach to the Travelling Salesman Problem*. Tech. Rep., Harvard University.

Durbin, R., and Willshaw, D.J. 1987. An analogue approach to the travelling salesman problem using an elastic net method. *Nature (London)* **326**, 689–691.

Hopfield, J.J., and Tank, D.W. 1985. Neural computation of decisions in optimization problems. *Biol. Cybernet.* **52**, 141–152.

Lawler, E.L., Lenstra., J.K., Rinooy Khan, A.H.G., and Shmoys, D.B. (eds). 1985. *The Travelling Salesman Problem*. Wiley, New York.

Kirkpatrick, S., Gelatt, C.D., Jr., and Vecchi, M.P. 1983. Optimization by simulated annealing. *Science* **220**, 671–680.

Kohonen, T. 1988. *Self-Organisation and Associative Memory*, 2nd Ed. Springer-Verlag, Berlin.

Terzopoulos, D., Witkin, A., and Kass, M. 1987. Symmetry-seeking models for 3D object recognition. *Proc. First Int. Conf. Computer Vision*, London, June 1987.

Willshaw, D.J., and von der Malsburg, C. 1979. A marker induction mechanism for the establishment of ordered neural mappings: Its application to the retinotectal problem. *Phil. Trans. R. Soc. Ser. B* **287**, 203–243.

22

Sorting with Self-Organizing Maps

Marco Budinich
Dipartimento di Fisica and INFN, Via Valerio 2,
34127 Trieste, Italy

A self-organizing feature map (Von der Malsburg 1973; Kohonen 1984) sorts n real numbers in $O(n)$ time apparently violating the $O(n \log n)$ bound. Detailed analysis shows that the net takes advantage of the uniform distribution of the numbers and, in this case, sorting in $O(n)$ is possible. There are, however, an exponentially small fraction of pathological distributions producing $O(n^2)$ sorting time. It is interesting to observe that standard learning produced a smart sorting algorithm.

Sorting n numbers requires at least $\lceil \log_2 n! \rceil$ comparisons and the "Heapsort" algorithm makes at worst $O(n \log n)$ steps. "Quicksort," faster on average, slows to $O(n^2)$ in the worst case (Knuth 1981; Aho 1974).

The standard Kohonen algorithm can sort: the n numbers to be sorted represent the patterns and there is a string of n neurons. The neurons start from random weights and "adapt" to the distribution of the input patterns during learning.[1] After learning each pattern is mapped onto a neuron and, scanning the neuron string, one gets a sorted list of the patterns.

Tests of a modified learning algorithm ($n \leq 10^5$) show that sorting time is fast and grows like $O(n)$ apparently violating the $\lceil \log_2 n! \rceil$ bound.

Disentangling this curious result is not easy given the stochastic nature of the algorithm so I examined a deterministic procedure carefully derived from it. It is conceivable that the results apply also to the neural net.

The basic idea is to put the n numbers in a histogram with n bins and to scan it: a bin with one number gives immediately its final position; a bin with k numbers iterates the procedure. In summary:

1. find minimum (m) and maximum (M) of the n numbers and save them;
2. put the $n - 2$ numbers in a histogram with n channels evenly distributed in $[m, M]$;

---

[1] Erwin (1992), Ritter (1992), and Csabai (1992) contain exhaustive analysis of learning; Budinich (1995) contains a simpler proof of ordering.

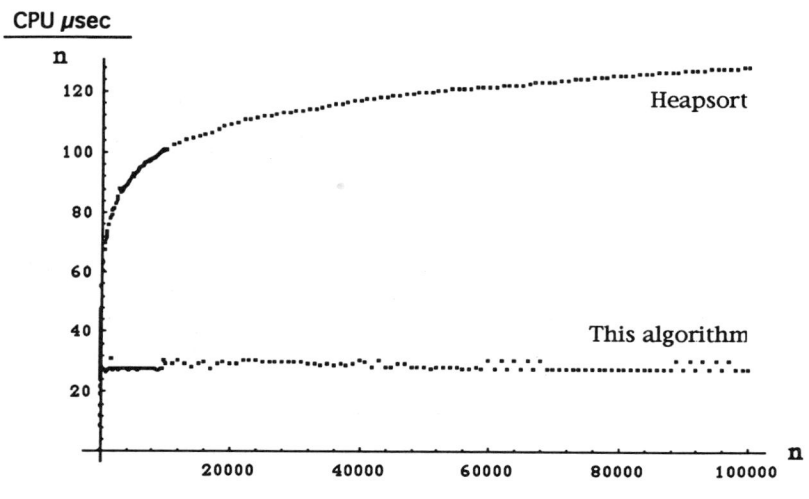

Figure 1: Comparison of unitary sorting time for uniformly distributed numbers.

3. scan the histogram taking the following actions depending on bin content k:

- if $k = 0$ skip the bin;
- if $k = 1$ append the content of the bin to the output list;
- if $k > 1$ recursively call the procedure for k numbers.

A slightly refined version of this algorithm produces the plot showing the sorting time per pattern for n up to 10^5 and for uniformly distributed numbers (Fig. 1). Sorting time is independent of n for this algorithm whereas it has the expected $\log n$ dependence for Heapsort.

Steps 1, 2, and 3 of the algorithm require αn steps after which, at most, βn patterns are still to be sorted: $0 \leq \beta \leq (n-2)/n < 1$ (the worst case has $n - 2$ patterns in one bin). The number of steps $S(n)$ needed to sort is

$$S(n) = \alpha n + S(\beta n) = \alpha n + \alpha \beta n + S(\beta\prime \beta n)$$

with

$$0 \leq \beta\prime \leq \frac{n-4}{n-2} < \beta < 1$$

taking $S(x) = 0$ for $x < 1$:

$$S(n) < \alpha n(1 + \beta + \beta^2 + \beta^3 + \cdots) = \frac{\alpha n}{1 - \beta}$$

With the upper limit for β we obtain an $O(n^2)$ trend whereas any distribution of the patterns giving constant β is sorted in $O(n)$. A combinatorial argument (due to E. Milotti) shows that the fraction of distributions giving at least one bin containing k or more numbers decreases exponentially with k.

This explains how the network algorithm sorts so quickly and it is amazing that learning of a self-organizing net adapts so well to the properties of the pattern distribution. One could argue that it is not so infrequent that nature has clever tricks to solve particular instances of problems that in general are difficult.

References

Aho, A. V., Hopcroft, J. E., and Ullmann, J. D. 1974. *The Design and Analysis of Computer Algorithms*. Addison-Wesley, Reading, MA.

Budinich, M., and Taylor, J. G. 1995. On the ordering conditions for self-organizing maps. *Neural Comp.* **7**(2), 284–289.

Csabai, I., Geszti, T., and Vattay, G. 1992. Criticality in the one-dimensional Kohonen neural map. *Phys. Rev. A* **46**(10), R6181–R6184.

Erwin, E., Obermayer, K. and Schulten, K. 1992. Self organizing maps: Ordering, convergence properties and energy functions. *Biol. Cybernet.* **67**, 47–55.

Knuth, D. E., 1981. *The Art of Computer Programming—Volume III Sorting and Searching*, 2nd ed. Addison-Wesley, Reading, MA.

Kohonen, T. 1984. *Self-Organisation and Associative Memory*. (3rd ed., 1989). Springer-Verlag, Berlin.

Ritter, H., Martinetz, T., and Schulten, K. 1992. *Neural Computation and Self Organizing Maps: An Introduction*, p. 303. Addison-Wesley, New York.

Von der Malsburg, Ch. 1973. Self-organising of orientation sensitive cells in striate cortex. *Kybernetik* **14**, 85–100.

Received January 18, 1994; accepted January 30, 1995.

Index

Note: Page numbers in bold indicate start of chapter. Figures, tables, and notes are designated f, t, and n, respectively.

Active data selection, 340
Adaptive-subspace self-organizing map. *See* ASSOM (adaptive-subspace self-organizing map)
Adelson, E. H., and J. R. Bergen, 150
Adiabatic approximation, 56, 65, 83
Ahmad, I. A., and P. Lin, 322
Alignment algorithms, 383
Amari, S., 55, 56, 58–60, 65
  cortical maps theory, 85
  neural map formation model, 88, 108, 120
Analytic models of map formation, 83
Andersen, P. et al., 156, 185, 186
Andrews, B. W., and D. A. Pollen, 33
Angéniol, B. et al., 408–409
Anisotropic effects on ocular dominance bands, 186, 191–193, 192f, 193f
Anitstropic map patterns, 156, 157f, 170t
Annealing process, 13, 241, 242f, 243f, 320, 411
  in stochastic model, 327, 328, 330–332
Arbitrary sigmoidal transfer function of neurons, 55
Areal geometry, 186. *See also* Geometric approaches; Ocular dominance
Artificial perception, 345. *See also* Cortical feature maps; Neural map formation models; Neurobiological modeling
ASSOM (adaptive-subspace self-organizing map), 345, 346, 358–359, 359f
  competitive learning, 349, 366–367
  formation of invariant feature-filters, 345, 346, 356, 363–367, 364f, 365f
  Gabor transformations, 345, 347, 350, 367
  learning algorithm, 355–356
  learning theory, 349–356
  objective functions, 351–352
  organizing power enhancement, 353–355, 359–360, 360f, 361f, 362f
  orthogonal projection, 347–348
  pattern recognition, 346–348
  transformation class recognition, 365–367
  translated speech signal, 356–357, 357f
  two-dimensional colored noise, 357–358, 358f
  wavelet transforms, 345, 367, 381
Atick, J. J., 20
Atick, J. J., and A. N. Redlick, 19, 20
Auscher, P., 28
Autocorrelation function, 149

Back-propagation learning, 249, 277–278
Barlow, H. B. et al., 369
Barrow, H. G., and H. J. Bray, 214
Barrow, H. G., H. J. Bray, and J. M. L. Budd, **213**
Batch processing of Kohonen algorithm, 311–313
Batch version vs. sequential application of GTM, 308
Bauer, H.-U., **185**
Bauer, H.-U., and B. M. Dow, 156, 163

Bauer, H.-U. et al., 117, 370
Bauer, H.-U., and K. Pawelzik, 194
Baxter, W. T., and B. M. Dow, structural model, 150t, 170t
Bayesian analysis of self-organizing map(s), 249, 270–271. *See also* VQ (vector quantization)
Bayesian probability theory, 39, 41
Bayesian self-organization. *See also* FMC (folded Markov chains); Information maximization model
  driven by prior probabilities distribution, 39, 41–45
  hidden Markov models, 49–50
  information maximization model, 39–41, 40f, 44, 45–47, 46f
  training of probabilistic encoders and, 249, 270–271, 277
Bayesian theories of visual perception, 39, 43–45, 50, 51, 74
Bayes' theorem, 43, 249, 253, 254, 256, 257, 258, 261, 272, 410
Becker, S., and G. E. Hinton, information maximization approach, 39–41, 40f, 42f, 44–47, 46f, 50
Behrmann, K., 117, 118
Bell, A. J., and T. J. Sejnowski, 12, 327, 369, 374, 381
Bienenstock, E., and C. von der Malsburg, 120
  neural mapping model, 85, 102, 109
Binary input-output functions of neurons, 55
Binocular vision, 39, 41–42, 142, 171t
Biological data, compared with color blob formation model, 230–232
Biological modeling. *See* Neurobiological modeling
Bishop, C. M., 295
Bishop, C. M., M. Svensén, and C. K. I. Williams, **291**, **327**. *See also* GTM (generative topographic mapping)

Blakemore, C., and R. C. van Sluyters, 157
Blasdel, G. G., 145f, 148
Blasdel, G. G. et al., 146
Blasdel, G. G. and G. Salama, 143, 148
Blind separation of sources. *See* Separable distributions
Blob formation models
  algorithmic, 108, 109, 110
  color blob formation model, 213, 225–227, 229–232
  probabilistic blob model, 88–90, 118, 119, 121–125
Borg, I., and J. Lingoes, 328
Boundary conditions, 132f, 153, 186
Braitenberg, V., 155
Braitenberg, V., and C. Braitenberg, 151–152, 155
  pinwheel model, 142, 150t, 151, 152f, 164f, 164, 168, 170t
Bruske, J., and G. Sommer, **385**
Budinich, M., **419**
  modified learning algorithm, 419–421, 420f
Buhmann, J. M., and H. Kühnel, 332, 351
Burr, D. J., 408

Cat
  cerebral cortex map, 327, 336–340, 337f, 338f, 339f
  ocular dominance bands in, 185–186
  visual cortex/system, 129, 156, 174, 195, 201, 338
CBL (correlation-based learning) models, 172–173
  Linsker, 150t, 166f, 167–168, 170t, 302
  Miller, 150t, 165f, 166f, 167–168, 170t, 171t, 215
  Miyashita and Tanaka model, 150t, 155, 166f, 167
  ocular dominance and, 173, 201–202
  ON/OFF competition model, 155, 165, 168, 173, 177

Index

simple-cell receptive fields, 201, 203f, 204, 210, 211
   symmetry assumption in, 202
Cell diversity, cortical, 28, 31f, 33, 36
Cells. *See also* LGN (lateral geniculate nuclei); Simple cells
   center surround retinal ganglion cells, 29
   color opponent cells, 30–33, 31f
   retinal/geniculate cells, 216f, 217t, 218f, 218, 224f
Cell structure in topology preserving map(s), 387
Center-surround structures, 3, 12f, 13–16, 15f
   circularly symmetric systems, 5–6, 6t, 8, 10
   energy criterion, 10, 11, 12f, 14t
   in simulations of Hebbian rules, 3, 10–16, 12f, 14t
   time development criterion, 10, 11–12, 12f
Cerebral cortex. *See also* Visual cortex/system
   in the cat (map of), 327, 336–340, 337f, 338f, 339f
Chemical marker–based models, 85
Chernjavsky, A., and J. Moody, 59
Chester, C. R., 60
Circularly symmetric systems. *See* Center-surround structures
Cities, touring. *See* Traveling salesman problem
Clark, J. J., and A. L. Yuille, 40, 44, 51
Cleveland, W. S., and S. J. Delvin, 319
C measure in mapping, 69, 70f, 70–71, 75–79, 76f, 77f, 116
CMF (cortical magnification factor), 55, 62
C neighborhood function, 313–314
Color blob areas, 35n, 35–36, 213–215, 228f
Color blob formation model, 213, 225–227, 229–232. *See also* Color vision

biological data compared with, 230–232
contrast/data variation, 229, 230
difference-of-gaussian processing, 217–218
geniculo-cortical projection in, 220–223, 222–223f
linear analysis, 227–229
luminance variation, 229
outputs, 217t, 218t, 218f, 220f, 220
receptive fields, 223–225, 224f
retinal/geniculate cells, 216f, 217t, 218f, 218, 224f
Color columns, 214
Color opponent cells, 30–33, 31f
Color vision. *See also* Color blob formation model; Probabilistic blob model
   color coding (DC development of), 229, 230
   cortical processing in, 219–221, 220f
   macaque striate cortex data, 144
   precortical processing, 215–218, 216f, 217t
   retino-cortical coding changes, 19, 32, 34f, 34–36, 35n
Combinatorial optimization, 407
Comparison of developmental models, 141
Competitive learning
   ASSOM, 349, 366–367
   Hebbian models, 149, 150t, 151, 153–154, 160, 166f, 170t, 171n, 172–173, 178
Competitive normalization, 85, 114–115
Computational map. *See* Cortical feature maps
Computational power or efficiency, 316, 340, 408, 409. *See also* Minimal wiring
   organizing power enhancement, 353–355, 359–360, 360f, 361f, 362f
Connectivity
   all-to-all models, 119
   from all-to-all to one-to-one, 84, 87–88

Connectivity (cont.)
  lateral in information maximization model, 130, 131
  lateral in neural map formation, 84, 86, 92
  neuronal output layer, 84
  one-to-one, 115
Conservative maps, 168, 170t
Constrained optimization
  introduced by coordinate transformations, 102–103
  in neural map formation, 83, 86–87, 91, 105, 119–121
Constraint function(s)
  functional aspects of term Q, 110–112, 119
  limitation constraint, 113
  neural map formation and, 86–87, 91, 97f, 103, 104t, 105
  penalty functions, 102, 104t
  role of, 203
  weight dynamics and, 96, 104t
Continuity principle, 151
Continuous mapping, 315
Coordinate transformation effects, 94–98, 95f, 99f, 102, 104t, 112–113, 119
Correlation-based learning models. See CBL (correlation-based learning) models
Cortex, early cortical, 21–22, 32, 36. See also Striate cortex; Visual cortex/system
Cortical cell diversity, 28, 31f, 33, 36
Cortical feature maps, 55, 144, 160–161, 208t. See also Visual cortical map models
  dynamic stability, 56
  existence of conditions, 56, 65–66
  formation of, 58–60
  magnification properties, 55, 56, 62, 64–65
  many-to-one mappings, 79–80
  models of, 55–56, 139, 149–151, 150t
  resolution properties, 56, 59, 60–64, 63f
  vector representation, 150, 151, 158–159, 168
  vertical cross-section, 63f
Cortical magnification factor (CMF), 55, 62
Cortical neurons, 19, 56, 205. See also Cells
Cortical processing
  in color vision, 219–221, 220f
  early, 21–22, 32, 36
Cortical response field, 58
Cost function, 69, 80, 249, 291. See also C measure in mapping
Covariance matrix theory, 8–10
Cross-validation methods, 277, 283
Curl free fields, 93, 94
Cytochrome oxidase, 35

Data analysis, unsupervised, 249
Data mining, 340
Data visualization, 78–79, 292, 297–298, 327–328, 369
  geometric approaches, 369, 408
Daubechies, I., 35, 345, 380, 381
Daugman, J. G., 222
DCS (dynamic cell structures). See also GCS (growing cell structures)
  DCS algorithm, 387
  supervised DCS-GCS, 390–391
  unsupervised DCS-GCS, 396–402, 397f
Dempster, A. P. et al., 283, 304, 332
Density network model, 307
DeSieno, D., 370
Developmental process, 173
Diao, Y.-C. et al., 156
Dimension reduction, 235, 236, 240. See also Minimal wiring
  kernel smoothing process and, 315
  minimal wiring and, 235–239, 237f, 238f, 239f, 240
Dynamic link matching, 85, 88, 89, 113–114
Dirac, P. A. M., 94
Dissimilarity values between data items, 328. See also MDS (metric multidimensional scaling)

Index

Diversity principle, 151, 153
Duda, R. O., and P. E. Hart, 328
Durbin, R., and D. J. Willshaw, 72–73, 80, 241, 411
Durbin, R., and G. Mitchison, 72, 75, 76f, 151, 153, 190, 195, 235
 on dimension reduction, 235, 236, 240
Durbin, R., R. Szeliski, and A. Yuille, **407**
Dynamic cell structures. *See* DCS (dynamic cell structures)
Dynamic link matching, 74–75, 105, 116
 neural map formation model, 85, 88, 89, 113–114

Early cortical processing, 21–22, 32, 36
Early visual cortex/system, 83, 214
 Hebbian learning models of, 215, 216f, 219–221, 220f
Eigenvectors analysis in simulations of Hebbian rules, 4–6, 6t, 7f, 14
Elastic matching, 116, 408
Elastic net approach to the traveling salesman problem, 407, 416
 probabilistic interpretation, 410–411
 scale parameter K, 407, 412f, 412–416
 tracking a minimum, 411, 412f
Elastic net model. *See* EN (elastic net) model
Emerson, R. C. et al., 150
EM (expectation-maximization) algorithm, 291, 295–297, 304, 307–308, 327, 330–332, 340. *See also* TMP (topographic mapping of proximity data)
Encoders, training of probabilistic, 249, 270–271, 277
Encoding, nearest neighbor, 251, 252f, 262
EN (elastic net) algorithm, 75, 76f, 76–77, 80, 185, 187, 189, 407
 GTM related to, 306

EN (elastic net) model, 150t, 153–154, 160, 162f, 163, 171t, 173, 178–179. *See also* Elastic net approach to the traveling salesman problem; Mitchison, G.
Energy-based matching, 408
Energy function, 85, 109, 120, 190, 411, 412. *See also* Objective function(s)
Entropy
 entropy maximization, 382
 maximum entropy principle, 327
Equipartition net (ICA), 375–381, 377f, 379f, 383
Ermentrout, G. B., and J. D. Cowan, 90
Erwin, E., and K. D. Miller, 202, 203, 205, 206, 210
Erwin, E., K. Obermayer, and K. Schulten, **141,** 168, 239, 304–305
Excitatory projections, 16
Expectation maximization. *See* EM (expectation-maximization) algorithm

Favardin, N., and V. Vaishampayan, 251
Feature extraction, 346
Feature selectivity, 156–158, 160–161, 171t
 in the macaque striate cortex, 172
Feature spaces, 235
Feature vectors, 150, 151, 158–159, 168
Feedforward activation, 130
Field, D. J., 20, 21f, 23, 28, 33
Filtered noise approach, 172
Filters
 in the early visual system, 21–22
 filter parameters, 153
 formation of invariant feature-filters (ASSOM), 345, 346, 356, 363–367, 364f, 365f
 Gabor filters, 34, 35
 oriented filters, 30–33, 61f
 spatial filters, 150, 213
 whitening filter, 35

Florence, S. L., and J. H. Kaas, 144
Flury, B. A., 317
FMC (folded Markov chains), 249, 253–255, 327
  full optimization of 2-stage FMCs, 272–275
  1-stage FMC, 255–260, 256f, 259f
  2-stage coupled FMC (multilayer SOM), 263–268, 264f, 267f, 269f
  2-stage FMC (SOM), 260f, 260–263, 263f, 328–330, 330f
Földiák, P., 346
Formation of invariant-feature filters. *See* ASSOM (adaptive-subspace self-organizing map)
Fractures, 144, 145f, 148f, 170t
Friedman, J. H., and W. Stuetzle, 316
Fruitzke, B., 386, 387, 389
Frontolimbic system, 338

Gabor filters, 34, 35
Gabor transformations, in ASSOM, 345, 347, 350, 367
Gaussian mixture model. *See* MAP (maximum a posteriori model)
GCS (growing cell structures), 386, 387, 389–391
  GCS-DCS, 387–388
  supervised DCS-GCS, 390–391
  unsupervised DCS-GCS, 396–402, 397f
GDM (generalized deformable models), 149, 150t, 162, 170t, 173, 277. *See also* MAP (maximum a posteriori model)
  compared with SOM algorithm, 281–283
  generalized self-organizing algorithm, 311, 319–320
Generalized deformable models. *See* GDM (generalized deformable models)
Generative topographic mapping. *See* GTM (generative topographic mapping)
Geniculo-cortical projection, 191f, 191, 201. *See also* LGN (lateral geniculate nuclei)
  in color blob formation, 220–223, 222–223f
Geometric approaches, 369, 408. *See also* Data visualization
Geometric effects on oriented ocular dominance bands, 185, 186
Geometric optimization, 129, 133–135, 137
Ginzburg, I., and H. Sompolinsky, 92
Global anistropic maps, 156
Global disorder principle, 149, 152–155, 154f, 170t
Global/local orthogonality, 142, 145, 146, 158, 160, 171t, 172
Golubitsky, M. et al., 378
Goodhill, G. J., neural map formation model, 106t, 110, 156, 215, 231
Goodhill, G. J., and D. J. Willshaw, 185, 186, 189, 190, 192
  elastic net (EN) model, 150t, 153–154, 160, 162f, 163, 171t, 173, 178–179
Goodhill, G. J. et al., 116, 192
Goodhill, G. J., and T. J. Sejnowsky, **69**
  C measure in topographic mapping, 69, 70f, 70–71, 75–79, 76f, 77f, 116
Goodman, C., and C. Shatz, 142
Götz, K. G., structural model, 150t, 152f, 170t
Graepel, T. et al., 332, 333
Graepel, T., and K. Obermayer, **327**, 328. *See also* Stochastic self-organizing map
Grajski, K. A., and M. M. Merzenich, 65
Grossman, A., and J. Morlet, 28
Growing cell structures. *See* GCS (growing cell structures)
GTM (generative topographic mapping), 291–297, 293f, 294f, 305f
  batch version vs. sequential application of, 308

Index

density network model (MacKay) related to, 307
EN (elastic net) algorithm related to, 306
GTM algorithm, 299–300
kernel vs. linear progression, 302–304, 304f
oil flow data results, 301f, 301
PSOMs (parameter self-organizing maps) related to, 306
SOM algorithm (Kohonen) related to, 302–306
toy problem results, 300f, 300
vector quantization and, 306–307

Hammersely-Clifford theorem, 44
Hand-digit representation, 64–65
Hardle, W., 320, 321
Hardy, G. H. et al., 71
Hastie, T., 318
Hastie, T., and W. Stuetzle, 318, 319
Häussler, A. F., and C. von der Malsburg, neural map formation model, 85, 93, 101, 108
Heapsort algorithm, 419, 420f
Hebbian learning, 83, 213
  competitive learning models, 149, 150t, 151, 153–154, 160, 166f, 170t, 171n, 172–173, 178
  Linsker's simulations of Hebbian rules, 3n1, 3–6, 6t, 7f, 8–16, 9f, 12f, 14t, 15f, 137
  models of the early visual system, 215, 216f, 219–221, 220f
Hebbian rules of synaptic modification, 56, 65, 85, 129, 131, 206
Held, R., 39
Helmholtz equation, 60
H function, 80
Hidden Markov models (HMMs), 41, 43–44, 49–50. See also Markov models
High-dimensional models, 118, 151, 175
  ON/OFF competition model, 155, 165, 168, 173, 177

SOM-h, 107t, 109, 116, 117, 150t, 151, 153, 161f, 167, 171t
High-low density representation, 369, 372
Hinton, G. E., and S. J. Nowlan, 232
"Historical" information, 130. See also Learning/learning rules
Hofmann, T., and J. Buhmann, 328
Hopfield, J. J., and D. W. Tank, 408
Horst, R. et al., 115
Hubel, D. H. et al., 144
Hubel, D. H., and T. N. Wiesel, 64
icecube model, 142, 150t, 151, 152f, 155, 170t
Hyperparameter selection for SOMs, 277, 278–280, 288
  experimental simulations, 283–287, 284f, 285f, 286f, 287f

ICA (independent component analysis), 327, 369, 372, 373f, 374–380, 375f, 376f, 379f, 380f
  equipartition net, 375–81, 377f, 379f, 383
  Voronoi partition, 372
Icecube structural model, 142, 150t, 151, 152f, 155, 170t
Imaging techniques, 142
Infomax. See Information maximization model
Information maximization model, 129
  Bayesian self-organization and, 39–41, 40f, 44, 45–47, 46f
  coarse-grained information rate, 133–135
  learning rules, 121, 130–131, 137
  magnification factor, 133, 135–136, 137
  neighbor-preserving map formation, 131–133, 132f, 137
  prior probabilities–based method compared to, 45–47, 46f, 50–51
  processing stage dynamics, 130–131, 137
  two-dimensional space in, 131, 133, 136

Information value assessment, 136–137
Information-theoretic optimization, 29
Input distributions, 369
Input-output layers
  input layer dynamics, 16, 92, 120
  neuronal input-output layers, 86, 87f, 89, 92–93
  output layer connectivity, 84
Input-output signals, maximizing information between, 129, 137
Intracortical interactions, 149, 192–193, 202
  color vision processing, 220–221
Invariant feature-filters formation, 345, 346, 356, 363–367, 364f, 365f
Inverse mapping, 137
Inverse probability, 261
Isoorientation contours, 146
Isotropic geometry effects on ocular dominance bands, 186, 188f, 189–191, 191f
Isotropic power spectrum, 153
Iterative kernel smoothing process, 313
Iterative spectral model, 150t, 154fa–b, 156, 157, 158–160, 166f, 168, 170t, 171t, 176–177

Jenkins, W. M. et al., 65
Joint visual cortical map models, 171t, 173
Jolliffe, I., 327
Jones, D. G. et al., 73

Kernel estimator, 303, 313
Kernel smoothing, 288
  self-organization as, 311, 315–316, 319–320
"Kinked" borders, 160, 172
Kirkpatrick, S. et al., 75, 411
Knudsen, E. I. et al., 55
Kohonen, T., 65, 80, 85, 131, 305, 351, 357, 408
  unsupervised learning, 345
  self-organizing feature map (SOFM), 369, 372
Kohonen, T., S. Kaski, and H. Lappalainen, **345**
Kohonen SOM algorithm, 116–118, 119, 185
  batch processing mode, 311–113, 322
  deficiencies of, 291–292
  as "feature map" algorithm, 121, 136
  GTM related to, 302–306
  interpretation in terms of functionals, 235, 236–239, 237f, 238f, 239f
  interpreted as a kernel smoothing process, 311
  Luttrell's cost function derived from, 249
  TMP algorithm related to, 327, 328, 332, 334, 340
Konen, W. et al., dynamic link matching, 85, 88, 89, 113–114
Konen, W., and C. von Malsburg, neural mapping model, 107t, 110, 112–113
Koornwinder, T, 380, 381
K scale parameter, 407, 412f, 412–416
Kulikowski, J. J., and P. Bishop, 33
Kullback-Leibler divergence, 43f, 43, 44–45, 47
Kushner H. J., and D. S. Clark, 352

Lades, M. et al., 116
Lagrangian multiplier method(s), 98–102, 136
Land, E. H., 230
Laplacian smoothing vs. kernel smoothing, 288
Latent variable models, 291, 292–295, 293f, 294f, 327. *See also* GTM (generative topographic mapping)
Lateral connectivity, 84, 86, 92, 130, 131
Lateral inhibition in cortical mapping, 56, 65
Lateral interaction/organization, 130, 142, 149

Index

Lawler, E. L. et al., 407
Layered neural networks, 65
  three-layered, 56–58, 57f
LBG algorithm, 316–317
Learning/learning rules. *See also*
  CBL (correlation-based learning)
  models; Hebbian learning;
  Kohonen SOM algorithm
  ASSOM learning algorithm, 349, 355–356, 366–367
  in the information maximization model, 121, 130–131, 137
  modified learning algorithm, 419–421, 420f
  network learning, 58
  parameter-schedule learning, 292
  stochastic learning, 48–50
  training patterns, 161f, 161
  unsupervised learning, 345
Lehky, S. R. et al., 150
LeVay, S., and S. B. Nelson, 144, 185
LGN (lateral geniculate nuclei), 73, 186, 191f, 205. *See also* Geniculocortical projection
  in color vision processing, 216, 218, 219, 220
Li, Z., and J. J. Atick, **19**, 20, 33
Lin, J., D. G. Grier, and J. D. Cowan, **369**
Linde, Y. et al., 312
  LBG algorithm, 316–317
Linear activity models, 92, 291
Linear correlation model, 92–93, 105, 108
  orientation and ocular dominance in, 204–205, 210–211
Linear cortical neurons, 19
Linear mapping, 3, 133, 134f, 168. *See also* Two-dimensional space(s)
Linear term L, 119
Linear zones, 144, 145f, 148f, 155, 170t
Lin, J., D. G. Grief, and J. D. Cowan, 369
Linked coordinates in models. *See also* CBL (correlation-based learning) models; Pinwheel structural model

Baxter and Dow model, 150t, 170t
Götz model, 150t, 152f, 170t
Linking functions, 159–160
Linsker, R., 120, **129**, 167. *See also*
  Information maximization model
  correlation-based learning model, 150t, 166f, 167–168, 170t, 215, 302
  neural map formation model(s) of, 92, 93, 106t, 108–109, 360
  simulations of Hebbian rules, 3n1, 3–6, 6t, 7f, 8–16, 9f, 12f, 14t, 15f, 137
Little, R. J. A., and D. B. Rubin, 307
Livingstone, M. S., and D. H. Hubel, 33, 148, 213, 214
L linear term, 119
Local cortical processing, 235
Local orthogonality, 142, 146, 158, 171t, 172
Local projection method, 345
Low dimensional models, 116, 117
  SOM-l, 148, 150t, 151, 153, 157f, 157, 160, 161f, 161, 171t, 173, 178, 186
Luminance variation, in color blob formation model, 229
Luttrell, S. P., 73, 74, 235, **249**, 332
  Bayesian analysis of self-organizing maps, 249, 251, 263, 268
  interpretation of Kohonen's algorithm, 235, 237, 238f, 250–251, 252, 262, 312

Macaque striate cortex, 142, 143–149, 145f, 146f, 147f, 148f, 155, 158
  color blob formation in, 214–215
  cortical map models compared to, 141, 150t, 158, 162, 164, 166f, 168, 169–175, 170–171t
  feature selectivity in, 172
MacKay, D. J. C., 277, 278, 279, 340
  density network model of, 307
MacKay, D. J. C., and K. D. Miller, **3**, 4, 9, 11, 13, 15, 85, 120

Magnification properties
  of cortical feature maps, 56, 64–65
  in the information maximization model, 133, 135–36, 137
magnification factor, 55, 62, 161
Malach, R., 213
Mallat, S., 35
Mammalian visual cortex/system, 141, 142, 367
MAP (maximum a posteriori model), 277–278, 281–283, 292, 305, 407, 411, 416
Mardia, K. et al., 303
Markov models. *See also* FMC (folded Markov chains)
  hidden (HMMs), 41, 43–44, 49–50
  Markov chain transition probabilities, 249
Marr, D., 40
Maximizing mutual information. *See* Information maximization model
Maximum entropy principle, 327
Maximum information preservation principle, 129–130
MDS (metric multidimensional scaling), 71–72, 76f, 76, 77, 78, 328
Miller, K. D., 16, 92, 142, 219, 231. *See also* ON/OFF competition model
  correlation-based learning model(s), 150t, 165f, 166f, 167–168, 170t, 171t, 215
  Hebbian-type model, 201–202
  on ocular dominance, 204, 206, 210
  ON/OFF competition model, 155, 165, 168, 173, 177
Miller, K. D., and D. J. C. MacKay, 114, 202, 206, 209, 210, 211
Miller, K. D. et al., neural map formation model, 107t, 109, 231
Minimal distortion, 73–74, 77f, 77–79, 251, 262
Minimal path length, 72–73, 76f
Minimal wiring
  dimension reduction, 235–239, 237f, 238f, 239f
  duality with self-organizing map (SOM), 235, 244

the gaussian case, 240–244
  objective function, 72, 73, 76f
  wire length interpreted as a functional, 235, 239–240, 242f, 243f, 244f
Minimization models, 186
Mitchison, G., 74, **235**
Mitchison, G., and R. Durbin, 72
Miyashita, M., and S. Tanaka, correlation-based model, 150t, 155, 166f, 167
Monkey. *See also* Macaque striate cortex
  ocular dominance bands in, 185–186, 192
  visual cortex of, 195
Monocular deprivation, 171t
Motor cortex, 84
Mulier, F., and V. Cherkassky, 282, **311**
  generalized self-organizing algorithm, 311, 319–320
Multiplicative normalization rule, 105
Multiscale representations, 33
Mumford, D., 45, 51

Nadaraya, É. A., kernel estimator, 303, 313
Najafi, H. L., and V. Cherkassky, 320
Nakayama, K., and S. Shimojo, 39
Neighborhood effects/interactions
  in ASSOM, 349
  nearest neighbor encoding, 251, 252f, 262
  receptive fields, 185, 189–191, 367
  in self-organizing systems, 320–321, 321f, 322
Neighborhood parameters, 292, 313–314, 317
Neighborhood preservation, 83, 131–133, 132f, 137
  neighborhood preservation hypothesis, 185, 194–195
Network architecture, 47, 216f, 348–349. *See also* Network models

Index

Network models, 55–56, 58, 65, 215, 311, 348–349. *See also* Neural map formation
 branch architecture network, 375f, 376f, 377f
 network architecture, 47, 216f, 348–349
 three-layered neural network model, 56–58, 57f, 65
Neural dynamics. *See also* Neural map formation; Weight dynamics
 coordinate transformation effects, 94–98, 95f, 99f, 102, 104t, 112–113, 119
 curl free fields, 93, 94
 objective functions, 85–86, 91, 93–96, 95f, 103, 104t, 105, 115–116
Neural map formation, 84f, 235
 collapsing or expanding maps, 121
 computational elements, 83, 235
 constrained optimization framework for, 83, 86–87, 91, 105, 119–121
 constraint function(s) and, 86–87, 91, 97f, 103, 104t, 105
 linear, 92–93, 105, 108
 nonlinear, 105, 109–110
Neural map formation models, 83, 103, 120
 Amari model, 88, 108, 120
 dynamic link matching model, 83, 85, 88, 89, 113–114
 Goodhill model, 106t, 110, 156, 215, 231
 Häussler and von der Malsburg model, 85, 93, 101, 108
 Konen and von Malsburg model, 107t, 110, 112–113
 Linsker's models, 92, 93, 106t, 108–109, 360
 Miller, K. D. et al. model, 107t, 109, 231
 model architecture, 86–87, 87f
 Obermayer et al. model, 107t, 109, 116–117
 tables of, 104t, 106–107t
 Tanaka model, 107t, 109–110, 150t, 155, 156

von der Malsburg model, 84–85, 92, 105, 106t, 108, 215
 Whitelaw and Cowan model, 106t, 108
Neural processing, early, 21–22, 32, 36
Neurobiological modeling, 78, 202–205, 207, 211, 215, 227, 292n1
 models vs. experimental data, 141, 150t, 158, 162, 164, 166f, 168, 169–175, 170–171t
Neurons
 binary, 55
 sigmoidal, 55
Niebur, E., and F. Wörgötter
 filtered noise approach, 172
 one-step spectral model, 150t, 151, 157, 158–159, 159f, 168, 170t, 175–176
Nodes, response properties, 129, 175
Nonlinear interactions, 140, 376
Nonlinear models, 105, 109–110, 153
 orientation and ocular dominance in, 204–205, 207, 209, 211
Nonlinear function (GTM), 292–295, 293f, 307–308
Nonparametric regression method, 311, 313–314, 314f
Normalization rules. *See* Weight normalization rules
Nowlan, S. J., 90, 115

Obermayer, K., 145f, 147f
Obermayer, K. et al.
 neural map formation model, 89, 107t, 109, 116–117
 probability blob location algorithm, 89, 109, 121–123
 self-organizing map (SOM) algorithm, 116–117
 SOM-h (high-dimensional model), 107t, 109, 116, 117, 150t, 151, 153, 161f, 167, 171t
 SOM-l (low-dimensional model), 148, 150t, 151, 153, 157f, 157, 160, 161f, 161, 171t, 173, 178, 186
Obermayer, K., and G. G. Blasdel, 145, 146, 148f, 148

Objective function(s)
  in ASSOM, 351–352
  C measure, 69, 70f, 70–71, 75–79, 76f, 77f, 116
  constrained optimization using, 83
  metric multidimensional scaling (metric MDS), 71–72, 76f, 76, 77, 78
  minimal distortion, 73–74, 77f, 77–79
  minimal path length, 72–73, 76f
  minimal wiring, 72, 73, 76f
  neural dynamics and, 85–86, 91, 93–96, 95f, 103, 104t, 105, 115–116
Object recognition, 21
Ocular dominance, 142, 144, 148f, 171t, 175. *See also* Orientation and ocular dominance
  correlation-based learning models and, 173
  formation of ocular dominance bands, 73, 146, 185, 186, 187–189, 188f
  instability conditions and, 185, 186, 195–197
  monocular deprivation, 171t
  ocular dominance bands in the cat, 185–186
  strabismus, 171t
Oil flow data results (in GTM), 301f, 301
ON-center and OFF-center inputs, 16
One-dimensional case(s), 22, 136, 190
One dimensional map, coupled, 369
1-stage FMC (folded Markov chains), 255–260, 256f, 259f
One-step spectral model, 150t, 151, 157, 158–159, 159f, 168, 170t, 175–176
On-line training prescription, 262
ON/OFF competition model, 155, 165, 168, 173, 177
Optical imaging/recording, 143, 145f, 156, 157, 159f

"Optimally topographic map," 69
Optimization. *See also* Constrained optimization
  Bayesian, 249–250, 253, 266–269
  combinatorial, 407
  geometric, 129, 133–135, 137
  information-theoretic, 29
  properties, 190
Ordered maps, generating, 129
Orientation
  correlations with cortical coordinates, 163–168, 166f
  deprivation, 156–158, 171t
  instability conditions and, 185, 186, 195–197
  ocular dominance bands and, 186, 193
  preference, 144, 147f, 156, 157, 158f, 175
  preference and ocular dominance bands, 186, 193
  selectivity and tuning, 121, 174, 206–207, 209
  specificity, 156, 157, 159f, 170t, 171t, 188
  symmetry-breaking, 31f, 31n, 33
Orientation mapping
  conservative maps, 168, 170t
  correlations with cortical coordinates, 163–168, 166f
  fractures, 144, 145f, 148f, 170t
  linear zones, 144, 145f, 148f, 155, 170t
  linked coordinates, 170t
  saddle points, 144, 145f, 146, 148f, 152, 170t
  singularities, 144, 145f, 146, 148f, 151, 155, 159–160, 170t, 172f
Orientation and ocular dominance, 186, 193
  constraints' role in, 206–207, 208t, 209–210, 211
  continuity principle, 151
  decoupling in symmetric CBL models, 201
  diversity principle, 151, 153
  global/local orthogonality, 142, 145, 146, 158, 160, 171t, 172

joint pattern development, 171t, 201, 204–205, 207, 209
"kinked" borders, 160, 172
  in linear correlation models, 204–205, 210–211
  in models compared to ma-caque data, 141, 144, 145, 149, 158, 161–163, 169f, 171t, 203
  in nonlinear models, 204–205, 207, 209, 211
  simple-cell receptive fields, 201, 203f, 204, 210, 211
  simulations of, 201, 206
  synaptic weights and, 206, 209, 211
Oriented striate cortex filters, 30–33, 61f
Orthogonal normalization rules, 96–98, 98f, 119
  derivation of, 98–102
Orthogonality
  global/local, 142, 145, 146, 158, 160, 171t, 172
  orthogonal vectors, 134f
  orthogonal projection in ASSOM, 347–348
OS (orientation selection) value, 206–207, 209
Output layer connectivity, 84
Output nodes, 130, 137
Outputs in color blob formation model, 217t, 218t, 218f, 220f, 220
Overview of developmental models, 141

Parameter adjustment, 43–44
Parameter effects
  on ocular dominance bands, 185
  in simulations of Hebbian rules, 8–10, 9f, 12f, 15f, 137
Parameter-schedule learning, 292
Parameter selection. *See also* Hyperparameter selection for SOMs
  in a nonlinear model, 298–299, 299f
Parameter self-organizing maps (PSOMs), 306
Parrot, visual processing in, 218f

Pattern models. *See* Spectral models; Structural models
Pattern recognition, 21, 346–348
Paul, D. B., 41, 49
PCA (principal component analysis), 327, 346
Penalty functions, 102, 104t
Perceptual pathway, 19–22, 129
Periodic boundary conditions, 132f, 153, 186
Piepenbrock, C., H. Ritter, and K. Obermayer, **201**, 203, 205
Pinwheel structural model, 142, 150t, 151, 152f, 164f, 164, 168, 170t
Poggio, T. et al., 40, 44
Posterior ectosylvian gyrus, 338–339
Power spectra, 147f, 153, 170t, 190, 193f
Precortical processing, 215–218, 216f, 217t
Preprocessing, visual, 215–218, 216f, 217t, 345
Presynaptic normalization, 105, 123
Primary visual cortex (V1), 83–84, 141, 201, 213
Principal curve algorithm, 311
  SOM algorithm related to, 318–319
Prior probabilities–based method, 39, 41–45
  compared to information maximization model, 45–47, 46f, 50–51
  implementation, 48–50
  maximum likelihood estimation, 49–50
Probabilistic blob model, 88–90, 118, 119, 121–125
Probabilistic encoders, 249, 270–271, 277
Probability density model, 307
Proximity data. *See* Stochastic self-organizing map (SOM)
PSOMs (parameter self-organizing maps), 306

Q term, functional aspects in neural map formation, 110–112, 119

Quadratic assignment problems, 79
Quicksort algorithm, 419

Receptive fields, 1, 26, 32, 55,
141, 150–151, 165–168, 172–173
  in color blob formation model,
    223–225, 224f
  computational advantages of, 19
  neighborhood interactions, 185,
    189–191, 367
  oriented, 3–16
  photoreceptive field properties of
    the retina, 22–25, 23n
  sensory receptor layer, 56
  simple-cell, 201, 203f, 204, 210, 211
  spatially disjoint, 47
Redlich, A. N., 41
Reggia, J. et al., 150
Regions. *See also* Separable
  distributions
  high and low density, 369–370
Relaxation dynamics, 56
Response properties of nodes, 129,
  175
Retinal cells
  ganglion cells, 29
  retinal/geniculate cells, 216f, 217t,
    218f, 218, 224f
  retinal neurons, 20n1
Retinal intensities patterns, 41–42f
Retinal photoreceptive field
  properties, 22–25, 23n
Retinal transformations, 19–20,
  20n1, 21f
  representations of, 25–30, 35
  translation group, 24–25
Retino-cortical changes
  in color vision, 19, 32, 34f, 34–36,
    35n
  correlations in map models, 163–
    168
  in the macaque cortex, 167
Retinotectal map, 83, 88
Retinotopy, 144, 194
Ritter, H., 251
Ritter, H. et al., 117, 315, 318
Ritter, H., and K. Schulten, 136, 186,
  187, 188, 195, 197, 239, 369, 372

Robbins, H., and S. Monro, 308, 351,
  352, 693
Rodrigues, J. S., and L. B. Almeida,
  316
Rojer, A. S., and E. L. Schwartz,
  spectral model(s), 150t, 151, 158–
  159, 160, 163, 168, 169f, 170t, 171t,
  172, 172f, 173
Rose, K. et al., 332
Ruderman, D. L., and W. Bialek, 23
Running blobs, 121
Rutkowski, L., 322

Saddle points, 144, 145f, 146, 148f,
  152, 170t
Scaling symmetry, 25–30
Scannell, J. W. et al., 336–337, 339
Second-order equations, 60, 121
Segmentation, 21
Sejnowski, T. J., 83, 92
Self-organization as a kernel
  smoothing process, 311, 315–316,
  319–320
Self-organizing map (SOM), 80,
  116–118, 185, 195. *See also*
  Bayesian self-organization;
  Kohonen SOM algorithm; *and by
  model or type*
  Bayesian analysis of, 249, 270–271
  combined with a local projection
    method, 345
  dynamics and formation of, 55
  extensions of, 327
  pruning and grouping algorithms,
    387
  sorting with, 419–421, 420f
Self-supervision theory, 249, 269f,
  269–271, 270f
  self-supervised multilayer SOMs,
    252–254, 263–268, 264f, 267f,
    269f
  unsupervised network notation,
    249, 250–251, 251t
Sensory deprivation simulation,
  157
Sensory processing, 129. *See also*
  Visual perception
Sensory receptor layer, 56

Index

Separable distributions
  faithful representation of, 369–370, 381–382
  modification of the one-dimensional SOM, 371–372, 382–383
Shannon, C. E., 129–130, 136
Shannon, C. E., and W. Weaver, 20
Shepard, R. N., 71
Sigmoidal transfer function of neurons, arbitrary, 55
Signals
  auto correlation of, 22
  input-output (maximizing information between), 129, 137
  leading bit vs. lower bit signal value, 136–137
  translated speech signals (ASSOM), 356–357, 357f
Silverman, B. W., 283
Similarity measures, 151
Simple cells
  "even-symmetric" and "odd-symmetric," 19, 28–30, 29f, 34–36
  receptive fields, 201, 203f, 204, 210, 211
Singularities, 144, 145f, 146, 148f, 151, 155, 159–160, 170t, 172f
Sirosh, J., and R. Miikkulainen, 150–151
Smirnakis, S. M., and A. L. Yuille, 39, 41
SOFM (self-organizing feature map), 369, 372
SOM. *See* Kohonen SOM algorithm; Self-organizing map (SOM); *and by model or type*
Somatosensory cortex/system, 84, 338
SOM-h (high-dimensional model), 107t, 109, 116, 117, 150t, 151, 153, 161f, 167, 171t
SOM-l (low-dimensional model), 148, 150t, 151, 153, 157f, 157, 160, 161f, 161, 171t, 173, 178, 186
Sorting with self-organizing maps, 419–421, 420f

Spatial filters, 150, 213. *See also* Color blob formation model
Spatially disjoint receptive fields, 47
Spatial relationships
  spatial patterns, 144, 146, 151
  striate cortex theory and, 19, 22–25, 29f
Spectral models, 149
  iterative model, 150t, 154fa–b, 156, 157, 158–160, 166f, 168, 170t, 171t, 176–177
  one-step model, 150t, 151, 157, 158–159, 159f, 168, 170t, 175–176
  Rojer and Schwartz model, 150t, 151, 158–159, 160, 163, 168, 169f, 170t, 171t, 172f, 172, 173
Speech signal, ASSOM translation, 356–357, 357f
Spline smoothing, 319–320
Stationary state models, 153
Stochastic learning, 48–50
Stochastic models, 278
  annealing process in, 327, 328, 330–332
Stochastic self-organizing map (SOM), 327
  first phase transition, 332–334
  numerical simulations, 334–336, 335f, 336
  TMP (topographic mapping of proximity data), 327, 328–334, 340
Strabismus, 171t
Striate cortex. *See also* Macaque striate cortex; Visual cortex/system
  in the cat, 73
  in the monkey, 33, 64–65, 73
  oriented filters, 30–33, 61f
  primate, 36, 213
  scaling group, 25–30
  theory of, 19, 22–25, 29f
Structural models, 149, 150t, 155, 157, 170t, 171t
  Baxter and Dow model, 150t, 170t
  Götz model, 150t, 152f, 170t
  icecube model, 142, 150t, 151, 152f, 155, 170t
  pinwheel model, 142, 150t, 151, 152f, 164f, 164, 168, 170t

Stryker, M. P. et al., 157
Surface distortion energy, 135
Sur, M. et al., 64
Swindale, N. V., 120, 144, 153, 186, 195
  iterative spectral model, 150t, 154fa–b, 156, 157, 158–160, 166f, 168, 170t, 171t, 176–177
Symmetric systems
  center-surround structures, 5–6, 6t, 8, 10
  "even-symmetric" and "odd-symmetric" simple cells, 19, 28–30, 29f, 34–36
Synapses, negative, 14
Synaptic connections. *See* Connectivity
Synaptic efficiencies (Hebbian rules), 55, 56, 65, 85, 129, 131, 206
Synaptic weights, 92, 206, 209, 211. *See also* Weight dynamics

Takiuchi, A., and S. Amari, 56
Tanaka, S., 120
  Miyashita and Tanaka correlation-based model, 150t, 155, 166f, 167
  models compared to experimental data, 150t, 155, 170t
  neural map formation model, 107t, 109–110, 150t, 155, 156
Tea trader model of neural development, 408
Telegraph equation, 60
Temporal sequences/events, 12f, 345, 346
Terzopoulos, D. et al., 408
Thalamic layer, 56, 65–66
Three dimensional vectors, 158–159
Three-layered neural network model, 56–58, 57f, 65
Three-layered recurrent network, 213
Tipping, M. E., and C. M. Bishop, 294, 327
TMP (topographic mapping of proximity data), 327, 328–334, 340. *See also* Stochastic self-organizing map

Tootell, R. B. et al., 144
Topographic mapping, 53, 69, 131, 408. *See also* Cortical feature maps; *and by model*
  C measure in, 69, 70f, 70–71, 75–79, 76f, 77f, 116
  generative (GTM), 291–297, 293f, 294f, 305f
  "optimally topographic map," 69
  of proximity data (TMP), 327, 328–334, 340
Torgerson, W. S., 71
Toy problem (GTM simulation), 300f, 300
Training patterns, 161f, 161
Transformation class recognition (in ASSOM), 365–367
Translation invariance assumption, 203
Traveling salesman problem, 72, 407–411, 408f, 416. *See also* Elastic net approach to the traveling salesman problem
Tresp, V. et al., 340
Trusk, T. C. et al., 213
Ts'o, D. Y., and C. D. Gilbert, 213, 214
Two-dimensional colored noise, ASSOM simulation, 357–358, 358f
Two-dimensional space(s), 161, 292, 367. *See also* Dimension reduction; Linear mapping
  dimension-reduction models, 163f
  in information maximization model, 131, 133, 136
2D-orientation preference, 221–222
2D vision, 30–33, 31n, 31f
2D-white noise, 172
2-stage FMC (folded Markov chains), 260f, 260–263, 263f, 328–330, 330f
  coupled (multilayer SOM), 263–268, 264f, 267f, 269f

Unifying objective function, 69
Unsupervised learning, 345. *See also* Learning/learning rules; Self-supervision theory

Index 439

Utsugi, A., **277**, 279, 280. *See also* Hyperparameter selection for SOMs

Vector quantization. *See* VQ (vector quantization)
Vector representation, 150, 151, 158–159, 168
Vertical cross-section of cortical map, 63f
Visual cortex/system, 141, 142, 367. *See also* Early visual cortex/system; Striate cortex; Visual cortex/system
  in the cat, 129, 156, 174, 195, 201, 338
  linear cortical neurons, 19
  in the monkey, 129, 174
  left- and right-eye inputs, 16
  in the monkey, 195 (*see also* Macaque striate cortex)
  orientation and ocular dominance models, 141
  primary (V1), 83–84, 141, 201, 213
Visual cortical map models. *See also* CBL (correlation-based learning) models; Cortical feature maps; Orientation and ocular dominance; Spectral models; Structural models
  anistropic map patterns, 156, 157f, 170t
  biases in feature preferences, 156–158, 160–161, 171t
  compared to data from a macaque striate cortex, 141, 150t, 158, 162, 164, 166f, 168, 169–175, 170–171t
  global disorder principle, 149, 152–155, 154f, 170t
  global/local orthogonality, 142, 145, 146, 158, 160, 171t, 172
  joint models, 171t, 173
  linking functions, 159–160
  properties of, 141, 143, 149–151, 150t, 155, 170–171t
Visual perception. *See also* Color vision; Retinal cells; Retinal transformations; 2D vision

Bayesian theories of, 39, 43–45, 50–51, 74
binocular stereo vision, 39, 41–42
early vision and self organization, 39
early vision and striate cortex theory, 21–22, 32, 36
Hebbian models of the early visual system, 215, 216f, 219–221, 220f
visual pathway, 19–22, 129
visual processing, 213, 345
von der Malsburg, C., 90, 219
  neural map formation model, 84–85, 92, 105, 106t, 108, 215
von der Malsburg, C., and D. J. Willshaw, 85, 114, 131
Voronoi partition, 372, 378, 379f, 381. *See also* Equipartition net (ICA)
Voronoi region, 311, 312–313
VQ (vector quantization), 256–260, 259f, 270–271, 271, 272, 312, 327
  GTM and, 306–307
  TVQ (total vector quantization), 332

Wallis, G. et al., 346
Watson, G. S., kernel estimator, 303, 313
Wavelets, 28, 35
  in ASSOM, 345, 367, 381
Waves, traveling, 121
Wehmeier, U. et al., 217
Weight dynamics, 103, 106–107t, 113, 115, 119, 120–121
  and constraint function(s), 96, 104t
  objective functions and, 95, 104t
  synaptic weights, 206, 209, 211
  weight growth, 83, 86–87, 88, 95–96, 104t, 119
Weight normalization rules, 83, 84, 87, 88, 91, 104t, 113
  effects of probabilistic blob model on, 123–126
  orthogonal normalization and, 96–102, 98f, 119
  soft vs. hard competitive normalization, 85, 114–115

Weight normalization rules (cont.)
  without objective function, 101–102
Weight vectors
  evolution of, 3n1, 3–4, 14
  representation of, 150
Whitelaw, D. J., and J. D. Cowan, neural map formation model, 106t, 108
Whitening filter, 35
Willshaw, D. J., and C. von der Malsburg, 87–88, 114
  tea trader model of neural development, 408
Wire length interpreted as a functional, 235, 239–240, 242f, 243f, 244f. *See also* Minimal wiring
Wiskott, L., and C. von der Malsburg, 97, 121
Wiskott, L., and T. J. Sejnowski, 75, **83**
World Wide Web, 340

Young, F. W., 71
Yuille, A. L., S. M. Smirnakis, and L. Xu, **39**, 51, 151, 277, 279. *See also* GDM (Generalized deformable models); Visual perception

Zhang, J., **55**